FUNDAMENTALS OF CLINICAL ENDOCRINOLOGY

REGINALD HALL, BSc, MD (Dunelm), FRCP

Professor of Medicine, University of Newcastle upon Tyne, and Physician to the Royal Victoria Infirmary, Newcastle upon Tyne

JOHN ANDERSON, MB, BS (Dunelm), FRCP

Senior Lecturer in Medicine, University of Newcastle upon Tyne, and Physician to the Royal Victoria Infirmary, Newcastle upon Tyne

GEORGE A. SMART, BSc, MD (Dunelm), FRCP

Director, British Postgraduate Medical Federation, Professor of Medicine, University of London, Honorary Consultant Physician, National Hospital for Nervous Diseases, London

MICHAEL BESSER, BSc, MD (London), FRCP

Professor of Endocrinology and Honorary Consultant Physician, St. Bartholomew's Hospital and Medical College, University of London

SECOND EDITION

PITMAN MEDICAL

First published 1969
Second edition 1974
Reprinted 1975

SIR ISAAC PITMAN AND SONS LTD
Pitman House, Parker Street, Kingsway, London WC2B 5PB
P.O. Box 46038, Banda Street, Nairobi, Kenya

SIR ISAAC PITMAN (AUST.) PTY LTD
Pitman House, 158 Bouverie Street, Carlton, Victoria 3053, Australia

PITMAN PUBLISHING CORPORATION
6 East 43rd Street, New York, NY 10017, USA

SIR ISAAC PITMAN (CANADA) LTD
495 Wellington Street West, Toronto 135, Canada

THE COPP CLARK PUBLISHING COMPANY
517 Wellington Street West, Toronto 135, Canada

Paperback edition: ISBN 0 272 00742 0

Printed in Great Britain at The Pitman Press, Bath
21.1402:81

£8-00

FUNDAMENTALS OF CLINICAL ENDOCRINOLOGY

Dr. Keith E. Evans.

[Consultant Physician,
Morriston Hospital, Swansea.]

PREFACE

This book does not aim to be comprehensive. It contains what the authors believe are the essentials of endocrinology. We make no apologies for the absence of photographs of patients suffering from gross acromegaly or myxoedema which have decorated endocrinology texts from time immemorial. Modern endocrinology is based on the diagnosis of early endocrine disease leading to the institution of effective treatment before permanent or crippling sequelae develop.

The text is aimed at senior medical students and postgraduates working for higher examinations both in medicine and surgery. We do not accept any clear distinction between the undergraduate and postgraduate phases of education, merely a shift in emphasis and, hence, this textbook is aimed at a broad medical audience. We have retained many chapters in conventional arrangement dealing with anterior pituitary, posterior pituitary, and thyroid but have tried at all stages to stress the interrelationships within the endocrine system. A number of chapters are included dealing with endocrine topics we think of special importance such as pregnancy, disorders of growth, and hormonal syndromes associated with neoplasms not derived from endocrine glands.

Diagnosis in clinical endocrinology has made great advances in recent years, particularly with the advent of radioimmunoassays of hormones, techniques that are replacing many of the indirect tests of endocrine function and the laborious and often imprecise bioassays. We have tried to provide sufficient detail in the text or appendix to help in the diagnosis of most endocrine syndromes. We have avoided the use of frequent references in the text, giving merely a few key articles and listing useful reviews.

Wherever possible we have tried to describe values in a meaningful way, the mean and standard deviation always being given where appropriate and when available. For many assays, however, such values have not only not been published, but they might well vary with the particular laboratory performing the estimation. Wherever possible the somewhat old-fashioned and not very informative method of giving a 'range' of values has been avoided. Readers are advised to find out for themselves the precise parameters of an estimation as obtained by the laboratory they use on a normal 'control' population and in disease states.

Dr John Gray contributed extensively to the chapter on Disorders of Sex Differentiation; Dr J. O'Riordan and Dr M. Peberdy kindly provided us with valuable material for the chapters on Parathyroid Glands and Calcium Metabolism and the Ovary respectively; Dr R. Wilkinson advised us on the section on aldosterone; the Departments of Medical Illustration and Photography of Newcastle University and St. Bartholomew's Hospital reproduced many of the illustrations and we particularly thank Mr R. Johnson and Mr D. Tredinnick; Dr C. H. Mortimer and Dr Peter Hunter gave invaluable help in proof-reading. We also wish to thank Pitman Medical Publishing Company and in particular Mr Stephen Neal and Mr Edward Summerson for their patience and co-operation in the production of this book.

Newcastle upon Tyne
and London, 1974

R. Hall
J. Anderson
G. A. Smart
M. Besser

CONTENTS

1

ANTERIOR PITUITARY

ANATOMY AND EMBRYOLOGY

The anterior and posterior parts of the pituitary gland have separate origins and function independently of one another. An upward evagination of the stomodaeum of ectodermal origin, Rathke's pouch, comes in contact with the infundibulum, a downgrowth from the floor of the diencephalon. Rathke's pouch then loses its attachment to the pharyngeal roof to form the anterior pituitary. From its upper part, cells proliferate to form the pars tuberalis, which partly encircles the pituitary stalk, while the portion in contact with the posterior pituitary is the poorly developed pars intermedia. The cells of the posterior pituitary develop from the infundibular process, becoming modified to form pituicytes. Many nerve fibres grow into the posterior pituitary via the pituitary stalk from the hypothalamic nuclei.

The human pituitary gland weighs about half a gramme; it is somewhat larger in the female, especially in parous women, and smaller in old age. Almost three-quarters of the weight of the gland is contributed by the anterior lobe. The pituitary lies in the sella turcica, a depression in the sphenoid, which is covered by a layer of dura mater, the diaphragma sellae, through which the pituitary stalk passes. The position of the diaphragma sellae on the lateral skull X-ray is usually indicated by the line joining the tuberculum sellae and the most anterior convexity of the posterior clinoid processes (Fig. 1.1). The size of the sella turcica is very variable in adults and, also, depends on age. Acheson (1956) defines the length of the pituitary fossa as the distance from the tuberculum sellae to the dorsum sellae, and the depth as the distance from the line joining these points to the lowest part of the sella (Table 1.1). A tube-film distance of three feet is specified, a lateral radiograph being taken with strict head positioning. Tumours in the pituitary fossa may initially declare themselves by erosion of the bony margins. The earliest changes are often asymmetrical so that a lateral X-ray of the fossa may show more than one contour to the floor. This 'double floor' appearance is often the first sign of the pituitary tumour and precedes frank ballooning of the sella.

TABLE 1.1 *Length and Depth of the Adult Pituitary Fossa*
(measured in mm)
(Acheson, R. M. (1956). 'Measuring the pituitary fossa from radiographs,' *Brit. J. Radiol.*, **29**, 76.)

	Male			Female		
	No.	Mean	S.D.	No.	Mean	S.D.
Length	80	13·5	1·8	49	13·3	1·4
Depth	80	7·2	1·2	49	7·1	1·1

Relations of the Pituitary. Above, the pituitary is related to the hypothalamus and the third ventricle, behind which are the mamillary bodies. Laterally, and above, lie the cavernous sinuses and optic tracts, and above and in front, the optic chiasm, which may be in contact with any part of the diaphragma sellae. The proximity of the gland to the optic pathways leads to visual disturbances if the gland enlarges beyond the sella turcica. The oculomotor nerves lie lateral to the edge of the pituitary fossa.

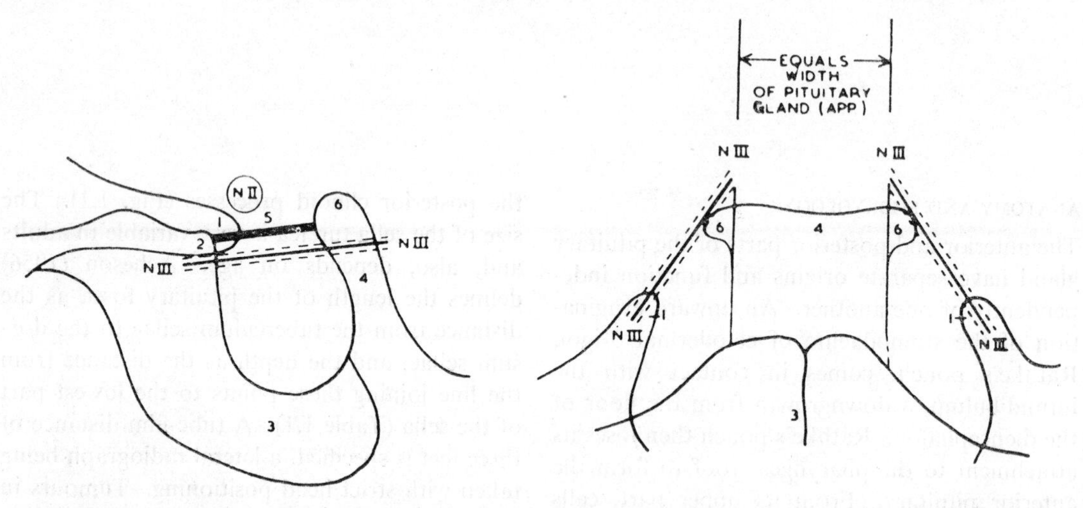

FIGURE 1.1 The pituitary fossa and its relationships (from Fraser and Joplin (1954), *Brit. J. Radiol.*, **32,** 527)

1 Anterior clinoid process
2 Tuberculum sellae
3 Sphenoid sinus
NII Optic chiasm
4 Dorsum sellae
5 Diaphragma sellae
6 Posterior clinoid process
NIII Oculomotor nerve

Blood Supply of the Pituitary Gland. A superior hypophyseal artery arises from each internal carotid in the middle cranial fossa and divides into anastomosing branches, which supply the pituitary stalk, and a separate 'artery of the trabecula' which enters the distal part of the gland. Inferior hypophyseal arteries from the internal carotids in the cavernous sinuses supply the posterior pituitary and branches which anastomose with the 'artery of the trabecula'. Branches of the superior hypophyseal artery to the pituitary stalk form capillaries which extend upwards into the median eminence and ramify around the hypothalamic centres and tracts from which they pick up the various chemotransmitters. These are carried to the anterior pituitary sinusoids by portal veins passing down the anterior surface of the stalk. The pituitary veins drain into the surrounding venous sinuses.

Microscopic Structure of the Anterior Pituitary. The glandular cells of the anterior pituitary are arranged in cords separated by wide vascular channels lined by reticulo-endothelial cells. They can be divided into chromophils and chromophobes by simple stains such as haematoxylin and eosin which are taken up by the secretory granules. The chromophobes usually have less cytoplasm than the chromophilic cells, which contain either acidophilic or basophilic granules. Some of the chromophobe cells may represent differentiating chromophils, and others degranulated chromophils. By the use of more elaborate histochemical staining methods, electron microscopy, and immunofluorescence techniques, separate types of cells can be identified for each of the anterior pituitary hormones.

The acidophils secrete growth hormone and prolactin. In animals, these hormones are secreted by distinct cells that have characteristic staining properties. In man, prolactin has only recently been shown to exist separately from growth hormone.

The basophils all contain periodic-acid-Schiff (PAS)-positive (red) granules, the source of the glycoprotein hormones TSH, FSH, and LH.

The chromophobe cells are fewer in number when complex staining techniques are used. Many contain light purple PAS-positive granules, which may be a source of ACTH and β-MSH, though these hormones may also be produced by certain types of basophils.

TABLE 1.2 *Principal Actions of Anterior Pituitary Hormones*

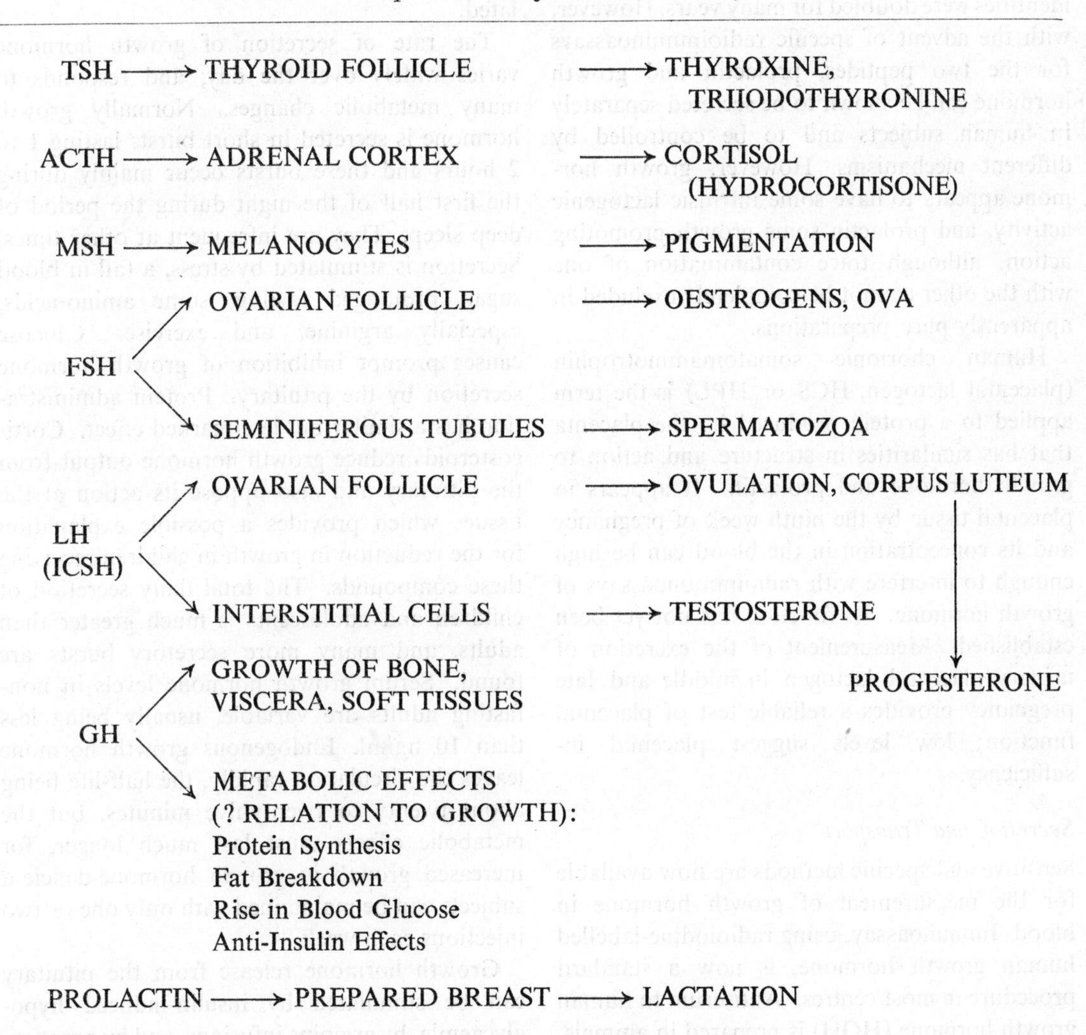

GROWTH HORMONE

Growth hormone makes up between 5 and 10 per cent of the dry weight of the human pituitary gland; it is a protein with a molecular weight of 21,000 consisting of 190 amino-acids. Clear evidence is now available that prolactin exists separately from growth hormone in man. Owing to similarities in structure and biological actions and the fact that prolactin is present in the human pituitary gland in much smaller quantities than growth hormone, their separate identities were doubted for many years. However, with the advent of specific radioimmunoassays for the two peptides, prolactin and growth hormone can be shown to be secreted separately in human subjects and to be controlled by different mechanisms. However, growth hormone appears to have some intrinsic lactogenic activity, and prolactin some growth promoting action, although trace contamination of one with the other cannot be completely excluded in apparently pure preparations.

Human chorionic somatomammotrophin (placental lactogen, HCS or HPL) is the term applied to a protein produced by the placenta that has similarities in structure and action to growth hormone and prolactin. It appears in placental tissue by the ninth week of pregnancy and its concentration in the blood can be high enough to interfere with radioimmunoassays of growth hormone. Its function has not yet been established. Measurement of the excretion of urinary placental lactogen in middle and late pregnancy provides a reliable test of placental function; low levels suggest placental insufficiency.

Secretion and Transport

Sensitive and specific methods are now available for the measurement of growth hormone in blood. Immunoassay, using radioiodine-labelled human growth hormone, is now a standard procedure in most centres. Antiserum to human growth hormone (HGH) is prepared in animals. Labelled HGH is incubated with anti-HGH in the presence of standard amounts of hormone or the serum to be assayed. The amount of HGH in the standard or unknown will vary the amount of labelled HGH bound to antiserum, since competition between them for binding to the antibody will occur. The free and bound HGH can then be separated and a standard curve produced, from which the amount of hormone in the serum specimen can be calculated.

The rate of secretion of growth hormone varies widely over the day, and responds to many metabolic changes. Normally growth hormone is secreted in short bursts lasting 1 to 2 hours and these bursts occur mainly during the first half of the night during the period of deep sleep. They are infrequent at other times. Secretion is stimulated by stress, a fall in blood sugar, prolonged fasting, some amino-acids, especially arginine, and exercise. Glucose causes prompt inhibition of growth hormone secretion by the pituitary. Protein administration has a similar but less marked effect. Corticosteroids reduce growth hormone output from the pituitary and also oppose its action at the tissues which provides a possible explanation for the reduction in growth in children receiving these compounds. The total daily secretion of children and adolescents is much greater than adults, and many more secretory bursts are found. Serum growth hormone levels in non-fasting adults are variable, usually being less than 10 ng/ml. Endogenous growth hormone leaves the circulation rapidly, the half-life being about twenty to twenty-five minutes, but the metabolic effects must last much longer, for increased growth in growth hormone-deficient subjects can be maintained with only one or two injections each week.

Growth hormone release from the pituitary can be stimulated by insulin-induced hypoglycaemia, by arginine infusions, and by pyrogen.

Hypoglycaemia and pyrogen also release ACTH but do not affect TSH or the gonadotrophins; arginine causes a rise in plasma insulin, possibly as a result of growth hormone release. The effects of growth hormone on the metabolism of carbohydrate and fat are discussed in Chapter 14.

The hypothalamus controls growth hormone synthesis and release by means of a humoral agent, growth hormone releasing-hormone, possibly a polypeptide similar to other hypothalamic hormones affecting anterior pituitary hormone formation. The metabolic factors affecting growth hormone release probably act largely at a hypothalamic level.

Growth hormone in blood appears to be transported in bound form but there is no agreement on the nature of the carrier protein, both albumin and an α_2-macroglobulin may be involved.

Metabolic Effects of Growth Hormone

The mechanism by which growth hormone produces its metabolic effects is not yet fully understood, but appears to involve the production of an intermediate or large polypeptide, somatomedin or the 'sulphation' factor, probably by the liver. This product appears to be related to growth of tissues.

Its effect on protein synthesis may, in part, be mediated by an increased transport of certain amino-acids into the cell, though the hormone can also stimulate protein synthesis in cell-free preparations. Growth hormone can still exert its effects when messenger-RNA synthesis is blocked by actinomycin and when new protein synthesis is inhibited by puromycin, so it is unlikely that the primary site of action of the hormone is on m-RNA. It may in some way affect the efficiency of the ribosomes, the site of protein synthesis.

CLINICAL EFFECTS OF GROWTH HORMONE

ACROMEGALY AND GIGANTISM

The increased secretion of growth hormone that may result from a pituitary adenoma leads to excessive body growth affecting both the skeleton and the soft tissues. Very rarely, this occurs prior to fusion of the epiphyses and results in gigantism. In adults, skeletal overgrowth is more obvious in the hands, feet, cranial sinuses, jaw, and supraorbital ridges, and soft tissue overgrowth is manifested in coarse features, thick skin and heel pads, and enlarged viscera. Gigantism and acromegaly may occur together in adolescents. The main clinical features in acromegaly are shown in Table 1.3.

The tumour is classically of the acidophilic type but is often chromophobe.

Local Effects of the Tumour

1. Headache
2. Enlargement of the sella turcica or erosion of its margins
3. Visual field defects, enlargement of the blind spot, papilloedema, optic atrophy, ocular palsies
4. Diabetes insipidus
5. Hypopituitarism

Associated Endocrine Features. The basal metabolic rate is increased in acromegaly, but this is usually a manifestation of growth hormone activity rather than hyperthyroidism. Non-toxic goitres are not uncommon but hyperthyroidism only occasionally occurs, probably on the basis of a multinodular goitre. Hypothyroidism may be a late result of destruction of pituitary thyrotrophic cells by the tumour, or a result of surgery or radiation to the pituitary.

Damage to the gonadotrophin-producing cells is a common occurrence in acromegaly and gigantism. The hypogonadism that results is responsible for the delayed closure of the epiphyses in gigantism, and for loss of libido and impotence in men, and infertility and decreased

TABLE 1.3 *Features of Active Acromegaly*

Clinical	%
Skin and subcutaneous tissue overgrowth	100
Skeletal overgrowth: skull vault, sinuses, supraorbital ridges, lower jaw producing prognathism, vertebrae producing kyphosis	100
Excessive sweating	60
Goitre—diffuse or multinodular	20
Clinical diabetes mellitus	12
Hypertension	14
Headache, visual field defects, acne, gynaecomastia with or without galactorrhoea, diabetes insipidus.	
Hypopituitarism: hypogonadism with infertility, impotence or decreased menstruation; ACTH or TSH deficiency.	
Biochemical	%
Resting plasma growth hormone above 10 ng/ml	100
Non-suppression of growth hormone to below 5 ng/ml during glucose tolerance	100
Urine calcium above 300 mg/24 hrs	50
Impaired glucose tolerance, 'chemical diabetes'	25

frequency of menstruation with reduced loss in women; it may also play a part in the osteoporosis occasionally seen. Persistent lactation (galactorrhoea) may be a feature of acromegaly or may precede it by many years.

Adrenal function is usually normal except in the late stages of the disease where progression of the tumour or therapy may damage the corticotrophin-producing pituitary cells. Hirsuties is not infrequent in women and may be due to the adrenal adenomas found in some patients with acromegaly, or to a direct action of growth hormone on hair follicles.

Diabetes insipidus is more likely to result from effects of hypothalamic damage due to upward extension of the tumour or to the effects of surgical or radiation treatment, than to destruction of the posterior pituitary. It may be masked by the presence of hypopituitarism when cortisol secretion is impaired because of the decreased solute load presented to the kidneys.

Overt diabetes mellitus occurs in about 12 per cent of acromegalics, and impaired carbohydrate tolerance is present on testing in an equal number. Growth hormone has anti-insulin effects and directly or indirectly appears to reduce the uptake and utilisation of glucose by muscle, causing increased insulin demands. This results in increased levels of immunoreactive insulin found in the blood of acromegalics prior to and during the early stages of diabetes. Pancreatic β-cell reserve may be adequate except in subjects with a hereditary predisposition to diabetes.

Multiple endocrine adenomas, functioning and non-functioning, may occur in acromegaly, affecting the parathyroid, thyroid, adrenal, and pancreas.

Other Clinical Features

Muscle and joint symptoms are frequent in acromegaly. Weakness is common, and synovial thickening, bony and cartilaginous overgrowth all predispose to arthritis. A wide joint space due to overgrowth of articular cartilage is a feature of the condition. Osteoporosis has many causes—hypogonadism, a negative calcium balance (the increased loss of calcium in the urine exceeds the increased absorption from the gut), muscle weakness, and inactivity. Acroparaesthesiae are common from compression of the median nerve in the carpal tunnel by overgrowth of bone and soft tissue. The heart is usually enlarged, and ischaemic heart disease and hypertension may contribute to congestive heart failure. Renal size, blood flow, and glomerular filtration rate are all increased. Some patients with acromegaly have pigmentation of the skin.

DIAGNOSIS OF ACROMEGALY AND GIGANTISM

In most patients, the diagnosis is obvious and the only problem is to determine the activity of the disease and to look for complications. The onset and rate of progress of the disease can often be determined by obtaining serial photographs from the patient. Increasing sizes of gloves, rings, and shoes may also be a useful guide. Hand and foot volumes can help in assessing the response to treatment. X-rays of the skull usually show enlargement of the sella turcica or erosion of its margins as well as the prominence of the jaw and supraorbital ridges. An air-encephologram may be required to demonstrate the extent of the suprasellar extension of the tumour. An assessment of soft tissue overgrowth, for example of the heel pad, can also be made by radiology, and the increased skin thickness can be measured with skin calipers. Urinary calcium excretion exceeds 300 mg/24 hr on a diet containing less than 500 mg calcium/day in about 50 per cent of patients. This effect of growth hormone on urinary calcium excretion requires the presence of the parathyroids. Elevation of the serum phosphate level is seen in a few patients but is not of much diagnostic help. Tests of carbohydrate metabolism may give useful indirect evidence of growth hormone hypersecretion. The glucose tolerance test is abnormal in one-quarter of patients.

The final confirmation of the diagnosis of acromegaly rests with the demonstration of an *elevated plasma growth hormone level* (normally less than 10 ng/ml, fasting and at rest) which *fails to suppress* normally (to less than 5 ng/ml) during an oral glucose tolerance test (*see* Appendix). It is important to exclude coexisting deficiency of gonadotrophins (*see* p. 27), TSH (Chapter 5), and of corticotrophin during an insulin tolerance test (*see* p. 29 and Appendix). However, in patients with elevated growth hormone levels larger doses of insulin than normal (for example 0·3 units/kg) have to be used in this test to reduce the blood sugar sufficiently—to less than 40 mg/100 mls, since these patients show insulin resistance.

Prognosis

Patients with active acromegaly have about twice the expected mortality rate, death usually being due to cardiovascular complications. For this reason the condition should be treated whenever there is evidence of activity on metabolic studies. Acromegaly rarely burns itself out although the progression of the changes in physical appearance may become static after several years. In such patients the growth hormone levels usually are still elevated and the metabolic consequences and the complications remain. Rarely the pituitary tumour may infarct and result in a spontaneous cure.

TREATMENT OF GIGANTISM AND ACROMEGALY

Ideally treatment should arrest the progress of the disease and cause improvement of the soft tissue and bony manifestations and metabolic abnormalities without the production of hypopituitaris.

Partial hypophysectomy is indicated for extrasellar extensions involving the visual pathways and should be followed by external radiation. Total hypophysectomy causes remission of the disease but is a very specialised technique necessitating permanent replacement therapy for hypopituitarism. In patients with large tumours total hypophysectomy is not always possible.

Conventional high voltage radiation therapy giving courses totalling 4,500 rad does not always cause clinical improvement, though progress of the disease may be halted. A satisfactory fall in growth hormone levels occurs in about half the patients but a partial biochemical and clinical response is seen in a higher proportion although the full effects may not be seen for three or four years. High energy heavy-particle radiation produces better results but the risk to vision is greater.

Needle application of radioactive seeds into the pituitary allows a greater dose of radiation to be given, and if judged correctly may improve the disease without producing hypopituitarism. Implants of ^{198}Au or ^{90}Y, or both, have been used, and satisfactory remissions produced. Yttrium-90 is at present the isotope of choice, seeds being inserted by a transnasal route so that most of the pituitary receives a dose of 50,000–150,000 rad, though a smaller dose may be considered in patients of childbearing age. Re-implantation may sometimes be necessary if a remission is not produced in a year or two. With this technique adequate remissions should be produced in more than 50 per cent of patients. The complications of this form of treatment are visual impairment caused by radiation, oedema or haemorrhage into the pituitary gland, diabetes insipidus due to damage to the hypothalamus and median eminence, cerebrospinal rhinorrhoea, which may lead to meningitis, and third nerve palsies.

When the growth hormone levels have returned towards normal, consideration of plastic surgery to the face especially the nose and eye lids, and partial resection of the mandibles to restore the occlusion of the teeth and improve facial appearance, is extremely important and often restores the patient's morale.

GROWTH HORMONE DEFICIENCY

PITUITARY DWARFISM

In the absence of growth hormone linear growth is impaired and bone maturation is delayed, though usually to a lesser extent. Growth hormone deficiency in the foetus does not lead to reduction in body length or weight at birth. The explanation for this finding is not clear; possibly maternal or placental growth-stimulating factors may be effective, and it has been suggested that under normal conditions growth *in utero* is little affected by hormones. Careful observations on children lacking growth hormone indicate that the growth impairment develops within a few months of birth, though most cases are not diagnosed until the age of two or three years.

Deficiency of growth hormone may be congenital or acquired.

Congenital hypopituitary dwarfism is usually recognised a year or two after birth. The children show a characteristic immaturity of appearance though the body proportions are in step with the chronological age. Height is more affected than skeletal maturity though both are impaired, and height is usually below the third percentile after the fourth year of life. Even in the absence of growth hormone growth in height continues at a slow rate, usually at less than 1 cm a year, and the duration of growth is also prolonged because of the delay in bone maturity. The cause of the condition is uncertain but may be due to a hypothalamic lesion preventing normal secretion of hypothalamic growth hormone-releasing hormone; pathological studies of the pituitary are rare but in some cases have shown a relative deficiency of eosinophils. It usually occurs sporadically, affecting predominantly males, but familial cases have been reported. Perinatal brain trauma is rarely responsible for pituitary damage.

Growth hormone deficiency may occur in isolation, but often there is also a deficiency of gonadotrophins causing failure of sexual development which may be partial or complete. Gonadotrophin deficiency is difficult to diagnose till the time of puberty as the normal levels in infancy are so low. Less frequently, thyroid-stimulating hormone and ACTH may be lacking. Hypoglycaemic attacks are probably due to secondary adrenal insufficiency, but growth hormone deficiency may play a part. In adult life, the pituitary dwarf retains childish immature features and normal body proportions. The bones are slender, the skin fine and, eventually, characteristically wrinkled. Muscular weakness and fatiguability are a result of poor muscular development.

Acquired hypopituitary dwarfism results from a wide variety of disease processes causing partial or complete hypopituitarism, e.g. craniopharyngioma, Hand-Schuller-Christian disease, eosinophilic granuloma, chromophobe adenoma, tuberculous meningitis, and trauma (*see* Table 1.5, p. 26). Local manifestations are usually obvious, such as calcification above the sella turcica in craniopharyngioma or tuberculous meningitis. The pituitary fossa may be abnormal on X-ray with pituitary tumours and intrasellar calcification may be due to a craniopharyngioma. Growth hormone deficiency is rarely an isolated finding in acquired hypopituitarism, and impaired secretion of other anterior pituitary hormones is often found.

DIAGNOSIS

The clinical features of hypopituitary dwarfism may suggest the diagnosis, in particular the fine skin, delicate features, and normal body proportions. Height is invariably less than the third percentile, and bone and teeth development is immature.

X-rays of the pituitary fossa are required to exclude a local lesion, and bone X-rays (usually the hand and wrist) are required to assess bone age. If there are visual field defects due to a pituitary lesion an air-encephalogram is required. Indirect assessment of growth hormone status by insulin sensitivity tests has now been replaced by direct measurement of growth hormone output by radioimmunoassay in response to insulin-induced hypoglycaemia (*see* Appendix). After a dose of soluble insulin of 0·1 unit/kg body weight given intravenously, serum growth hormone levels often exceed 50 ng/ml within the next two hours. If hypoglycaemia is adequate (the lowest blood glucose level falling below 40 mg/100 ml accompanied by a little sweating), normal children should show a rise in growth hormone level to more than 20 ng/ml. The patient should not be left unattended during an insulin tolerance test, which should be terminated with glucose and hydrocortisone if serious manifestations of hypoglycaemia develop. The patient should be given a meal at the end of the test and kept under observation in hospital for several hours. Very occasionally normal children fail to respond to hypoglycaemia with a rise in growth hormone levels. If the hypoglycaemia has not been adequate and there has been no response the test should be repeated using a larger dose of insulin e.g. 0·15 or 0·2 units/kg. Before concluding that there is deficiency of growth hormone output it is wise to demonstrate that there is no rise also in response to intravenous arginine infusion, or during the second or third hour after administration of 1 mg subcutaneous glucagon (*see* Appendix). Growth hormone is normally secreted as the blood sugar falls again, having risen after glucagon administration. Some clinicians screen their dwarfed patients for growth hormone deficiency by taking blood after physical exercise, or at intervals for two hours after a drink of Bovril (*see* Appendix). If the growth hormone level is over 20 ng/ml growth hormone deficiency can be excluded.

Laron *et al.* (1966), observed that the insulin response to the infusion of arginine was reduced in certain patients with dwarfism who had signs of growth hormone deficiency but had high serum concentrations of immunoreative HGH. He postulated that this syndrome is due to an inherited defect of growth hormone synthesis which results in an immunologically active but biologically inactive hormone being secreted from the pituitary. The inactive hormone is presumably released in response to arginine but is unable to stimulate pancreatic insulin release. Recent studies by Merimee *et al.* (1968) on African pygmies suggest that their short stature may be due to subresponsiveness to normal growth hormone—a tissue defect.

Clinical and laboratory evidence of deficiency of other pituitary hormones should be sought and this topic is dealt with in the section on hypopituitarism (*see* p. 25). The differential diagnosis of pituitary dwarfism from delayed onset of adolescent growth and development, primordial dwarfism, gonadal dysgenesis, and other varieties of dwarfism will be considered in Chapter 4, Disorders of Growth.

TREATMENT OF PITUITARY DWARFISM

The main object of treatment is to increase the height of the patient and to correct deficiencies of other hormones as necessary. Shortness of stature has many adverse psychological effects on the individual, being particularly poorly tolerated in the female. Parental anxiety is ever present and the whole clinical situation needs handling with particular tact and discretion. As supplies of human growth hormone increase so does the need for early and critical diagnosis. It has been postulated that the full use of pituitaries from every possible autopsy would permit treatment of about 1,000 children in this country.

Before treatment with growth hormone can be considered, deficiency of the hormone should be proved by growth hormone assay during adequate insulin-induced hypoglycaemia or arginine infusion. X-rays of the lower femoral and upper tibial regions should be performed to confirm that the epiphyses are not yet fused. This is usually so except when gonadal function is normal or when the patient has been treated with sex hormones to increase sexual development or to induce menstruation. It is usual to observe the patient for a year to demonstrate lack of linear growth, since particularly after operation in the region of the hypothalamus, normal growth may be seen in the absence of measurable growth hormone. This phenomenon is unexplained. Such children usually have pathologically excessive hunger due to hypothalamic damage and are fat.

When selected for growth hormone therapy on the basis of these criteria, natural human growth hormone is usually given in a dose of five or ten milligrams twice weekly. Growth hormone causes retention of nitrogen, phosphorus, sodium, potassium and chloride, and excretion of calcium in the urine rises. Blood urea falls and the fasting blood sugar rises. With this treatment it is possible to bring pituitary dwarfs to adult heights after several years, the rate of linear growth increasing two- to fourfold. Treatment with sex hormones should be withheld as long as possible since they increase the rate of bone maturity as well as accelerating increase in height. Corticosteroid dosage should be kept to the minimum since cortisol antagonises some of the effects of growth hormone, in particular its effect on growth. Thyroxine replacement should be adequate.

When growth hormone is in short supply some selection of patients is inevitable, but no rigid criteria can be given. In general, patients with progressive lesions or those who will be unlikely to cooperate in a full course of therapy might be considered unsuitable. Ideally, the sooner treatment is begun the better while there is still growth potential. In some patients, antibodies to growth hormone can be detected in the circulation soon after beginning therapy. High titres of antibodies may interfere with the effects of the hormone, and growth ceases, but low titres of antibodies do not appear to be detrimental and tend not to be a problem with highly purified preparations. Anabolic steroids and the sex hormones can cause some acceleration of growth in pituitary dwarfs but because of the enhanced bone maturity the ultimate height of the patient may be reduced.

PROLACTIN

Prolactin is the lactogenic hormone, whose main action is to initiate and sustain lactation. In most species, growth hormone and prolactin can easily be separated, but this has proved difficult in man. There is, however, now no doubt that prolactin is present as a separate protein in human pituitaries and blood.

Assay of Prolactin

Prolactin can induce milk secretion in cultured breast tissue from rabbits and this has been used as a bioassay for the hormone. It is more sensitive than the older assay based on the increase in the weight of the pigeon crop. Now more specific radioimmunoassays for prolactin have been developed which differentiate it clearly from growth hormone.

Secretion and Action

The secretion of prolactin by the pituitary is normally kept under tonic inhibition by secretion of a prolactin inhibitory hormone. This is formed in the hypothalamus, is stored in the median eminence and is secreted into the portal capillaries of the pituitary stalk to reach the anterior pituitary cells. Cessation of secretion of prolactin inhibitory hormone allows prolactin secretion. Normally plasma prolactin levels are less than 20 ng/ml and show a circadian rhythm, the highest levels being found during the night. Prolactin secretion is high in the neonate, accounting for the common 'witch's milk' of the new born, and in the mother during breast feeding and there is a reflex secretion during stimulation of the breast. It is also secreted during stress.

In animals, prolactin causes milk secretion in the mammary gland that has already been primed by other hormones. Oestrogens and progesterone are required for proliferation of the mammary ducts and alveoli. Cortisol must also be present for the ovarian steroids to be fully effective. Milk secretion into the alveoli and terminal ductules results from the action of prolactin but oxytocin is required to cause contraction of the myoepithelial cells of the alveoli and ductules forcing milk into the larger ducts and cisterns. Although prolactin has a definite effect on the corpus luteum in lower species, this action does not appear to be present in man. Corpora lutea following ovulation induced by FSH and HCG in hypophysectomised women have a normal life span.

Prolactin has many metabolic effects on different tissues, similar to those of growth hormone. It causes nitrogen, potassium and phosphate retention, and hypercalcuria. A hyperglycaemic effect occurs in the hypopituitary subject, and in pituitary dwarfs animal prolactin can cause an increase in linear growth. The action of prolactin at a molecular level is not yet defined but it has been demonstrated to stimulate protein synthesis *in vitro*.

Prolactin secretion is probably maintained by the stimulus of suckling, afferent nervous pathways from the breast traversing the spinal cord to reach the posterior median eminence.

GALACTORRHOEA

OVERPRODUCTION OF PROLACTIN

Irritation of the thoracic-spinal nerve segments after thoracotomy or herpes zoster can initiate persistent lactation, presumably by stimulation of the afferent pathway for prolactin release. Various drugs such as reserpine, chlorpromazine and other centrally-acting drugs may cause lactation, probably by inhibiting hypothalamic centres which normally secrete prolactin inhibitory factor. A variety of diseases in the pituitary-hypothalamic region can also initiate or prolong lactation (Table 1.4).

Persistent lactation without suckling, may occur spontaneously or follow pregnancy. Such patients are not infrequently found to have a pituitary tumour, and even if there is no enlargement of the sella turcica careful follow up is indicated. The amenorrhoea that usually occurs is due to lack of gonadotrophin secretion which is a common accompaniment of hyperprolactinaemia. Prolonged lactation may also occur in women who have never been pregnant due to a similar mechanism. Galactorrhoea may occur in association with chromophobe,

TABLE 1.4 *Common Causes of Galactorrhoea and Hyperprolactinaemia*

1. *Centrally-acting drugs:*
   phenothiazines including some antihistamines;
   oral contraceptives;
   reserpine;
   methyldopa;
   haloperidol;
   tricyclic antidepressants.
2. *Hypothalamic disease and pituitary stalk lesions:*
   tumours, granulomas, meningitis.
3. *Pituitary tumours:*
   otherwise non-functioning tumours;
   acromegaly;
   Cushing's disease.
4. *'Ectopic' prolactin secretion:*
   lung tumours.
5. *Primary hypothyroidism (rare):*
   ? due to increased TRH secretion which causes both TSH and prolactin release.
6. *Chest wall injury:*
   trauma;
   surgery;
   herpes zoster.

basophil, and eosinophil adenomas of the pituitary. Rarely, it occurs in men. A variety of eponyms has been applied to the various syndromes associated with amenorrhoea and galactorrhoea. They serve no useful purpose since one syndrome may develop into the other and all are due to hyperprolactinaemia. Acromegaly or Cushing's disease may be found, or may develop, in patients who present with galactorrhoea. Galactorrhoea with or without amenorrhoea may complicate or follow oral contraceptive medication.

Treatment of Inappropriate Lactation

The hyperprolactinaemia and galactorrhoea disappear if any precipitating drug can be stopped. In the presence of pituitary or hypothalamic disease, radiation, oestrogen or clomiphene therapy usually do not work. Recently treatment with the new ergot alkaloid, 2-brom-α-ergocryptine has been shown to reduce elevated prolactin levels, stop the galactorrhoea and usually to restore gonadotrophin secretion to normal. Sometimes l-dopa therapy may improve hyperprolactinaemia and inhibit milk production.

UNDERPRODUCTION OF PROLACTIN

This is the cause of failure of lactation in post-partum pituitary necrosis and other causes of pan-hypopituitarism. In patients with selective failure of gonadotrophin production, e.g. as a result of anorexia nervosa, lactation but not menstruation may follow pregnancy induced by gonadotrophin therapy.

CORTICOTROPHIN (ACTH) AND MELANOCYTE-STIMULATING HORMONES (α- AND β-MSH)

Human ACTH is a single chain polypeptide of 39 amino-acids, with a molecular weight of approximately 4,500. It has been completely synthesised, and the amino-acid sequences essential for ACTH action have been characterised. The first 'amino-terminal' 24 amino-acids of ACTH are required for its actions on the adrenal cortex, to promote synthesis of corticosteroids—mainly cortisol (hydrocortisone) in man, but also some corticosterone—and to increase the blood flow through the gland (Fig. 1.2). The melanocyte-stimulating hormones α- and β-MSH are peptides closely related to the steroidogenic 1-24 portion of the ACTH molecule. α-MSH has 13 amino-acids and the sequence is identical to the first 13 amino-acids of ACTH. Specific radioimmunoassay studies suggest that α-MSH is only found in the pituitary gland and does not appear to circulate in the blood. Its functional significance is unknown. Human β-MSH contains 22 amino-acids, of which numbers 11 to 17 are the same as 4 to 10 of ACTH and α-MSH. β-MSH circulates in the blood and appears to be secreted under all circumstances together with ACTH, and indeed it is synthesised in the same basophilic cells of the anterior pituitary. β-MSH has little trophic effect on the adrenal cortex, and ACTH has only 3 per cent of the pigmentary activity of β-MSH. The increased pigmentation associated with diseases in which ACTH secretion is excessive, for example primary adrenocortical insufficiency, Addison's disease, is due to the parallel secretion of β-MSH which stimulates the melanocytes of the skin, most characteristically in the exposed parts of the body, the genitalia, pressure points and the buccal mucosa.

The function of the non-steroidogenic 'carboxyl-terminal' portion of the ACTH molecule, amino-acids 25 to 39, is unknown. It is within this portion that the differences lie between ACTH of different species, although such differences are small. Several 'extra-adrenal' actions of ACTH have been demonstrated *in vitro*, and some have been ascribed to this C-terminal part of the molecule. However, there is no reliable evidence to suggest that these actions are important in man.

Secretion and Transport. ACTH release from the pituitary is mediated by specific polypeptides produced in the hypothalamus, especially in the median eminence, which reach the anterior pituitary by way of the local portal circulation. These corticotrophin-releasing factors (CRF) have been designated α-CRF and β-CRF. The β-CRF resembles vasopressin and is the more active; α-CRF, which can be further separated into α_1- and α_2-CRF, has a structure similar to α-MSH. It is still uncertain whether they represent the true CRF. The hypothalamic centres are, in turn, controlled by brainstem and suprahypothalamic centres. Distinct hypothalamic sites are responsible for the response to high and low circulating steroid levels in a negative feedback system and to stressful stimuli, e.g. surgical operations, hypoglycaemia or fever.

ACTH MOLECULE

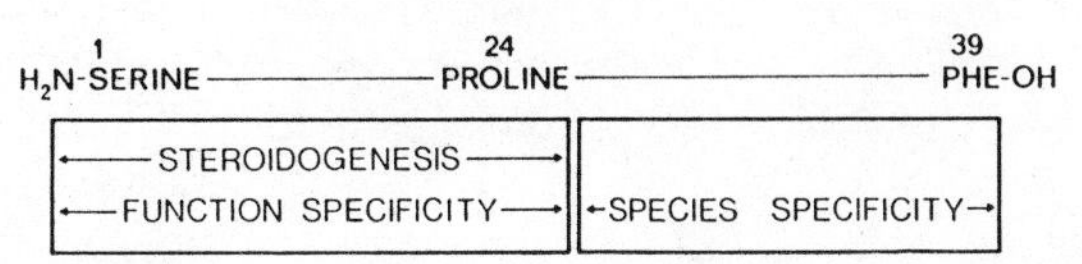

FIGURE 1.2 Diagrammatic representation of the 39 amino-acids of ACTH showing the 'N-terminal' steroidogenic and 'C-terminal' species-specific portions of the molecule. The amino-acid sequence of α-MSH is the same as 1 to 13 of ACTH, and β-MSH has the sequence 11 to 17 in common with 4 to 10 of ACTH.

There is also a circadian rhythm of ACTH secretion initiated by the hypothalamus which leads to changes in cortisol output from the adrenal—the plasma cortisol is at its peak about the time of waking, at its lowest about the time of retiring and normally begins to rise at about 3 a.m. Disturbances of the rhythm occur in Cushing's syndrome, heart failure, depressive illness, and other forms of stress, but not in Addison's disease. The situation is well summarised by Cope (1964) who concludes: 'the corticotrophin-release mechanism does not consist of a single centre responding to stimulant, inhibitory, or stressful stimuli but a much more complex situation is involved in which each of these forms of influence is capable of exerting its own effect independently of the others and probably through a separate chain of events.'

The concentration of ACTH in the circulation can be determined by bioassay and by radioimmunoassay procedures. In man, the normal level in venous blood between 8.0 and 10.0 a.m.

ranges from 10 to 70 pg/ml of plasma. The changes in circulating ACTH that have been seen in various clinical situations are shown in Fig. 1.3. ACTH disappears rapidly from the circulation with a half-time of five to twenty minutes.

Metabolic Effects of ACTH and MSH. Many theories have been offered to explain the action of ACTH on the adrenal cortex but none is fully adequate. Synthesis of cortisol and some corticosterone is stimulated and adrenal weight and vascularity increased. Koritz (1968) has postulated that ACTH, via cyclic 3′5′ AMP, affects the mitochondrial membrane, increasing the rate of removal of pregnenolone from the mitochondria. All the subsequent reactions of steroidogenesis except 11-hydroxylation occur outside the mitochondria, hence the rate of formation of steroids depends on the availability of pregnenolone. Again, pregnenolone inhibits

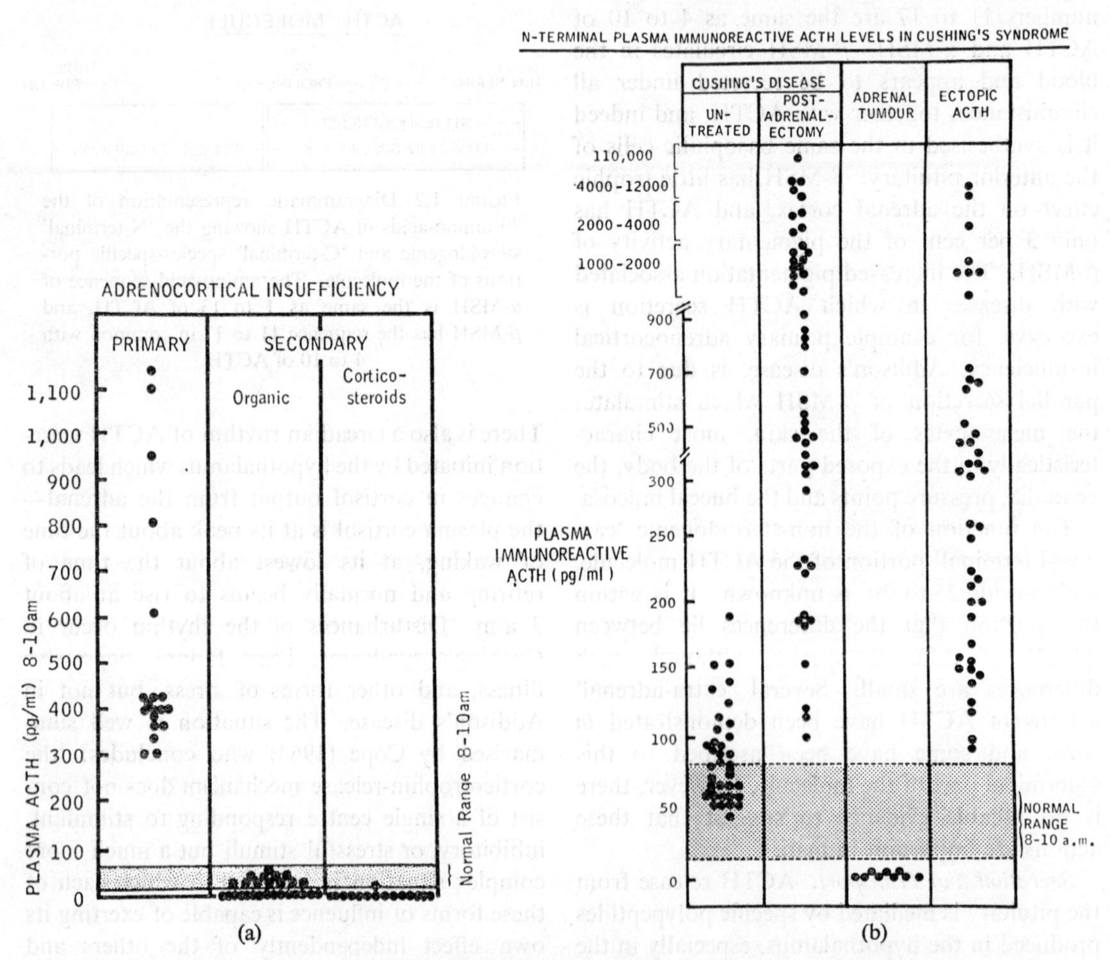

FIGURE 1.3 Plasma ACTH concentrations, measured by radioimmunoassay in conditions of adrenocortical insufficiency and Cushing's syndrome. Some patients with pituitary or hypothalamic disease have been normal basal ACTH levels but cannot increase the secretion in response to stress.
(Fig. 1.3*a*. from Besser, G. M., (1972), *Medicine*, Number 1, page 105, by permission of Medical Education (International) Ltd., and Fig. 1.3*b*. from Besser, G. M., and Edwards, C. R. W. (1972), *Clinics in Endocrinology and Metabolism*, *1*, 473, by permission of W. B. Saunders Ltd.).

the transformation of cholesterol to 20α-hydroxycholesterol, the first reaction in its own formation, and removal of pregnenolone from the mitochondrion will reduce this inhibition. Certainly the first step in the action of ACTH is to attach itself to specific membrane receptors on the surface of the adrenocortical cell and activate the cyclic AMP mechanism. Further studies on the mechanism of action of ACTH should indicate whether this proposed scheme is a valid one.

ACTH also has numerous extra-adrenal actions which have been documented in adrenalectomised animals, but not, as yet, in patients. In man, the only effect so far proved to be of clinical significance is the melanocyte-stimulating action which causes the pigmentation seen in some patients with Cushing's disease, Addison's disease and in congenital adrenal hyperplasia. Increased pigmentation is frequent when plasma ACTH levels exceed 500 pg/ml. However since β-MSH is always secreted in excess along with ACTH, and it is much more pigmenting than ACTH, β-MSH would seem to be the hormone principally responsible for the pigmentation. In animals, MSH causes dispersal of melanin granules in the melanocytes, thereby causing darkening of the skin. Such dispersal of granules may occur in man but MSH may also act by stimulating melanin formation.

CLINICAL EFFECTS OF ACTH

OVERPRODUCTION OF ACTH

Increased production of ACTH by the pituitary can occur in response to a fall in plasma cortisol resulting from adrenal disease, or because of some derangement in the pituitary-hypothalamic mechanisms controlling ACTH release. In the former case, if the plasma cortisol is not restored to normal by the increased ACTH acting on the adrenal cortex, a further rise in circulating ACTH will occur. An elevated plasma ACTH and β-MSH may then cause increased pigmentation of the skin. If the adrenals are intact, increased secretion of ACTH caused by pituitary-hypothalamic disease will produce Cushing's disease because of the overproduction of cortisol. The term Cushing's syndrome should be used to include all the abnormalities that result from sustained inappropriate elevation of plasma corticosteroids. 'Cushing's disease' should be restricted to that form caused by excessive secretion of pituitary ACTH. The condition resulting from prolonged overdosage with corticosteroids for treatment differs in no way from that produced by overproduction of cortisol from the adrenal cortex.

In clinical practice, 70 to 80 per cent of cases of Cushing's syndrome are associated with pituitary-dependent adrenocortical hyperplasia, and 20 to 30 per cent are due to adrenal or extra-adrenal tumours. Occasional cases of adrenal hyperplasia occur in response to ACTH-like peptides produced by various malignant tumours, especially bronchogenic carcinomas.

The main defect in Cushing's disease associated with bilateral adrenal hyperplasia probably lies in the hypothalamus. In such patients the control of ACTH secretion is abnormal, high levels of the trophic hormone being produced regardless of the high level of circulating cortisol and the normal circadian rhythm is abolished. The increased ACTH secretion cannot easily be reduced by exogenous steroids, as occurs in normal subjects. In Cushing's disease, much higher doses of cortisol-like steroids, e.g. dexamethasone 2 mg every six hours, are required to reduce ACTH production. The response of the hypothalamic centres to a fall in plasma cortisol is usually intact since administration of metyrapone, which blocks cortisol synthesis, usually causes a rise in ACTH production and adrenal stimulation. Further evidence for a hypothalamic abnormality in Cushing's disease is seen in the response to insulin-induced hypoglycaemia. This stress acting through hypothalamic and possibly higher levels, normally causes pituitary ACTH release and adrenal stimulation. In Cushing's disease the response to hypoglycaemia is lost. This suprapituitary abnormality causing stimulation of the pituitary may be responsible for the pituitary tumours associated with Cushing's disease, which may occur pre- or post-adrenalectomy, the incidence being approximately 30 per cent. They are most commonly composed of chromophobe cells and, less frequently, basophils. Rarely they may be malignant. The presence of these tumours is usually heralded by an increase in skin pigmentation, similar to that seen in Addison's disease but of much greater intensity. Some of the patients have enlargement of the sella turcica, and the tumours causing this are usually chromophobe adenomas. The tumours respond in part to the normal feedback mechanisms, the output of ACTH being partially suppressed by high doses of dexamethasone. However, in a number of cases the plasma ACTH is found to be higher than in other patients with Cushing's disease. The tumours also produce β-MSH, since elevated levels of MSH in plasma and urine have been described. Earlier suggestions that the tumours were less frequent after partial adrenalectomy have not been substantiated. The occurrence of such tumours in Cushing's disease after adrenalectomy is likely to be a result of the natural course of the disease, though it is possible that the fall in cortisol levels produced by adrenalectomy may accelerate their rate of growth. If the disease originates at pituitary or hypothalamic levels it would seem reasonable to direct the treatment to the pituitary. Hypophysectomy by surgery, yttrium-90 or external radiation treatment is not always successful in curing the disease, and ACTH-secreting pituitary remnants are sometimes difficult to eradicate. However, pituitary irradiation at the time of total adrenalectomy usually prevents the progressive pigmentation and enlargement of the fossa. Further discussion of Cushing's syndrome will be found in Chapter 6.

UNDERPRODUCTION OF ACTH

This will result in decreased secretion of cortisol and adrenal androgens. ACTH production is usually a late function to be lost in pituitary disease and is therefore almost always associated with gonadotrophin and growth hormone deficiency and often also by TSH deficiency. Very rarely an isolated deficiency of ACTH production may be seen with maintenance of other trophic hormone production but it would seem that such cases are more likely to be due to hypothalamic disease. Patients with solitary ACTH deficiency have exhibited weakness, hypoglycaemia and weight loss. Decreased axillary and pubic hair growth may occur in female patients. In these patients, primary adrenal disease must be excluded by demonstrating a normal response to ACTH. The diagnosis of deficiency of pituitary ACTH production will be considered in the section on hypopituitarism (*see* p. 25).

GONADOTROPHINS

The human pituitary secretes two gonadotrophins, follicle-stimulating hormone (FSH) and luteinising hormone (LH), alternatively named interstitial-cell stimulating hormone (ICSH) in the male. In certain species, including the rat, prolactin has a luteotrophic action and can be regarded as a third gonadotrophin, but in man the corpus luteum can be maintained without the action of prolactin.

Assays

Pure preparations of the gonadotrophins have been obtained only very recently. In the past insensitive bioassays have mainly been used in the estimation of gonadotrophins in blood and urine or pituitary extracts, but recently more sensitive radioimmunoassays have been developed for both FSH and LH.

Bioassay for FSH. 1. Ovarian follicle growth in hypophysectomised immature rats. This is a specific test for FSH but is too laborious for clinical use. 2. Augmentation tests. These depend on the increase in ovarian weight of intact, immature rats or mice previously treated with excess human chorionic gonadotrophin (HCG). HCG augments the action of FSH on the ovary and eliminates the effects of any LH in the test material since the action of HCG is similar to that of LH.

Bioassay for LH. 1. The ventral prostatic weight test in hypophysectomised immature male rats is specific for LH but too laborious for routine use. 2. The ovarian ascorbic acid depletion test using intact immature pseudopregnant rats is a satisfactory method of assay for LH. The animals are pretreated with gonadotrophin from pregnant mares' serum, followed by chorionic gonadotrophin. The sensitivity of the test can be increased by measuring depletion of cholesterol.

Non-specific Bioassays. The mouse uterus test is the most widely used assay. Extracts of test urine are injected into immature mice for several days and the amount required to produce a 100 per cent increase in uterine weight contains one mouse unit. This method measures the combined effects of FSH and LH and provides a clinically useful index of total gonadotrophin activity. The magnitude of response depends on the relative proportions of FSH and LH in the specimens as well as their absolute amounts, so it is difficult to express the results in quantitative terms. The result can be converted to appropriate international reference standards by comparison with control preparations. In most assays, careful extraction of urine is required to remove toxic materials, and to concentrate the hormones.

Immunoassays. Immunoassays are now available for LH and FSH in blood and urine. LH can easily be assayed in men and non-pregnant women because of its ability to cross-react with antiserum to human chorionic gonadotrophin (HCG). A radioimmunological technique is used based on the competition between HCG or LH in the sample and ^{131}I-labelled HCG for binding sites in antisera to HCG. These tests do not distinguish between LH and HCG but since HCG is normally absent in non-pregnant subjects, LH can be measured. More specific radioimmunoassays for LH utilise anti-LH antisera and ^{131}I-labelled LH. Specific anti-FSH sera now available show little or no cross-reaction with LH. Many of the earlier gonadotrophin antisera were not very specific and showed cross-reaction with each other and with TSH. Radioimmunoassays for FSH and LH now give results that correlate well with those of bioassays.

Standards

The field of gonadotrophin assays has been confused by variations in methodology and standards. Different extraction procedures on urine or blood samples and the different strains of animals used in the assays have made it difficult to compare results from individual laboratories. Again, standard preparations have varied, and results expressed in relation to standards from other species are not always valid in man. Radioimmunoassays require their own standards and the relationships with the results of bioassays need to be worked out for each individual system. Urinary gonadotrophins are assayed against an International Reference Preparation (IRP) of human urinary menopausal gonadotrophin (HMG) but pituitary or blood gonadotrophin assays should use a reference standard derived from purified pituitary LH and FSH since gonadotrophins in the urine have different characteristics from those in blood or the pituitary and presumably represent partially degraded material.

FOLLICLE-STIMULATING HORMONE (FSH)

FSH is a glycoprotein with a molecular weight of about 30,000, containing approximately 8 per cent of carbohydrate. Sialic acid is an integral part of the molecule. It is doubtful whether full purification of FSH has yet been achieved. The primary follicle of the ovary develops to the fluid-filled vesicular stage under the action of FSH, which also stimulates granulosa cell proliferation, plays some part in oestrogen biosynthesis, and increases oestrogen production. In the male, FSH increases spermatogenesis and seminiferous tubule development.

LUTEINISING HORMONE (LH, ICSH)

LH is also a glycoprotein with molecular weight in the region of 30,000. It has a high cystine content. The hormone induces ovulation, stimulates oestrogen production by the theca interna, and initiates and maintains the corpus luteum. In the male, LH stimulates the interstitial or Leydig cells to produce androgens and, therefore, has a secondary role in maturation of spermatocytes and in the development of secondary sexual characteristics.

HUMAN MENOPAUSAL GONADOTROPHIN (HMG)

In human blood the gonadotrophin levels increase after the gonadal failure which results in the menopause. This gonadotrophin is excreted in the urine and may be extracted for therapeutic use. One such preparation—Pergonal—has been used to stimulate ovulation.

CHORIONIC GONADOTROPHIN (HCG)

HCG is produced by the human placenta and by ovarian, testicular and uterine tumours of trophoblastic origin. It has a close functional and structural relationship to LH and is predominantly luteinising in function. Its molecular weight is about 30,000 and its carbohydrate content is 30 per cent. A simple reliable pregnancy test has been developed based on the detection of HCG in the urine of pregnant women by immunological techniques. Both haemagglutination inhibition and complement fixation tests have been used. Peak levels occur about the ninth week of pregnancy, followed by low levels in mid-pregnancy and a second smaller peak in the third trimester. In certain cases of threatened abortion a fall in level of HCG may give a warning of impending placental failure. High levels of HCG are found in certain trophoblastic tumours and hormone assay can be used as an index of the effectiveness of therapy.

Secretion and action of gonadotrophins is dealt with in Chapter 7.

GONADOTROPHIN LEVELS IN SERUM

There appear to be no circadian changes in LH or FSH but there are spontaneous fluctuations in each suggesting that they are secreted in surges lasting one to two hours at a time. Serum LH levels show a very large peak prior to ovulation and are raised in post-menopausal women. Serum FSH levels are higher in the follicular phase of the menstrual cycle, decline prior to the LH peak, show a secondary rise which may coincide with the LH peak and then gradually rise during the luteal phase. Levels of FSH are more variable than LH throughout the cycle. In post-menopausal women FSH levels are markedly elevated.

THE FEEDBACK MECHANISM

The mechanism controlling the release of gonadotrophin is still poorly understood. Both FSH- and LH-releasing factors (FSH-RF, LH-RF) were found in early work using extracts of the stalk median eminence region of the hypothalamus. However, only one pure peptide hormone has been isolated from these hypothalamic extracts. This hormone contains 10 amino-acids and studies with the synthetic material has shown that although it causes the pituitary to release large amounts of LH, some FSH is also released. This hormone has therefore been provisionally called the LH/FSH-releasing hormone. Whether there is also a second, predominantly FSH-releasing hormone, is not yet known but it seems possible that the complex sequence of hormonal secretion which occurs during the menstrual cycle could result from the interaction of the circulating gonadal steroid concentrations and midbrain influences, on the secretion of one gonadotrophin-releasing hormone and its action on the anterior pituitary cells. The nature of the negative feedback mechanism acting in the pituitary-gonadal axis is complex and inadequately documented in man. The rising oestrogen levels during the follicular phase may inhibit FSH but trigger the release of the ovulatory surge of LH. Release of LH is later suppressed by progesterone in the presence of oestrogens. In males gonadotrophin secretion is relatively constant. Testosterone appears to activate the negative feedback mechanism for LH whereas FSH secretion may be influenced by an as yet unidentified hormone secreted by the seminiferous tubules. Decreased sensitivity of the hypothalamic receptor sites to the negative feedback of gonadal steroids may account for the development of puberty. Levels of steroid secreted by the immature gonads become incapable of inhibiting FSH and LH production and puberty ensues.

CLINICAL APPLICATIONS OF GONADOTROPHIN ASSAYS

The most valuable application of the gonadotrophin assays is in determining whether gonadal failure is due to pituitary or hypothalamic disease or a disorder affecting the gonads themselves. In 'primary' gonadal failure, following castration or in chromosomal abnormalities such as Turner's syndrome or Klinefelter's syndrome, gonadotrophin levels are high whereas in gonadal failure secondary to anterior pituitary or hypothalamic disease gonadotrophin levels are low or undetectable. In adults with pituitary or hypothalamic disease gonadotrophin production usually fails early and the finding of normal gonadotrophins in the blood or urine is strong evidence against a diagnosis of hypopituitarism. In females with primary or secondary amenorrhoea, gonadotrophin estimations are particularly helpful. Clomiphene, a drug with anti-oestrogen actions, attaches itself to gonadal steroid receptors in the hypothalamus, and causes secretion of the gonadotrophins. It can be used to confirm a suspected diagnosis of hypopituitarism in men or women since the serum LH should normally rise during administration of clomiphene in a dose of 2 or 3 mg/kg body weight (*see* Appendix). Absence of this rise confirms hypopituitarism but may also be found in severe anorexia nervosa. Unfortunately the drug has to be given for at least 7 days for this test.

Patients with seminoma of the testis sometimes excrete large amounts of gonadotrophin indistinguishable from HMG. Before puberty, gonadotrophin levels are low but in girls they rise in the year prior to puberty. Positive results are not usually found in boys before the age of thirteen years. After the menopause, raised gonadotrophin excretion occurs, but in old age (above seventy years) in both sexes the levels fall.

Certain types of bronchogenic carcinoma with hypertrophic pulmonary osteoarthropathy and gynaecomastia secrete gonadotrophins resembling FSH, which may account for the raised oestrogen levels found in the urine in these cases.

CLINICAL USES OF GONADOTROPHINS

Primary or secondary amenorrhoea may be due to lack of secretion of pituitary gonadotrophins or to ovarian failure. The latter cause can be confirmed by the finding of high blood or urinary gonadotrophins. Low pituitary gonadotrophin secretion can result from clinically obvious pituitary or hypothalamic disease, but in most cases no other abnormality can be detected. Such patients usually present with secondary amenorrhoea and infertility and serum gonadotrophin levels which do not respond to clomiphene. In early cases the uterus may be normal or small, the endometrium proliferative or inactive, the ovaries normal in size, and oestrogen excretion may fluctuate. In later cases the uterus is small, the endometrium inactive or atrophic, the ovaries small, and oestrogen and pregnanediol excretion is low.

Ovulation and, hence, restoration of fertility can be induced in patients with hypopituitarism by treatment with human FSH and HCG. The object of such therapy is to cause ovulation and produce urinary excretion of oestrogens and progesterone which simulate those occurring in a normal cycle. FSH may be obtained from human pituitaries or from urine (human menopausal gonadotrophin, HMG—Pergonal). Best results are obtained with FSH preparations which also contain LH activity. The total dose is divided into three equal injections over five days and followed on the eighth day with 4,500 IU of HCG. The total dose of FSH is increased each month till ovulation occurs, as shown by a rise in urinary oestrogens and, later, of pregnanediol. Pregnanediol is a major metabolite of progesterone and its excretion indicates the formation of a functioning corpus luteum and therefore of ovulation. By careful regulation of dosage of FSH and urinary assays of steroid hormones the main complications of therapy, overstimulation of the ovary and multiple ovulation, can be avoided. Over-dosage with FSH or LH or undue sensitivity of the patient may cause a 'hyperstimulation syndrome', comprising massive ovarian enlargement, abdominal discomfort, ascites, pleural effusion, thromboembolic phenomena, and death. By careful selection of patients, ovulation and subsequent pregnancies can often be produced. The pregnancies are sometimes complicated by abortion or placental failure, and scrupulous ante-natal care is required. Further work is required to define optimal dosage schedules of FSH preparations. In panhypopituitary patients treated in this way menstruation may not occur till two weeks after HCG administration, suggesting that only a single luteotrophic stimulus is needed at the time of ovulation and that prolactin is not an essential luteotrophic factor in man.

HMG can be used to demonstrate that amenorrhoea is due to primary ovarian failure, when no rise in oestrogen excretion can be produced. It can also be used along with HCG to stimulate spermatogenesis in the hypophysectomised male. There are many causes of male infertility but in appropriate cases, where gonadotrophin excretion is low, HMG and HCG may rarely restore fertility.

Clomiphene is ineffective in stimulating gonadotrophin secretion in women with organic hypopituitarism. However, in women with secondary amenorrhoea without pituitary or hypothalamic lesions, clomiphene in doses of 50–150 mg daily for five days can cause ovulation. Administration of HCG seven days after the clomiphene may help to produce ovulation. Ovarian enlargement occurs in some cases, and minor effects, including hot flushes, blurring of vision, and nausea and vomiting, are occasionally seen. If clomiphene has not been effective after 3 to 6 courses given at monthly intervals HMG should be tried. In normal males, clomiphene produces a generalised increase in steroid output, especially of oestrone. Its role in male infertility is not yet precisely defined.

Patients with the polycystic ovary syndrome show a variable response to HMG or clomiphene. Some show a marked rise in urinary oestrogens, others fail to respond. Courses of FSH and HCG, or clomiphene, can induce ovulation in some patients with this disorder. Regular menstruation and fertility can sometimes be restored by clomiphene, bromergocryptine or pituitary gonadotrophins in patients with galactorrhoea (*see* p. 12).

Thyroid-stimulating Hormone (*TSH*)

This hormone is dealt with in Chapter 5.

PITUITARY TUMOURS

Pituitary tumours may be situated in or above the sella turcica, depending on their size and extent of growth as well as on the particular cells from which they arise. Tumours may develop from cells of the anterior lobe, the posterior lobe, or from epithelial remnants of the cranio-pharyngeal duct. Small asymptomatic pituitary adenomas are found in one-quarter of pituitary glands examined at autopsy. Clinically significant pituitary tumours make up about 10 per cent of all intracranial neoplasms. Anterior lobe tumours are classified according to the character of their secretory granules—acidophil, basophil, and chromophobe—but more than one cell type may occur in a particular tumour. The normal anterior lobe contains about 52 per cent chromophobe cells, 37 per cent eosinophils, and 11 per cent basophils. Chromophobe tumours are four times commoner than those arising from chromophil cells, the incidence being chromophobe adenomas 79 per cent, eosinophilic adenomas 15 per cent, and basophil adenomas 6 per cent.

Chromophobe adenomas are rare in childhood and occur with about equal frequency in the sexes. Familial cases have been reported and there may be an association with parathyroid adenomas and pancreatic islet-cell tumours. Histologically there is a wide variation in granularity but usually large granules are lacking. The cells often contain fine PAS-positive granulation; they may become very large and locally invasive, but distant metastases are extremely rare.

Eosinophil adenomas have a similar age and sex distribution to the chromophobe variety. Mixed tumours containing eosinophil and chromophobe cells are common. In some cases of acromegaly and gigantism eosinophil hyperplasia may be present.

Basophil adenomas are rarely large enough to cause expansion of the pituitary fossa. They occur in about 20 per cent of patients with Cushing's disease and may in some cases antedate the disease or develop after adrenalectomy. A review of the histology of 43 cases of pituitary tumours associated with Cushing's disease showed 28 to be chromophobes, only 9 basophil, 1 eosinophil and 5 mixed basophil-chromophobe; 12 of these were malignant (Nelson and Sprunt, 1965). Crooke observed a constant change in the pituitary basophils in Cushing's syndrome whether primarily of pituitary or adrenocortical origin. This consisted of replacement of most of the cytoplasmic granules by a hyaline homogeneous material. When an adenoma is present the tumour basophils are spared, whereas those of the rest of the gland are affected. Crooke's hyaline change represents the reponse of pituitary ACTH-producing basophils to a raised level of circulating cortisol.

Primary tumours of the posterior pituitary are rare; astrocytomas, ganglioneuromas, and tumours made up of cells resembling pituicytes have been reported.

Craniopharyngiomas are the commonest tumour in the pituitary area in children and adolescents. In about half the cases symptoms arise before the age of fifteen years. The tumours are most often situated above the sella and make up about 4 per cent of all intracranial tumours. They may be entirely cystic or partly solid, and cholesterol crystals are numerous in the cyst fluid. Histological appearances of the craniopharyngioma are variable, ranging from groups of columnar cells on a basement membrane to squamous cells with cornified areas that are often calcified.

Tumours of the optic chiasm, hypothalamus, third ventricle, mid-brain, and pineal may all affect the pituitary-hypothalamic region. Secondary tumours from breast, lung, and other sites and various reticuloses may also involve the area.

CLINICAL MANIFESTATIONS

The clinical manifestations of pituitary tumours depend on:

(*a*) local consequences of a space-occupying lesion
(*b*) hormonal changes

(*a*) LOCAL EFFECTS OF PITUITARY TUMOURS

Headache
Visual disturbances
Cranial nerve palsies
Hypothalamic syndromes
'Pituitary apoplexy'
Radiological findings

Headaches are a frequent complaint of patients with pituitary tumours though their location and severity are variable. They are probably caused by traction on the diaphragma sellae, adjacent dura and neighbouring blood vessels.

Loss of vision is a common complication of pituitary tumours indicating that the tumour or the expanded sellar diaphragm are pressing on the optic chiasm or, less frequently, on the nerves or tracts. The commonest visual defect is a bitemporal hemianopia caused by pressure on the lower crossing central fibres of the chiasm, with sparing of the uncrossed lateral fibres. The first defects are in the upper temporal quadrant and they may be associated with enlargement of the blind spot and loss of colour vision, especially for red. The nature of the visual defect depends on the relation of the pituitary fossa to the chiasm which normally lies directly on the diaphragma sellae, and to the direction of growth of the tumour. Anterior, posterior, superior, and lateral deviations of the chiasm occur as anatomical variations, so the types of defect produced vary considerably and indeed the pituitary tumour often expands asymmetrically. When displaced upwards the optic nerves may be compressed against the posterior communicating arteries. Optic atrophy is common but papilloedema is rare. The visual fields should always be checked by confrontation in the routine clinical examination and exact plotting of the central fields using a Bjerrum screen is essential, especially to follow the progress of visual defects. Field plotting using both red and white objects is important since early abnormalities are often only detectable in the red fields.

Cranial nerve palsies are uncommon. Occasionally the third, fourth and sixth nerves and the olfactory nerves or tracts can be affected.

Suprasellar lesions, especially craniopharyngiomas, may produce abnormalities from pressure on various hypothalamic centres. Although obesity and disturbances of sleep such as somnolence, narcolepsy, and cataplexy can occur, diabetes insipidus is by far the commonest manifestation of hypothalamic disease. The management of diabetes insipidus may be particularly difficult if there is concomitant damage to the centres controlling thirst. The centres controlling appetite may be affected producing increased or decreased appetite and obesity or emaciation. Damage to the hypothalamic centres transmitting chemical mediators to the anterior pituitary can cause impaired pituitary secretion of growth hormone, TSH, ACTH, and the gonadotrophins. Further extension of the tumour may lead to internal hydrocephalus with raised intracranial pressure and its clinical sequelae.

Haemorrhage into a pituitary tumour sometimes causes acute pituitary insufficiency with loss of vision. Small infarcts of tumours leading to cystic degeneration are common and if extensive may produce an appearance of an 'empty fossa' on air encephalography, i.e., air passes into an enlarged pituitary fossa which contains only little pituitary tissue. There may be surprisingly normal pituitary endocrine function despite the 'empty fossa'.

Pituitary tumours cause erosion of the walls of the sella, and the enlargement is visible on skull X-rays. Acidophil tumours involve, particularly, the region of the anterior clinoids since the eosinophil cells are mainly distributed in the superior lateral part of the pituitary. The anterior and posterior clinoid processes become eroded, thin and indistinct on X-ray. Almost half the patients with chromophobe adenomas show a double contour of the pituitary fossa on lateral skull X-rays, due to asymmetrical expansion of the tumour and this is usually the first abnormality seen. Confirmation that the double contour of the sella is due to asymmetrical enlargement is easily obtained by tomograms in either the sagittal or coronal planes. Ballooning of the floor of the sella is another common feature. The degree of suprasellar extension of the tumour can be assessed by air encephalography. The normal dimensions of the pituitary fossa have been listed. Abnormal calcification above or within the dorsum sellae usually indicates a craniopharyngioma but can result from previous tuberculous meningitis. Care must be taken not to confuse para-sellar calcification in the carotid arteries with true fossa calcification.

(*b*) HORMONAL CHANGES

These result either from deficient hormone secretion (*see* next section) or over-production. Growth hormone overproduction occurs predominantly with tumours of the eosinophilic variety and usually leads to acromegaly, for the tumours do not often develop before adult life; if they do, they may produce gigantism. Rarely, spontaneous infarction of the tumour may arrest its activity and cause panhypopituitarism but this rarely occurs from expansion of the tumour alone although lesser degrees of hormone deficiency are common. Most cases of so-called 'burnt out' acromegaly have raised circulating growth hormone, and the apparent inactivity is presumably due to an equilibrium between tissue growth response and growth hormone levels. The metabolic complications remain however.

Apparent prolactin overproduction can result from either chromophobe or acidophilic adenomas and the prolonged or spontaneous lactation that results may herald acromegaly or Cushing's syndrome. Patients with the galactorrhoea and amenorrhoea syndrome should always be carefully followed up with periodic skull X-rays in case a pituitary tumour develops. Hypothalamic damage may cause inappropriate lactation by removal of the normal inhibitory hypothalamic influence.

Primary adrenal disease and extra-adrenal malignancy account for no more than 20 per cent of all cases of Cushing's syndrome. As mentioned previously, only 20 per cent of the remaining patients have clinically significant pituitary tumours, usually of the chromophobe variety. Basophilic tumours are found in some of the remaining cases, but they are not usually large enough to cause radiological abnormalities. The presence of a pituitary tumour is usually heralded by the development of skin pigmentation of the Addisonian variety, resulting from the excessive ACTH and β-MSH they secrete. Cushing's syndrome occurring in the absence of primary adrenal disease or non-endocrine tumours and conventionally called Cushing's disease (*see* p. 148) may result from some functional abnormality of the hypothalamus. Overproduction of ACTH resulting from pituitary or hypothalamic disease is dealt with in the section on ACTH.

Overproduction of vasopressin has been described in association with acromegaly. The reason for this occurrence is not clear and requires further documentation. It may be due to minor degrees of underproduction of ACTH causing secondary hypoadrenalism. Increased levels of vasopressin are known to result from cortisol or thyroid hormone deficiency and respond to replacement therapy. Most commonly, inappropriate secretion of ADH results from malignant tumours, especially of the bronchus, and leads to dilutional hyponatraemia and hypochloraemia (*see* Chapter 20). Reduced ADH output is uncommon in tumours of the anterior lobe but is more often found after pituitary operations. Suprasellar tumours, especially craniopharyngiomas, frequently cause diabetes insipidus.

TREATMENT OF PITUITARY TUMOURS

Pituitary tumours can be treated by surgical hypophysectomy, by radiotherapy, by cryosurgery or by combinations of these procedures.

Surgical hypophysectomy by the trans-frontal or trans-nasal approaches gives good results but special experience and skill are required to avoid leaving a rim of pituitary tissue. Visual field defects are usually an indication for surgical decompression of the optic chiasm. Craniopharyngiomas are compatible with long survival even when complete surgical removal of the tumour is not possible. Aspiration of the cyst contents often causes remarkable improvement.

Complete ablation of the pituitary by *radiation* requires several hundred thousand rads and this is not possible by conventional external radiation when the dose should not usually exceed 4,500 rad since at higher dose levels damage to the optic pathways may occur. External radiation often halts progress of adenomas causing acromegaly and in about 50 per cent of patients causes regression of the soft tissue and bone changes and marked lowering of growth hormone levels. Chromophobe adenomas respond well to external radiation alone, and up to 75 per cent freedom from recurrence over four years can be expected. Intrasellar chromophobe tumours are adequately treated by this method and it can also be used in patients unsafe for operation because of the large size of the tumour or their poor general condition. For patients with pituitary adenomas who present with visual defects, decompression of the chiasm combined with post-operative radiotherapy is a satisfactory form of treatment.

Pituitary radiation can also be carried out by implanting radioactive seeds into the gland. By this means a larger dose of radiation can be given to the pituitary while the dose to adjacent parts is kept at a low level. Before this method is decided upon air encephalography should be carried out to determine the extent of any suprasellar extension. In most clinics, extension of the tumour beyond the pituitary fossa is regarded as a contra-indication to implantation. Yttrium-90 (half-life 2·54 days) is the isotope preferred at present because it emits only beta rays of intense (2·2 meV) but local effect. Gold-198 (half-life 2·69 days) has also been used but it emits gamma rays of greater penetration. The radioactive material is inserted into the pituitary under X-ray screening control, the implanting needle being inserted either by trans-nasal or trans-ethmoidal routes. Yttrium-90 is usually implanted as two rods, one on either side of the mid-line. Precise placement and dosimetry are needed to produce adequate pituitary ablation and prevent radiation damage to the optic chiasm or to the diaphragm sellae, which can produce cerebrospinal rhinorrhoea. Hydrocortisone cover is not needed unless there is evidence of impaired ACTH output. Antibiotics are given to cover the implant procedure, and the dangerous complication of meningitis should be looked for especially in cases with cerebrospinal rhinorrhoea. Patients with CSF rhinorrhoea should be given long-term chemotherapy with sulphamezathine 0·5 G twice daily, and if the condition persists plugging of the holes by the trans-nasal route may be required. One advantage of implantation is that histological examination of the contents of the pituitary fossa is often possible. Further implantation may be required in some cases. If adequate X-ray screening facilities are available implantation may be the treatment of choice for most types of pituitary tumour, in the absence of visual impairment. Growth hormone secreting adenomas, and secretory and non-secretory chromophobe adenomas may be treated in this way but whether the long term results are better than those following external irradiation remains to be demonstrated. By careful regulation of radiation dosage the tumour may be treated without causing hypopituitarism. Restoration of normal pituitary function without the need for replacement therapy can sometimes be achieved in patients with Cushing's disease. Doses of the order of 20–50,000 rad are usually required in acromegaly. Pituitary ablation by implantation of Yttrium-90 is also used for the treatment of particular types of diabetic retinopathy and certain patients with metastatic breast carinoma. Occasionally disseminated prostatic carcinoma may respond.

HYPOPITUITARISM

Hypopituitarism can result from any one of a variety of lesions causing destruction of the anterior pituitary or the hypothalamus. Occasionally, failure of one or more hormones develops without demonstrable organic disease in the area.

Postpartum pituitary necrosis was previously the commonest cause of hypopituitarism but this complication is much less frequent with improvement in obstetric practice. The pituitary gland is hyperplastic at the end of pregnancy, and hypotension following haemorrhage at this time may cause spasm of the infundibular arteries which, if prolonged, causes necrosis of the anterior lobe. Varying degrees of pituitary damage can occur, and it has been estimated that if more than 30 per cent of the gland is preserved the condition is asymptomatic. The commonest spontaneous cause of hypopituitarism is now a pituitary tumour, particularly the chromophobe adenoma in the adult (Nieman *et al.*, 1967) and craniopharyngiomas in children. Iatrogenic hypopituitarism is also common as a result of surgical or radiotherapeutic damage to the pituitary for malignant, diabetic, or pituitary disease. The main causes of hypopituitarism are shown in Table 1.5. Isolated deficiencies of individual pituitary hormones may occur and these are most probably due to a hypothalamic defect resulting in absent releasing hormone secretion. Gonadotrophin or growth hormone deficiency are the most common.

Deficiency of posterior lobe hormones does not commonly result from pituitary tumours or other diseases confined to the pituitary fossa unless these have been treated, usually by operation, when some degree of hypothalamic damage is frequent. Hypothalamic disease often presents with deficiency of vasopressin, which will be considered fully in Chapter 2.

The clinical picture of hypopituitarism depends on:

(*a*) The degree of pituitary failure;
(*b*) the pattern of failure among the various trophic hormones;
(*c*) the presence of symptoms and signs arising from increased tension in the sella or from a space-occupying lesion in the region of the pituitary.

The rate of onset and progression of the disease and the age and sex of the patient are also important.

Deficiencies of single hormones may occur and can easily be mistaken for disease of the target organ. A good response to the administration of the trophic hormone usually indicates that the disease is at the pituitary level. Partial hypopituitarism is much commoner than total loss of all secretions; gonadotrophin and growth hormone secretion both tend to be impaired early with gonadotrophin secretion usually going first; these are followed by ACTH, TSH and, finally vasopressin. In patients with hypothalamic dysfunction, diabetes insipidus is more common, and patients with slowly progressive lesions in the pituitary-hypothalamic region may present with diabetes insipidus which improves when anterior pituitary damage becomes sufficient to impair ACTH output. This improvement may be due to lowering of glomerular filtration rate caused by cortisol deficiency. Diabetes insipidus recurs when treatment with adrenal steroids is given.

Hypopituitarism should be considered in the differential diagnosis of *coma*. The factors

TABLE 1.5 *Aetiology of Hypopituitarism*

1. *Pituitary tumours*
   Pituitary adenomas especially of the chromophobe variety, eosinophil adenomas, craniopharyngiomas.

2. *Malignant disease*
   Secondary carcinomas especially from breast and lung. Local cerebral tumours, e.g. meningioma, glioma of the optic chiasma.

3. *Infectious diseases*
   Tuberculous basal meningitis, syphilis, encephalitis.

4. *Granulomatous diseases*
   Sarcoidosis, other granulomas that sometimes affect the thyroid and adrenals as well, causing a 'multiglandular syndrome', Hand-Schuller-Christian disease, eosinophilic granuloma.

5. *Vascular disease*
   Postpartum necrosis, severe haemorrhage with hypotension, diabetes mellitus, cranial arteritis, pituitary apoplexy, vascular malformations.

6. *Iatrogenic*
   Surgical hypophysectomy for pituitary tumours, breast carcinoma or for diabetic retinopathy. Radiation either by conventional radiation (usually insufficient to cause hypopituitarism without prior damage by surgery or pituitary disease), yttrium implantation, selective failure of TSH or ACTH production after prolonged therapy with thyroid hormone or adrenal steroids.

7. *Trauma*
   After head injury.

8. *Secondary to hypothalamic disease* (this is usually associated with diabetes insipidus)
   Craniopharyngiomas and other tumours. Rarely may also produce pathological hunger and obesity, or loss of appetite and severe malnutrition.

9. '*Functional*' *hypothalamic disorders*
   Secondary to malnutrition and usually producing reversible hypogonadotrophic hypogonadism: anorexia nervosa, starvation, malabsorption syndromes.

responsible for coma in hypopituitarism vary but include hypoglycaemia, sodium depletion, water intoxication, cerebral anoxia, hypothyroidism, and hypothermia. Untreated, the patients are particularly *susceptible to stresses* of all kinds—infections, surgery and anaesthetics. *Hypoglycaemia* and *insulin sensitivity* also occur in a variety of clinical conditions, e.g. adrenocortical insufficiency and malnutrition. In hypopituitarism, insulin sensitivity results from deficiencies of growth hormone and cortisol production, and poor food intake sometimes may play a part. In hypopituitary dwarfs deficient in growth hormone, the increased insulin sensitivity can be corrected by administration of growth hormone. Although weight loss may occur in hypopituitary patients, extreme emaciation should always suggest a diagnosis of anorexia nervosa, for patients with hypopituitarism are usually of normal weight (Sheehan and Summers, 1949).

CLINICAL FEATURES

TABLE 1.6 *Clinical Features of Anterior Pituitary Hormone Deficiency*

Gonadotrophins	*In children*, selective failure without growth hormone deficiency (hypogonadotrophic hypogonadism) causes normal or increased height, and eunuchoid habitus with delayed puberty. Anosmia may be associated. *In men* there is decreased libido, impotence, aspermia, decreased size and softening of the testes, and some loss of pubic, axillary, facial, and body hair. *In women* there is decreased libido, amenorrhoea or oligomenorrhoea, atrophy of the genitalia, reduced body hair, sometimes decrease in breast size. Menopausal symptoms do not occur. In both sexes there is characteristic fineness and excessive wrinkling of the skin, especially of the face (growth hormone deficiency may also be involved).
Growth hormone	Dwarfism and delayed skeletal development in children. No obvious features in adults but may contribute to fine skin and insulin sensitivity. Viscera are small.
Prolactin	Failure of lactation is often the first sign of post-partum pituitary necrosis.
Thyrotrophin	*In children* hypothyroidism causes growth retardation. Hypothyroidism *in adults* may be indistinguishable from that due to primary thyroid disease, though swelling of the subcutaneous tissues is usually less prominent. Lassitude, cold intolerance, dryness of the skin, and prolongation of tendon reflexes occur.
Adrenocorticotrophic hormone	Features of hypoadrenocorticism usually of insidious onset, e.g. asthenia, nausea, vomiting, postural hypotension, hypoglycaemia, collapse, and coma.
Melanocyte-stimulating hormone	Characteristic pallor of the skin. Depigmentation of the areolae of the breasts. Patients tan less after exposure to sunlight.

Anaemia is less marked than the pallor of the patient would suggest. A moderate normocytic normochromic anaemia reflecting marrow hypofunction is correctable by replacement therapy. Electrolyte regulation is less affected than in patients with Addison's disease since aldosterone secretion is maintained in ACTH deficiency. *Hyponatraemia* is common, being more often due to water intoxication than to sodium loss. Water diuresis is impaired in cortisol insufficiency but there is usually no increased sodium loss in hypopituitarism because aldosterone secretion is not affected. Children with hypopituitarism usually present with *short stature*, and evidence of hypogonadism develops later. The habitus is normal but they have an immature appearance and bone X-rays reveal retarded skeletal development. Such patients may continue to grow very slowly till the third or fourth decade until the epiphyses eventually fuse spontaneously or as a result of sex hormone therapy.

DIAGNOSIS OF HYPOPITUITARISM

A diagnosis of hypopituitarism depends on demonstration of clinical and laboratory evidence of pituitary hormone deficiency and, if possible, of the underlying cause of the disorder. Measurement of the levels of the pituitary hormones in blood and of the 24-hour output in urine, ideally under conditions that would be expected to stimulate their increased secretion, is the absolute method of assessment of pituitary function. With the development of radioimmunoassays routine estimation of pituitary hormone levels is now available to assist in the assessment of gonadotrophin and growth hormone secretion. Deficiency of pituitary target organ secretion can be taken to indicate pituitary disease if a lesion of the target organ is ruled out by its response to trophic hormone administration, e.g. in deficiency of ACTH or TSH. Raised levels of pituitary trophic hormone indicate the presence of secretory pituitary tumours or disease of the target organs. However, basal levels of pituitary or target organ hormones are not infrequently maintained, deficiencies being revealed only by dynamic tests that indicate impaired pituitary reserve capacity.

Tests should then be directed to finding a possible cause of pituitary-hypothalamic damage. X-rays of the sella may reveal a double floor, enlargement, ballooning, or erosion of the posterior clinoids. Calcification in the region is often due to a craniopharyngioma or to previous tuberculous meningitis. Possible sources of secondary deposits should always be looked for, and a chest X-ray is essential. Plotting of the visual fields with red and white objects may give evidence of extra-sellar extension of a pituitary tumour. Air encephalography is indicated if there is a field defect, to determine the extent of the tumour.

The clinical features exhibited by the patient may suggest the nature of the trophic hormone deficiencies. Investigations should then define precisely the hormone deficiencies and, where possible, the reserve capacity of the pituitary.

Growth Hormone Deficiency

Growth hormone deficiency in children leads to shortness of stature and retarded bone development. Undue insulin sensitivity is partly attributable to reduced growth hormone secretion, and so is the lowered fasting blood sugar.

Circulating growth hormone levels are low in many fasting normal subjects, so tests involving stimulation of growth hormone output are required. The resting level of serum growth hormone as determined by radioimmunoassay is usually less than 10 ng/ml unless sampling coincides with a spontaneous secretory burst. Insulin-induced hypoglycaemia stimulates the hypothalamic centres affecting pituitary growth hormone release. In normal persons growth hormone levels exceed 20 ng/ml during a standard insulin tolerance test providing the hypoglycaemia is 'adequate', that is the blood sugar falls to less than 40 mg/100 ml and the patient sweats (*see* Appendix). Plasma fatty acids fall during the growth hormone secretion but this is a poor indicator of response. Although patients with hypopituitarism tend to be more sensitive to insulin, measurement of blood glucose alone during the insulin test is of little help in making a diagnosis. Since occasional normal patients may respond to adequate insulin-induced hypoglycaemia with a growth hormone level of only 10 to 20 ng/ml the diagnosis of growth hormone deficiency should be accepted only if the inadequate response to hypoglycaemia is confirmed when the test is repeated, or if inadequate secretion is also seen during arginine infusion or glucagon stimulation. Screening procedures for growth hormone deficiency include measuring plasma growth hormone levels after muscular exercise or Bovril administration (*see* Appendix and p. 9).

Gonadotrophin Deficiency

Gonadotrophin deficiency occurs early in pituitary disease and, in adults, estimation of blood or urinary gonadotrophins before and during clomiphene administration (*see* p. 19) is a useful index of hypopituitarism. Normal levels of gonadotrophins in a patient suspected of hypopituitarism should always call for review of the diagnosis, though isolated deficiencies of other hormones can rarely occur. Before puberty, gonadotrophin levels are normally low and are of little diagnostic value. High levels of gonadotrophins indicate that hypogonadism is due to primary disease of the gonads. Low levels of ovarian and testicular hormones in the blood or urine occur in hypopituitarism as well as in disease of the target organs but they rise when the pituitary hormone is given (as HMG or HCG) if hypopituitarism is present, and should be measured during the appropriate stimulation test (*see* Appendix). Vaginal smears and endometrial biopsy may confirm the lack of oestrogens where assays are not available. The response in urinary oestrogens and, later, of pregnanediol output after HMG and HCG can be used to distinguish primary ovarian failure from pituitary-hypothalamic disease. In men plasma testosterone will rise after HCG if pituitary hypothalamic disease is present.

Thyrotrophin Deficiency

Radioimmunoassays of TSH are now becoming available for routine clinical use. Basal levels are low and are of little help in the diagnosis of hypopituitarism. Raised levels of TSH in the blood indicate that hypothyroidism is due to thyroid disease. Pituitary TSH deficiency is usually indicated by clinical and laboratory evidence of hypothyroidism in the absence of primary thyroid disease or a raised TSH level. To distinguish primary hypothyroidism from hypopituitarism it is necessary to test the response of the thyroid to TSH if serum TSH assays are not available. Since some patients with longstanding hypopituitarism are unable to respond to a single injection of TSH it is best to give at least three daily injections of 10 units TSH before estimating the rise in 24-hr thyroidal ^{131}I uptake and the serum PBI or thyroxine (*see* Appendix). The presence of circulating thyroid antibodies is evidence of thyroid disease but autoimmune thyroiditis is common and may therefore coexist with pituitary disease.

ACTH Deficiency

ACTH assays are not available for routine use. Raised plasma ACTH levels occur when the adrenals are damaged and, also, as a result of certain types of pituitary tumour in Cushing's disease. Reduced ACTH output is usually demonstrated by a reduced output of adrenal cortisol and 'androgens', which can be corrected by ACTH administration.

The urinary excretion of adrenocortical 'androgens' (usually measured as 17-oxosteroids) and of cortisol and its metabolites (measured as 17-hydroxycorticosteroids) is lowered in hypopituitarism. Total 17-hydroxycorticosteroid excretion in normal adult males of average weight and height average 11 mg/24 hr (range 5 to 21 mg). The corresponding values in women are, mean 9 mg/24 hr (range 4 to 17 mg). Urinary 17-oxosteroids are derived largely from the adrenal cortex (almost entirely in the female and about two-thirds in the male). In men between the ages of 20 and 40 years most values lie between 12 and 17 mg/24 hr (*see* Chapter 6). Most patients with hypopituitarism excrete <6 mg/24 hr, and very low values (<1 mg/24 hr) are frequent.

Plasma fluorogenic corticosteroids (cortisol and corticosterone) are usually determined by the Mattingly procedure in clinical practice. The mean plasma 'cortisol' level between 9 and 10 a.m. after an overnight fast in normal adults is $12{\cdot}7 \pm 2{\cdot}9$ μg/100 ml (Nieman *et al.*, 1967) with a range of 6·8 to 20·2 μg. In hypopituitarism, the 9 a.m. value is often low. In patients with a low steroid output, adrenal disease can usually be ruled out by assessing the rise in plasma 'cortisol' 30 and 60 minutes after injection of the synthetic ACTH preparation, Synacthen (250 μg intramuscularly: *see* Appendix). In some patients with hypopituitarism a normal response is obtained, indicated by an increment of >7 μg/100 ml of plasma 'cortisol' to a maximum above 18 μg/100 ml. If a negative result is obtained, a course of ACTH must be given (3 days of 1 mg Synacthen-Depot intramuscularly daily). A rise in plasma cortisol, improvement in the results of the 'Synacthen test' and a rise in urinary 17-OHCS and 17-OS occurs and the output of the former should exceed 30 mg/24 hr by the third day of the test.

The response of the entire hypothalamic-pituitary-adrenal axis to stress can be tested by

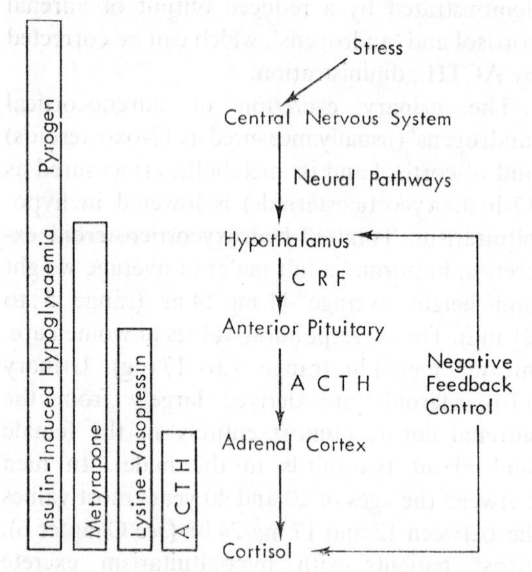

FIGURE 1.4 Diagram of the tests for the mechanisms controlling the secretion of cortisol (after Landon, J., James, V. H. T., and Stoker, D. J. (1965))

administration of insulin to produce hypoglycaemia or pyrogen and determining the subsequent rise in plasma 'cortisol' level. If the plasma cortisol rises to above 20 μg/100 ml the patient does not require hydrocortisone replacement. Metyrapone, which causes a transient lowering of the plasma cortisol, can also be used to assess the response of the pituitary-adrenal system (Cope, 1965). Lysine vasopressin (Gwinup, 1965) has recently been used to test the integrity of the pituitary ACTH producing mechanism but the precise site of action of this compound in man is not yet known (Fig. 1.4). Pyrogen and lysine vasopressin tests are now rarely used since the insulin tolerance test gives the relevant information, that is whether or not replacement therapy is required, with less discomfort for the patient. Details of these tests are given in the Appendix.

DIFFERENTIAL DIAGNOSIS

Malnutrition from any cause may simulate hypopituitarism but it is the syndrome of *anorexia nervosa* that is most often confused with hypopituitarism. This disorder usually occurs in adolescent girls or young women, in the absence of any demonstrable organic disease. Progressive weight loss, often initiated by a period of slimming, is characteristic of the condition. The patients may have been rather plump in the past and the desire to lose weight becomes an obsession which cannot be controlled. They develop abnormal body images thinking they are overweight when in fact they are very thin. Restless activity tends to hasten the loss of weight. A history of earlier feeding difficulties and the existence of problems associated with psychological maturation such as tomboyishness, lack of social confidence, and the presence of a domineering mother are often found. The patients deny concern about their loss of weight and are typically evasive about the amount of food eaten. They often eat high protein diets with green vegetables but avoid carbohydrates. They complain of nausea and vomiting if forced to eat and frequently take purgatives. Amenorrhoea is almost invariably present and occasionally precedes the onset of weight loss; it may persist for several years even when normal weight is restored. Emaciation may be extreme, and oedema of the legs from hypoproteinaemia may develop, especially after refeeding and the inevitable extra sodium loading. In contrast to hypopituitarism, the pubic and axillary hair are normal and the body may be covered with a fine growth of lanugo hair particularly over the back. If starvation is prolonged, death may occur from intercurrent infection if the patient is not carefully supervised. In severe cases the pulse rate and blood pressure may be low and the fasting blood sugar and metabolic rate decreased.

Hormonal abnormalities may occur as a result of malnutrition but the only pituitary function consistently affected is gonadotrophin secretion. In emaciated patients, gonadotrophins are reduced and refeeding causes an increase in production. A rise in gonadotrophin output on refeeding can be associated with an increased output of 17-hydroxycorticosteroids (17-OHCS) and 17-oxosteroids. Refeeding also causes alterations in proportions of urinary oestrogens, greater amounts of oestriol being excreted. Urinary 17-oxosteroids are often lowered but 17-OHCS are more often normal and plasma cortisol levels may even be raised. The urinary steroid abnormalities are not due to corticosteroid deficiency but to a change in their metabolism so that less steroid is extracted in the organic solvents used to estimate urinary steroids, While insulin sensitivity is increased in anorexia nervosa, growth hormone levels usually respond normally to hypoglycaemia and the pituitary-adrenal response to metyrapone is normal. Hormone therapy is not required and mild cases respond well to firm but sympathetic handling on an outpatient basis. If rapid improvement does not occur, supervised feeding in hospital should be arranged. Chlorpromazine therapy lessens the patient's anxiety, and tube feeding may be needed. With gain in weight confidence in eating returns, although careful and continued follow up is necessary to prevent relapses. Amenorrhoea may persist, and other neurotic reactions may be seen in later life.

The lack of skin pigmentation usually allows hypopituitarism with adrenocortical insufficiency to be separated from Addison's disease. Occasionally, hypothyroidism due to hypopituitarism may simulate myxoedema, but in the latter axillary and pubic hair loss is less, the skin is thicker, and amenorrhoea is not common. In doubtful cases cortisol should be given along with l-thyroxine until the diagnosis is clarified. A premature menopause occasionally raises the possibility of hypopituitarism but such patients have normal body hair and experience hot flushes. Hypogonadism due to gonadal disease can be distinguished by gonadotrophin assays.

TREATMENT OF HYPOPITUITARISM

Treatment should be directed to the cause of the hypopituitarism in the first instance, but in some cases no detectable cause can be ascertained. Patients with dwarfism can be treated with growth hormone, but in adults of normal height this hormone confers no obvious benefit. Careful investigation is always required to define the pattern of trophic hormone deficiency. Gonadotrophin therapy with human FSH and HCG can induce ovulation and allow pregnancy to occur, and in males with pituitary deficiency such treatment may restore fertility. When ovulation is induced by clomiphene, HCG may help to prolong the span of the corpus luteum. Substitution therapy with cyclical oestrogens and progestogens can induce withdrawal bleeding and improve breast development as well as conferring psychological benefit and protecting the bones from osteoporosis (*see* Chapter 7). In men, androgen therapy with testosterone (Testoral, 10 to 40 mg sublingually daily) or testosterone injections (Sustanon 250, 1 ml i.m. each three to four weeks) can improve gonadal function and development. If basal corticotrophin output is normal, cortisol maintenance therapy may not be required, but impaired cortisol response to insulin induced hypoglycaemia indicates that cortisol cover is needed under conditions of stress. Maintenance therapy in patients with deficient basal ACTH production is preferably given as cortisol rather than cortisone, since the latter has to be converted to cortisol, mainly in the liver, before becoming metabolically active, and both absorption and conversion are variable. Even with cortisol, blood levels are often variable from patient to patient and it is necessary to monitor the patient's corticosteroid levels on replacement therapy when a particular regime is started. Most commonly patients require cortisol in a dose of 20 mg on waking and 10 mg at suppertime. Plasma corticosteroids peak 30 to 60 minutes after oral cortisol and ideally the peak plasma concentration should reach between 25 and 35 μg/100 ml after the morning dose and then fall slowly to between 6 and 8 μg/100 ml before the evening dose, after which a peak of 15 to 20 μg/100 ml is reached. The dose of cortisol should be adjusted until these levels obtain; sometimes an extra 10 mg dose is needed at mid-day but occasionally very high levels may be seen in patients receiving only 30 mg per day of cortisol. A mineralocorticoid such as fludrocortisone is not required in patients with hypopituitarism since aldosterone secretion is maintained in the absence of ACTH. During minor stresses 20 mg cortisol is given orally each 6 or 8 hours. During major stress hydrocortisone hemisuccinate is given intramuscularly, 100 mg each 6 hours. A 'steroid card' should always be carried by the patient indicating full details of his therapy and if possible the patient should wear a bracelet or necklace giving the diagnosis of hypopituitarism and reference to a hospital or particular doctor (*see* Appendix). If hypothyroidism is also present, thyroxine treatment will be required in a dose of 0·1 to 0·2 mg each day. Care should be taken not to begin treatment with thyroxine before cortisol therapy is initiated. In patients with coma resulting from hypopituitarism emergency treatment includes intravenous administration of hydrocortisone hemisuccinate, and dextrose saline and correction of hypothermia where required. Triiodothyronine acts more rapidly than 1-thyroxine and may be used with caution where necessary starting with a dose of 2·5 μg, each eight hours, administered down a stomach tube if necessary, but not by injection, and doubling after 24 hours. Spontaneous improvement of hypopituitarism can occur when the condition is mild, and pregnancy has been reported with further amelioration due to the pituitary hypertrophy of pregnancy.

REFERENCES

Anterior Pituitary and General References

Besser, G. M. (1972), *Medicine* (Part 2), 'The Hypothalamus and Pituitary' (Bayliss, R. I. S., and Hall, R., Eds). London: Medical Educational (International) Ltd., p. 97.

Fraser, R., and Joplin, G. F. (1959). *Brit. J. Radiol.*, **32,** 527.

Greenwood, F. C., and Landon, J. (1966). *J. Clin. Path.*, **19,** 284.

Growth Hormone

Daughaday, W. H. (1970). *New Engl. J. Med.*, **282,** 1430.

Grant, D. (1973). *Clin. Endocrinol.*, **1,** 387.

Editorial (1973), *Brit. med. J.*, **1,** 188.

Laron, Z., Pertzelan, A., and Mannheimer, S. (1966). *Israel J. Med. Sci.*, **2,** 152.

Wright, A. D., Hill, D. M., Lowry, C., and Fraser, T. R. (1970). *Quart. J. Med.*, **29,** 1.

Tanner, J. M., Whitehouse, R. H., Hughes, P. C. R., and Vince, F. P. (1971). *Arch. Dis. Childh.*, **46,** 754.

ACTH (MSH)

Abe, K., Nicholson, W. E., Liddle, G. W., Island, D. P., and Orth, D. N. (1969). *J. Clin. Invest.*, **48,** 1580.

James, V. H. T., and Landon, J. (Eds) (1968). 'The Investigation of Hypothalamic Pituitary-Adrenal Function.' Cambridge: Cambridge University Press.

Landon, J. (1968). J. Roy. *Coll. Physicns. Lond.*, **2,** 289.

Liddle, G. W., Island, D., and Meador, C. E. (1962). *Rec. Prog. Horm. Res.*, **18,** 125.

Gonadotrophins

Cargill, C. M., Ross, G. T., and Hoshimi, T. (1969). *J. Clin. Endocrinol.*, **29,** 12.

Anderson, D. C., Marshall, J. C., Young, J. L., and Fraser, T. R. (1972). *Clin. Endocrinol.*, **1,** 127.

Prolactin

Besser, G. M., and Edwards, C. R. W. (1972). *Brit. med. J.*, **2,** 280.

Besser, G. M., Parke, L., Edwards, C. R. W., Forsyth, I. A., and McNeilly, A. S. (1972). *Brit. med. J.*, **3,** 669.

Forsyth, I. A., Besser, G. M., Edwards, C. R. W., Francis, L., and Myres, R. P. (1971). *Brit. med. J.*, **3,** 225.

Forsyth, I. A., and Edwards, C. R. W. (1972). *Clin. Endocrinol.*, **1,** 293.

2

POSTERIOR PITUITARY

The neurohypophysis or posterior lobe of the pituitary consists of three parts, the median eminence, the infundibular stem, and the infundibular process or neural lobe. It is composed of nerve cells and their fibres, neuroglia, blood vessels, and supporting connective tissue. Nerve fibres reach it from the supraoptic and paraventricular nuclei (SON and PVN) ending in close apposition to capillaries. The cells of the SON and PVN are neurosecretory, synthesising oxytocin, vasopressin and neurophysin, which pass down their nerve fibres, to be stored and released from the posterior lobe. It is likely that the SON is mainly responsible for the synthesis of vasopressin, and the PVN for oxytocin, though it is not yet known whether individual neurones secrete one or both hormones. The SON and PVN, their nerve fibres, and the neurohypophysis can be considered as one functional hypothalamo-neurohypophyseal system (HNS).

Vasopressin

Vasopressin (antidiuretic hormone) is, like oxytocin, a cyclic octapeptide with a molecular weight of about 1,000 consisting of an S—S bonded ring of five amino-acids and a tail of three amino-acids (Fig. 2.1). Arginine vasopressin is the antiduretic hormone in man and other mammals, apart from the pig, the peccary and the hippopotamus where lysine vasopressin is found. Lysine vasopressin is more stable than arginine vasopressin and, since its synthesis was achieved, its main uses have been in the treatment of diabetes insipidus and in testing the integrity of the anterior pituitary by causing release of ACTH and hence cortisol. The close chemical similarity of vasopressin and oxytocin explains the overlap of their biological actions.

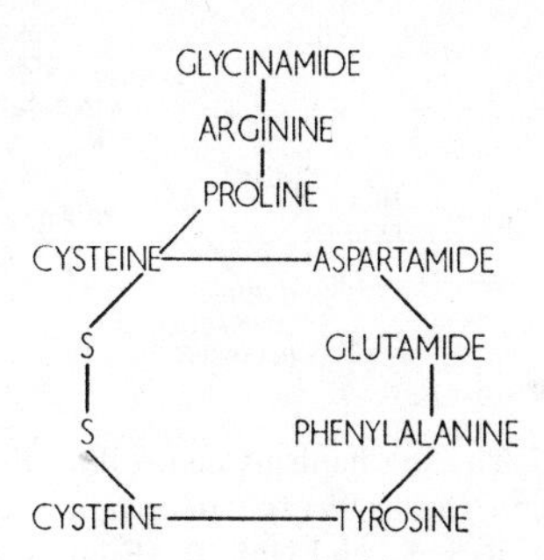

FIGURE 2.1 Arginine vasopressin

Basic amino-acids (lysine or arginine) in position 8, and a phenylalanine group in position 3, increase antidiuretic activity.

The main actions of vasopressin are to promote the renal tubular reabsorption of water and to stimulate smooth muscle contraction, though it is unlikely that it has any physiological role in the maintenance of blood pressure. In pharmacological doses it causes pallor, coronary vasoconstriction, and contraction of smooth muscle in the gut.

Vasopressin exerts its antidiuretic action on the distal part of the nephron by increasing the osmotic permeability of the distal tubular and collecting duct cells. The hormone acts at the level of the cell membrane where it can be considered to increase the mean pore diameter. It has been suggested that vasopressin may also act on sodium transport from the ascending limb of the loop of Henle, accounting for the build up of sodium concentration in the renal medulla, but this action has not yet been demonstrated. The disulphide linkage of the peptide may be the means of attachment to the target organ since blockage of these groups prevents the fixation and action of the hormone.

Each day some 70 to 100 litres of fluid, iso-osmotic with plasma, are filtered by the glomeruli. Of the filtered water, 85 per cent is reabsorbed passively by the proximal tubule along with the active reabsorption of solutes, especially sodium and chloride, without the aid of vasopressin. The urine, therefore, remains iso-osmotic with plasma. The long U-shaped loops of Henle form a counter-current concentrating system in which the ascending limb actively transports sodium to the interstitial fluid of the renal medulla, rendering this region hypertonic and the urine reaching the distal tubule hypotonic. In the absence of vasopressin, the distal tubules and collecting ducts are impermeable to water, and hypotonic urine is produced in large amount. Vasopressin, by increasing the permeability of these segments of the nephron to water permits the water to pass from the hypotonic tubular fluid and pass along the concentration gradient. The renal tubules may be unresponsive to vasopressin because of a genetic defect or as a result of potassium depletion, hypercalcaemia, or amyloidosis.

Release of vasopressin results from a rise in plasma osmolality and from a fall in plasma volume. The osmoreceptors are located somewhere in the vascular bed supplied by the internal carotid artery, possibly in an adjacent but separ-

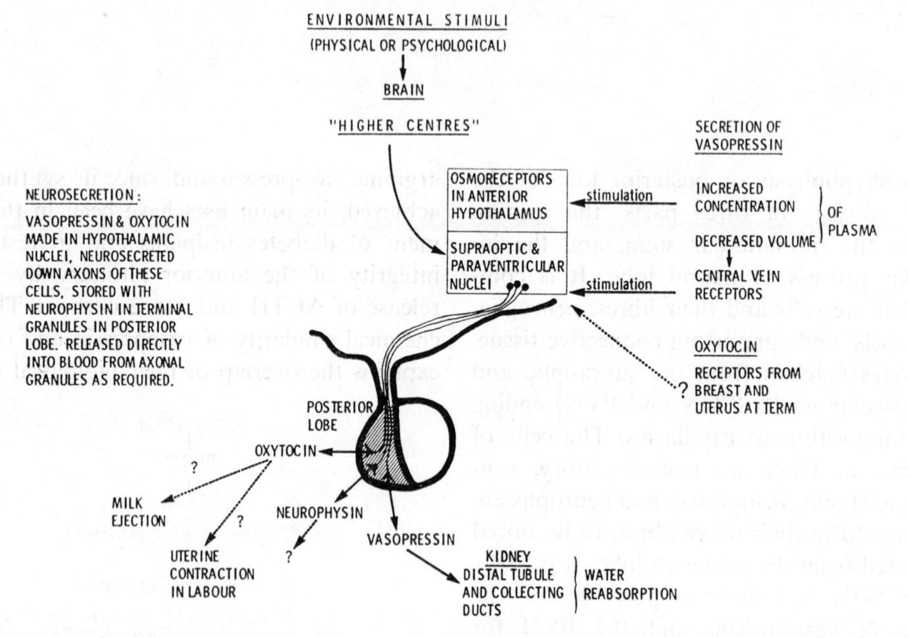

FIGURE 2.2 The mechanisms controlling the secretion of the hormones of the posterior lobe of the pituitary. The question marks denote uncertain mechanisms (from Besser, G. M. (1972), *Medicine* (Part 2), Bayliss, R. I. S., and Hall, R. (Eds), p. 108. London: Medical Education (International) Ltd.).

ate area from the SON. Reduction of plasma volume appears to stimulate vasopressin release even if the plasma is hypo-osmolar. Again, the site of the volume receptors has not been accurately determined but probably they are in the great veins of the thorax. Emotional factors are potent triggers for vasopressin release as are nicotine, morphine, and ether; alcohol has the opposite effect.

VASOPRESSIN DEFICIENCY (DIABETES INSIPIDUS)

Deficient production of vasopressin or failure of the renal tubules to respond results in the passage of large volumes of dilute urine. As a consequence of the polyuria the patient is thirsty and drinks more.

1. *Cranial Diabetes Insipidus.* In about one third of patients with this condition the cause is either a primary or secondary tumour in the area. Pituitary tumours do not cause diabetes insipidus unless there is a suprasellar extension, surgical or X-ray interference, since the median eminence or hypothalamus must be involved. Removal of the posterior lobe alone only results in temporary diabetes insipidus. Craniopharyngioma is the commonest primary suprasellar tumour causing diabetes insipidus. Metastatic carcinoma from the breast or lung, large primary tumours of the pituitary or meningiomas and gliomas in the region of the hypothalamus may also produce vasopressin insufficiency.

In another third of cases there is no apparent cause for the diabetes inspidus and such cases maybe familial. Although viral or 'degenerative' causes have been suggested, it seems likely that some such cases will eventually be shown to result from metabolic disturbance in the neurosecretory system.

A further third result from a variety of lesions, including trauma, Hand-Schuller-Christian syndrome, sarcoidosis and other granulomas, syphilis, basal meningitis, encephalitis or the rare cerebral reticulosis, microgliomatosis cerebri. After head injury, usually when there has been a fracture of the base of the skull, the polyuria may not be present for several days and may be followed by an interval of apparent improvement lasting a further few days. The diabetes insipidus which follows head injury or neurosurgical trauma is of variable severity and usually remits by the end of a year and often within a few weeks.

2. *Nephrogenic Diabetes Insipidus.* The renal tubules may fail to respond to vasopressin because of a genetic defect, transmitted as a sex-linked recessive, the polyuria occurring in male infants six to eight weeks after birth. This is presumed to be due to a metabolic error resulting from failure of the nephron adenyl cyclase system to be stimulated by normally secreted vasopressin. Potassium depletion, hypercalcaemia, amyloidosis and other forms of acquired renal disease also cause polyuria unresponsive to vasopressin and must be excluded.

CLINICAL FEATURES

Polyuria and polydipsia are the main complaints, and sleep is often disturbed. Attempts to limit the volume of urine by fluid restriction lead to intolerable thirst and dehydration. The urine output varies, often being in the region of five litres but occasionally as much as twenty litres each day. There may be evidence of a space-occupying lesion in the region of the pituitary. In patients without evidence of organic disease the symptoms may develop acutely and the patient may be able to give the precise date and, sometimes, the hour at which symptoms began.

The symptoms of polyuria and thirst in a patient with cranial diabetes insipidus will disappear and the urine may be concentrated if the pituitary or hypothalamic lesion progress to produce anterior pituitary deficiency since adequate circulating corticosteroids are required to excrete a water load. Before testing for the presence of diabetes insipidus plasma cortisol should be measured and adequate replacement given if necessary.

DIAGNOSIS

This is often obvious from the clinical context, e.g. the polyuria that follows head injury or pituitary operations. Chronic renal failure often causes polyuria, possibly due to an osmotic diuresis induced by the load of urea presented to a limited number of nephrons, and chronic pyelonephritis sometimes causes renal tubular defects and polyuria. Examination of the urine for albumin, casts, pus cells, and organisms, and plasma urea and electrolyte estimations will indicate renal disease. In chronic renal disease the urine osmolality is fixed at about 285 m Osm/kg whereas in most instances of diabetes insipidus the urine is very dilute with an osmolality of less than 200 m Osm/Kg. In diabetes mellitus, polyuria with a high urine specific gravity results from the osmotic diuresis produced by glucose. Serum potassium and calcium estimations will usually indicate polyuria caused by hypokalaemia and hypercalcaemia. When these diseases have been excluded and the polyuria confirmed, the diagnosis usually lies between diabetes insipidus and compulsive water drinking (psychogenic polydipsia). In the latter, there is an initial increased water intake with secondary polyuria. Such compulsive water drinkers are usually women with some psychological abnormality. Normal or only marginally impaired vasopressin output or action can be demonstrated by the tests outlined below, and administration of vasopressin does not improve the symptoms in these patients, continued drinking sometimes causing water intoxication, whereas in patients with impaired vasopressin output correction of the deficiency is always beneficial. The very rare nephrogenic diabetes insipidus does not respond to vasopressin.

Since vasopressin cannot be routinely assayed in the blood, its effects are assessed by tests that normally stimulate its output. A rise in plasma osmolality, which normally stimulates increased vasopressin output, can be induced by administration of hypertonic saline or by fluid deprivation. Saline infusion is not without risks as it may precipitate heart failure, and it may also cause an osmotic diuresis and, thus, no alteration in urine flow. Nicotine stimulation either by injection or from cigarette smoking may cause vomiting or sweating and is often unreliable. Neither the hypertonic saline test nor nicotine administration give more valuable data than the routine water deprivation test properly conducted.

The 8-*hour fluid deprivation test* is the most satisfactory for routine use (Dashe *et al.*, 1963) and is preferred by the authors. In normal subjects, the initial plasma osmolality reported was 285 ± 4·4 mOsmol/kg of water and the final value after 8 hours fluid deprivation was 286 ± 5·5 mOsmol/kg. The urine concentration rose from 756 to 1,496 mOsmol/kg, and the urine/plasma osmolality ratio for the last hour of the test was 3·8 ± 0·9. In diabetes insipidus, all thirteen cases studied showed a plasma osmolality of 300 mOsmol/kg or more by the end of the test, the final concentration exceeding the initial by an average of 12 mOsmol/kg. Less concentrated urine was secreted, and the mean urine/plasma ratio over the last hour was 0·93. In psychogenic polydipsia the initial serum osmolality ranged from 270 to 288 mOsmol/kg and did not change during the test; the urine/plasma ratio was normal. Close supervision of the patients during this test is required and it should be done during the day. The details and precautions to be adopted are given in the Appendix. Urine osmolality must be measured rather than flow rate since a severely dehydrated patient may drop his glomerular filtration rate and therefore urine flow, without concentrating the urine. If the patient has been receiving pitressin tannate-in-oil it must be stopped 48 hours before testing and 8 hours withdrawal is needed if lysine vasopressin nasal spray has been used.

Estimations of plasma osmolality without fluid deprivation can help in the diagnosis of diabetes insipidus, for in this condition the level is raised, whereas in psychogenic polydipsia values lower than normal are found. Low values may also be seen if a patient with diabetes insipidus is overtreated with vasopressin.

If urine concentration does not occur during the water deprivation test, the patient should be give 5 or 10 units of pitressin tannate intramuscularly. Concentration of urine now confirms the diagnosis of cranial diabetes insipidus. If the patient is a child the dose must be reduced accordingly.

TREATMENT

Whenever possible the underlying disease should be treated, though surgical interference in the pituitary region may aggravate or initiate diabetes insipidus. Dehydration is an important risk in diabetes insipidus, especially if fluid intake is inadequate because of investigations, mental abnormality, damage to the adjacent thirst centre or other reasons, hence adequate fluid should always be given.

Cranial diabetes insipidus is treated with vasopressin. Vasopressin is available either in the natural form as pitressin, derived from pig and beef posterior pituitaries, or as synthetic lysine-vasopressin. Recently a more potent synthetic analogue of vasopressin, DDAVP, has been developed which has a longer length of action.

Pitressin, soluble posterior pituitary powder, only acts for three to four hours after injection, and has to be used in a modified long-acting form, pitressin tannate in oil. Administered intramuscularly or subcutaneously in a dose of 5 or 10 units, it lasts between 1 and 3 days and is best given last thing at night. Patients rarely like the injections and the technique of administration is critical. The active ingredients tend to settle at the bottom of the ampoule so that the supernatant oil may be injected without any active material. This is the commonest cause of apparently inactive pitressin. To give it correctly, stand the pitressin ampoule in a container and pour boiling water over it, and allow to stand for 3 minutes. Then shake vigorously for a full minute before drawing the contents into the syringe. Check that the ampoule contains no residual powder and then immediately inject the oil with the suspended pitressin tannate.

Lysine vasopressin nasal spray contains the synthetic polypeptide in a concentration of 10 units/ml. It is much more convenient than pitressin in oil but only works for about 4 hours. Two sprays up each nostril are given as often as necessary; each spray delivers approximately 5 units. It is only effective in mild cases and occasionally causes nasal irritation.

At one time pitressin powder was given as a nasal snuff but it often produced chronic rhinitis, bronchospasm and occasionally pulmonary fibrosis and now should never be used.

Chlorpropamide, a sulphonylurea normally used as an oral hypoglycaemic agent in diabetes mellitus, is also very effective in cranial diabetes insipidus. It appears to cause a marked increase in the renal tubular sensitivity to vasopressin. With the exception of the most severe cases, small normally ineffective amounts of vasopressin continue to be secreted in patients with cranial diabetes insipidus. Such patients respond dramatically to chlorpropamide and the thirst and polyuria subside without the need for pitressin. In the few patients whose symptoms are not fully controlled, the addition of intermittent lysine vasopressin spray often suffices. The dose, given once daily, is 100 to 350 mg, unless the patient also has diabetes mellitus—surprisingly not uncommonly associated with idiopathic diabetes insipidus—in which case the daily dose may be increased to 500 mg. There is often a delay of about 3 days before the drug is fully effective. Care must be taken to avoid hypoglycaemia which may occur particularly at night. Carbohydrate foods should be spread evenly throughout the day and some must be taken last thing at night. Hypoglycaemia is most likely to occur in children and in patients with anterior pituitary dysfunction and it is essential to ensure that ACTH secretion is normal or that adequate replacement is given. Idiopathic diabetes insipidus is the variety most likely to respond, and post-hypophysectomy patients the least likely. Unfortunately chlorpropamide has an 'Antabuse' effect, so that patients may flush and have a headache after alcohol. Although unpleasant they prefer this to the need to inject pitressin. The anticonvulsant, *carbamazepine* is also said to be effective in diabetes insipidus although the precise dose requirements and mechanism of action are not clear.

DDAVP (desamino-cys^1-d-arginine^8-vasopressin) is a newly introduced synthetic analogue of arginine vasopressin, the structure of which is modified so that the antidiuretic activity is increased many times compared with natural vasopressin, without any increase in pressor activity. Furthermore its rate of destruction in the circulation is greatly slowed since it is less susceptible to enzymic degradation. It is active by intranasal administration. 10 to 20 μg are needed in adults, and about 5 μg in children, once or twice a day. When generally available this material will undoubtedly prove to be the most acceptable form of treatment for all types of cranial diabetes insipidus. *Nephrogenic diabetes insipidus* cannot be treated with vasopressin or chlorpropamide. Since polydipsia is marked, adequate water intake is required sufficient to maintain the plasma osmolality between 275 and 295 mOsmol/kg. Unfortunately this often entails such a large fluid intake that the child fails to eat adequately and growth may be retarded. The urine volumes may be so large that the bladder distends and even a hydroureter or hydronephrosis may occur. Useful improvement in the polyuria may be achieved using diuretics such as bendrofluazide or the long acting polythiazide. A suitable daily dose of polythiazide in a child would be about 1 mg/day. It is essential to ensure that hypokalaemia does not occur and oral potassium supplements are required and sometimes the potassium sparing diuretic, triampterine, must be added (for example, 25 to 50 mg two or three times daily). The mechanism whereby diuretics work in nephrogenic diabetes insipidus is unknown although sodium depletion may be involved.

VASOPRESSIN EXCESS

Dilutional hyponatraemia is found either when vasopressin secretion from the hypothalamus and pituitary continues despite a reduction in plasma tonicity, or because a tumour of non-endocrine origin starts synthesising and secreting vasopressin 'ectopically'. The former situation usually occurs in association with lung infections such as pneumonia, an abscess, pleural effusion or tuberculosis and the mechanism is quite unknown. It may also occur with any intracranial pathology, myxoedema or indeed most serious illnesses. It probably accounts for most cases of what used to be called the 'sick cell syndrome'. Ectopic vasopressin secretion most often occurs from an oat cell carcinoma of the bronchus. Such vasopressin secretion is 'inappropriate' because it continues despite a hypotonic or dilute plasma, the urine being concentrated and the resultant water rentention leading to dilution of the electrolytes. The serum sodium is usually less than 120 meq/litre although the total body sodium is commonly normal. The urine volume may be small and its osmolality is at least twice that of the plasma.

Severe symptoms due to hyponatraemia usually appear when the plasma sodium falls to below 100 meq/litre. Somnolence, depression, confusion and anorexia occur and as the sodium concentration falls towards 100 meq/litre convulsions and coma may ensue. Oedema is rare. Treatment is simple; the patient's intake of water must be reduced to somewhat less than the volume of urine passed per day, usually to the region of 500 ml/day. The serum sodium and other electrolytes rapidly rise and the patient's general condition improves equally quickly. Extra potassium may be required for a few days, but sodium supplements are not required as there is no overall sodium deficit, merely dilution. Only if coma or convulsions occur should saline be given, as 500 ml of 3 per cent sodium chloride for the acute emergency. Mineralocorticoids are not required. The serum sodium will remain normal if the underlying condition can be corrected or treated. If this is not possible then the fluid intake should be adjusted so that the serum sodium and body weight remain steady.

If pigmentation is present, coincidental ectopic ACTH and MSH production should be suspected; if hypercalcaemia due to malignant disease is also present, this may block the ectopic vasopressin action and the dilutional hyponatraemia will only be seen when the serum calcium is reduced with treatment. The 'ectopic' hormone syndromes are discussed in Chapter 20.

OXYTOCIN

Oxytocin is an octapeptide similar in structure to vasopressin with which its biological properties overlap (Fig. 2.3). The actions of oxytocin are largely confined to the uterus and to the

```
              GLYCINAMIDE
                   |
                LEUCINE
                   |
                PROLINE
               /
CYSTEINE ---------------- ASPARTAMIDE
   /                          \
  S                         GLUTAMIDE
  |                             |
  S                         ISOLEUCINE
   \                           /
CYSTEINE ---------------- TYROSINE
```

FIGURE 2.3 Oxytocin

breast in animals, but it is not clear what role this hormone plays in man.

UTERINE ACTIONS

The uterus is more sensitive to oxytocin during the follicular stage of the cycle and stimulation of uterine contraction may aid the transport of spermatozoa to the Fallopian tubes. During human pregnancy and labour oxytocin is difficult to detect except during very brief bursts of uncertain significance, even using the most sensitive and specific radioimmunoassays; however the hormone is present in the pituitary and hypothalamus of men and women. During pregnancy oxytocin levels maybe balanced by a rise in oxytocinase and progesterone. The role of oxytocin in the induction of labour is still controversial but the uterus is certainly very sensitive to oxytocin at the end of pregnancy particularly if prostaglandin E or $F_2\alpha$ is also given and, at term, labour can be induced by their administration alone or in combination. Oxytocin acts on the myometrial cell membrane, rendering it more permeable to potassium, lowering the membrane potential, and increasing excitability. From experiments on rabbits it has been suggested that mechanical dilatation of the uterus, cervix or vagina reflexly stimulates oxytocin release and, hence, uterine contractions. In women with diabetes insipidus and hypothalamic disease labour is usually normal.

BREAST ACTIONS

Ejection of milk from the breast is due to a neurohumoral reflex. Afferent stimuli from the nipple during suckling travel along sensory pathways via the spinal cord to the hypothalamus. Oxytocin is subsequently released from the pituitary and transported to the breast where it stimulates contraction of myoepithelial cells around the alveoli, causing milk ejection. The latent period of thirty seconds between the onset of suckling and milk release is largely due to the time involved in oxytocin release and transport. There is some controversy as to whether oxytocin itself initiates the release of prolactin necessary for the maintenance of lactation, for, although suckling is required to maintain lactation, it is not essential to postulate that this effect is mediated by oxytocin. Drugs such as reserpine and chlorpromazine, which can induce prolactin-secretion, actually inhibit the release of oxytocin that normally follows suckling. Secretion of prolactin during lactation is probably maintained by the removal of hypothalamic inhibition.

Oxytocin excess or deficiency has not yet been associated with any disease process though oxytocin has been isolated from some non-endocrine tumours.

REFERENCES

Besser, G. M. (1972). *Medicine* (Part 2), 'The Hypothalamus and the Pituitary' (Bayliss, R. I. S., and Hall, R., Eds). London: Medical Educational (International) Ltd., p. 106.

Chard, T., and Edwards, C. R. W. (1972). *Modern Trends in Endocrinology*, **4,** 102, 'The Hypothalamus and the Posterior Pituitary' (Prunty, F. T. G., and Gardiner-Hill, H., Eds). London: Butterworths, p. 102.

Dashe, A. M., Cramm, R. E., Crist, C. A., Habener, J. F., and Solomon, D. H. (1963). *J. Amer. med. Assn.*, **185,** 699.

Price, J. D. E., and Lauener, R. W. (1966). *J. clin. Endocr.*, **26,** 143.

3

HYPOTHALAMUS

The major role of the hypothalamus is to act as an integrating centre, co-ordinating short-term autonomic responses with more delayed alterations in the activity of the endocrine system. It is concerned with the regulation of pituitary function, sexual activity, body temperature, and water and calorie balance.

ANATOMY

The hypothalamus lies at the base of the brain, beneath the thalamus, connected to the pituitary gland below by the pituitary stalk (Fig. 3.1). It includes the lateral walls of the lower part of the third ventricle and, laterally, it is related to the optic tracts, the ansa lenticularis, the globus pallidus, the internal capsule, and the inferior part of the thalamus. Anteriorly it reaches to just in front of the optic chiasm, and posteriorly to the rear end of the mamillary bodies.

Blood Supply. The hypothalamus receives its arterial supply from the circle of Willis. The anterior cerebral arteries and anterior communicating artery supply the anterior hypothalamus; the middle hypothalamus receives blood from the posterior communicating arteries; the posterior hypothalamus is supplied from the bifurcation of the basilar artery and the posterior cerebrals. The blood supply to some of the more important nuclei has been defined. The supraoptic nucleus is supplied by the posterior communicating, the posterior cerebral, the anterior cerebral, and the internal carotid arteries. The paraventricular nucleus receives blood from the anterior cerebral, internal carotid, and posterior communicating arteries. It is of interest that the supraoptic nucleus is supplied by the richest capillary bed of any group of neurones in the nervous system.

Veins draining the hypothalamus enter the venous circle lying above the circle of Willis which, in turn, empties into the basal vein and reaches the vein of Galen. Other veins leave the capillary plexuses in the median eminence stalk region to pass down the pituitary stalk to the capillary sinusoids of the anterior lobe of the pituitary. These veins connecting two capillary beds are referred to as portal veins and they are the major route by which the hypothalamus affects the anterior pituitary gland.

Neural Connections. Although much is known about the neural connections of the hypothalamus, the functions of the various pathways is poorly understood. Afferent fibres pass to the hypothalamus from the pyriform cortex, the hippocampus, the anterior thalamus, and medial parts of the mid-brain. Efferent fibres run from the hypothalamus to these areas and to the posterior pituitary by the hypothalamo-hypophysial tract.

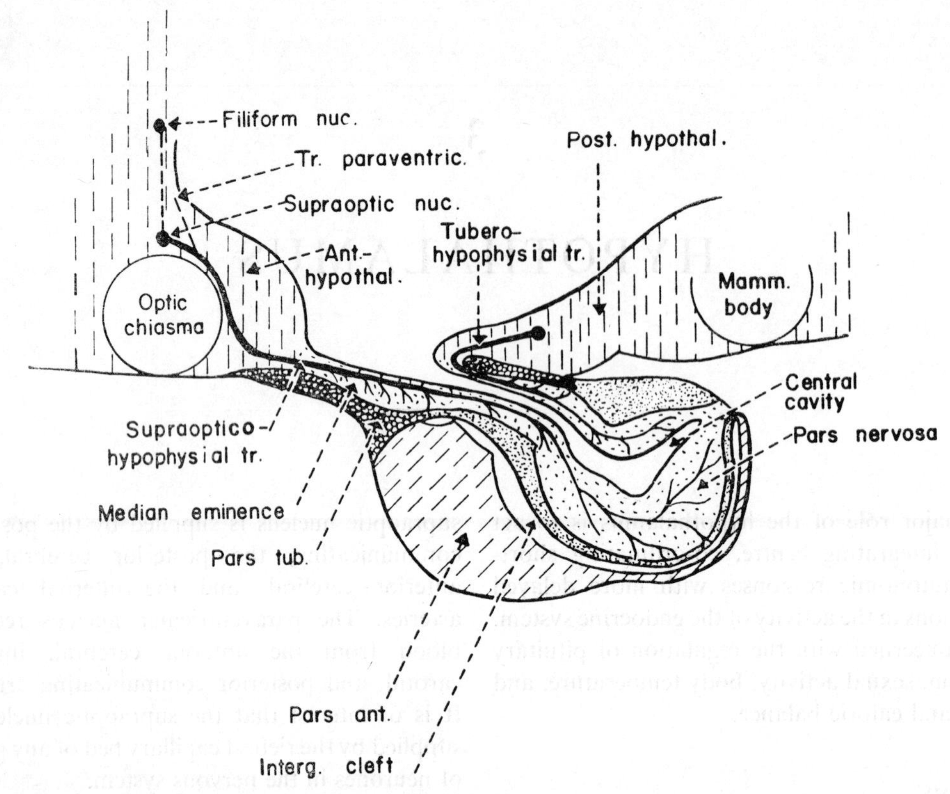

FIGURE 3.1 Sagittal section through hypothalamus (diagrammatic) (from *Textbook of Endocrinology* (1968), Ed. Williams, by permission of W. B. Saunders Co.).

HYPOTHALAMIC CENTRES

Although many nuclear groups can be recognised in the hypothalamus, little progress has been made in attributing functions to most of them. In man, the pathological processes that affect the hypothalamus are rarely confined to a single nuclear group (except in diabetes insipidus where, very often, all other hypothalamic and pituitary functions are normal). The groups of neurones that make up the hypothalamus can be delineated on the basis of anatomical, physiological, and neurochemical criteria.

With the exception of the supraoptic and paraventricular nuclei concerned with posterior pituitary activity, and the ventro-medial nuclei involved in satiety, it has not been possible to designate functional activity to anatomically recognised centres in man.

Diseases involving the hypothalamus may selectively involve certain 'centres' concerned in physiological reactions. For example, after severe head injury the only evidence of impaired hypothalamic function may be failure of response to a metyrapone-induced fall in plasma cortisol. Anatomical localisation of this centre and of all others involved in the control of pituitary ACTH output is remarkably lacking.

By the use of histochemical techniques it can be shown that some groups of neurones in the hypothalamus are cholinergic or dopaminergic while others are adrenergic. Even in a single anatomical site different physiological effects can be elicited by different chemical stimuli, suggesting overlap of functional areas. Injection of adrenaline into the lateral hypothalamus of the rat causes increased food intake, whereas a cholinergic drug (carbachol) increases water intake. The supraoptic nuclei are cholinergic and can be stimulated to produce vasopressin by the administration of nicotine, which has a cholinergic action. Drugs such as reserpine, which deplete hypothalamic catecholamine stores, can cause lactation.

At present, only the supraoptic nuclei are capable of definition on anatomical, physiological, and neurochemical criteria. They can be recognised histologically, local stimuli, (e.g. hypertonic saline) increase their hormonal output, and they function as cholinergic neurones, capable of stimulation by cholinergic drugs.

HYPOTHALAMIC CONTROL OF THE ANTERIOR PITUITARY

There are no neural connections between the hypothalamus and the anterior pituitary. The stalk median eminence region of the hypothalamus influences the pituitary by humoral agents which are released into its capillary bed and pass down the portal veins to the sinusoids bathing the cells of the anterior lobe. These humoral agents can be extracted from the median eminence and their injection stimulates or inhibits release of the appropriate pituitary hormones. They are present in tiny amounts and are thought to be small molecular weight polypeptides. Distinct hypothalamic nuclei are likely to be responsible for the synthesis of the various regulatory hormones, which are then stored in the median eminence to be released as required, pass down the capillary vessels of the stalk and then to act on the cells of the anterior pituitary. The influence of higher centres and the midbrain control of any circadian periodicity of the anterior pituitary hormones appears to act by modifying the secretion of these hypothalamic hormones. The negative feedback mechanism operates so that the circulating level of target gland hormone either alters the secretion of the hypothalamic hormones, or interferes with their action at the pituitary cell level (Fig. 3.2). In most cases the hypothalamic site of action appears to be the more important for feed-back control; however in the case of TRH (thyrotrophin-releasing hormone), the hypothalamic hormone controlling secretion of TSH, the circulating levels of tri-iodothyronine

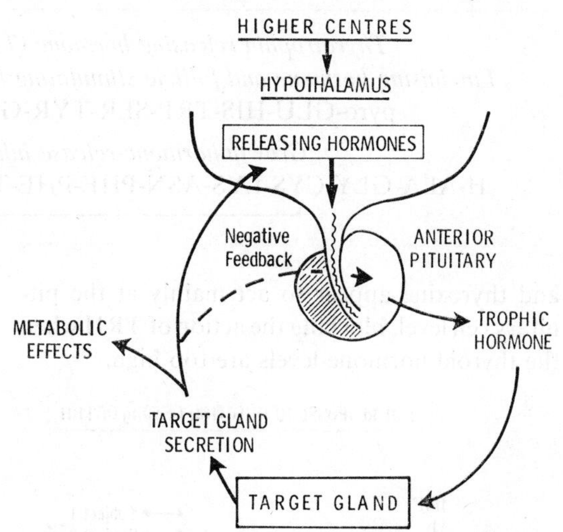

FIGURE 3.2 Diagrammatic representation of the relationships between the hypothalamic regulatory hormones and their actions on the pituitary. Secretion, or inhibition of tonic secretion, of specific trophic hormones occurs, which in turn influences secretion of the target organ hormones. These target hormones may modify pituitary hormone secretion via the feedback control mechanism either at the hypothalamic level or by interfering with the action of the regulatory hormones on the pituitary cells.

TABLE 3.2 *Known Hypothalamic Regulatory Hormones or Factors Acting on the Anterior Pituitary Cells*

Releasing hormones (RH) or releasing factors (RF) for:	
Thyrotrophin	TRH*
Luteinising hormone Follicle stimulating hormone	LH/FSH-RH
Growth hormone	GHRF
Corticotrophin	CRF
Prolactin	PRF

* TRH has intrinsic prolactin releasing activity but a separate PRF exists.

Inhibitory Hormones (IH) or inhibitory factors (IF) for:	
Prolactin release	PIF
MSH release	MIF
Growth hormone release	GR-IH

TABLE 3.3 *Structures of Identified Hypothalamic Hormones*

Thyrotrophin releasing hormone (TRH): pyro-GLU-HIS-PRO-NH_2

Luteinising hormone and follicle stimulating hormone-releasing hormone (LH/FSH-RH): pyro-GLU-HIS-TRP-SER-TYR-GLY-LEU-ARG-PRO-GLY-NH_2

Growth hormone-release inhibitory hormone (GR-IH): H-ALA-GLY-CYS-LYS-ASN-PHE-PHE-TRP-LYS-THR-PHE-THR-SER-CYS-OH

and thyroxine appear to act mainly at the pituitary cell level, blocking the action of TRH when the thyroid hormone levels are too high.

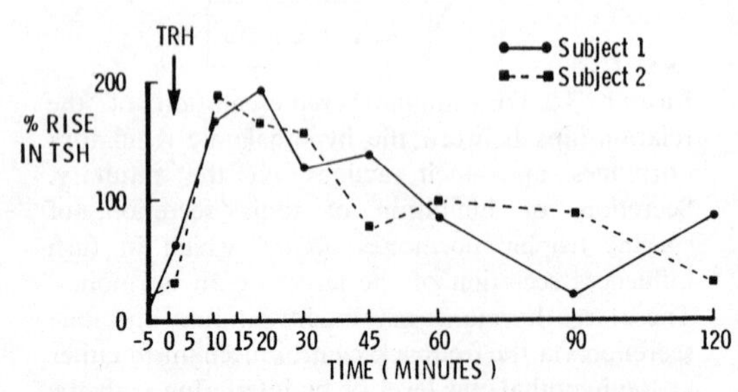

FIGURE 3.3 Change in serum TSH concentration after intravenous TRH in two normal subjects.

Originally these hypophysiotrophic substances were recognised by demonstrating that different extracts of sheep, bovine or pig hypothalami could modify the release of the hormones of the anterior pituitary *in vitro* or *in vivo*, either causing stimulation or inhibition of hormonal secretion. They were therefore called releasing or inhibitory 'factors'. Recently however three have been fully identified, their structures ascertained and the compounds synthesised and used in experimental and clinical situations. It has become the convention to call the fully identified substances releasing or inhibitory 'hormones'; the details are shown in Tables 3.2 and 3.3. It is clear that the releasing hormones not only cause secretion of the trophic hormones from the anterior pituitary cells, but also stimulate their synthesis within these cells. While these hormones must be secreted into the pituitary stalk capillary blood in extremely low concentrations, they can sometimes be detected in the general circulation, e.g. CRF after stress in hypophysectomised animals, and LH/FSH-RH at the times of the mid-cycle LH peak in the menstrual cycle.

Thyrotrophin Releasing Hormone (*TRH*)

Intravenous administration of as little as 10 μg of this synthetic peptide will cause the serum TSH

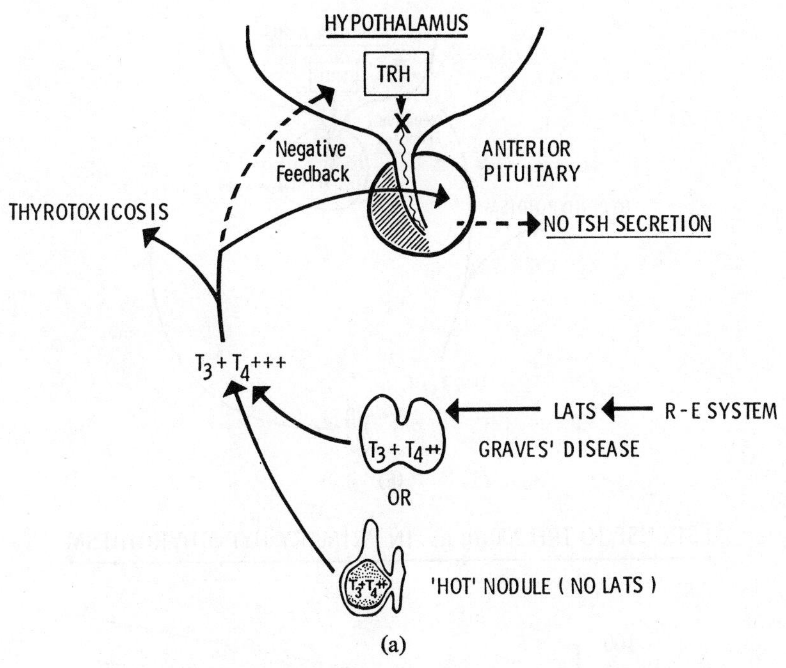

(a)

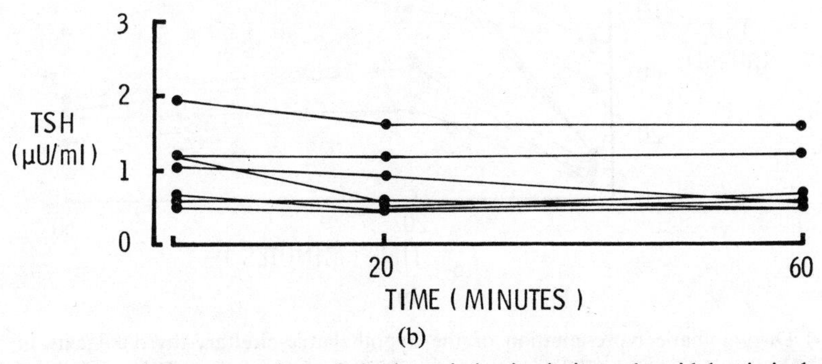

(b)

FIGURE 3.4 (*a*) Diagrammatic representation of the hypothalamic-pituitary-thyroidal axis in hyperthyroidism due either to Graves' disease or an autonomous thyroid nodule. TRH secretion, and the TSH response to TRH, are impaired.
(*b*) Absent serum TSH responses to 200 μg i.v. TRH in patients with thyrotoxicosis.

levels to rise within two minutes but doses of 50 μg and above give consistent responses (Fig. 3.3). Since elevated thyroid hormone concentrations both interfere with the action of TRH on the pituitary cells and also impair hypothalamic TRH secretion, TSH secretion is markedly reduced in thyrotoxicosis (Fig. 3.4*a* and 3.4*b*) after a standard dose of TRH; conversely in myxoedema due to primary thyroid disease, there is excessive TRH secretion and an increased TSH response to administered TRH (Fig. 3.5*a* and 3.5*b*). These responses to TRH have proved most valuable in clinical practice and will be discussed further in Chapter 5. The

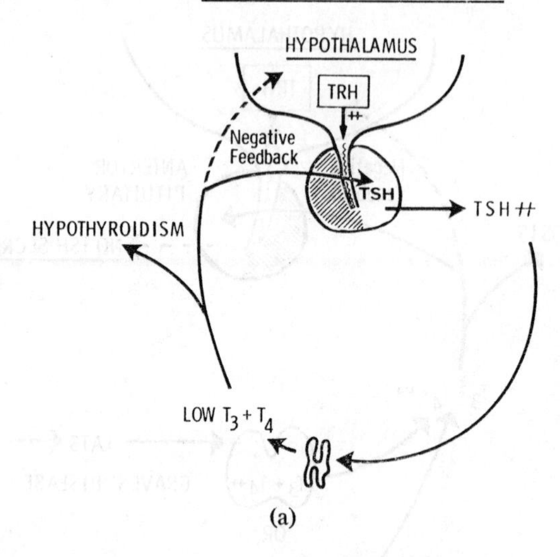

(a)

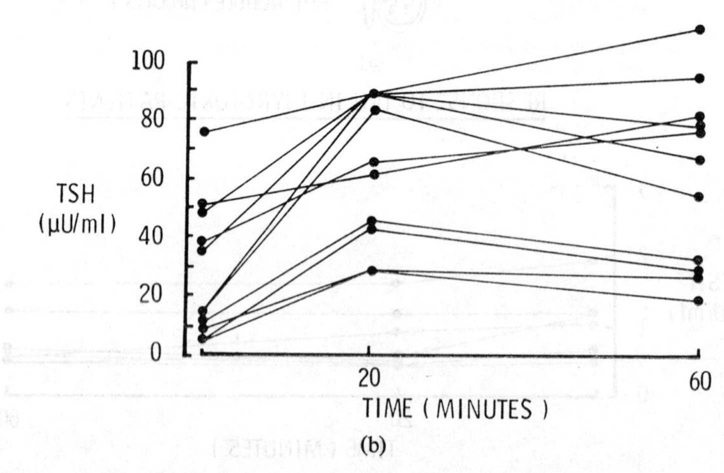

(b)

FIGURE 3.5 (*a*) Diagrammatic representation of the hypothalamic-pituitary-thyroidal axis in primary hypothyroidism. TRH secretion, and the TSH response to TRH, are increased—a TSH level above 20 μU/ml after TRH is excessive.
(*b*) Excessive serum TSH responses to 200 μg i.v. TRH in patients with primary hypothyroidism. Note that the vertical scale is different from Fig. 3.4 (*b*).

use of TRH in assessment of hypothalamic and pituitary disease has proved less valuable than in primary hypothyroidism or thyrotoxicosis. An absent TSH response to 200 μg TRH given intravenously is always seen when a patient is frankly hypothyroid due to a pituitary lesion, but an impaired pituitary TSH secretion may be seen even though the patient is still euthyroid. Presumably the pituitary TSH reserve is reduced but adequate for the time being. A characteristic 'hypothalamic' type of response has been described which is usually only seen when hypothalamic lesions are present but the pituitary is intact. In response to the standard 200 μg intravenous injection, with blood sampling for serum TSH levels at 0, 20 and 60 minutes (*see* Appendix), normal subjects show higher TSH values at 20 than 60 minutes. With hypothalamic lesions however the response is delayed, the 60 minute value being higher than that at 20 minutes, although the 20 minute level may be low or within the normal range.

Luteinising Hormone and Follicle Stimulating Hormone—Releasing Hormone (LH/FSH-RH)
Although the original studies suggested that there would be two separate hypothalamic hormones for the gonadotrophins, only one, a decapeptide (Table 3.3), has been isolated so far. This appears to cause release of both LH and FSH (Fig. 3.6), although the effect on LH is much greater than on FSH. Experience with the LH/FSH-releasing hormone is, as yet, much more limited than with TRH. However early evidence suggests that although the level of circulating gonadal steroids can modify the action of the decapeptide on differential pituitary gonadotrophin release, it is unlikely that all the cyclical secretory activities can be explained on the basis of only one gonadotrophin releasing hormone. It seems most likely that another with predominant FSH releasing activity will be found. Furthermore it seems clear that LH/FSH-RH is essential for synthesis of the gonadotrophins as well as for inducing their release.

Early clinical work indicates that this compound will be of great value in clinical endocrinology. Most hypogonad patients with organic pituitary disease as well as those with anorexia nervosa can be made to secrete both LH and FSH with the synthetic decapeptide. It is clear

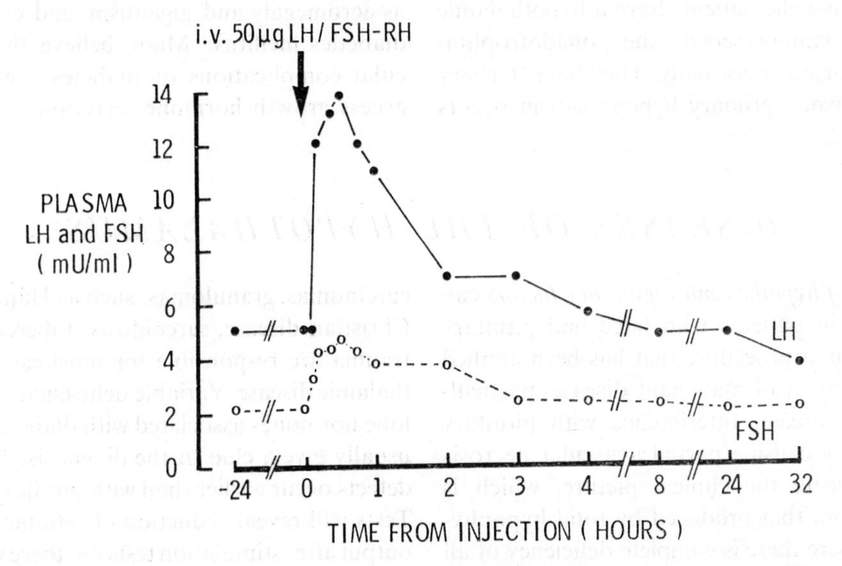

FIGURE 3.6 Change in serum luteinizing hormone (LH) and follicle stimulating hormone (FSH), after 50 μg of synthetic LH/FSH-RH given intravenously to a normal subject.

that this material will prove to be a valuable treatment for hypogonadotrophic male and female patients. Since it is synthetic it will be much cheaper to use than natural human gonadotrophins. Investigation of patients with so called 'isolated gonadotrophin deficiency' has shown that most secrete LH and FSH after administration of LH/FSH-RH, indicating that in these patients the pituitary gonadotrophs are intact but that the patients have a hypothalamic defect and cannot secrete the gonadotrophin-releasing hormone normally. They have 'tertiary hypogonadism'; primary hypogonadism occurs with intragonadal disease, and in secondary hypogonadism the pituitary is diseased.

Growth hormone release-inhibitory hormone (GR-IH). This 14 amino-acid peptide powerfully inhibits growth hormone release in normal patients and in acromegalics. It was discovered in 1973. It holds out great promise for the effective medical treatment of disorders associated with excess growth hormone secretion such as acromegaly and gigantism, and even perhaps diabetics mellitus. Many believe that the vascular complications of diabetes are related to excess growth hormone secretion.

DISEASES OF THE HYPOTHALAMUS

Deficiency of hypothalamic regulatory factors can be studied in patients who have had pituitary stalk section, a procedure that has been applied to the treatment of malignant disease, particularly of the breast. Interference with pituitary blood supply causing partial avascular necrosis will complicate the clinical picture, which is different from that produced by total hypophysectomy where there is complete deficiency of all anterior lobe hormones. After stalk section thyroid and adrenal function are reduced, but to a lesser extent than after pituitary removal. The normal feedback control (*see* below) of TSH and ACTH output is impaired. Basal gonadotrophin output may continue but there is no cyclical variation and menstruation is invariably absent. The patients do not respond to clomiphene. Growth hormone output is reduced and is unaffected by alterations in blood glucose level. In some patients lactation begins, a result of withdrawal of the usual hypothalamic inhibition of pituitary prolactin production. Tumours or granulomas that damage the pituitary stalk can cause a similar syndrome.

Deficient production of hypothalamic hormones may result from any hypothalamic disease. Tumours, particularly craniopharyngiomas, chromophobe adenomas, pinealomas, secondary carcinomas, granulomas, such as Hand-Schüller-Christian disease, sarcoidosis, tuberculosis, and trauma are responsible for most cases of hypothalamic disease. Variable deficiencies of anterior lobe hormones associated with diabetes insipidus usually give a clue to the diagnosis. Visual field defects occur earlier than with pituitary tumours. Tests will reveal reduction of pituitary hormone output after stimulation tests but there will usually be pituitary hormone secretion in response to the appropriate releasing hormone. Although alterations in calorie balance, temperature control and normal sleep rhythm may occur, they are not observed in the majority of patients with hypothalamic disease. Pathological hunger due to hypothalamic damage is most commonly seen after neurosurgical treatment of craniopharyngiomas. Such patients may continue to grow despite absent growth hormone secretion until they are dieted, when they may stop growing. The cause of this phenomenon is not known.

Many diseases attributed to the hypothalamus cannot stand critical scrutiny. Most boys with so-called Fröhlich's syndrome of obesity and hypogonadism are normal obese boys with late or delayed puberty. The syndrome of metabolic craniopathy is vague and ill-defined. The Laurence-Moon-Biedl syndrome of obesity, hypogonadism, mental retardation, atypical retinitis pigmentosa, and polydactylism is probably a true recessively inherited disease involving the hypothalamus.

Overproduction of hypothalamic releasing factors is responsible for certain diseases, though this conclusion must remain tentative until direct estimation of these compounds is possible in man. Increased output of CRF is likely to be the aetiological factor in most patients who have Cushing's disease due to bilateral adrenal hyperplasia. Even the pituitary tumours that are found in some 10 per cent of these patients could be the result of longstanding overstimulation by CRF. Early production of gonadotrophin releasing hormones, causing premature release of pituitary gonadotrophins, is likely to be the cause of true precocious puberty. This is seen in some patients with Albright's syndrome of polyostotic fibrous dysplasia of bone, in which there may also be localised areas of skin pigmentation. Most cases of precocious puberty in girls are 'idiopathic', and no local lesion of the hypothalamus can be demonstrated. In boys there is usually a local cause for precocious puberty, e.g. a hypothalamic or 'pineal' tumour.

FEEDBACK CONTROL OF THE ANTERIOR PITUITARY

The hypothalamus is involved in the feedback control of pituitary output of TSH, ACTH, and the gonadotrophins.

TSH. The output of TSH from the pituitary shows a reciprocal relationship with the level of circulating thyroxine and triiodothyronine. This effect may be mediated at both a pituitary and hypothalamic level though experimental confirmation is lacking in man. The feedback mechanism is responsible for the low levels of TSH in the circulation in conditions of hyperthyroidism due to a toxic adenoma of the thyroid where the adenoma is autonomous, and in Graves' disease where the thyroid overactivity is the result of an extrapituitary agent, such as the long-acting thyroid stimulator (LATS). When thyroid hormone production is lowered as a result of drugs, (e.g. carbimazole, iodide, perchlorate), or because of a genetically determined enzyme defect, pituitary TSH output is increased and is responsible for the goitre that is the usual accompaniment of these diseases. Very rarely, the prolonged stimulus of thyroxine deficiency causes such pituitary hypertrophy that there is enlargement of the pituitary fossa. These cases can be distinguished from patients with hypothyroidism resulting from a pituitary tumour by the finding of high levels of TSH in the blood, with an excessive response to TRH and failure of the thyroid gland to respond to injections of TSH. Overproduction of TSH as a result of pituitary or hypothalamic disease is very rare. Underproduction of TSH is a common finding in pituitary and hypothalamic disease and may rarely occur as a solitary defect of TSH formation, an abnormality more likely to be due to a hypothalamic defect. In these patients, despite the hypothyroidism there is secretion of TSH after TRH is given, although the response is 'delayed'.

ACTH. Low levels of cortisol stimulate pituitary ACTH release, which causes a compensatory increase in adrenocortical output. The centre involved in this feedback control is in the hypothalamus, and may be damaged by severe head injury or tumours in this region. Integrity of the feedback mechanism can be tested by the use of metyrapone. This drug interferes with 11-hydroxylation in the adrenal cortex and reduces the level of circulating cortisol. In normal circumstances pituitary ACTH output is increased and adrenocortical steroid formation is stimulated. The steroids produced, unlike cortisol, are not hydroxylated in the 11-position, but can be measured as 17-hydroxycorticosteroids in the urine.

The high levels of ACTH and of β-MSH, which are secreted in response to low cortisol levels, are responsible for the skin pigmentation found in Addison's disease where the adrenal cortex is relatively or absolutely unresponsive to ACTH.

High levels of cortisol reduce pituitary ACTH output by a different control system from the low-cortisol feedback mechanism. Integrity of these pathways is tested for by administration of dexamethasone to which the centres respond but which does not interfere with the estimation of cortisol or its metabolites in the blood or urine. Abnormalities in the 'high cortisol centre' are seen in Cushing's disease with bilateral adrenal hyperplasia, and in some cases of head injury involving the hypothalamus.

Low levels of ACTH result from overproduction of cortisol by adrenocortical adenomas or carcinomas. This has clinical significance because the low circulating ACTH level results in atrophy of the opposite adrenal, which can be observed at operation. Postoperative hypoadrenalism may follow removal of a secreting tumour even if the remaining gland is stimulated with ACTH. Various factors, including pyrogen and hypoglycaemia, also stimulate ACTH output. Although the hypoglycaemic stimulus acts mainly at a hypothalamic level and is impaired in the presence of hypothalamic disease, the site of action of pyrogen is still poorly understood. Pyrogen-induced fever can be abolished by an antipyretic without stopping the steroid response.

An excess of ACTH can also activate the receptors of the negative feedback mechanism, diminishing the formation of CRF and the level of ACTH. This process has been termed the 'short feedback loop'. Its significance in man is unknown.

Excess cortisol reduces CRF secretion by the hypothalamus, the 'long feedback loop', but also interferes with the action of CRF on the pituitary cells.

Gonadotrophins. Animal experiments have provided direct evidence that the action of oestrogens on the hypothalamus is to inhibit pituitary output of FSH and LH. Indirect evidence of possible inhibition of gonadotrophin formation by oestrogens is seen in the amenorrhoea that occasionally follows withdrawal of the oral contraceptive. This may be accompanied by prolactin secretion and galactorrhoea. Progesterone action on the hypothalamus is indicated by the rise in body temperature that occurs during the luteal phase of the menstrual cycle and during the early part of pregnancy. Lowered sex steroids resulting from oophorectomy or the menopause stimulate pituitary FSH and, to a lesser extent, LH output, and the vasomotor instability associated with menopausal hot flushes may result from a combination of oestrogen deficiency and gonadotrophin excess. The drug clomiphene stimulates ovulation; although its mechanism of action is not fully worked out, present evidence suggests that it acts as an anti-oestrogen at the hypothalamic level, thereby stimulating pituitary gonadotrophin output. One of its side effects is the occurrence of hot flushes.

When investigating the cause of amenorrhoea the principles of the feedback control are applied. Amenorrhoea due to an early menopause or ovarian failure is accompanied by high levels of pituitary gonadotrophins which can be estimated by one of the many assay procedures. Amenorrhoea due to pituitary or hypothalamic disease is the result of lowered levels of gonadotrophins. The amenorrhoea that precedes or follows psychogenic anorexia, particularly the syndrome of anorexia nervosa, produces an apparent secondary hypothalamic abnormality. While the patient is underweight, her gonadotrophin production is diminished, the level rising as her weight increases as a result of treatment. Plasma growth hormone and cortisol levels are usually high before treatment. Amenorrhoea due to anorexia nervosa may be prolonged even after satisfactory weight gain, but ovulation and conception can be produced by clomiphene or pituitary gonadotrophin therapy, and a normal pregnancy maintained.

PUBERTY

Long before puberty, the gonads and secondary sexual tissues are capable of response to appropriate hormonal stimuli, and normal feedback control of gonadotrophin output can be demonstrated. Present evidence suggests that the pituitary is under hypothalamic restraint prior to puberty and that the main factor involved in the initiation of puberty is a reduction in hypothalamic sensitivity to the sex steroids. Hypothalamic disease, as mentioned previously, can remove this normal inhibitory control and allow the precocious onset of puberty. This true precocious puberty must be distinguished from the pseudo-precocious puberty caused by overproduction of sex-steroids in congenital adrenal hyperplasia and testicular or ovarian tumours. Here there is development of the secondary sexual characteristics but gonadotrophin output is inhibited, the testes remain small, and cyclical menstruation and fertility do not occur.

CYCLICAL HYPOTHALAMIC ACTIVITY

The output of certain pituitary hormones varies with the time of day, the time of month, with the emotional state of an individual, and with his environmental conditions. There is a circadian rhythm of ACTH output which is lost in diseases affecting the hypothalamus and in Cushing's syndrome. Output of ACTH and, hence, of cortisol is highest between 6·00 and 9·00 a.m. and lowest about 12 midnight. Serial estimations of plasma cortisol during the 24-hour period show abolition of the normal circadian rhythm in patients with Cushing's syndrome, whereas in obese patients the normal circadian rhythm is retained—obesity is only very rarely a manifestation of organic hypothalamic disease.

Cyclical production of the gonadotrophins FSH and LH are responsible for menstruation but the factors involved in the variation of pituitary gonadotrophin output during the menstrual cycle are still largely unknown. There is little doubt that ovulation is produced by a surge of LH but the stimulus to this is obscure. Functional hypothalamic abnormalities are likely to be involved in the menstrual disorders associated with obesity, emotional upsets, and the polycystic ovary syndrome. The lowered thyroid activity seen in tropical climates and the converse in colder regions is mediated by alterations in pituitary TSH formation almost certainly following readjustment at a hypothalamic level.

HYPOTHALAMIC CONTROL OF BODY TEMPERATURE

Severe damage to the anterior hypothalamus in man by trauma, encephalitis, or tumours may cause hyperthermia due to loss of the normal heat dissipating mechanisms. Animal experiments also indicate that the anterior hypothalamus and adjacent pre-optic region are involved in the control of body temperature. Neurones in this region are sensitive to alterations in temperature of the blood perfusing them, a rise in temperature causing an increased rate of discharge and a fall decreasing the rate. By their action, heat loss or retaining mechanisms are initiated by autonomic reflexes on a short-term basis and probably by alterations in thyroid activity and, hence, of metabolic rate over the long-term. The remarkably constant body temperature maintained under a wide variety of metabolic and environmental conditions testifies to the efficiency of this homeostatic mechanism.

Fever is the result of an altered setting of the hypothalamic thermostat, most probably due to the influence of pyrogens released by leucocytes or bacteria. Variations about the new set-point can still be achieved by altering the environmental temperature. Pyrogens may act directly on the hypothalamic cells or indirectly by causing release of monoamines, the nature of which vary from species to species. Another manifestation of hypothalamic damage in man may be wide variations in body temperature, independent of that of the environment.

HYPOTHALAMIC REGULATION OF CALORIE BALANCE

Hypoglycaemia, acting on hypothalamic receptors, causes the release of pituitary growth hormone and ACTH. The metabolic processes initiated by these hormones compensate for the fall in blood sugar. Growth hormone mobilises an alternative energy supply in the form of free fatty acids while ACTH releases cortisol which, along with growth hormone, antagonises insulin action on muscle and itself causes increased conversion of amino-acids into glucose. The rate of fall in blood sugar as well as the absolute level reached are important in causing the hypothalamic response, and the peripheral manifestations depend largely on the rate of fall. Autonomic reactions and catecholamine release, causing pallor, sweating and tachycardia, also occur with a rapid drop in blood sugar. Conversely, a rise in blood sugar reduces growth hormone output; this forms the basis of an important test for acromegaly, where growth hormone cannot be suppressed to low levels by glucose administration during a standard glucose tolerance test.

Animal experiments indicate that the hypothalamus contains a lateral 'feeding centre' and a medial 'satiety centre'. Damage to the former causes aphagia and adipsia and separate cholinergic and adrenergic neurones in this area may be responsible for these effects. Damage to the ventro-medial 'satiety centre' causes overeating and obesity, the overfeeding ceasing when a certain increment of weight has been achieved. The nature of the stimulus to the satiety centre is still uncertain; it is unlikely to be either the absolute levels of blood glucose or free fatty acid although changes in the rate of utilisation of glucose may be of importance. A humoral agent has also been suggested.

Severe anorexia or obesity may rarely occur as a result of hypothalamic disease in man, but as mentioned before, most patients who present with either of these conditions are not suffering from hypothalamic disease, which is suspected very much more frequently than can be proven.

HYPOTHALAMIC REGULATION OF WATER BALANCE

This has been dealt with in Chapter 2. It should be mentioned that diabetes insipidus is the commonest presentation of hypothalamic disease. In progressive diseases affecting the hypothalamus, e.g. secondary carcinoma, diabetes insipidus, which can normally be compensated for by excessive fluid intake, may get out of control. It is postulated that a hypothalamic thirst centre has been involved in the disease process, causing fluid intake to fall, leading to marked dehydration and elevation of serum sodium and chloride levels which can be lowered to normal by careful manipulation of fluid intake and by vasopressin therapy.

REFERENCES

Hypothalamus

Brown-Grant, K., and Cross, B. A. (Eds) (1966). *Brit. med. Bull.*, **22**, No. 3.

James, V. H. T., and Landon, J. (Eds) (1968). *The Investigation of Hypothalamic-Pituitary-Adrenal Function.* Cambridge: Cambridge University Press.

Reichlin, S. (1963). *New Eng. J. Med.*, **269**, 1182, 1246, 1296.

Reichlin, S. (1967). *Amer. J. Med.*, **43**, 477.

TRH

Ormston, B. J., Garry, R., Cryer, R. J., Besser, G. M., and Hall, R. (1971). *Lancet*, **11**, 10.

Hall, R., Ormston, B. J., Besser, G. M., Cryer, R. J., and McKendrick, M. (1972). *Lancet*, **i**, 759.

LH/FSH-RH

Besser, G. M., McNeilly, A. S., Anderson, D. C., Marshall, J. C., Harsoulis, P., Hall, R., Ormston, B. J., Alexander, L., and Collins, W. P. (1972). *Brit. med. J.*, **3**, 267.

Marshall, J. C., Harsoulis, P., Anderson, D. C., McNeilly, A. S., Besser, G. M., and Hall, R. (1972). *Brit. med. J.*, **4**, 643.

GR-IH

Hall, R., Besser, G. M., Schally, A. V., Coy, D. W., Evered, D., Goldie, D. J., Kastin, A. J., McNeilly, A. S., Mortimer, C. H., Tunbridge, W. M. G., Phenekos, C., and Weightman, D. (1973). Lancet, **ii**, 581.

4

DISORDERS OF GROWTH

Normal growth in height and size results from an interplay of many intrinsic and extrinsic factors on the 'innate' genetically determined capacity for growth of the body cells. The relationship of growth to development is well summarised by Greulich and Pyle (1959):

> 'Growth manifests itself by an increase in mass and volume as disclosed by an increase in weight and by changes in external dimensions as the child advances in age; development is the expression of those processes by means of which he becomes progressively more mature. While growth and development proceed concomitantly in the normal child, they are to some degree potentially independent processes *and are under different hormonal and metabolic controls*. This is clearly evident in such contrasting pathological states as precocious puberty and marked hypogonadism or eunuchoidism.'

Although growth in height is most easily observed, alterations in skeletal proportions, maturation of the features, dental development and skeletal maturation must all be taken into account. The ultimate height attained depends not only on the rate of linear growth but on its duration, thus the actual height at a given age should always be assessed in the light of the bone maturity or bone age.

The factors that influence growth in height vary at different times. *In utero* hormonal factors have little effect, and the intrauterine environment appears to overcome the effects of many disorders that later cause stunting of growth. In congenital adrenal hyperplasia, where adrenal androgens are present in excess, neither body length nor skeletal maturation are significantly advanced at birth, though, later, both are increased and skeletal maturation proceeds at a greater rate, causing the ultimate height to be below average. In Turner's syndrome there is considerable growth retardation, which mainly occurs after birth. The mean height of adult women with this condition is at least 15 per cent below normal, whereas the birth length of children with Turner's syndrome is only about 7 per cent less than average. In cretinism, the birth length is also usually normal in the presence of markedly retarded skeletal maturation and epiphyseal dysgenesis. Factors that interfere with placental function or in some way impair the intrauterine environment may cause growth retardation even with a fetal life of normal duration. Maternal disease, smoking habits, uterine size, pre-eclamptic toxaemia, and high altitude environments may all effect fetal size.

After birth, the rate of growth is slowed, the 'innate' growth stimulus decreases, and hormonal regulation begins to play a part. In the first year of life a baby increases its birth length by 50 per cent, while in the second and third years the rate falls to 16 per cent and 10 per cent respectively. Thyroid hormone is essential for normal growth after birth, and cretins are always short. Growth hormone, contrary to previous belief, affects growth within a few months of birth though the slowing of growth in hypopituitary dwarfs is rarely recognised till the second or third year of life. Androgens, and possibly oestrogens, are responsible for the adolescent growth spurt, but when present in excess they accelerate maturation faster than linear growth.

In normal girls there is a fairly constant relationship between the menarche and the period of maximum growth. The maximum annual increment of growth in height usually occurs in the year preceding the menarche. By the time menarche occurs the growth rate has already begun to decelerate, principally due to fusion of the epiphyses of the long bones of the lower limbs. Similarly, in normal boys, the changes of puberty are preceded or accompanied by the maximum growth in height. It is possible to forecast with some accuracy the time of the menarche by the degree of skeletal maturation in childhood. Children with advanced 'bone age' have an earlier menarche.

Temporary interference with growth when it is most rapid—*in utero* and, possibly, during the first year of life—may result in permanent reduction of stature. In later childhood temporary interference with growth, e.g. by an infection, is usually followed by a compensatory period of rapid growth—'catch-up growth.'

Bone maturation, which is measured as 'bone age' or 'dental age', is under different hormonal control from linear growth. The effect of different hormones on these processes is shown in Table 4.1.

TABLE 4.1 *Effect of Hormones on Linear Growth and Bone Maturation*

Hormone	Linear growth	Bone maturation
Growth hormone	++	+
Thyroid hormone	+	++
Androgens and oestrogens	+	++
Glucocorticoids	−	+

+ indicates increase − indicates decrease

EVALUATION OF GROWTH

1. *Height*. Charts relating height to age give an indication of the rate of growth and compare it with normal. The charts prepared by J. M. Tanner and R. H. Whitehouse (University of London, Institute of Child Health, for the Hospital for Sick Children, Great Ormond Street, London) are in general use. Persons whose height falls below the third centile or above the 97 centile certainly warrant further investigation but changes in rate of growth are also important.

2. *Skeletal Proportions*. The lower segment measured in the standing position is the distance from the top of the symphysis pubis to the floor. The upper segment is obtained by subtracting the lower segment from the total height. At birth, the ratio of upper segment to lower segment is about 1·7 :1. Since the limbs grow more rapidly than the trunk, this ratio decreases, and by the age of ten or eleven years reaches unity and remains there. Hypothyroid dwarfs retain infantile proportions, unlike hypopituitary and other types of dwarf (except those due to skeletal abnormalities) whose skeletal proportions correspond more closely with their chronological age. Measurement of the span is also helpful since it largely reflects the length of the arms. In normal adults the span is similar to the height, whereas in eunuchoidism both span and lower segment are increased.

3. *Weight*. In children, the relation of weight to age can be obtained from Tanner's charts;

in adults, a suggested scheme is shown in Appendix F. It is important to realise that these charts should never be interpreted rigidly as there is a considerable variation in bone structure and lean body mass. In adults, where obesity has developed in later life, it is often helpful to aim to reduce the patient's weight towards his weight as a young adult. It is obvious that if impaired growth is due to malnutrition, weight is likely to be reduced to a greater extent than height.

4. *Maturation of Features.* Facial appearance is an important guide to skeletal maturity. Growth of the bridge of the nose during infancy is impaired in hypothyroidism and accounts for the characteristically immature face of the cretin. Hypopituitary dwarfs do not usually show the lengthening of nose and jaw that occurs at normal puberty and their appearance is thus somewhat juvenile.

5. *Bone Maturation.* 'Bone age' can be determined from Table 4.2 and Fig. 4.1, which show the extent of skeletal maturation at different ages. For accurate assessment of bone age the reader is referred to the *Radiographic Atlas of Skeletal Development of the Hand and Wrist* by W. W. Greulich and S. I. Pyle (1959), where X-ray films of the hand and wrist can be compared with plates depicting the degree of skeletal development of healthy children at different ages. They give tables of standard deviations from which the probability of deviation from normal can be determined. A skeletal age more than two standard deviations from the mean makes it highly probable that the child is abnormally advanced or retarded.

6. *Dental Development.* Development of the primary and secondary dentition is affected by the same factors as bone maturation. The times of calcification and eruption of the deciduous and permanent dentition are shown in Table 4.3.

DIAGNOSIS OF CAUSE OF SHORT STATURE (Table 4.4)

Most patients with short stature are not suffering from any endocrine disease. The cause can usually be determined by the clinical features and a few investigations (Table 4.5). Particular attention should be paid to the family history of growth and development, the patient's birth weight and length when they are available, the pattern of growth in height and epiphyseal development, facial features and secondary sexual characteristics, dental development, body weight, appetite and nutrition, infections and previous diseases, and intelligence. Examination should include recording of the present height, lower segment, span, body weight, skull circumference, and assessment of body configuration, e.g. neck webbing, cubitus valgus, shortness of metacarpals, body fat, evidence of systemic disease, sexual maturation—in particular body hair distribution, breast development, testicular and penile size. The urine should always be tested for albumin and sugar, and a full blood count and ESR determined. Routine X-rays usually include skull and chest and those required for assessment of bone age or chromosomal abnormalities. Additional investigations depend on the findings.

1. *Constitutional Delay in Growth and Adolescence.* Most patients with short stature fall into this category. They probably represent the lower tail of the normal distribution curve. Birth weight and length are usually normal but throughout childhood height is below average and epiphyseal development is similarly retarded. Puberty and its attendant growth spurt are delayed but the growth is prolonged because of late epiphyseal fusion. It is helpful to grade pubic hair growth, genital maturity and breast development by standard photographs (*see* Appendix B). Without treatment such patients usually attain 'normal' height and development. Often there is a strong family history of delayed growth and adolescence. When there is psychological disturbance because of the delayed puberty it is sometimes justifiable to initiate puberty with its concomitant growth spurt by hormone treatment, although this plan of action should only rarely be entered upon before the age of 15 years. A six week course of

TABLE 4.2 *Time of Appearance of Epiphyseal Ossification Centres* (after Maresh, by permission of Lange Medical Publications)*

HAND AND WRIST

Age (Yr//month†) Percentile (boys)			Epiphyseal centres (see Fig. 4.1)	Age (Yr//month†) Percentile (girls)		
5	50‡	95		5	50‡	95
Birth	0//2·5	0//4	Capitate	<term¶	0//2·25	0//4
Birth	0//3·5	0//6	Hamate	<term¶	0//2·5	0//5
8//8	1//0	2//0	Distal radius	0//6	0//10	1//6
1//0	1//6	2//0	Prox. III carpal	0//9	0//11	1//3
1//0	1//6	2//0	Prox. II, IV carpal	0//9	0//11	1//6
1//3	1//6	2//3	Metacarpal II	0//9	0//11	1//6
1//0	1//6	2//3	Distal I carpal	0//9	1//0	1//6
1//3	1//9	2//6	Metacarpal III	0//9	1//0	1//6
1//6	2//0	2//6	Metacarpal IV	1//0	1//3	1//9
1//6	2//0	2//6	Prox. V carpal	1//0	1//3	2//0
1//6	2//0	2//6	Middle III, IV carpal	1//0	1//3	2//0
1//6	2//3	3//0	Metacarpal V	1//0	1//6	2//0
1//6	2//3	3//0	Middle II carpal	1//0	1//6	2//0
1//0	2//3	4//6	Triquetrum	1//0	1//6	3//0
2//0	2//3	3//0	Metacarpal I	1//6	1//6	2//6
2//6	3//0	3//6	Proximal I carpal**	1//3	1//9	2//6
2//6	3//6	5//0	Middle V carpal**	1//6	2//0	3//3
1//6	4//0	5//6	Lunate**	2//6	3//0	4//0
3//6	5//3	6//6	Greater multang.**	2//6	4//0	5//6
3//6	5//3	6//6	Lesser multang.**	2//6	4//0	5//6
4//0	5//3	7//0	Navicular**	3//0	4//0	6//6
6//0	7//0	8//0	Distal ulna	5//0	5//6	7//0
10//0	11//0	13//0	Pisiform	7//6	8//0	10//6

* Compiled from data obtained from the Harvard Growth Study, Fels Institute, Brush Foundation, and the University of Colorado Child Research Council.

† E.g., 1//3 = 1 yr 3 months.

‡ 50th percentile and mean are approximately the same in most studies.

¶ <term = before term.

** Centres which are most variable in time and order of appearance.

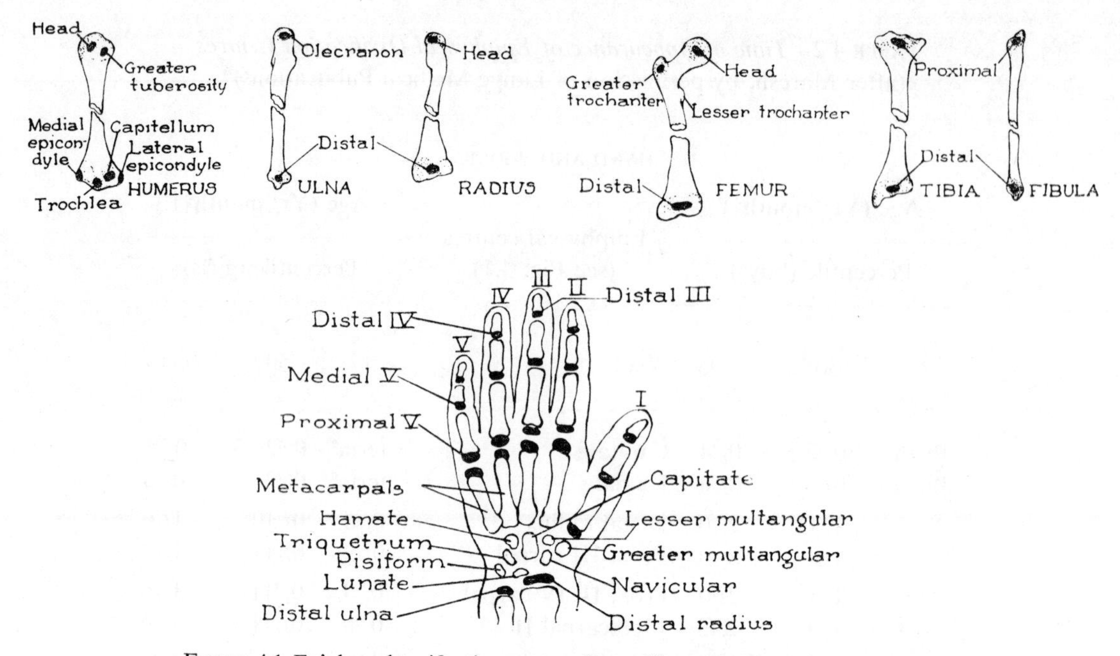

FIGURE 4.1 Epiphyseal ossification centres (from Silver, Kempe and Bruyn, 1965)

EXTREMITIES (excluding Hand and Wrist)

<term¶	<term¶	2 wks	Distal femur	<term¶	<term¶	1 wk
<term¶	<term¶	2 wks	Prox. tibia	<term¶	<term¶	1 wk
<term¶	2 wks	6 wks	Tarsal cuboid	<term¶	1 wk	2 wks
Birth	3 wks	0//2	Head of humerus	Brith	2 wks	0//1
0//3	0//4	0//9	Distal tibia	0//2	0//3	0//8
0//4	0//5	0//10	Head of femur	0//3	0//4	0//8
0//5	0//7	1//6	Capit. of humerus	0//3	0//5	1//0
0//7	1//0	2//0	Gr. tuber. humerus	0//4	0//8	1//6
0//8	1//0	2//0	Distal fibula	0//8	0//9	1//6
2//6	3//6	4//6	Gr. troch. femur	2//0	2//6	4//0
3//0	4//0	5//6	Prox. fibula	2//0	2//6	4//6
3//6	5//0	7//6	Prox. radius	3//0	4//0	6//0
4//6	6//0	8//0	Med. epicond. humerus	3//0	3//6	6//0
7//6	10//0	12//0	Trochlea of humerus	6//0	8//0	10//0
8//0	10//6	12//0	Prox. ulna	6//6	8//0	9//6
10//0	12//0	13//0	Lat. epicond. humerus	8//0	9//6	11//0

TABLE 4.2 (*Continued*)

TABLE 4.3 *Times of Calcification and Eruption of Deciduous and Permanent Teeth* (By permission of Lange Medical Publications)

Primary or Deciduous Teeth

	Calcification		Eruption*		Shedding	
	Begins at	Complete at	Maxillary	Mandibular	Maxillary	Mandibular
Central incisors	4th fetal month	18–24 months	6–10 months (2)	5–8 months (1)	7–8 yr	6–7 yr
Lateral incisors	5th fetal month	18–24 months	8–12 months (3)	7–10 months (2)	8–9 yr	7–8 yr
Cuspids	6th fetal month	30–39 months	16–20 months (6)	16–20 months (6a)	11–12 yr	9–11 yr
First molars	5th fetal month	24–30 months	11–18 months (5)	11–18 months (3)	9–11 yr	10–12 yr
Second molars	6th fetal month	36 months	20–30 months (7)	20–30 months (7a)	9–12 yr	11–13 yr

Secondary or Permanent Teeth

	Calcification		Eruption*	
	Begins at	Complete at	Maxillary	Mandibular
Central incisors	3–4 mth	9–10 yr	7–8 yr (3)	6–7 yr (2)
Lateral incisors	Max. 10–12 mth Mand. 3–4 mth	10–11 yr	8–9 yr (5)	7–8 yr (4)
Cuspids	4–5 mth	12–15 yr	11–12 yr (11)	9–11 yr (6)
First Premolars	18–24 mth	12–13 yr	10–11 yr (7)	10–12 yr (8)
Second Premolars	24–30 mth	12–14 yr	10–12 yr (9)	11–13 yr (10)
First Molars	Birth	9–10 yr	$5\frac{1}{2}$–7 yr (1)	$5\frac{1}{2}$–7 yr (1a)
Second Molars	30–36 mth	14–16 yr	12–14 yr (12)	12–13 yr (12a)
Third Molars	Max. 7–9 yr Mand. 8–10 yr	18–25 yr	17–30 yr (13)	17–30 yr (13a)

* Figures in parenthesis indicate order of eruption. Many otherwise normal infants do not conform strictly to the stated schedule.

TABLE 4.4 *Causes of Short Stature*

1. '*Constitutional*' delay in growth and adolescence
2. *Familial short stature*
3. *Low birth-weight shortness of stature*
   (*a*) Intrauterine infections
   (*b*) Autosomal chromosomal anomalies
   (*c*) Recognised syndromes
   (*d*) Unrecognised syndromes
   (*e*) Abnormal pregnancy
4. *Nutritional*
   (*a*) Deficient intake for social, economic, psychological or other reasons
   (*b*) Malabsorption syndromes
   (*c*) Others, e.g. familial diabetes insipidus (poor intake)
   glycogen storage disease
   protein loss
   cystinuria (poor absorption and excessive loss)
   (*d*) Chronic infections
5. *Disease of a major organ*
   (*a*) Congenital heart disease, especially cyanotic variety
   (*b*) Chronic renal disease
   (*c*) Chronic pulmonary disease
   (*d*) Chronic hepatic disease
   (*e*) Chronic central nervous system disease
   (*f*) Chronic infections
   (*g*) Anaemia
6. *Sex chromosome abnormalities*
   Turner's syndrome
7. *Skeletal diseases*
   (*a*) Congenital—phocomelia
   (*b*) Hereditary
      (i) Primarily affecting bones, e.g. chondrodystrophies (achondroplasia)
      (ii) Affecting other tissues as well, e.g. Hurler's syndrome, diastrophic dwarfism (Walker *et al.*, 1972) Laurence-Moon-Biedl syndrome, Ellis-van Creveld syndrome, pseudo- and pseudo-pseudo-hypoparathyroidism
      (iii) Resulting in bone disease
      Vitamin D resistant rickets, hypophosphatasia
8. *Miscellaneous disorders*
   Progeria, Leprechaunism (Donahue's syndrome), Bird-headed dwarfs, Silver's syndrome, and Cockayne's syndrome (Danowski, 1965)
9. *Endocrine disorders*
   Pituitary dwarfism
   Hypothyroidism
   Cushing's syndrome
   'Congenital adrenal hyperplasia'
   'Sexual precocity'
10. *Emotional deprivation*

TABLE 4.5. *Diagnosis of Important Varieties of Short Stature*

	Constitutional delay in growth and adolescence	Familial short stature	Pituitary dwarfism	Hypothyroid dwarfism	Turner's syndrome
Family history	Positive	Positive	Usually negative	Negative	Usually negative
Birth weight and height	Normal	Reduced	Normal	Normal	Slightly reduced
Pattern of growth	Rather slow from birth	Slow from birth	Slow from few months after birth	Slow from birth	Slow from birth
Epiphyseal development	Moderate but not progressive retardation	Almost normal	Progressive retardation	Marked retardation	Within normal but wide variation
Features	Immature but later normal	Mature	Immature	Infantile	Often characteristic
Puberty	Late but eventually normal	Normal	Usually delayed unless solitary growth hormone deficiency	Delayed	Usually no signs except in mosaics
Serum cholesterol	Normal	Normal	Raised	Raised	Normal
Growth hormone level	Normal	Normal	Low	Normal	Normal
Gonadotrophin level (after puberty)	Normal	Normal	Low unless solitary growth hormone deficiency	Normal or may be raised	Raised

human chorionic gonadotrophin is given by intramuscular injection in a dose of 4000 IU twice weekly.

2. *Familial Short Stature.* This is common although it is not necessarily genetic in origin since environmental factors which affect parents may also affect children. Before birth growth is mainly determined by the intrauterine environment and to some extent by the mother's but not the father's height. Apart from a baby's sex, growth *in utero* is little affected by genes. However during the first two years of life growth is under genetic control and a child assumes a rate of growth which follows the same curve until puberty. There is a correlation between a child's height and the mean height of both parents (mid-parental height) which increases from 0·2 at birth to 0·5 at two years. Special growth

charts have been produced by Tanner from which it is possible to assess whether a child's height is normal in relationship to its parents. Children with familial shortness of stature are otherwise well. Sometimes the birth weight is less than average, and weight is appropriate for height. The height curve advances below and parallel to the third centile. Bone age is usually retarded but not markedly so. No treatment is necessary or indeed possible, but psychological support may be indicated.

3. *Low Birth Weight Shortness of Stature.* Most babies who are born before term, but who are of appropriate weight for their gestational age will continue to grow normally after birth and are not short in later childhood. Likewise the majority of babies who are underweight at birth for their gestational age tend towards the mean during childhood. However some short children do have a history of a birth weight which is low for their gestational age. There are two major reasons for this situation. Firstly the baby may have some abnormality before and/or after birth which impairs growth, for example an infection or some chromosomal or genetic anomaly. Secondly there may have been some abnormality of the intrauterine environment which has impaired subsequent growth potential. This might be a short-lived insult in early pregnancy causing a congential abnormality as well as the growth defect, or a prolonged cause of growth restraint in later pregnancy.

Parkin (1972) recognises at least five different clinical groups in this category:

(*a*) *Intra-uterine infections* such as rubella or toxoplasmosis, may damage the fetus leaving the stigmata associated with the infection as well as growth failure. Serological evidence of the infection may be present during the first year of life.

(*b*) *Autosomal chromosomal anomalies* usually cause multiple physical abnormalities as well as stunted growth (Smith, 1967, Hamerton, 1971).

(*c*) *Recognised syndromes* of which there are many, may be characterised by a low birth weight (Smith, 1967).

(*d*) *Unrecognised syndromes* are quite common and may be associated with a wide variety of major or minor congenital abnormalities such as an odd facies, ptosis, an incurved fifth finger or a high-arched palate.

(*e*) *Abnormal pregnancy* in which there is an unhealthy placenta, for example maternal hypertension, may cause low birth-weight dwarfism.

The diagnosis is based on a low birth-weight for gestational age and a height which remains below the third centile. Bone age is almost invariably retarded but endocrine investigations are normal. There is no specific therapy.

4. *Nutritional.* Nutritional causes should often be suspected from the clinical findings of ill health and malnutrition, and the family and social background is helpful. Brain damage may affect appetite, and mental retardation inhibit the development of normal eating habits. Malabsorption syndromes must always be excluded in any dwarfed child without obvious cause by jejunal biopsy, faecal fat estimation and other tests. In diabetes insipidus food intake may be reduced because of impaired appetite resulting from the excessive fluid intake. Patients may also recognise that the more food they eat the more urine they pass and consciously or subconsciously limit their intake. In glycogen storage disease, carbohydrate is not available for normal metabolism, and gluconeogenesis supplies much of the glucose required. In various amino-acidurias defective absorption of specific amino-acids may occur along with excessive loss in the urine. In kwashiorkor, lack of protein is a potent cause of growth stunting.

These patients are thin and their weight is further below the third centile than their height. The age of onset and subsequent growth curves are related to the cause and its time of occurrence. Bone age is retarded in proportion to the stunting in height.

5. *Diseases of Major Organs.* Congenital heart disease may be associated with growth retardation, especially if there is cyanosis. Many factors are probably involved, e.g. tissue anoxia, diminution of peripheral blood supply from a

sub-optimal cardiac output, respiratory infections or concomitant abnormalities such as Turner's syndrome. A dramatic growth spurt may follow correction of the defect.

There are many reasons why growth is retarded when chronic renal disease is present, e.g. from anorexia, acidosis, anaemia, sodium depletion and infection. In chronic pyelonephritis in children, growth retardation may overshadow more local manifestations. Similarly, chronic pulmonary disease may inhibit growth presumably by virtue of anoxaemia, infections, or anorexia. Mental retardation is also associated with shortness of stature—the more severe the mental defect the greater is the degree of shortness. It is important to note that to impair growth systemic diseases must be severe. If the patient appears well, if the physical examination is normal, if no abnormalities can be detected on urinalysis, measurements of the blood urea and plasma bicarbonate and the chest X-ray, it is unlikely that shortness is caused by disease of a major organ.

6. *Sex Chromosome Abnormalities.* Many abnormalities of the sex chromosomes are associated with shortness of stature. Turner's syndrome (karyotype 45/XO) is always associated with reduction in linear growth. It can be suspected by the somatic abnormalities that usually accompany it, e.g. webbing of the neck, cubitus valgus, coarctation of the aorta and lymphoedema, to mention but a few. Buccal smears usually indicate that the woman is chromatin negative, but mosaicism (XO/XX; XO/XXX) may cause the buccal smear to be chromatin positive (*see* Chapter 13). In this case, blood or skin cultures for chromosome analysis may be required. Sexual development is nearly always impaired, but in mosaics breast development may occur, height may be less stunted, and a few instances of successful pregnancies have been reported. The characteristic skeletal malformations that can be shown radiologically may give a clue to diagnosis—rounding of the medial femoral condyle, short fourth metacarpal, reduced carpal angle, and many other changes.

7. *Skeletal Diseases.* Skeletal deformities are usually so characteristic as to be easily recognised on clinical or radiological examination. Conditions such as achondroplasia and Morquio's disease affect bone primarily; the Hunter-Hurler syndrome, diastrophic dwarfism and the Ellis-van Creveld syndrome affect bone and other tissues; other disorders result in bone disease such as vitamin D resistant rickets and hypophosphatasia.

8. *Miscellaneous Disorders.* Many syndromes have been described, usually characterised by peculiar types of disproportionate growth. Some may have underlying chromosomal or metabolic abnormalities but there is little virtue in cataloguing their numerous features. Details of the main ones are shown pictorially in monographs by Smith (1967) and (1970). It is important to make a precise diagnosis because this gives information about the patient's future intelligence and helps in genetic counselling. Some syndromes such as de Lange's are associated with severe mental retardation whereas in others such as Silver's, the intellect is normal.

9. *Endocrine Disorders*

Pituitary dwarfism is dealt with in Chapter 1. Genetic disorders of endocrine glands leading to shortness of stature are comprehensively reviewed by Rimoin and Schimke (1971). The growth-promoting action of GH may, at least in part, be mediated by a protein termed the sulphation factor (SF) produced largely by the liver. Levels of SF are not reduced unless there is GH deficiency except in the group of children described by Laron *et al.*, (1971). These patients had familial shortness associated with raised serum GH levels measured by radioimmunoassay and low SF levels which may be due either to a general tissue unresponsiveness to GH or to a specific defect in SF production.

The subject of growth hormone treatment for one to seven years in 100 children with growth hormone deficiency, low birth-weight, inherited smallness, Turner's syndrome and other complaints is reviewed by Tanner *et al.*, (1971).

Hypothyroidism is a not uncommon cause of dwarfism. The earlier the onset of hypothyroidism the more marked is the deficit of skeletal length and maturation. The proportion of the upper and lower segments remains infantile, the naso-orbital configuration is immature, and dental development is delayed. Bone age is retarded even more than height. X-rays of different parts of the skeleton should be taken, depending on the patient's age, as they may give a clue to the time of onset of the hypothyroidism and may reveal epiphyseal dysgenesis, an appearance said to be pathognomonic of the condition. It may only appear after the start of therapy but then only in centres which should already have appeared. The epiphysis is misshapen with irregular margins and fragmentation. The clinical and laboratory diagnosis of hypothyroidism is considered in Chapter 5.

Cushing's syndrome, in which the level of circulating cortisol is raised due to pituitary, adrenal or malignant disease or by cortisol administration, is always accompanied by growth retardation in children. Linear growth and skeletal maturation are both affected. High cortisol levels reduce GH release and also impair its peripheral action.

Congenital Adrenal Hyperplasia. The stimulus of excessive androgens causes increased linear growth and skeletal maturation after birth, and the ultimate height is usually reduced. The aim of therapy is to restore the circulating cortisol level, thereby reducing ACTH and, hence, androgen production. This procedure usually slows down skeletal growth, but only rarely is average height attained.

Sexual precocity whether due to 'true' precocious puberty or to androgen or oestrogen-secreting tumours is associated with excessive skeletal growth and maturation. Ultimate height is reduced and juvenile body proportions with relatively short legs may be seen (*see* Chapter 12).

10. *Emotional Deprivation.* This is an important cause of failure to thrive in the early years and of shortness of stature. Deprivation of food may be associated, but emotional deprivation alone may lead to a temporary hypothalamic disturbance with impaired release of growth hormone and sometimes also of corticotrophin from the anterior pituitary. Emotional disturbance may be obvious with a voracious appetite, stealing of food, thirst and offensive stools. Social assessment reveals gross disorders of the child's family relationships and environment. Facial appearance, behaviour and intellect are immature, and the abdomen protuberant. Bone age is retarded in proportion to the reduced height. Responses of GH and ACTH to appropriate stimuli are deficient but return to normal after the child has spent some time in a secure environment, when the growth rate increases rapidly. It is important to exclude a malabsorption syndrome to which the condition bears some clinical similarities. Treatment requires improvement in the child's emotional environment, usually away from home in the first instance. Psychiatric and social assistance is often needed for the parents.

TREATMENT OF SHORT STATURE

The treatment of short stature depends upon its cause. Whenever possible the responsible defect should be remedied, e.g. correction of a congenital cardiac defect, treatment of a chronic urinary infection or improvement of the diet. In patients with constitutional delay in growth and adolescence no therapy is usually needed. When puberty has not started by 15 to 16 years the adverse psychological effects may force the physician's hand, and in boys a course of chorionic gonadotrophin may initiate penile and testicular development which progress into normal puberty. In girls, cyclical oestrogen-progesterone therapy may be indicated if puberty has not developed by 16 to 17 years, and the puberty growth spurt will then ensue. Withdrawal of therapy may later be followed by spontaneous normal menstruation in 'late developers'. No therapy affects the ultimate height of congenital dwarfs. Pituitary dwarfs respond well to growth hormone except patients who develop high levels of antibodies (*see* Chapter 1, p. 10). Hypothyroid dwarfs may attain normal height and development with thyroxine therapy in full dosage. Androgens and anabolic steroids have been used to accelerate growth in height in many varieties of short stature but it is generally agreed that skeletal maturation is always accelerated and it is doubtful whether in the long term height is increased.

DIAGNOSIS OF CAUSE OF TALL STATURE (Table 4.6)

1. *Constitutional Tall Stature.* Most children who are brought for advice about tall stature are not suffering from detectable endocrine disease. They may represent the upper end of the normal distribution of height just as children with constitutional delay in growth and adolescence reflect the lower end of the distribution curve. Very often there is a family history of tallness in one or both parents. Their ultimate height can often be predicted by assessment of bone age. If this is advanced, their ultimate height may not be excessive (*see* the Tables by Bayer and Bayley, 1959, for prediction of final height on the basis of skeletal maturation).

TABLE 4.6 *Causes of Tall Stature*

1. Constitutional
2. Overnutrition
3. Brain damage
4. Arachnodactyly and other syndromes
5. Hormonal
   (*a*) Gigantism
   (*b*) Sexual precocity
   (*c*) Eunuchoidism
   (*d*) Hyperthyroidism

2. *Overnutrition.* Obese children are often taller than average for their age, bone maturity is also advanced, and puberty may occasionally occur earlier. Most children who become obese have a normal birth weight. It is not uncommon for the onset of obesity to follow some emotional upset, e.g. admission to hospital for tonsillectomy. Overnutrition is probably responsible for the increased growth. In Copenhagen, obese children were not taller than their contemporaries, possibly because nutrition in all the children studied was optimal and overnutrition would produce no additional effect. Support for this view comes from studies of children from the professional classes, where obesity is not associated with increased growth. Weight loss is usually associated with slowing down of bone growth and maturity. The heavier, longer children born to diabetic or prediabetic mothers may result from excessive insulin release from the child's pancreas. Hubble (1965) makes the point that, if overnutrition is associated with shortness of stature, then some cause of growth retardation should be looked for, e.g. Turner's syndrome or hypothyroidism.

3. *Brain Damage.* Some children are overweight at birth and continue to grow rapidly in height with skeletal maturation lagging only slightly behind. There is often a history of difficult labour and birth trauma, and the child may be mentally retarded. The cause of the increased growth is not known but it may be the result of brain damage. One variety is associated with clumsiness and is termed cerebral gigantism.

4. *Arachnodactyly* (*Marfan's Syndrome* and other syndromes). Patients with Marfan's syndrome are usually above average height. They may

be recognised by the numerous skeletal and somatic anomalies present, e.g. high arched palate, dislocated lenses, long fingers and patellar ligaments, and kyphoscoliosis. The excessive length of the metacarpals has been used to derive a metacarpal index $\left(\frac{\text{length}}{\text{width}} > 8{\cdot}4 \text{ is abnormal}\right)$ which is increased in this condition. Again, the lower segment is usually longer than the upper segment because of the overgrowth of the lower limbs. Neither of these measurements necessarily differentiate arachnodactyly from gigantism. Arachnodactyly, being a congenital and often familial anomaly, usually manifests itself at an early age. Many patients are seen who have some 'Marfanoid' features but cannot be regarded as having 'true' Marfan's syndrome.

Children with some chromosomal syndromes, XXY or XYY, may be above average height. In the former at least this may be partly due to androgen deficiency.

5. *Hormonal* (*a*) *Gigantism* (see Chapter 1). Gigantism in adolescence is often associated with stigmata of acromegaly but is much rarer than the adult syndrome. Growth hormone levels are raised and there is insulin resistance. The pituitary fossa is not always enlarged, and eosinophilic hyperplasia is sometimes seen rather than an eosinophilic adenoma. It should present no major difficulty in diagnosis since growth hormone levels are not raised in constitutionally tall children.

(*b*) *Sexual Precocity* (*see* Chapter 12). Precocious sexual development with 'true' precocious puberty can be differentiated from precocious sexuality resulting from excessive androgen or oestrogen production. Overproduction of sex hormones is due either to tumours of testes, ovaries or adrenals or to congenital adrenal hyperplasia. In both varieties of sexual precocity linear growth and bone maturation are rapid, and although early height may be above average the ultimate height is reduced.

(*c*) *Eunuchoidism*. Hypogonadism from any cause can produce an increase in linear growth due to delayed fusion of epiphyses, as long as growth hormone output is not impaired.

(*d*) *Hyperthyroidism*. An increase in growth rate associated with advanced bone age is seen in hyperthyroid children.

TREATMENT OF TALL STATURE

Constitutional tall stature does not usually call for any specific therapy apart from reassurance of the parents and patient. A prognosis as to the ultimate height can sometimes be made by assessment of the degree of bone maturity. In some girls, however, the excessive height may be socially embarrassing and an effort should be made to slow down the rate of growth. Cyclical oestrogen-progesterone therapy before the age of twelve years will cause withdrawal bleeding and breast development, and by accelerating bone maturation may reduce the ultimate height. After the age of twelve years such therapy has little effect. The treatment of gigantism is dealt with in Chapter 1, and sexual precocity in Chapter 12.

REFERENCES

Bayer, L. M., and Bayley, N. (1959). *Growth Diagnosis.* Univ. Chicago Press.

Danowski, T. S. (1965). *Outline of Endocrine Gland Syndromes.* Baltimore: Williams & Wilkin Company, Chapters 76 and 77.

Greulich, W. W., and Pyle, S. I. (1959). *Radiographic Atlas of Skeletal Development of the Hand and Wrist,* 2nd Edition. London: Oxford University Press.

Hamerton, J. L. (1971). *Human Cytogenetics,* Vol. II, *Clinical Cytogenetics.* London: Academic Press.

Hubble, D. (1965). 'Disorders of growth,' in *Recent Advances in Paediatrics*, 3rd Edition (Ed. Douglas Gairdner). London: Churchill Ltd., Chapter 8, p. 190.

Laron, Z., Pertzelan, A., Karp, M., Kowaldo-Silbergeld, A., and Daughaday, W. H. (1971). *J. clin. Endocr.*, **33,** 332.

Parkin, M. (1972). 'Disorders of growth,' in *Medicine*, No. 2 (R. I. S. Bayliss and R. Hall, Eds), p. 118.

Rimoin, D. L., and Schimke, R. N. (1971). *Genetic Disorders of the Endocrine Glands.* Saint Louis: The C. V. Mosby Company.

Smith, D. W. (1967). 'Compendium on shortness of stature', *J. Pediat.*, **70,** 463.

Smith, D. W. (1970). *Recognisable Patterns of Human Malformation.* London: Saunders.

Tanner, J. M., Whitehouse, R. H., Hughes, P. C. R., and Vince, F. P. (1971). *Arch. dis. Childh.*, **46,** 745.

Walker, B. A., Scott, C. I., Hall, J. G., Murdoch, J. L., and McKusick, V. A. (1972). *Medicine*, The Williams and Wilkins Co., **51,** 41.

Wilkins, L. (1962). 'The influence of the endocrine glands upon growth and development,' in *Textbook of Endocrinology*, 3rd Edition (R. H. Williams, Ed). London: W. B. Saunders Co., Chapter 15, p. 908.

Wilkins, L. (1965). *The Diagnosis and Treatment of Endocrine Disorders in Childhood and Adolescence*, 3rd Edition. Springfield, Illinois: C. C. Thomas.

5

THYROID

EMBRYOLOGY, ANATOMY, AND PHYSIOLOGY

The thyroid gland can be recognised in human embryos by the end of the first month after conception when the embryo is 3·5 to 4 mm in length. It is derived from the mid-line endoderm of the pharynx between the first and second branchial pouches. A diverticulum is formed, enlarges, descends, and eventually loses contact with the pharynx. The course of descent is indicated by the thyroglossal duct which occasionally persists, opening on to the tongue at the foramen caecum. Thyroid tissue may eventually be found anywhere between the base of the tongue and the normal thyroid position. The pyramidal lobe, an upward extension of the isthmus of the thyroid, is a residue of the thyroglossal duct, and not infrequently it can be traced for two or three inches on one or other side of the larynx in the adult. Part of the lateral lobes of the thyroid is also derived from the fourth branchial pouch from the ultimobranchial bodies. This tissue is the origin of the parafollicular or 'C-cells' in the thyroid which secrete calcitonin (*see* below).

The thyroid gland, situated in the lower neck, consists of two lobes connected by an isthmus that crosses the front of the second and third tracheal rings. A fibrous capsule which invests the gland is connected with the pretracheal fascia. Blood supply to the gland is derived largely from the superior thyroid arteries (from the external carotids) and from the inferior thyroid arteries (from the subclavians). A rich capillary network surrounds each follicle, and veins are derived from a perifollicular plexus. The thyroid is richly supplied with lymphatics.

In the adult, the thyroid is the largest endocrine gland, weighing about 20 g in this country. Microscopically it is composed of spherical follicles with a diameter of between 50 and 500 μ whose walls consist of a single layer of epithelial cells with their apices directed towards the lumen of the follicle and their bases towards a basement membrane. The follicles are bound together in groups of about forty to form lobules, each supplied by an end artery. Within each follicle is a substance known as colloid, largely made up of proteins, especially the iodinated glycoprotein thyroglobulin (MW 650,000). Each 19S thyroglobulin molecule contains 115 tyrosine residues and consists of four 8S subunits which are iodinated during and after aggregation to form the complete molecule. The thyroid also contains albumin-like 4S iodoproteins containing mainly mono- and diiodotyrosine. In certain thyroid disorders these 4S proteins are released and contribute to the PBI but not to thyroxine. The two thyroid hormones, thyroxine and triiodothyronine are stored in the colloid as part of the thyroglobulin molecule, and these hormones can be released only when thyroglobulin is broken down by enzymes.

Because the thyroid hormones contain large

amounts of iodine, adequate dietary intake of iodine is essential for their synthesis. Iodine in the diet is largely derived from sea fish and from milk (especially in winter) and from eggs and iodised salt. In calculating dietary iodine intake from tables the losses incurred in preparation must be allowed for. The average intake of iodide

A third hormone has also been isolated from the human thyroid, and named calcitonin because of its action on calcium metabolism. The hormone is formed in the parafollicular or 'C-cells'. Injections of calcitonin lower the serum calcium and phosphate levels in certain situations but its role in calcium homeostasis

HO–(ring, I at 3)–CH2-CH(NH2)-COOH

3-monoiodotyrosine

HO–(ring, I at 3 and 5)–CH2-CH(NH2)-COOH

3:5-diiodotyrosine

HO–(ring, I at 3')–O–(ring, I at 3 and 5)–CH2-CH(NH2)-COOH

3:5:3'-triiodothyronine
or triiodothyronine or T_3

HO–(ring, I at 3' and 5')–O–(ring, I at 3 and 5)–CH2-CH(NH2)-COOH

3:5:3':5'-tetraiodothyronine
or thyroxine or T_4

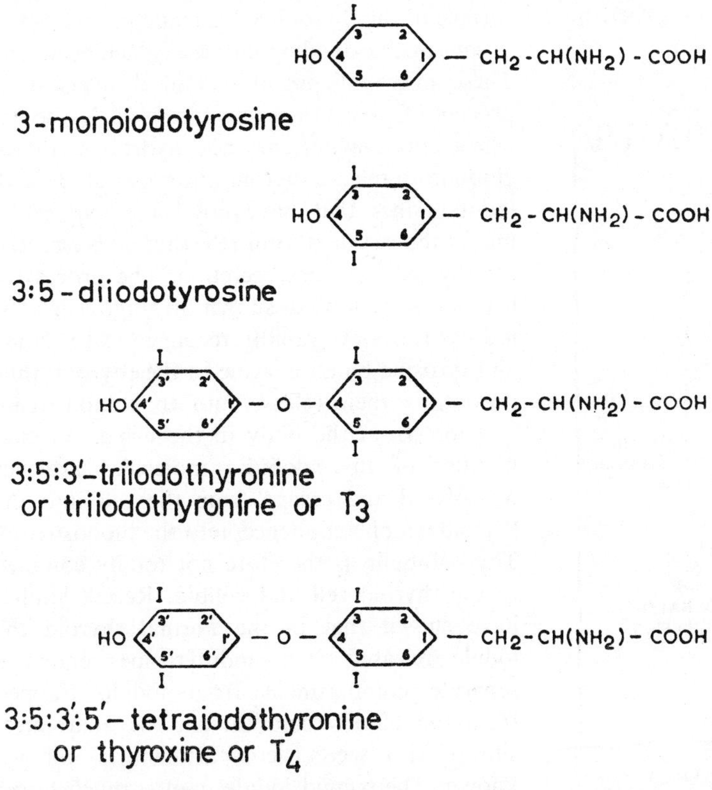

FIGURE 5.1 Thyroid hormones and their precursors

in the United Kingdom is between 100 and 150 μg each day. Iodides are readily absorbed from the stomach and upper small bowel but are present in only very small amounts in the circulation. The range of plasma iodide levels is wide and depends on geographical locality, e.g. in Glasgow, levels range from 0·04–0·57 μg/100 ml (Wayne *et al.*, 1964). About two-thirds of the iodide in the blood is excreted in the urine and one-third is trapped by the thyroid. Some 95 per cent of the body's iodine stores are situated in the thyroid, the remainder circulating as hormone in the blood and tissues.

remains to be established. Further details of the hormone will be found in Chapter 18.

The normal human thyroid gland is able to concentrate iodide from the blood at a rate of about 2 μg/hr but the ability to trap iodide is not unique to the thyroid. Iodide also appears in high concentration in the saliva, gastric juice, and in the milk of lactating women, but none of these tissues is able to use the trapped iodide to form thyroid hormones and, so far as we know, this function does not serve any useful purpose. Active transport of iodide occurs at the basal cell membrane and is an energy-requiring process involving cell-membrane bound adenosine triphosphatase. The iodide trapped by the thyroid is converted to thyroid hormones by a complicated series of enzymatic reactions that are as yet not fully understood. Before the iodide can be used for hormone synthesis it must first be oxidised to some active form by a peroxidase enzyme system, plus hydrogen peroxide, generated by oxidation of TPNH by a

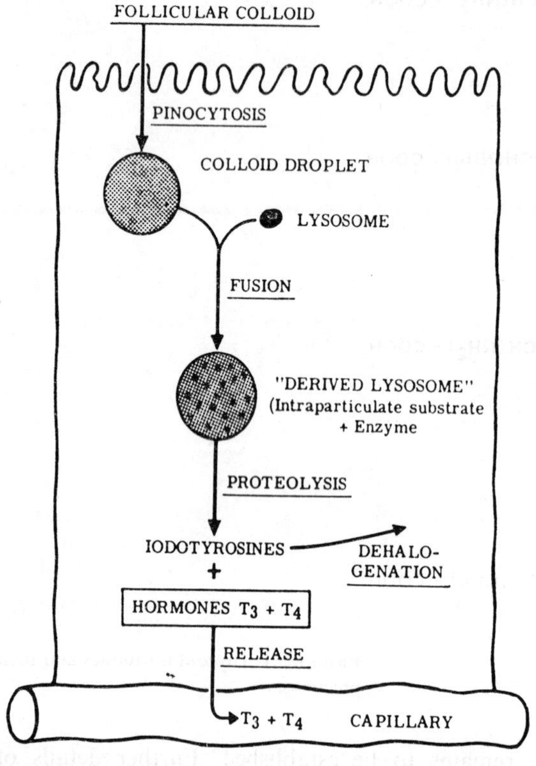

FIGURE 5.2 The process of thyroid hormone secretion

flavoprotein which can be auto-oxidised to produce H_2O_2. Methimazole specifically inhibits the peroxidation of iodide and it is this reaction which is responsible for the therapeutic action of the drug. Oxidation of iodide occurs very rapidly, with the result that the thyroid contains very little free iodide and most of the iodide in the gland is found in thyroid hormones or their immediate precursors. The active form of iodine combines with molecules of the amino-acid tyrosine attached to thyroglobulin to form monoiodotyrosine and diiodotyrosine. Two molecules of diiodotyrosine then couple together to form thyroxine, and one molecule of monoiodotyrosine and one of diiodotyrosine form triiodothyronine (Fig. 5.1). Hormone containing molecules of thyroglobulin are then stored in the colloid till required. The apical surface of the thyroid cell is made up of a series of microvilli extending into the follicular lumen. These microvilli engulf colloid droplets by a process of pinocytosis and fuse with lysosomes whose proteolytic enzymes hydrolyse thyroglobulin to release thyroid hormones along with iodotyrosines that have not been coupled. A microtubule system within the thyroid is essential for thyroid hormone secretion. The process of thyroid secretion is shown in Fig. 5.2. The iodotyrosines are rapidly reconverted to iodide and tyrosine by an enzyme in the thyroid, thus preventing their release into the bloodstream and loss from the body in the urine. A small number of thyroglobulin molecules are not hydrolysed and escape from the cell into the thyroid lymph and, hence, into the bloodstream. Thyroglobulin is therefore not totally confined to the thyroid cell and colloid. Recent studies have shown that in the normal thyroid the iodide released from iodotyrosines enters a separate compartment from iodide trapped from the bloodstream though the anatomical site of this second compartment is not yet known. The second iodide pool is much larger than the first and turns over more slowly.

PITUITARY-HYPOTHALAMIC CONTROL

The complicated series of enzymatic reactions in which iodine is trapped and converted to thyroid hormones is under the control of thyroid-stimulating hormone (TSH) secreted by the pituitary gland. If for any reason the blood concentration of free thyroid hormone falls an increased secretion of TSH stimulates the thyroid to produce greater amounts of thyroxine and triiodothyronine. Increased levels of these hormones cause a shut-down of TSH production which decreases hormone synthesis by the thyroid till the normal blood free hormone level is restored. Thyroid hormones act directly on the anterior pituitary to influence the release of TSH. Synthesis and release of TSH from the thyrotroph cells of the anterior lobe is mediated by the tripeptide pyroglutamyl-histidyl-proline-amide, the thyrotrophin-releasing hormone (TRH). Increased circulating levels of thyroid hormones, acting by some protein intermediate, inhibit the action of TRH on TSH release; hence serum TSH levels are low in hyperthyroidism. TRH is synthesised over a wide area of the hypothalamus and is stored in the median eminence, from which it is released into the portal veins passing down the pituitary stalk to the anterior lobe. There is preliminary evidence in animals that thyroxine may increase TRH synthesis but the significance of this is unknown. Again preliminary animal experiments suggest that inhibition of deiodination of T4 to T3 prevents the blocking effect of T4 on TRH-mediated TSH release. implying that T4 itself is metabolically inert and requires conversion to T3 before it is effective.

THYROID-STIMULATING HORMONE (TSH)

TSH is a glycoprotein, molecular weight 28,000 which consists of two non-identical polypeptide units designated α and β. The α-subunit has a very similar if not identical structure to the α-subunits of the other glycoprotein hormones, LH, FSH and HCG, and is biologically inactive. The β-subunit differs markedly from those of the other glycoproteins, although there are some sequences in common, and it has only slight biological activity.

Secretion of TSH (vide infra) is under the control of TRH from the hypothalamus and of circulating T4 and T3. There is good evidence for a circadian rhythm of TSH production, probably mediated by TRH, increased levels occurring some two hours or more after the onset of sleep, peaking between 2 and 4 a.m.

Almost every metabolic process in the thyroid that has been investigated can be stimulated by TSH. Iodide trapping, formation of thyroid hormones and their release are all increased by TSH as are most of the processes of intermediary metabolism within the gland, e.g. glucose oxidation, ribonucleic acid synthesis and phospholipid formation. The mechanism of action of TSH on the thyroid is still uncertain but the following sequence is acceptable at present. TSH binds to a hormone receptor on the thyroid cell membrane (LATS may also attach itself to this site, *see* p. 108). This leads to activation of the enzyme adenyl cyclase which then converts adenosine triphosphate (ATP) to cyclic adenosine monophosphate (cyclic AMP). The processes by which cyclic AMP mediates the effects of TSH on the thyroid are not yet fully understood, but it seems likely that cyclic AMP activates a protein kinase which then phosphorylates a variety of proteins thereby causing activation or inactivation of their functions.

CIRCULATING THYROID HORMONES

The hormones released from the thyroid are rapidly bound to proteins in the plasma, the intensity of the binding being indicated by the very small proportion of the hormones in the unbound state. Only 0·024 per cent (2 ng per 100 ml) of thyroxine and 0·36 per cent (0·43 ng per 100 ml) of triiodothyronine are present in the free form, yet all the regulating mechanisms are concerned to maintain the levels of free hormones. Since it has been shown that the metabolic activity of T3 is about four times that of T4, by weight, it is evident that the contributions of free T4 and free T3 would be about equal in biological activity.

Three proteins are known to bind thyroid hormones; in order of decreasing affinity they are thyroxine-binding globulin (TBG), thyroxine-binding prealbumin (TBPA), and albumin. These account for about 60 per cent, 30 per cent and 10 per cent respectively of the thyroxine binding capacity of serum, although the precise amount of hormone bound to each protein in the circulation is unknown, since all the methods of

TABLE 5.1 *Abnormal Protein-binding Capacities*

(Reproduced by permission of Dr K. Sterling)

	Increased	Decreased
Thyroxine-binding globulin	Pregnancy	Nephrotic syndrome
	Myxoedema	Marked hypoproteinaemias
	Genetic	Severe illness
	Hepatic disease (rare)	Genetic
	Acute porphyria	Hepatic disease (rare)
	Analbuminaemia	Uncompensated acidosis
		Endocrine disease:
		Acromegaly
		Thyrotoxicosis
		Cushing's syndrome
	Drug therapy:	Drug therapy:
	Oestrogens including the contraceptive pill	Anabolic steroids
	Phenothiazines (prolonged)	Androgens
	Clofibrate	Diphenylhydantoin
		Tetrachlorthyronine
		Corticosteroids (massive)
Thyroxine-binding prealbumin	Analbuminaemia	Severe illness or trauma
	Endocrine disease:	Endocrine disease:
	Acromegaly	Thyrotoxicosis
	Cushing's syndrome	
	Drug therapy:	Drug therapy:
	Corticosteroids (massive)	Dinitrophenol
		Salicylates

analysis are prone to artefacts. The affinity of T3 for TBG is two- to sixfold less than that of T4 for TBG. T3 does bind to TBPA with an affinity similar to that for albumin. Since the concentration of albumin is about 200 times greater than that of TBPA in serum, it is obvious that more T3 will be bound to albumin than to TBPA. All three binding proteins are not essential for survival since persons born without TBG do not suffer from any ill effects. It is interesting that as one ascends the animal kingdom the complexity of the thyroxine-binding proteins increases. Fishes and birds lack TBG but show thyroxine binding to albumin, and only mammals possess thyroxine-binding globulin.

What then is the function of the thyroid hormone-binding proteins? By restricting the level of free hormone in the circulation they prevent its loss by way of the liver and kidneys. They regulate the rate of delivery of free hormone to its intracellular sites of action and degradation, buffering the effects of alterations in thyroid secretion or tissue degradation of hormone. It might also be asked what is the need for more than one thyroid hormone-binding protein? TBG appears to act as a stable, relatively inert, reservoir of hormone while TBPA provides a labile, rapidly available supply of hormone in stressful situations. In any severe acute illness there is a rapid decrease in thyroxine bound to TBPA, which has been shown to result from a decreased blood level of the protein. Decreased synthesis of the protein or increased degradation could account for the reduced blood levels. Recent evidence suggests that impaired synthesis of the protein is responsible, and it seems possible that this mechanism provides the rapid source of thyroxine necessary for the body's defence against illness. The lower intensity of binding of triiodothyronine explains its rapidity of action and peripheral turnover. In birds, which lack TBG, the speed of action of thyroxine and triiodothyronine is the same.

Abnormal binding capacities of TBG and TBPA are caused by many diseases and drugs as well as genetic defects. These conditions are summarised in Table 5.1. In general, alterations of thyroid hormone-binding protein capacities

TABLE 5.2 *Clinical and Biochemical Findings in Patients with Familial Alterations of TBG*

Condition	Thyroid status	Serum T4	Residual binding capacity	Free T4 index	Daily degradation T4	Fractional turnover rate T4	Half-life T4	Distribution space T4
TBG deficiency	Eu	Low	'Hyperthyroid value'	Normal	Normal	High	Short	High
TBG increase	Eu	High	'Hypothyroid value'	Normal	Normal	Low	Long	Low

do not affect the thyroid status of the individual since a normal free thyroxine level is maintained by the feedback mechanism.

Table 5.2 shows the results of thyroid function tests and thyroxine kinetic studies in patients with TBG deficiency and in those with increased TBG. Both conditions are familial with X-linked inheritance. Three family types may be recognised in affected males: TBG deficiency, low TBG capacity and high TBG capacity. Only females are heterozygous, having values intermediate between affected males and normals, overlap in heterozygotes being commonest in families with low TBG. Oestrogens do not increase TBG in patients with TBG deficiency although heterozygotes do respond with an increase in TBG capacity. This group of patients is euthyroid with a normal level of free thyroxine (FT4) and normal daily degradation of T4, achieved by an altered turnover rate compensating for the wide variation in the extrathyroidal T4 pool. Refetoff *et al.*, (1972) have suggested that all TBG abnormalities in man described so far are X-chromosome-linked and manifested by quantitative variations in the serum concentration of an apparently structurally unaltered TBG. Mutations at a single locus controlling TBG synthesis could then explain the entire spectrum of genetic TBG abnormalities in man.

METABOLISM OF THYROID HORMONES

About 10 per cent of the thyroxine secreted each day is excreted in the bile, largely as free thyroxine but also conjugated as the glucuronide. Hormone not excreted in this way is deiodinated in the periphery, the iodide released being recycled by the thyroid or excreted in the urine. Although the concentration of T4 in the tissues is lower than the free level in serum, the reverse is true for T3 suggesting either differential trapping or conversion of T4 to T3 at tissue level. The major sites of T4 metabolism are the liver and muscle where inactivation occurs by deiodination, oxidative deamination and conjugation. In the liver the main site of metabolism is the smooth endoplasmic reticulum. Some current estimates of kinetic parameters for thyroxine and triiodothyronine are shown in Table 5.3.

There is good evidence for the peripheral conversion of T4 to T3 although the sites of this process, its extent, and the factors which control it, are poorly understood. Some studies suggest that about one-third of the T4 metabolised each day is deiodinated to T3. Assuming an average T4 degradation of 79 μg per day, about 22 μg of T3 would be produced daily from T4. If about 33 μg of T3 are degraded each day, then only about 11 μg would be secreted directly

TABLE 5.3 *Current Estimates of Kinetic Parameters for T4 and T3* (Larsen, 1972)

	Serum concentration (μg/litre)	Distribution volume (litres)	Turnover rate (day-1)	Total extrathyroidal hormone (μg)	Metabolic clearance (μg day-1)	Free hormone %	Free hormone ng/100 ml
T4	84·2	9·4	0·100	790	79	0·024	2·0
T3	1·20	37·3	0·726	45	33	0·36	0·43

from the thyroid. The extent of T3 secretion and peripheral conversion from T4 in thyroid and other diseases is not clear. It remains possible that T3 is the metabolically active thyroid hormone and that T4 is merely an inactive precursor.

BIOLOGICAL ACTIONS OF THYROID HORMONES

The best known action of thyroid hormones is their ability to stimulate oxygen consumption, usually measured as an increase in basal metabolic rate (BMR). This emphasis is probably derived from the fact that measurement of the BMR was the first test of thyroid function available to physicians. Thyroid hormones are essential for normal growth and development, both overall body growth and maturation of specific tissues being affected. The dwarfism associated with lack of thyroid function in cretins is a good example of the effect of thyroxine deficiency on body growth. Induction and acceleration of metamorphosis in the frog is one of the more dramatic actions of thyroid hormone. Removal of the thyroid gland from a tadpole prevents it developing into a frog, but at any time metamorphosis can be produced by treatment with thyroid hormone.

Yet these gross effects on growth and development are the reflections of alterations in metabolism of carbohydrates, proteins, and fats. Indeed, a vast literature has accumulated relating qualitative and quantitative changes in almost every body constituent to thyroid hormone levels. Unfortunately, many experiments were carried out with very large doses of thyroid hormone and these probably bear little relation to normal physiology since it is well known that physiological and pharmacological levels of the hormones can have opposite effects on biochemical processes. In view of the multiple actions of thyroid hormones, recent work has been directed, so far without success, to finding a primary effect that would explain all the other actions.

Thyroid hormones alter the number and structure of the mitochondria and reduce the efficiency of oxidative phosphorylation. They cause increased transcription of messenger RNA, probably via cyclic AMP. As a result there is an increase in protein synthesis in mitochondria and microsomes which allows the increase in cell respiration. Many sites in the cell respond to thyroid hormones in responsive tissue—the nucleus, endoplasmic reticulum and mitochondria. In addition many other metabolic processes are accelerated, e.g. protein breakdown in collagen, carbohydrate and lipid turnover, and calcium mobilisation from bone. A number of the actions of thyroid hormones are compatible with increased sensitivity of β-receptors to catecholamines, e.g. the tachycardia of hyperthyroidism. These effects can be suppressed by β-adrenergic blocking agents. There does not appear to be an increased production of catecholamines in hyperthyroidism.

LABORATORY DIAGNOSIS OF THYROID DISEASE

The laboratory tests used in the diagnosis of thyroid disease can be divided into two groups:

A. Those measuring the level of thyroid function;
B. Those indicating the cause of thyroid dysfunction.

Practical details of the tests will be found in Appendix C. Normal values are shown in Table 5.4.

Thyroid iodide clearance and estimations of absolute iodide uptake are usually reserved for patients presenting diagnostic difficulties. While the PBI is a routine test in most laboratories it is liable to many errors, particularly that of iodide contamination, and greater use is being made of resin uptake or other similar tests that are independent of iodide administration. The $PB^{131}I$ requires a larger tracer dose of radioiodine and is raised in hyperthyroidism and disorders associated with a low intrathyroidal iodine pool.

TABLE 5.4 *Normal Values for Thyroid Function Tests*
(Authors' Laboratories)

Test	Mean and Normal range	
1. Thyroid iodide trap tests:		
Radioiodine uptake (% dose)		
At 6 hours	<45	
At 24 hours	>20	
Radioiodine clearance (ml/min) between one and two and a half hours	23	10–45
Absolute iodine uptake (μg/hr)	2·2	0·5–6·0
2. Thyroid hormone release tests:		
PBI (μg/100 ml serum)	5·4	4·0–8·2
$PB^{131}I$ (% dose/l serum, 48 hr)		<0·3
Residual binding capacity (Thyopac-3)	1·06	0·95–1·17
Free T4 index (calculated from above)	6·17	3·7–8·6
T3 (ng/ml serum)	1·26	0·79–1·73
T4 (μg/100 ml serum)	9·1	5·5–13·5
Urinary T4 (μg/24 hr)	7·8	3·8–11·8
Urinary T3 (μg/24 hr)	2·9	1·9–3·9

A. TESTS MEASURING THE LEVEL OF THYROID FUNCTION

1. Thyroid iodide trap tests;
2. Thyroid hormone release tests;
3. Peripheral tissue response tests.

1. THYROID IODIDE TRAP TESTS

The thyroid uptake of radioiodide is the most widely used test of thyroid function. In most laboratories the isotope ^{131}I is used because this is a powerful γ-emitter and its half-life of eight days makes it convenient for clinical use. The dose of radiation given in the tracer dose may be reduced by using the isotope ^{132}I (half-life 2·3 hours) or Technetium-99^{m} (^{99m}Tc, half-life 6 hours) but because of the short half-lives of these isotopes they must be administered intravenously and only early uptake measurements are possible. When radioiodine tests are deemed necessary in patients in whom the radiation must be kept to an absolute minimum, e.g. infants or pregnant women, ^{132}I or ^{99m}Tc should be used.

Another way of assessing the trapping of iodide by the thyroid is to measure the thyroid clearance rate of iodide (*see* Appendix), which is the quantity of radioiodine taken up by the thyroid per unit time divided by the mean plasma activity over the time considered. The thyroid iodide clearance is a better index of iodide trapping than the iodide uptake, to which it has a complicated non-linear relationship. The thyroid and kidney compete for the iodide in the plasma, and the higher the renal clearance the lower is the thyroid clearance; thus, later thyroid clearance and uptake measurements will be more affected by renal clearance.

The amount of a dose of radioiodine taken up will also depend on the level of plasma inorganic iodide (PII), which, in turn, depends on the extrathyroidal iodide pool. The PII determines the dilution of the radioisotope since for practical purposes the tracer dose contains a negligible amount of iodine. The higher the level of PII the smaller the amount of radioiodide that will be taken up by the thyroid and vice versa. When carrying out the thyroid radioiodine uptake test it is assumed that the PII is not unduly high or low, but it should be noted that alterations in the PII can be produced by the dietary intake of iodine and by many drugs, X-ray media, shampoos, hand creams, etc. that contain iodine (*see* Appendix).

Early thyroid uptake measurements, up to six hours after administration of the dose, are preferable for the diagnosis of hyperthyroidism, later measurements at twenty-four hours are more reliable in the diagnosis of hypothyroidism. Late measurements of radioiodide uptake in hyperthyroidism may miss the early peak because of rapid discharge of labelled thyroid hormone from the gland. The values for uptake measurements will vary in different parts of the world, depending on the iodine intake and, to a lesser extent, on instrumentation. In Newcastle upon Tyne, using a six-hour radioiodine uptake the lower 95 per cent confidence limit for thyrotoxic patients is 55 per cent.

^{99m}Tc is trapped like iodide by the thyroid but there is no significant organic binding. Twenty minutes after intravenous injection there is a good correlation between the thyroid uptakes of radioiodine and of ^{99m}Tc and both isotopes give a good index of thyroid iodide trapping when used in this way. Because of its short half-life, ready availability and radiation characteristics ^{99m}Tc is also of value in thyroid scanning. Its uptake by the thyroid can be measured by scanning techniques or by a standard scintillation counter (Van't Hoff *et al.*, 1972). This provides a rapid, simple method for the diagnosis of hyperthyroidism giving a much lower radiation dose to the thyroid than radioiodine and allowing accurate correction for extrathyroidal neck activity. Tests can be repeated at short intervals and are very reproducible. The twenty minute uptake of intravenously administered ^{99m}Tc is valuable in the assessment of thyroid function in patients receiving antithyroid drugs, in children and when necessary during pregnancy and to determine thyroid suppression by T3.

In patients in whom measurements of thyroid radioiodine uptake and thyroid clearance give equivocal results it is sometimes necessary to determine the absolute uptake of iodide (AIU) by the thyroid.

2. THYROID HORMONE RELEASE TESTS

The rate of release of thyroid hormone from the gland can be measured by administering a dose of radioiodine, blocking further utilisation of iodine by an antithyroid drug, and then counting the radioactivity over the gland each day. This test is not in routine use because it is too laborious and involves administration of drugs.

Serum Protein-Bound Iodine

The serum protein-bound iodine (PBI) is one of the most useful tests of thyroid function. PBI measurements are more precise and less expensive than most direct measurements of serum thyroxine available at present particularly as the test is readily automated. The test depends on the fact that thyroxine, and to a lesser extent triiodothyronine, are loosely bound to protein and are precipitated along with the plasma proteins. The PBI estimation may be invalidated by the intake of large amounts of iodine unless the serum is routinely passed through a column to remove inorganic iodine. Some X-ray contrast media contain iodine in a form that is bound to protein, and the effects of a cholecystogram may last for more than a year. Drugs such as salicylates and the hydantoin group (phenytoin) compete with thyroxine for binding sites on thyroxine-binding proteins and cause a lowering of the PBI. The level of thyroxine-binding protein is raised by oestrogens, e.g. in the contraceptive pill or during pregnancy, and lowered by androgens or by renal loss in the nephrotic syndrome. Such alterations in the level of TBG affect the PBI without altering the level of thyroid function, which depends on the concentration of free thyroid hormone. If care is taken to elicit a full drug history the PBI is still a useful test of thyroid function.

Serum Thyroxine

Serum thyroxine can be measured by saturation analysis techniques using the thyroxine-binding protein contained in pooled human serum as the specific binding agent (Ekins *et al.*, 1969) or by chemical methods after separation by column chromatography (e.g. Bio-Rad T4 column test). A variety of kits is available for estimation of serum T4, e.g. Thyopac-4 (Amersham); they are simple to use but rather more expensive than the PBI and usually less precise. Serum T4 estimations are subject to similar errors as the PBI when there are alterations in the levels of TBG, but are not affected by iodine contamination. In hyperthyroid patients PBI values are often found to be higher than those of T4 owing to the presence of other iodinated proteins in the circulation.

Serum Triiodothyronine

Measurements of serum T3 are difficult because of the very low concentration of this hormone in the circulation and also as a result of the relatively high concentration of T4. Radioimmunoassays for T3 have been made possible by the production of antisera which are highly specific for T3. Competition between the antibodies and TBG for T3 during the assay have been overcome by the use of agents such as salicylates, diphenylhydantoin, or thyroxine which block the binding of T3 to serum proteins. Extraction of T3 from serum has also been used to deal with the problem of competition between TBG and antibodies to T3. Table 5.5 shows a comparison of T3 and T4 concentrations in various clinical conditions.

In normal subjects, iodine depletion is a major cause of an increased serum T3/T4 ratio, and this can be reversed by iodide repletion. Increased T3/T4 ratios in iodine deficiency may not be associated with a measurable rise of TSH, although this may be due to lack of assay sensitivity. Alternatively iodine deficiency might cause an increase in T3 synthesis by some intrinsic thyroid mechanism. In general there is a good correlation between the serum concentrations of T3 and T4, a notable exception being the syndrome of T3 toxicosis (Evered and Hesch, 1973). Raised total serum T3 levels in patients with TBG elevation and lowered levels in those with reduction of TBG confirm the role of TBG in the transport of T3. Similarly salicylates reduce both T3 and T4 levels in the serum by competition for binding sites on TBG. During pregnancy T3 levels increase but cord serum and neonatal urine show a markedly reduced T3 concentration. It is possible that the low T3 level in the baby at birth is one factor in triggering the marked rise in serum TSH which occurs shortly after birth.

In hypothyroidism T3 values are lowered but there is some overlap with the normal range. Some patients with mild hypothyroidism have T3 levels in the normal range, so a normal T3 level cannot be used to exclude hypothyroidism. However a lowered T3 level is strong evidence for the presence of significant thyroid failure.

In hyperthyroidism T3 values are raised and there is remarkably little overlap with the normal range. As described later occasional patients with hyperthyroidism have raised T3 levels in the presence of a normal serum T4. A raised serum

T3 level can also be seen in some apparently euthyroid patients with thyroid nodules or ophthalmic Graves' disease. Serum T3 measurements provide a sensitive index of acute changes in thyroid hormone secretion, for example in response to antithyroid therapy.

TABLE 5.5 *Comparison of T3 and T4 Concentrations in Various Clinical Conditions* (Larsen, 1972) (by permission of the author and the Editors of *Metabolism*)

Clinical status	No.	T3* ng/ml	T4* μg/100 ml	T4/T3 (by weight)
Euthyroid				
Male, normal TBG	18	1·18 ± 0·27	7·6 ± 1·5	67 ± 4
Female, normal TBG	24	1·06 ± 0·20	7·6 ± 1·5	73 ± 3
Idiopathic raised TBG	7	1·80 ± 0·24	15·7 ± 4·7	88 ± 9
Idiopathic lowered TBG	3	0·63 ± 0·14	3·6 ± 0·2	58 ± 6
Pregnant (at delivery)	8	1·64 ± 0·47	14·2 ± 3·2	91 ± 11
Cord serum	8	0·53 ± 0·15	13·3 ± 3·7	260 ± 32
Receiving thyroxine	9	1·54 ± 0·47	13·2 ± 3·6	89 ± 7
Hyperthyroid	39	5·16 ± 3·89	23·2 ± 8·9	53 ± 3
Hypothyroid (primary)	34	0·42 ± 0·29	2·4 ± 1·0	88 ± 14

* S.D.

Residual Binding Capacity (*Resin uptake or thyroid hormone binding tests*)

This test is based on measurements of the unoccupied binding sites on thyroid hormone binding proteins (TBP). The more thyroxine present the more saturated will be the TBP and the fewer binding sites will be unoccupied. Conversely when little thyroxine is present more unoccupied sites will be available. When labelled T3 or T4 is added to serum, the amount taken up by the TBP will depend on the unoccupied binding sites. Addition of some material which adsorbs thyroid hormone, e.g. a resin or sephadex will result in uptake of the unbound thyroid hormone by the material which can then be counted to give the resin uptake. In certain kits, e.g. 'Thyopac-3' (Amersham) the supernatant is counted rather than the resin and the results are the reciprocal of the resin uptake: low values are observed in hyperthyroidism and high values in hypothyroidism. The test is influenced both by the amount of thyroid hormone and the total amount of TBP. An increase in TBP as a result of pregnancy or oestrogen therapy produces hypothyroid values in the residual binding capacity test but the PBI and total T4 levels will be raised. A decrease in TBP as seen in the nephrotic syndrome or as a result of androgen therapy produces results in the hyperthyroid range but in these conditions the PBI and total T4 levels will be low. The residual binding capacity test depends on the uptake of labelled T3 and is sometimes termed the T3 uptake test; this terminology is best avoided since it leads to the residual binding capacity test being confused with the direct estimation of serum T3.

Free Thyroxine

The free thyroxine concentration can be measured directly by equilibrium dialysis methods but these are too cumbersome for routine use. The product of the serum PBI or T4 and the residual binding capacity (measured by resin uptake) gives a value that is independent of TBP. This product is termed the free thyroxine index and shows a remarkably close correlation with the free thyroxine concentration obtained by equilibrium dialysis or gel filtration. Normal values are obtained for the free thyroxine index in the presence of altered levels of TBP and it is widely used as the most reliable simple test of thyroid function.

Effective Thyroxine Ratio

The effective thyroxine ratio (ETR) is a new *in vitro* method which combines serum thyroxine and residual binding capacity measurements in one kit. The method is rapid and relatively simple, providing similar information to the free thyroxine index.

Urinary Thyroxine and Triiodothyronine

Measurements of urinary T4 and T3 might be expected to reflect the circulating content of the free non-protein bound hormones just as the urinary 'free cortisol' excretion is related to unbound plasma cortisol levels. Total urinary T4 is measured by competitive protein-binding and T3 by radioimmunoassay after extraction with ethyl acetate; T4 excretion ranges from 3·8 to 11·8 μg per 24 hours (mean value of 7·8 μg) and T3 excretion from 1·9 to 3·9 μg per 24 hours (mean value 2·9 μg) in euthyroid subjects and normal values are observed during pregnancy, oestrogen administration and in hypoproteinaemic states. Raised values were found in hyperthyroidism and low values in hypothyroidism (Chan and Landon, 1972, Chan *et al.*, 1972). Without extraction, Burke *et al.* (1972) found lower values of unconjugated free T4, mean 2·0 μg per day (range 0·54–3·90) in normal subjects. Similarly they observed lower values for immunoassayable T3—0·8 μg per day (range 0·33–1·91) in normal subjects. Further investigation is required to assess the value of urinary measurements in clinical practice.

3. PERIPHERAL TISSUE RESPONSE TESTS

The final test to indicate whether the tissues have been exposed to increased or decreased levels of thyroid hormone is the therapeutic trial of an antithyroid agent or of thyroid hormone. In hyperthyroidism it is usually possible to reach a firm diagnosis by careful clinical assessment and the tests previously mentioned, and a therapeutic trial is rarely required to confirm the diagnosis. In some cases of hypothyroidism all routine tests of thyroid function are normal yet the patient improves with replacement therapy. This is to be expected in a graded phenomenon like hypothyroidism where there is a continuous range from slightly diminished thyroid function to complete thyroid deficiency.

Tests based on the peripheral action of thyroid hormone are sometimes useful when routine thyroidal radioiodine and PBI estimations are interfered with by drugs, by various diseases, or by pregnancy. They also give an indication of the severity of the disease. Many of the tests described are non-specific and have been poorly validated in clinical practice. The tests that will be considered are tyrosine tolerance, serum creatine phosphokinase, tendon reflex duration, serum cholesterol, basal metabolic rate, the electrocardiogram, the red cell sodium, the radioimmunoassay of thyroid-stimulating hormone and the thyrotrophin-releasing hormone test.

(a) Tyrosine Tolerance

Fasting plasma tyrosine is raised in hyperthyroidism and lowered in hypothyroidism. After a tyrosine load, plasma levels rise higher than normal in hyperthyroidism and lower in hypothyroidism.

However estimation of fasting plasma tyrosine gives similar results to a tyrosine tolerance test but about one-third of hyperthyroid patients have plasma tyrosine levels within the normal range. The rest is therefore not a useful addition to the routine diagnosis of hyperthyroidism and has no value in the diagnosis of hypothyroidism.

(b) Serum Creatine Phosphokinase

Serum enzyme levels have been studied in hypo- and hyperthyroid patients. An inverse relationship between serum creatine phosphokinase and thyroid activity has been reported. Such a relationship has not been reported for other serum enzymes. The cause of the altered serum enzyme levels in thyroid disease is not known, but it may, in part, represent release of the enzyme from muscle. This estimation is of little value in the diagnosis of hyperthyroidism except to draw attention to concurrent muscle disease if the level is high. Even in hypothyroidism, where raised levels are also found, some 33 per cent of results are within the upper 95 per cent confidence limits. Where routine thyroid function tests are not possible the enzyme estimation may occasionally be useful. The level is also raised in myocardial infarction, polymyositis, muscular dystrophies, muscle trauma, or major surgery.

(c) Tendon Reflex Duration

Measurement of the duration of the Achilles tendon reflex can be used as an index of thyroid function. The test is of little value in the diagnosis of hyperthyroidism and many hypothyroid patients have results within the normal range. It is the patients with obvious hypothyroidism who tend to have the longest reflexes, and in the mildly hypothyroid patient in whom there is diagnostic difficulty the tendon reflexes are either in the upper normal range or only slightly prolonged. This limits the diagnostic value of the test. Measurement of the tendon reflex duration can be helpful in assessing the effectiveness of treatment, and with adequate therapy the tendon reflex time falls within the normal range.

Prolongation of tendon reflexes has also been reported in obesity, arteriosclerosis, sarcoidosis, neurosyphilis, myasthenia gravis, hypokalaemia, gross oedema, diabetes mellitus, and Parkinson's disease. Some of the patients with these conditions who were reported to have prolonged reflexes may well have been mildly hypothyroid, hence further critical observations are required. Shortening of tendon reflexes has been reported in dystrophia myotonica and in response to large doses of salicylates, dexamphetamine, steroids and oestrogens.

(d) Serum Cholesterol

The serum cholesterol is lowered in hyperthyroidism and raised in hypothyroidism. The overlap with normal is so wide that the test has little diagnostic value in hyperthyroidism. Even in hypothyroidism, where Wayne (1960) found 81 per cent of his patients had values over 300 mg/100 ml, the estimation is not very helpful, since raised values are found in many other conditions and in some apparently normal persons. In many patients with pituitary hypothyroidism normal serum cholesterol values are found.

(e) Basal Metabolic Rate (BMR)

Estimation of the BMR is still a useful test of thyrotoxicosis or hypothyroidism though because of its inaccuracies and the time taken to carry out the test it is rarely used. Oxygen consumption is measured in the resting patient after an overnight fast. It is assumed that under these conditions the R.Q. is 0·85 and that the consumption of one litre of O_2 corresponds to the liberation of 4·83 calories. Results are expressed as a percentage difference between the estimated result and a standard value for persons of the same age, sex, and surface area, using the Robertson and Reid standards. To eliminate anxiety, sedation is desirable and close duplicate estimations must be obtained on consecutive days. A correction factor for obesity can be applied; depot fat has a low rate of O_2 consumption so that obesity causes an increase in surface area without a proportional increase in O_2 consumption. Oedema and ascites cause a similar error. Despite these precautions the BMR of some 10 per cent of thyrotoxic patients falls within the normal range, though there is a fall in their BMR after therapy. The BMR is lowered in anorexia nervosa, malnutrition, hypoadrenalism and hypothermia, and raised in heart failure, pyrexia, phaeochromocytoma, and leukaemia.

With meticulous supervision the BMR remains a useful test for the diagnosis of hypothyroidism and hyperthyroidism.

(*f*) *Electrocardiogram*

The ECG is abnormal in most severe cases of hypothyroidism but in mild cases no abnormality may be detected. The changes consist of bradycardia, flattening or inversion of T waves, and decreased amplitude of the R wave. Some of these features may occasionally be due to a pericardial effusion, which can occur in myxoedema. The findings are often non-specific but their significance becomes apparent with their improvement after thyroid hormone medication, and in children this can be used as a rapid diagnostic test. Sandler (1959), in a carefully controlled study, did not find any specific abnormalities in hyperthyroidism apart from left ventricular hypertrophy and increased QRS duration.

(*g*) *Red Cell Sodium*

In hyperthyroidism the rate of exchange of sodium inside the red cell with the potassium outside is reduced, hence the red cell sodium is increased. Goolden *et al.* (1971) have shown that 90 per cent of hyperthyroid patients have results above the normal range. Although hypothyroid patients have low red cell sodium levels discrimination from normal is poor. The test is somewhat inconvenient for routine use since the cells must be separated from the plasma without delay.

(*h*) *Thyroid-Stimulating Hormone Immunoassay*

Specific radioimmunoassays for TSH are now widely available (Hall, 1972). Current assays lack sensitivity and are in general unable to separate low levels from the normal range. Normal TSH levels are probably <1 μU per ml of MRC Standard A which is below the sensitivity of most assays. Most sensitive immunoassays record mean values for TSH of 1–2 μU per ml with an upper limit of normal of about 4 μU per ml. There are no significant differences in TSH levels in men, women or children. In the elderly TSH levels are rather higher and in the neonatal period there is a transient sharp rise of TSH.

Hypothyroidism. The major clinical value of TSH measurements lies in the diagnosis of hypothyroidism due to primary thyroid disease (*see* p. 102). A raised TSH level does not necessarily imply clinical hypothyroidism but it does indicate patients at risk for symptomatic hypothyroidism. Patients with non-specific symptoms compatible with hypothyroidism who have a raised TSH level despite normal routine thyroid function tests warrant a careful therapeutic trial with thyroxine. In general the higher the TSH level the more likely is the patient to have symptomatic hypothyroidism. A normal TSH level excludes hypothyroidism on the basis of thyroid disease, hence TSH levels are very useful as a screen for possible thyroid failure, particularly in persons subjected to destructive therapy to the thyroid or with a family or personal history of organ-specific autoimmune disease.

Hyperthyroidism. Only very rarely is hyperthyroidism due to overproduction of TSH from the pituitary. In the majority of subjects with hyperthyroidism TSH levels are low or undetectable, but because of limitations in the sensitivity of current assays these values cannot be readily separated from normal. However, the TSH assay can be used to aid in the diagnosis of hyperthyroidism. Patients with hyperthyroidism fail to show a rise in TSH in response to TRH (vide infra).

Non-toxic goitre. Most patients with non-toxic goitres have normal TSH levels. The finding of a raised TSH level in such a patient implies some degree of thyroid failure and the patient is usually suffering from autoimmune thyroid disease or more rarely is receiving some goitrogen or has a dyshormonogenetic goitre.

(*i*) *Thyrotrophin-Releasing Hormone Test*

TRH can be used as a test of thyroid function (Ormston *et al.*, 1971) and as a test of pituitary-hypothalamic function with regard to TSH (Hall *et al.*, 1972). The response to TRH can be monitored by measuring serum TSH, T4 or T3 levels after intravenous or oral TRH. In the authors' standard TRH test, blood is taken for basal TSH, PBI, T4 and T3 measurements and 200 μg of synthetic TRH is administered rapidly intravenously in 2 ml of solution. Blood is removed at 20 minutes (peak TSH level), 60 minutes (to detect a delayed TSH response) and, if required, at three hours (peak T3 level) and at six hours (peak T4 level). A normal range for TSH response should be established for each sex in each laboratory performing the TSH immunoassay (*see* Fig. 5.3 and Table 5.6). No major side-effects have resulted from TRH but cological doses of corticosteroids and by chronic administration of levodopa; an increased response results from oestrogen treatment in men, from large doses of theophylline and after overtreatment with antithyroid drugs. Before assessing the TRH response in treated patients it is important to withdraw T4 for three weeks and T3 for two weeks.

Hypothyroidism. Patients with hypothyroidism

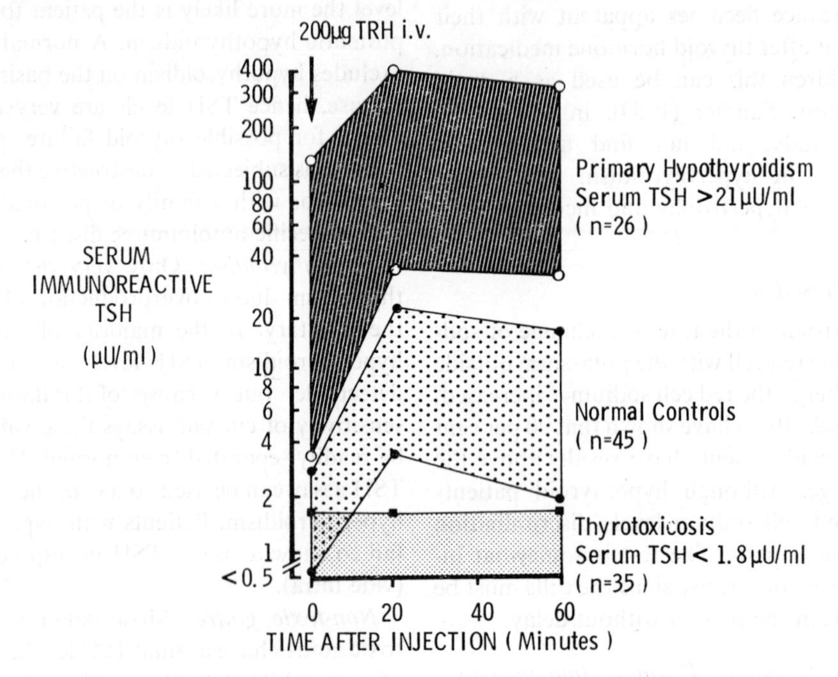

FIGURE 5.3 Serum TSH response to TRH in normal controls and in patients with thyrotoxicosis and primary hypothyroidism (values to right of figure refer to levels 20 min after TRH)

minor side effects, which are trivial and transient, are common. These include nausea, flushing and a sudden desire to pass urine. They are only observed after administration of the rapid intravenous bolus of TRH and are probably due to stimulation of plain muscle of the gastro-intestinal and genito-urinary tracts.

Normal Subjects. Females show a greater response than males because of the effect of circulating oestrogens. Age does not appear to have any major effect on the response. A variety of drugs alter the TSH response to TRH—reduction is caused by T4 and T3, by pharma-

have elevated basal levels of TSH and an exaggerated and prolonged rise of TSH in response to TRH but no change in circulating thyroid hormone levels. Where the basal TSH level is borderline or only minimally elevated the enhanced TRH response can provide evidence for some degree of thyroid failure. The TRH test is also useful in separating pituitary from thyroid causes of hypothyroidism. A patient with hypothyroidism due to disease of the pituitary fails to respond to TRH whereas a patient with hypothyroidism resulting from hypothalamic disease may show a normal response.

Hyperthyroidism. Because of the suppressive action of the increased circulating levels of thyroid hormones on the anterior pituitary, there is suppression of the TSH response to TRH. This is a dose-dependent phenomenon and some patients with mild hyperthyroidism do show a response (usually blunted) to very large intravenous or oral doses of TRH. However in the authors' experience no patient with proven hyperthyroidism has yet responded to a small (200 μg) dose of intravenous TRH. The TRH test is of particular value in separating patients with mild hyperthyroidism from those who are euthyroid—a normal response to TRH excluding hyperthyroidism. However, the converse is not true, not all of those who fail to respond to TRH are hyperthyroid. Other causes of an absent or impaired TSH response to TRH include some patients with:

- Ophthalmic Graves' disease
- Graves' disease, euthyroid after therapy
- Autonomous thyroid adenoma
- Multinodular goitre
- Patients receiving thyroxine or triiodothyronine
- Patients with Cushing's syndrome (spontaneous or iatrogenic)
- Hypopituitarism
- Patients receiving levodopa

The TRH test can now replace the T3 suppression test since it is safer, quicker and does not require the administration of a radioisotope. Patients who fail to suppress with T3 fail to respond to TRH. Like the T3 suppression test, the TRH test is helpful in the diagnosis of unilateral exophthalmos, the majority of patients with ophthalmic Graves' disease show some abnormality of response to TRH.

TABLE 5.6 *TSH Response to 200 μg TRH given Intravenously* (Ormston *et al.*, 1971)

		TSH μU per ml Men	TSH μU per ml Women	Significance of difference
Basal	Mean	1·6	1·4	Not
	Range	<0·5–2·8	<0·5–2·7	significant
20 minute	Mean	9·5	13·5	p<0·001
	Range	3·5–15·6	6·5–20·5	
60 minute	Mean	6·8	9·8	p<0·001
	Range	2·0–11·5	4·0–15·6	

B. TESTS INDICATING THE CAUSE OF THYROID DYSFUNCTION

1. Triiodothyronine suppression test;
2. TSH stimulation test;
3. Perchlorate discharge test;
4. Plasma proteins, flocculations and ESR;
5. Thyroid antibody tests;
6. Thyroid biopsy.

1. TRIIODOTHYRONINE SUPPRESSION TEST (*see* Appendix)

Triiodothyronine suppresses pituitary TSH output and, therefore, reduces the thyroid radioiodine uptake in normal patients. In Graves' disease, hyperthyroidism is due to stimulating factors other than TSH which are unaffected by triiodothyronine. Triiodothyronine does not lower the radioiodine uptake in hyperthyroid patients with Graves' disease, in some cases of Graves' disease when hyperthyroidism has remitted or if ophthalmic Graves' disease is present, in autonomous thyroid adenomas and in some multinodular goitres. Suppression of radioiodine uptake by triiodothyronine is very strong evidence against the presence of hyperthyroidism though failure to suppress may indicate past or present hyperthyroidism or the other conditions listed above. The test is useful in distinguishing the high radioiodine uptake of iodine deficiency from that of hyperthyroidism. Care must be taken when carrying out this test in elderly patients since if they are toxic and therefore do not suppress their thyroid hormone output, the administered T3 may precipitate atrial fibrillation, angina or heart failure.

2. TSH STIMULATION TEST (*see* Appendix)

Administration of TSH increases thyroid radioiodine uptake in normal persons and in those with hypothyroidism secondary to pituitary disease. Patients referred for assessment of thyroid function who are on treatment with thyroid hormone can be tested in this way without withdrawal of therapy. For many years the TSH stimulation test has been regarded as the absolute criterion for establishing the presence of impaired thyroid reserve. However critical evaluation of the standard TSH stimulation test has demonstrated a normal response in about 50 per cent of patients with mild hypothyroidism. It seems that a significant increase in thyroidal radioiodine uptake can be produced by the very large and unphysiological dose of TSH used even in the face of mild thyroid failure.

3. PERCHLORATE DISCHARGE TEST (*see* Appendix)

This test is used in the diagnosis of the commonest variety of dyshormonogenesis—the organification defect. A similar defect is often present in Hashimoto's disease and after treatment with certain types of goitrogens including some antithyroid drugs. After administration of radioiodine, perchlorate is given and the activity over the gland followed. Perchlorate blocks further trapping of iodide, and unbound radioiodide and iodide diffuse out of the gland if the organification process is defective. A fall in radioactivity over the gland can then be detected.

4. PLASMA PROTEINS, FLOCCULATION TESTS, AND ESR

Abnormalities of serum proteins, flocculation tests, and the ESR are found in Hashimoto's disease, myxoedema, and some cases of Graves' disease. The raised IgG and abnormal flocculation tests may be helpful in the diagnosis of autoimmune thyroiditis when full antibody studies are not available. The ESR is rarely raised in 'simple' non-toxic goitre but is elevated in many patients with myxoedema and Hashimoto's disease. Surprisingly high values, occasionally up to 90 mm/hour may be seen. Hypothyroidism is also a cause of raised CSF protein, and thyroid antibodies can be detected in the spinal fluid. While neither the raised CSF protein nor the elevated ESR are very helpful in diagnosis, an awareness of these findings sometimes prevents a patient being subjected to unnecessary and unpleasant investigations.

5. THYROID ANTIBODY TESTS

Many methods have been devised for detecting thyroid antibodies but only those in routine clinical practice will be considered. Antibodies to thyroglobulin can be detected by a precipitin test, by a latex fixation test, and by the tanned red cell (TRC) test with increasing order of sensitivity. Antibodies to a microsomal component of the thyroid cell can be detected by a complement-fixation test (CFT). Antibodies to thyroglobulin, the microsomal component, and a second colloid antigen CA2 can all be detected by immunofluorescence procedures, which will not be dealt with here.

Thyroglobulin Antibody Tests. A line of precipitation develops in the agar between an extract of thyroid gland containing thyroglobulin and the serum of some patients with Hashimoto's disease containing high levels of antibodies. The Ouchterlony plate technique or a micro variation can be used to demonstrate this reaction which usually takes a few days to develop. A positive test is indicative of extensive autoimmune thyroiditis. The latex fixation test is a rapid slide test for antibody to thyroglobulin. A suspension of polystyrene latex particles coated with thyroglobulin is aggregated by antibody to thyroglobulin. A rapid result can be obtained but the test is less sensitive than the TRC test.

The TRC test is similar in principle to the latex test. Red cells treated with tannic acid pick up thyroglobulin and can then be agglutinated by antibody to thyroglobulin. A commercial preparation from Burroughs Wellcome is now available. The test is very sensitive and positive results can be obtained with serum dilutions of several millions in some cases.

Microsomal Antibody Tests. Antibodies to thyroid microsomes can be detected by complement fixation tests, details of which vary in different laboratories. Non-organ specific complement fixing antibodies are found in various diseases, and the thyroid specificity of a positive result should always be confirmed by obtaining a negative result with an extract of another organ, usually liver.

Diagnostic Importance of Thyroid Antibody Tests

Thyroid antibody tests can aid in diagnosis and prognosis in three main clinical situations: non-toxic goitre, suspected hypothyroidism, and suspected hyperthyroidism.

(*a*) *Non-toxic Goitre.* Thyroid antibody tests are helpful in the diagnosis of non-toxic goitre since the titre of antibodies correlates approximately with the extent of the lymphocytic thyroiditis. A positive precipitin test, a positive TRC test at 1/2000 serum dilution or more or a positive CF test at 1/32 or more (in the authors' laboratories) are indicative of the extensive autoimmune thyroiditis of Hashimoto's disease. Only three per cent of patients with Hashimoto's disease have negative TRC and CF tests. Strongly positive antibody tests are usually found in the subacute variety of autoimmune thyroiditis which mimics De Quervain's thyroiditis because of the pain and tenderness in the gland. Table 5.7 shows the incidence of thyroid antibodies in some thyroid diseases.

TABLE 5.7 *Thyroid Antibodies in Various Thyroid Diseases*

	Positive antibody tests		
	Precipitin	CFT	TRC
Autoimmune thyroiditis (Hashimoto's disease)	70%	92%	90%
Myxoedema	18%	57%	65%
Graves' disease	2%	40%	57%
'Simple goitre'	0%	8%	27%
Thyroid cancer	4%	10%	28%

These figures are the averages from a number of large series.

(*b*) *Suspected Hypothyroidism.* Positive thyroid antibodies in a patient with suspected hypothyroidism is evidence of an autoimmune thyroiditis, the 'severity' of which depends partly on the titre of antibodies. Patients with TRC tests positive in a titre greater than 1/1,000 can be considered to be at risk for the development of hypothyroidism or other diseases of the organ-specific autoimmune group. Screening of families in which one member is affected by autoimmune thyroid disease allows other affected members who are at risk for goitre or hypothyroidism to be recognised. In patients with hypothyroidism the finding of thyroid antibodies is evidence against pituitary disease but hypopituitarism and 'primary' hypothyroidism can coexist. Some cases of idiopathic hypopituitarism could have an autoimmune basis though the evidence for this is scanty at present.

(*c*) *Suspected Hyperthyroidism.* Since many patients referred to hospital clinics with suspected hyperthyroidism have, in fact, a psychiatric disorder, thyroid antibody tests are useful in selecting those with thyroid disease. High levels of antibodies correlate with a high incidence of postoperative hypothyroidism and are a relative contra-indication to operative treatment. Some patients with early autoimmune thyroiditis have high thyroidal radioiodine uptakes and a raised PB ^{131}I. Hyperthyroidism may be diagnosed in error, but the high level of antibodies should alert the clinician to the presence of autoimmune thyroiditis, and the euthyroid state can be confirmed by the TRH test or the T3 suppression test.

6. THYROID BIOPSY

The authors consider that needle biopsy of the thyroid is rarely indicated. Thyroid antibody tests are sufficient to indicate the severity of the autoimmune thyroiditis in most cases. When carcinoma is suspected, even in the presence of strongly positive antibody tests, exploration of the neck should be carried out taking open biopsies from any suspicious areas. A drill biopsy of the thyroid sampling such a small fragment of the gland may give misleading results.

NON-TOXIC GOITRE AND HYPOTHYROIDISM

If the thyroid gland fails to secrete enough thyroid hormone for the body's needs the condition of hypothyroidism develops. Before overt hypothyroidism occurs there may be a period when TSH stimulation of the gland is just sufficient to produce adequate amounts of thyroid hormone, but the thyroid reserve capacity is lost. The usual effect of TSH stimulation of the thyroid is to produce a goitre and, apart from neoplasms, most goitres can be considered to result from the action of TSH on a thyroid that has failed to produce sufficient thyroid hormone. Sometimes the increased function and increased cell mass that results from TSH stimulation is enough to correct the hormone deficiency leading to a 'goitre with compensated thyroid function'. On other occasions, especially if there is marked curtailment of thyroid hormone production, compensation is inadequate and goitrous hypothyroidism results. The term non-toxic goitre is used to describe all goitres resulting from interference with thyroid hormone formation. The factors that determine whether or not goitre develops in response to hormone deficiency are poorly understood. From these considerations it is evident that correction of the hormone deficiency will remove the TSH stimulus to the gland, which should then decrease in size. When the goitre is of longstanding and nodular or cystic, however, the situation may be irreversible. Removal of goitres without correction of the hormone deficiency will often be followed by recurrence of the thyroid enlargement.

Non-toxic goitre and/or hypothyroidism may result from the following disease processes:

1. Iodine deficiency;
2. Congenital defects in the enzymes involved in hormone synthesis (dyshormonogenesis);
3. Acquired defects in enzyme action caused by drugs (goitrogens);
4. Autoimmune thyroiditis;
5. Riedel's thyroiditis.

1. IODINE DEFICIENCY

In certain parts of the world, particularly isolated mountainous areas far from the sea, iodine intake is low enough to interfere with thyroid hormone formation. The usual result is a goitre with compensated thyroid function but, less often, hypothyroidism with or without goitre is found. When a high proportion of the population has a goitre the cause is usually iodine deficiency or, less frequently, goitrogens. In most endemic goitre areas the major aetiological factor is iodine deficiency. The evidence for this is summarised below:

(*a*) The soil, water and food iodine content is low;
(*b*) The plasma inorganic iodide is low and the thyroidal radioiodine uptake is high;
(*c*) The urinary excretion of iodide is low;
(*d*) Administration of iodine over a period reduces the incidence of goitre in such a region.

In the United Kingdom iodine intake is variable from area to area and in different individuals. Since most of the iodine in the diet is derived from sea food and milk, especially in the winter, and from iodised salt, the iodine intake will vary greatly with a person's dietary habits. Again, the loss of iodine in the urine or faeces may vary from time to time, e.g. there is an increased renal clearance of iodide during pregnancy. Sensitivity to iodine deficiency may also vary, certain persons responding with a goitre and others compensating adequately without an increase in thyroid size. In Glasgow, some 90 per cent of goitres studied were not due to dyshormonogenesis, drugs or autoimmune thyroiditis. The term 'simple goitre' was used to describe this group. Measurements of the intake of iodine, the plasma inorganic iodide, the radioiodine uptake, and the urinary excretion of iodide all tended to support the view that this group of patients was iodine deficient. Those patients with raised radioiodine uptakes had the clearest evidence of iodine deficiency. In patients with 'simple goitre' in whom tests are normal and there is no good evidence of iodine deficiency, protagonists of the iodine deficiency hypothesis fall back on the unassailable assumption that such patients developed their goitres in response to previous iodine deficiency. Many workers have sought, but few have found, convincing evidence that enzyme deficiencies are responsible for the syndrome of 'simple goitre'. Analysis of the goitres has tended to show increased amounts of iodotyrosines compared with iodothyronines and a high monoiodotyrosine/diiodotyrosine ratio, but these findings are non-specific and can be produced by iodine deficiency or by goitrogens. Patients with endemic goitre may maintain a euthyroid state with raised circulating levels of TSH and T3 but low T4 levels.

2. DYSHORMONOGENESIS

At present, six separate intrathyroidal defects have been demonstrated that interfere with thyroid hormone production. Although it is postulated that these diseases are due to defects in various enzymes, the evidence for this is usually indirect. These types of thyroid defect have a number of features in common. They are inherited, most often as a Mendelian recessive, causing goitre and often hypothyroidism which usually present in childhood. Removal of the goitre is invariably followed by recurrence of thyroid enlargement unless thyroid hormone is given. The thyroid is hyperplastic and, in some instances, this hyperplasia is sufficiently gross to simulate malignancy. These enzyme defects are uncommon and make up only a small proportion of all cases of non-toxic goitre. The types of defect are listed below:

(*a*) Iodide trap defect;
(*b*) Organification group of defects;
(*c*) 'Coupling' defect;
(*d*) Dehalogenase defect;
(*e*) Iodoprotein group of defects;
(*f*) Protease defect.
(*g*) Other defects.

(*a*) *Iodide Trap Defect*. This is the rarest type of dyshormonogenesis. It causes goitre and hypothyroidism because the thyroid is unable to concentrate iodide from the circulation. The defect is also found in the salivary glands and stomach. The thyroid radioiodine uptake is low and the salivary/plasma and gastric juice/plasma ratios of radioiodine approach unity, whereas in normal persons saliva and gastric juice show twenty to forty-fold concentration of iodine compared with plasma. Treatment with iodide in large amounts corrects the intrathyroidal iodine deficiency, the goitre and the hypothyroidism.

(*b*) *Organification Group of Defects*. This is the commonest intrathyroidal enzyme defect. Familial goitre due to defective iodide organification has been grouped into three types which are probably genetically distinct:

1. The most severe defect, associated with goitrous cretinism, apparently due to complete lack of thyroid peroxidase activity.
2. The syndrome of non-toxic goitre and normal hearing in which there is a genetic alteration in the protein structure of the peroxidase which prevents normal binding of the prosthetic group with the apoenzyme present in the gland.
3. Pendred's syndrome of congenital nerve deafness and goitre where the patient is usually euthyroid. Thyroid tissue from these patients shows no deficiency of iodide peroxidase or tyrosine iodinase activity, nor is there any defect in the site where the prosthetic group interacts with the enzyme. There appears to be a separate defect in the iodination mechanism in Pendred's syndrome, perhaps involving the production of hydrogen peroxide.

Tests on these patients reveal a high radioiodine uptake, particularly one to six hours after the tracer dose, with a subsequent fall of radioactivity in the gland. If 600 mg of potassium perchlorate are given by mouth one hour after a tracer dose of radioiodine there is a rapid fall in radioactivity over the gland—further trapping is abolished and the unbound radioiodine diffuses out of the thyroid. Some patients are euthyroid despite a low serum T4 and measurement of the serum T3 has revealed raised levels. This is presumably a compensatory mechanism to intrathyroidal iodine deficiency and also possibly to TSH stimulation. Treatment with thyroid hormone corrects the hypothyroidism and the goitre but does not affect the mental retardation or nerve deafness. It is usually assumed that the mental retardation has resulted from the hypothyroidism *in utero* but, like the nerve deafness, it may be an independent accompanying feature.

(*c*) '*Coupling Defect*'. A group of patients has been described with goitrous hypothyroidism, a high thyroidal radioiodine uptake, and a low ratio of iodothyronines to iodotyrosines in the thyroid. It has been postulated that deficiency of a hypothetical enzyme coupling iodotyrosines to iodothyronines on the thyroglobulin molecule is responsible but the evidence for this is scanty. In all cases where the stable iodine concentration of the thyroid was measured it was found to be remarkably low, and an equally plausible explanation is that only a few of the tyrosine molecules on thyroglobulin are iodinated and, hence, the chance of coupling of two iodotyrosine molecules to form an iodothyronine is much reduced.

(*d*) *Dehalogenase Defect*. This defect has been extensively studied by McGirr and his colleagues in Glasgow in a family of tinkers of Irish extraction. Mental retardation, goitre and hypothyroidism are the presenting features. The thyroid traps iodide rapidly but there is a release of radioactivity from the gland over the first twenty-four hours. There is good evidence that the thyroid and other tissues are deficient in an enzyme that breaks down iodotyrosines to release iodine. This enzyme is essential for the iodine economy of the thyroid, since iodotyrosines are normally released when thyroglobulin is broken down to liberate thyroxine and triiodothyronine. In the absence of the dehalogenase enzyme, iodotyrosines escape from the thyroid into the circulation and are excreted in the urine, the kidney like the thyroid being deficient in the dehalogenase system. This results in a loss of iodine to the body, and the goitre and hypothyroidism are the result of the iodine deficiency. Correction of the iodine deficiency leads to reduction in the goitre, and the normal production of thyroid hormone is restored. It is conceivable that minor degrees of this defect could be masked by a high iodine intake and made manifest by an iodine-deficient diet. This is a good example of the interplay of inherited and environmental factors in the genesis of disease.

(*e*) *Iodoprotein Group of Defects*. In its most severe form this defect causes goitrous hypothyroidism associated with release of an abnormal iodinated albumin from the thyroid. The glands of these patients contain large amounts of iodoalbumin but very little thyroglobulin. While the commonest iodoprotein is one having the characteristics of iodoalbumin, other iodoproteins corresponding to a prealbumin and to globulins have been described. The fundamental nature of these defects is not known. Characteristically, the thyroid radioiodine uptake is high and the radioactivity of the gland remains high for several days. Extraction of plasma with acid butanol twenty-four to forty-eight hours after a large tracer dose of radioiodine (50–500 μCi) fails to remove most of the radioactivity, indicating the presence of a butanol-insoluble iodinated protein, whereas normally at least 90 per cent of the protein bound ^{131}I in plasma at that time interval is in thyroid hormone, which is readily removed by several extractions with acid butanol.

From the authors' experience in the North of England this type of defect has been found to underlie a number of 'simple goitres'. There is often a family history of thyroid disease, and the pattern of inheritance of this type of defect more closely resembles a Mendelian dominant than any other. The raised, sustained radioiodine uptake gives a clue to the diagnosis, which is confirmed by the discrepancy between PB ^{131}I and BE^{131}I (protein-bound ^{131}I and butanol-extractable ^{131}I) or of PB^{127}I and BE^{127}I. Thyroid hormone medication causes a prompt reduction in the size of the thyroid. It should be noted that iodoproteins other than thyroglobulin are also found in the thyroid and in the circulation in patients with autoimmune thyroiditis, hyperthyroidism, thyroid cancer and adenoma.

(*f*) *Protease Defect*. McGirr has described a patient with a large goitre that contained iodothyronines but lacked protease activity. It was postulated that there was a defect of thyroid protease activity, impairing the release of thyroid hormones from thyroglobulin and causing the thyroid to liberate partially digested fragments of thyroglobulin into the circulation.

(*g*) *Other Defects*. A variety of other thyroid and peripheral tissue defects have been described, many on inadequate scientific evidence. Familial goitre with hypothyroidism or euthyroidism can be associated with high circulating levels of free and total thyroid hormones, normal TBG and raised or normal TSH. It has been postulated that the explanation for these findings is an increased resistance to thyroid hormone in the tissues including the pituitary gland.

3. GOITROGENS (*see* Appendix)

Goitrogens are substances that interfere with the synthesis of thyroid hormones, and the resultant goitre is mediated by TSH action. Usually, compensation is adequate and the enlarged hyperplastic gland is able to synthesise normal amounts of thyroid hormone. If treatment with the goitrogen is prolonged or the goitrogenic action of the drug is high, hypothyroidism may develop. Rarely, goitrogens can cause hypothyroidism without thyroid enlargement.

Goitrogens in the diet are unlikely to be a frequent cause of goitre. In various parts of the world milk has been found to contain goitrogens the cow has eaten. These are often present in apparently insignificant amounts, and convincing evidence of a clinical effect is still not available at the present time. Unknown goitrogens acting alone or synergistically with iodine deficiency could yet be responsible for some cases of 'simple goitre' in the UK.

Antithyroid drugs used in the treatment of hyperthyroidism are, of course, goitrogenic, but many drugs given for diseases unrelated to the thyroid have, as a side effect, a goitrogenic action. Goitrogens can be divided into two groups*, depending on the mechanism by which they interfere with thyroid hormone formation. The inorganic ions perchlorate, thiocyanate, and nitrate interfere with trapping of iodide by the thyroid, possibly because they have a similar molecular volume to the iodide ion. Potassium perchlorate is the only drug in this group to have found popularity in the treatment of hyperthyroidism though it is now no longer the drug of choice. Since these drugs interfere with iodide-trapping their antithyroid effect can be overcome by increasing iodide intake. Many drugs interfere with the iodination of tyrosine and some of these may also affect the conversion of iodotyrosines to iodothyronines and the peripheral breakdown of thyroid hormones, though their precise mechanism of action is unknown. The commonly used antithyroid drugs carbimazole, methyl and propyl thiouracil, and methimazole are all thioureylene derivatives having the grouping —NH—C=(S)—NH—. Substituted benzene derivatives like phenylbutazone, para-aminosalicylates, and resorcinol are much weaker goitrogens and act in a similar manner to the thioureylenes. The sulphonylurea antidiabetic drugs tolbutamide and, possibly, chlorpropamide may have a mild antithyroid action in man. Iodine in excess taken as such or in cough mixtures or in the proprietary asthma medication Felsol† interferes with the organification process and also with the release of thyroid hormone from the gland. Patients with autoimmune thyroiditis seem to be particularly sensitive to the action of iodides.

All goitrogens, apart from iodine, will lower the thyroidal iodine stores because less iodide is able to enter the thyroid or because unbound iodine leaves the gland. In addition, the normal stores of thyroid hormone bound to thyroglobulin in the colloid will be depleted. Withdrawal of the goitrogen allows the hyperplastic gland to renew its synthesis of thyroid hormone, causing a rapid uptake of iodide for this purpose. The plasma inorganic iodide level falls and can only be restored by iodine in the diet, the time taken depending on the iodine content of the diet. If radioactive iodine tests are carried out while the plasma inorganic iodide is low there will be a high uptake of the isotope by the gland as in any iodine-deficiency state. This sequence of events is important if radioiodine tests are used to assess the level of thyroid function after antithyroid drugs. The high radioiodine uptake might suggest increased thyroid activity but measures of absolute iodide uptake will be normal once the gland stores of iodine have been restored.

During or following goitrogen administration more T3 relative to T4 may be secreted so that a patient may be euthyroid with a low circulating PBI or T4 level.

4. AUTOIMMUNE THYROIDITIS

The term autoimmune thyroid disease is used to define the group of conditions characterised by the presence of circulating thyroid antibodies although it does not imply that these antibodies necessarily have any causal relationship to the thyroid disorder. It includes Hashimoto's disease, its atrophic variant myxoedema, and Graves' disease. In all these diseases antibodies to thyroid tissue are found in the circulation and there is a variable degree of lymphocytic infiltration of the thyroid gland.

Hashimoto's disease is characteristically found in middle-aged women but any age group may be affected. There is a marked female preponderance of the clinical disease, a sex ratio of about 15:1 being usual. The patient may complain of thyroid enlargement, and hypothyroidism can occur at any time (*see* hypothyroidism in the adult, p. 99). In the subacute variety of

* Lithium, used in the treatment of manic-depressive disorders, has been shown to have an antithyroid action. It decreases the rate of secretion of iodide and thyroid hormone from the thyroid and inhibits peripheral hormone degradation.

† Iodopyrine in Felsol is a compound of phenazone and iodine, and both of these components have been demonstrated to have an antithyroid action.

the disease, pain and tenderness of the gland may be prominent. The thyroid shows diffuse lymphocytic infiltration with lymphoid follicles, many plasma cells, and disruption of thyroid follicles. Some of the follicular cells are enlarged and eosinophilic in appearance—the so-called Askanazy cells. Patients with myxoedema present with symptoms of hypothyroidism, and in a typical case no goitre can be felt. The thyroid histology resembles that seen in Hashimoto's disease though fibrosis is more marked and cellular infiltration scanty. Cases intermediate between Hashimoto's disease and myxoedema are seen in which a small firm thyroid can be felt on careful palpation.

Circulating antibodies to thyroid can be found in most patients with Hashimoto's disease and myxoedema, though titres are usually lower in the latter. Antibodies are directed against thyroglobulin, a second antigen termed CA2 in the colloid, and against thyroid microsomes. The antigens and the tests used to detect antibodies are shown in Table 5.8.

TABLE 5.8 *Thyroid Antigens and Antibody Tests*

Antigen	Tests used to Detect Antibody
Thyroglobulin	Precipitin test Tanned red cell test Immunofluorescence (fixed sections)
Second colloid antigen (CA2)	Immunofluorescence
Thyroid microsomes	Complement fixation (CFT) Immunofluorescence (unfixed sections) Cytotoxic action of serum on thyroid tissue culture

Antibodies to thyroid similar to those found in Hashimoto's disease and myxoedema are present in 85 per cent of patients with Graves' disease though the titres are usually lower than in either of the former conditions. About five per cent of patients with Graves' disease have high levels of antibodies in the circulation, and in this group the thyroid shows extensive lymphoid thyroiditis in addition to hyperplasia. Again, LATS is found in the majority of patients with Graves' disease if sufficiently refined tests are used. This substance is known to be an IgG molecule produced by lymphocytes and is likely to be a thyroid antibody with thyroid-stimulating properties.

Autoimmune thyroid diseases may be classified as follows:

1. Hashimoto's disease
   (*a*) Fibrous variant (90 per cent precipitin positive, high titre CFT);
   (*b*) Hypercellular variant;
      (i) oxyphilic (4 per cent precipitin positive, high titre CFT);
      (ii) non-oxyphilic (low titres antibodies);
2. Myxoedema (12 per cent precipitin positive).
3. Focal lymphocytic thyroiditis (low titres antibodies).
4. Graves' disease (5 per cent precipitin positive).

Apart from LATS, none of the other antibodies have been shown to have any direct effect on the thyroid gland *in vivo*. It is likely that some common defect associated with thyroid autoimmunity is present in all of the patients with autoimmune thyroid disease. Any of the diseases can affect members of the same family, and antibodies can be detected in some apparently normal persons, indicating the presence of subclinical disease. It now seems likely that the ability to form thyroid antibodies is under polygenic control and is of moderate heritability (Hall *et al.*, 1972).

The prevalence of thyroid antibodies in the general population is shown in Table 5.9. Several workers have shown a correlation between circulating thyroid antibodies and lymphocytic infiltration of the thyroid, the higher

TABLE 5.9 *Prevalence of Thyroid Antibodies in the Normal Adult Population*

	Thyroglobulin antibodies* (by tanned red cell test) %	Cytoplasmic antibodies** (by complement-fixation test) %	Both antibodies	Either antibody
Men	0·7	0·7	0·3	1·7
Women	0·5	5·4	0·25	6·1

* Titres of 1/20 or more considered positive.
** Titres of 1/32 or more considered positive.

the titre of antibodies the greater the extent of the lymphoid thyroiditis. Only a small proportion of persons with diffuse thyroiditis in the general population have any complaint though careful examination may reveal the presence of a small, firm, goitre. The factors responsible for the development of overt thyroid disease are not understood.

Autoimmune thyroid disease in which antibodies to thyroid can be detected is one of the group of organ-specific autoimmune diseases that includes pernicious anaemia, some cases of atrophic gastritis that may be associated with iron deficiency anaemia, autoimmune Addison's disease, and some cases of idiopathic hypoparathyroidism. In these diseases antibodies are formed to constituents of particular organs, e.g. the parietal cells of the stomach and intrinsic factor in pernicious anaemia. Rarer associations of the organ-specific autoimmune diseases include premature ovarian failure (associated particularly with autoimmune Addison's disease), diabetes mellitus especially the insulin-dependent, juvenile-onset type (associated particularly with pernicious anaemia and autoimmune thyroid disease), renal tubular acidosis, fibrosing alveolitis and chronic hepatitis. At the other end of the spectrum are the non-organ specific diseases characterised by systemic lupus erythematosus, where antibodies are formed to various body constituents, e.g. cell nuclei. Only rarely is there any overlap between the two groups, though certain disorders such as Sjögren's syndrome appear to occupy an intermediate position having a clinical association with thyroiditis and with rheumatoid arthritis. In Sjögren's syndrome, antibodies are formed to thyroid, to duct tissue of salivary glands and, also, to cell nuclei (antinuclear factor). In juvenile thyroiditis the increased incidence of antinuclear factor suggests the presence of a more widespread immunological disturbance. All of these diseases show a marked female preponderance. The organ-specific autoimmune diseases tend to overlap both in an individual patient and in a family, and the presence of one of these diseases should always alert the clinician to the possibility of another developing. Some five per cent of patients with myxoedema have pernicious anaemia. Vitiligo, which consists of patchy areas of depigmentation of the skin surrounded by areas of increased pigmentation, is associated with all the organ-specific autoimmune diseases. Segmental vitiligo, hypopigmented rings surrounding dark naevi (halo naevi), leucotrichia, premature graying of the hair, and alopecia areata are all, like typical vitiligo, associated with this group of diseases.

The fundamental defect responsible for the occurrence of the organ-specific autoimmune diseases is unknown (*see* p. 106, aetiology of Graves' disease). Calder *et al.* (1972) have demonstrated circulating lymphocytes sensitised to various thyroid components—thyroglobulin, mitochondria and microsomes, in a high proportion of patients with Hashimoto's disease. Inhibition of leucocyte migration caused by mitochondria was non-organ-specific, similar findings have also been observed in diabetes mellitus. It seems most likely that the destructive process involving the thyroid in Hashimoto's disease and myxoedema is due primarily to the sensitised lymphocytes but humoral antibodies may also be involved by causing adherence of non-sensitised lymphocytes to thyroid tissue and adding to cell damage (cytotoxic action of the complement-fixing microsomal antibody).

5. RIEDEL'S THYROIDITIS

This is an extremely rare cause of thyroid enlargement, and it may be symmetrical or asymmetrical. It is characterised by dense fibrosis that may extend beyond the confines of the thyroid to affect adjacent tissues. The aetiology is unknown, but it is probably one variety of a group of conditions characterised by dense fibrous tissue deposition. The term multifocal fibrosclerosis may be used for the group which includes mediastinal fibrosis, hilar fibrosis, retroperitoneal fibrosis, sclerosing cholangitis, ligneous perityphlitis and orbital pseudotumour. The thyroid is extremely hard, pressure symptoms are common, and carcinoma is usually suspected. Treatment is to remove as much of the affected tissue as required to relieve pressure effects. Hypothyroidism may develop before or after surgical intervention.

CONGENITAL GOITRE AND HYPOTHYROIDISM

If a goitre is present at birth it is likely that the mother has been taking some goitrogen during pregnancy, e.g. iodides, or antithyroid drugs given for hyperthyroidism. The goitre usually regresses over a few months, a process that can be accelerated by administration of thyroid hormone.

Dysgenesis of the thyroid is a common cause of hypothyroidism in children. It may be due to absence of the thyroid or to maldevelopment, which is often associated with maldescent. Although it was formerly assumed that most sporadic cretins were athyroidic, scanning of the neck has shown that there is often a small functioning thyroid remnant somewhere in the midline of the neck. Of 51 cases of nongoitrous hypothyroidism of childhood investigated by Hutchinson and McGirr, 27 had a definite ectopic thyroid, 11 were possibly ectopic, 11 were athyroidic and 2 were hypopituitary. An ectopic thyroid can be demonstrated by scanning the neck after a dose of radioiodine. The level of plasma protein-bound ^{131}I twenty-four or forty-eight hours after the dose may be raised because the small thyroid remnant is synthesising hormone at a rapid, albeit inadequate rate, and there is a low intrathyroidal iodine pool.

CLINICAL ASPECTS OF GOITRE

The incidence of goitre varies in different parts of the world, an endemic goitre area being defined as one in which more than 10 per cent of the population show thyroid enlargement. Criteria for the presence of a goitre vary from centre to centre and the main problems are to decide the degree of thyroid enlargement that is to be considered abnormal and to allow for observer variation. The authors would agree with Trotter that the lobes of the normal thyroid gland are not palpable, though the isthmus can usually be felt as a band across the trachea. In the United Kingdom the upper weight of the normal thyroid is about 25 g. The degree of thyroid enlargement can be classified according to Kilpatrick *et al.* (1963).

	On inspection	On palpation
Stage 0	Not visible	Not palpable
Stage 1	Not visible	Palpable but less than 40 g
Stage 2	Visible	Palpable but less than 40 g
Stage 3	Visible	Palpable and more than 40 g

There is less observer variation in the reporting of visible glands than in those where the gland is palpable but not visible. Pads of fat in the lower neck may simulate a goitre but do not move on swallowing. Swellings in the neck that move on swallowing are usually thyroid in origin though some carcinomas or partly retrosternal goitres are fixed.

In North-East of England some 9 per cent of women and 1 per cent of men in the general population show significant thyroid enlargement (Stages 2 or 3). Many persons with Stages 1 or 2 thyroid enlargement are unaware that they have a goitre. It is important in the assessment of patients referred to hospital with goitre to bear in mind the various reasons for referral. Goitres found incidentally at routine examination should not always be mentioned to the patient. The physician must first decide whether further investigations or treatment are justified, bearing in mind the frequency of thyroid enlargement in the population. There is always a temptation to relate a patient's complaints to the swelling in her neck, especially if her symptoms in any way resemble those of hyperthyroidism. Some patients referred with suspected hyperthyroidism are found to be suffering from psychiatric disorders, especially anxiety states, the home doctor often having been misled by the coincidental goitre. The patient or her friends may notice the swelling in the neck and the patient may seek medical advice about it. Often she is afraid about the possibility of cancer and will be relieved to have this fear brought into the open. Local symptoms from a goitre are uncommon, and enormous goitres can be tolerated with remarkably little disability. The pressure effects depend on the position of the gland as well as on the degree of enlargement. When this is wholly or partly retrosternal, common symptoms are difficulty in swallowing and shortness of breath. Audible higher pitched expiration is a useful sign of significant tracheal compression. Feelings of a lump in the throat or choking feelings are more often manifestations of anxiety than of the goitre itself.

Pain or tenderness in the thyroid may be localised to one area, usually in a palpable nodule or be diffuse and associated with generalised enlargement of the gland. Sudden pain in a nodule is most likely to be the result of haemorrhage into a cyst or adenoma or rarely to a focal area of autoimmune thyroiditis or an early thyroid carcinoma. Diffuse mild pain, is often due to autoimmune thyroiditis whereas severe pain is more likely to be related to de Quervain's thyroiditis. Pyogenic infections of the thyroid are very rare as are granulomatous infiltration by tuberculosis, syphilis or sarcoidosis. A rapidly-infiltrating anaplastic carcinoma or a lymphoma of the thyroid may be painful. Reidel's thyroiditis may also be associated with discomfort in the gland.

The duration of the goitre is important; obviously a longstanding goitre is less likely to be malignant than one that is enlarging rapidly. A history of enlargement of the goitre during pregnancy is relevant since there is often spontaneous regression afterwards. A detailed list of all drugs being taken should be drawn up, special reference being made to those with a goitrogenic action. Family histories are particularly helpful—a familial goitre in an adult is more likely to be due to autoimmune thyroiditis, and in a child, dyshormonogenesis or thyroiditis. If the patient or a member of her family suffers from pernicious anaemia her goitre is probably due to autoimmune thyroiditis. The other organ-specific autoimmune diseases are so uncommon that they are rarely found in patients presenting with goitres. Questions are then directed to ascertaining the patient's level of thyroid function. Symptoms of hyperthyroidism will be discussed later. Most patients presenting with goitre are, in fact, euthyroid and their symptoms are often the result of a concomitant psychiatric disorder. Symptoms of hypothyroidism will be considered later, but it should be stressed that these are often mild and so slow in developing that the patient may feel they are merely due to natural ageing.

Examination should be directed to the goitre and to determining the level of thyroid function. The patient should be asked to swallow with the neck extended, and the movement of the thyroid observed. Both lobes of the thyroid and the isthmus should be palpated, preferably with the patient sitting or standing. The consistancy is graded soft, firm, or hard, and the surface smooth, finely nodular, or nodular. Asymmetry is important since malignant goitres are rarely symmetrical. The thyroid gland in Hashimoto's disease is usually symmetrical, firm and finely nodular, but there are many exceptions. Thyroid size can be graded as mentioned previously; confirmation of the previous clinical assessment should be obtained at operation whenever possible. The pyramidal lobe should be looked for—it forms a firm band on one or other side of the larynx. Enlargement signifies some diffuse process affecting the thyroid gland. Palpation and auscultation may reveal increased vascularity of the gland, usually a sign of present or past hyperthyroidism. The vascular murmur should not be confused with an aortic systolic murmur or a venous hum, which is higher pitched and continuous and abolished by occluding the internal jugular veins. Tracheal displacement should be determined, especially in asymmetrical nodular goitres. A search should be made for lymph nodes in both anterior and posterior triangles. Enlarged lymph nodes may be due to carcinoma, thyroiditis, or some coincidental disease. Enlargements in the mid-line above the thyroid may be thyroglossal cysts, which frequently become infected, or thyroid tissue which has not descended normally. Before removing such a lump it is best to confirm, by scanning, that the thyroid is present in the normal position below.

INVESTIGATION

X-rays of the neck can give information as to the type of goitre. Large areas of *calcification* are seen in some longstanding multinodular goitres, and fine scattered calcification is present in a certain type of thyroid carcinoma. *Tracheal compression* should be looked for in the lateral as well as the antero-posterior view. A retrosternal goitre may be visible as a *superior mediastinal enlargement*.

Special investigations to determine whether the goitre is due to dyshormonogenesis, goitrogens or to autoimmune thyroiditis are dealt with elsewhere. In 'simple goitre', investigations are not usually very helpful. Some patients will show a raised thyroid radioiodine uptake, and detailed iodine studies in this group indicate iodine deficiency. In other patients, the tests are completely normal and one can regard the aetiology either as unknown or to have been due to previous iodine deficiency.

Tests to determine the level of thyroid function should always be performed even if the patient is apparently clinically euthyroid. Minor degrees of thyroid dysfunction may be impossible to recognise clinically yet their presence may help in diagnosis and their correction benefit the patient. For example a patient with a goitre who is found to have evidence of thyroid failure can usually be diagnosed as suffering from autoimmune thyroiditis or more rarely have an acquired (goitrogens) or congenital defect in thyroid hormone synthesis. Again the recognition of mild hyperthyroidism in a patient who was apparently euthyroid with a nodular goitre and atrial fibrillation can lead to effective treatment of the complication. Normal conventional tests of thyroid function are not sufficient to rule out minor thyroid dysfunction. Hyperthyroidism can be eliminated by finding a normal TSH response to TRH, normal thyroid suppressibility with T3 and a normal serum or urinary T3 level. Hypothyroidism can easily be eliminated by finding a normal serum TSH level or if this value is borderline, a normal TSH response to TRH. Fig. 5.4 shows the steps in the diagnosis of a patient presenting with a goitre.

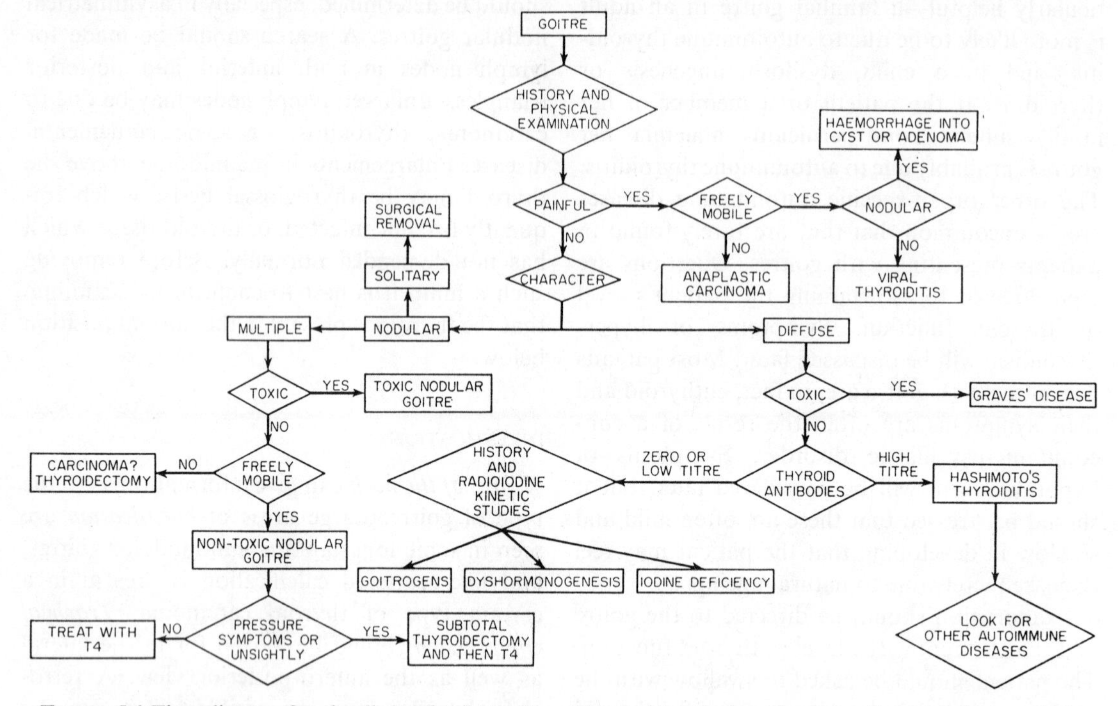

FIGURE 5.4 Flow diagram for the diagnosis of a goitre. Diagnostic steps are shown as diamond shapes which represent simple yes/no decisions, the rectangular shapes representing diagnoses or the management of a particular diagnosis (from *Medicine*, *Endocrine Diseases*, 1972, by permission of the Editorial Director, Dr Simon Campbell-Smith, and of Dr R. I. S. Bayliss)

TREATMENT

It is impossible to be dogmatic about the treatment of non-toxic goitre, but if hypothyroidism is present replacement with thyroid hormone is necessary (*see* below).

Goitres due to dyshormonogenesis can be reduced in size with thyroxine, bearing in mind that a child may require the full adult dose. The aim of therapy is to suppress pituitary TSH output, which allows the goitre to regress. Suppression of thyroid ^{131}I uptake to values of less than 10 per cent of the dose at six or twenty-four hours will confirm that an adequate dose of thyroxine is being given. In those cases of dyshormonogenesis in which there is an abnormal iodide trap or an organification defect, suppression tests will not be helpful. The iodide trap type of defect and that due to deficiency of the dehalogenase enzyme respond, as one might expect, to treatment with iodides, e.g. 5 mg twice daily of potassium iodide.

Goitres due to drugs can be reduced with thyroxine if it is necessary to continue the goitrogenic agent. Alternatively, stopping the drug is usually followed by a decrease in thyroid size. The process of involution can be accelerated with a course of thyroxine.

Goitres due to autoimmune thyroiditis may require no therapy if they are small and the patient is euthyroid. If the patient is worried about the goitre and/or if it is of substantial size, treatment with full doses of thyroxine usually causes a decrease in the size of the goitre in a few months; though where fibrosis is marked it may be many months before a change is evident. When the goitre is large and pressure effects point to the possible need for surgery it is worth trying the effect of a course of prednisone (initial dose 20 mg daily) in addition to thyroid hormone as this may cause a more rapid reduction in gland size, thus sparing the patient an unnecessary operation. Thyroid hormone should always be continued permanently since withdrawal is usually accompanied by recurrence of the goitre, and hypothyroidism can develop insidiously at any time. Surgery is indicated in patients with Hashimoto's disease in whom there is any suspicion of malignancy. This possibility is raised by:

1. Asymmetrical thyroid enlargement especially if a scan reveals an area of decreased uptake (a 'cold area');
2. Excessive hardness of the thyroid;
3. Marked pressure effects especially hoarseness;
4. Failure of diminution in gland size with full doses of thyroid hormone;
5. Presence of cervical lymphadenopathy.

When operation is carried out, a frozen section is examined from any suspicious area. If carcinoma is confirmed, then as radical a thyroidectomy as possible is usually indicated. If thyroiditis only is found it is customary to carry out a partial thyroidectomy and afterwards treat the patient with thyroid hormone. Most patients explored will be found to have thyroiditis rather than carcinoma but operation is justifiable for the above indications even if thyroid antibody tests show strongly positive results.

The treatment of 'simple goitre' depends on many factors, and the physician must bear in mind the reason for referral and take special note of the patient's psychiatric state. A small goitre, soft and symmetrical found incidentally will not usually require any therapy and the patient can be firmly reassured. A multinodular goitre is very rarely malignant and, unless there has been a recent rapid increase in size and if the gland is small and not worrying the patient, it can usually be left alone and the patient observed in six months or a year to confirm there has been no change. In a nodular goitre, the indications for surgical intervention are very similar to those that make operation desirable in Hashimoto's disease. A large goitre that is causing a patient concern, is cosmetically disfiguring, or is causing pressure effects may justify surgery and, afterwards, a small dose of thyroxine reduces the risk of recurrence. In some simple goitres treatment with thyroxine in full doses causes a reduction in size and the goitre does not always recur after cessation of therapy. The more nodular the goitre the less the chance of a response to thyroid hormone. If the patient has a single nodule in the thyroid a scan is very helpful. Nodules that take up radioiodine are very rarely malignant. It is sound policy to remove all 'cold nodules', especially those in which there has been a recent increase in size. The incidence of malignancy in a single thyroid nodule is difficult to assess because of the variable selection of patients. Overall, it is likely to be about 10 per cent, with higher figures in children and men. Most of the non-malignant single nodules will, at operation, be found to be the only clinically detectable nodule in a multinodular gland or to be cysts or poorly functioning adenomas.

CLINICAL ASPECTS OF HYPOTHYROIDISM

CLASSIFICATION OF CAUSES

1. Endemic cretinism
2. Dyshormonogenesis
3. Goitrogens
4. Autoimmune thyroiditis—
   Hashimoto's disease
   Myxoedema
5. Dysgenesis—
   Athyreosis
   Maldevelopment (ectopic thyroid)
6. Thyroid damage—
   Surgery
   Radiation
7. Pituitary or hypothalamic disease impairing the release of thyrotrophin-releasing hormone (TRH) or of thyroid-stimulating hormone (TSH).

ENDEMIC CRETINISM

The occurrence of endemic cretinism is geographically determined, it is found wherever goitre is highly endemic in regions such as the Himalayas, New Guinea, the Andes and the Congo. It is possible to recognise two major components in the syndrome of endemic cretinism (Querido, 1971).

1. Damage to the central nervous system
   Mental retardation
   Perceptive deafness
   Neuromotor retardation
   Brain stem damage
2. Hypothyroidism of varying severity

The underlying pathology of the nervous system damage is largely unknown. However carefully controlled studies using iodised oil suggest that iodine administration prior to conception is capable of preventing endemic cretinism. It seems that iodine *per se* is necessary for the development of the central nervous system in some process independent of the presence of thyroid hormone. Two different factors are probably involved in the pathogenesis of the hypothyroidism—(*a*) destruction of thyroid tissue as shown in the Congo studies and (*b*) severe iodine deficiency which leads to a shortage of iodine available for thyroid hormone synthesis. Both factors may operate in the same area and in the same patient.

Although iodine deficiency constitutes the main aetiological factor in endemic goitre and cretinism other factors may also be involved in certain areas. In parts of the Congo with similar degrees of iodine deficiency a marked variation in goitre prevalence is observed. In the goitrous region larger quantities of cassava are eaten and the urinary excretion of thiocyanate (which reflects the presence of natural goitrogens) is higher. There is also some evidence that fluoride might act as a goitrogen in areas of iodine deficiency.

There is no doubt that the best method of preventing endemic goitre is by prophylactic administration of iodine either in the form of iodised oil given intramuscularly, as iodised salt or by the addition of potassium iodate to bread. In some areas an increased prevalence of hyper thyroidism follows on iodine prophylaxis (Jod–Basedow phenomenon).

MYXOEDEMA

Although cretinism had been described by Paracelsus (1493–1541), it was not until the end of the nineteenth century that the possibility of an analogous 'cretinoid' condition in adults occurred to Hilton Fagge (1871). To Fagge's contemporary at Guy's Hospital, Sir William

Gull, belongs the credit for shortly afterwards describing the first case (Gull, 1874). Four years later the term myxoedema was coined to describe the characteristic non-pitting subcutaneous swelling, which was considered to contain some fifty times the normal amount of mucin (Ord, 1878). Despite criticism at the time and subsequently (e.g. Halliburton, 1893; Wayne, 1960), chiefly on the grounds that it describes only one and by no means the most constant feature, 'myxoedema' has become attached to the whole syndrome of primary thyroid deficiency in adults. An attempt by Osler (1898) to bestow eponymous glory on Gull met with little success, nor has the more accurate but less euphonious 'hypothyroidism' supplanted the earlier term.

Semon (1883) first discerned the relationship between myxoedema and the thyroid gland. His hypothesis that cretinism, myxoedema, and cachexia strumipriva (a term used to describe a syndrome resulting from thyroidectomy) were due to one and the same cause, namely thyroid deficiency, was disbelieved at first but came to be accepted after a committee appointed by the Clinical Society of London to study the disease published its report in 1888, a document that also contained an admirable description of the clinical features.

For the introduction of 'as perfect a form of therapy as any known to medicine' (Means, 1948) physicians are indebted to George R. Murray, Professor of Comparative Pathology at Newcastle upon Tyne. Early in 1891, at a meeting of the Northumberland and Durham Medical Society, Murray outlined his idea of treating myxoedema with hypodermic injections of an extract of sheep's thyroid. Later the same year he was able to report a brilliantly successful outcome in the first case (Murray, 1891a, b).

HYPOTHYROIDISM IN THE ADULT

Incidence. No reliable estimates are available of the overall incidence of myxoedema, but that it is by no means a rare disease in temperate countries is a matter of common experience. In the United Kingdom, it has been thought to be significantly more frequent in Northern England and Scotland than in the South. Women, especially multiparae, are affected about four times more often than men. Although the condition can appear at any time of life, the usual age at diagnosis is in the region of forty years. There is an undoubted familial association, which is referred to later.

Pathology. The thyroid itself shows a variable degree of atrophy and fibrosis. Histological examination of the remnant has usually revealed, in addition to fibrotic replacement of the parenchyma, changes of chronic thyroiditis resembling, except in volume and intensity, those of Hashimoto's disease. These consist of focal accumulations of lymphocytes and plasma cells, metaplasia of residual follicles, and sparse, poorly staining colloid associated with occasional multi-nucleated giant cells. Elsewhere, particularly in the skin, tongue, and vocal cords, there is deposition of the mucoid substance after which the condition is named. The material, which is extracellular and associated with mast cell proliferations, consists of acid mucopolysaccharides in combination with protein. The heart is usually enlarged and there is a significant degree of coronary atheroma. In longstanding cases of early onset, pituitary enlargement, visible on skull X-ray, presumably results from the long-standing stimulus to TSH secretion.

Clinical Features. It is now clear that hypothyroidism is a graded phenomenon and it is clinically convenient to define various grades of thyroid failure based on the clinical features, the serum TSH level and the presence of circulating thyroid antibodies (Evered and Hall, 1972).

Overt hypothyroidism or myxoedema is characterised by major symptoms of thyroid hormone deficiency—mental and physical sluggishness, intolerance of cold, constipation, and gain in weight. The appearance and behaviour of the patient on examination are characteristic. Thought and movement are retarded, speech is slow, and the voice has a hoarse, croaking quality. The skin is rough and dry, often with a distinct yellowish tint; peripheral cyanosis is usually evident in the lips, ears, and extremities, and accounts in part for the malar flush which is part of the typical myxoedema facies. In the hands, Raynaud's phenomenon may provide further evidence of peripheral circulatory insufficiency. The generalised non-pitting thickening of subcutaneous tissue, which gives the condition its name, is variable in degree, but is usually obvious as puffiness around the eyes where it confers a characteristic 'nephrotic' appearance. The hair is dry, brittle, and sparse, and tends to come out easily. Too much reliance should not be placed on thinning of the outer thirds of the eyebrows, since this is by no means uncommon in normal people. Menorrhagia is typical in middle-aged women although primary or secondary amenorrhoea may be presenting features in younger patients. Perceptibly delayed relaxation of the tendon jerks is a characteristic and helpful sign, and one that rapidly remits with adequate therapy. Apart from this, and the presence of some degree of bradycardia, detailed systemic examination is of no great help in establishing the diagnosis. It is a clinical truism that myxoedema is recognised either at first sight or not at all.

The actual presentation, moreover, may fail to conform to the textbook pattern. Presenting features which, though not uncommon, have sometimes proved deceptive include: faecal impaction due to intense and prolonged constipation; perceptive deafness (some degree of which occurs in 40 per cent of all cases); angina pectoris; and anaemia of normochromic, iron-deficiency or megaloblastic type (due to concomitant pernicious anaemia). A common error is to treat a patient for 'endogenous depression' without recognising myxoedema as the underlying cause, while psychotic manifestations ('myxoedematous madness'), which can cause behaviour to be the opposite of that expected in myxoedema—noisy, quarrelsome, and even violent—have occasionally led to confinement in mental hospitals. It should be remembered that patients with myxoedema are accident-prone and may gain their first opportunity for expert advice in the casualty department.

The condition must always be considered in the differential diagnosis of coma, especially when there is hypothermia; this complication occurs characteristically in elderly subjects living alone with inadequate protection against the cold. It is particularly dangerous to administer phenothiazines such as chlorpromazine to elderly hypothyroid patients since these drugs may lower the body temperature and precipitate coma. Occasionally, compression by myxoedematous tissue of the median nerve in the carpal tunnel leads the patient to seek advice for tingling and numbness in the fingers. Muscular aches and pains may be a prominent feature, especially in hypothyroidism following thyroidectomy or radioiodine ablation of the thyroid gland. Very rarely, a patient presents with stiff, aching and swollen muscles, and is found to have signs of myotonia (Hoffman's syndrome). A variety of central nervous system disorders have been described including epilepsy, drop attacks, dementia, cerebellar ataxia and a peripheral neuropathy, all of which may in large part recover with thyroxine treatment. However it is vital to exclude concomitant deficiency of vitamin B_{12} which is a not uncommon association of autoimmune thyroiditis.

Mild hypothyroidism presents many diagnostic problems since the symptoms are usually minor and non-specific. Tiredness, depression, puffiness of the face, swelling under the eyes, hair loss, dryness of the skin or constipation may be present singly or in any combination. Such symptoms are common in the middle-aged and elderly and are usually not associated with thyroid disease. Suspicion of hypothyroidism in the appropriate clinical context is the key to diagnosis. A family history of thyroid or other organ-specific autoimmune disease, the presence of a goitre or vitiligo or a history of previous destructive therapy to the thyroid should all alert the clinician to the possibility of thyroid failure.

Subclinical hypothyroidism (compensated

euthyroidism) is an asymptomatic state in which reduction of thyroid activity has been compensated for by an increased TSH output to maintain a euthyroid state (Evered and Hall, 1972).

Autoimmune thyroid disease without disturbance of thyroid function is quite common. Such patients are asymptomatic and have normal serum TSH levels.

The natural history of subclinical hypothyroidism and of autoimmune thyroid disease without thyroid failure is poorly understood. Some patients in these categories do undoubtedly progress to symptomatic hypothyroidism, but the frequency and time-course of this occurrence is unknown. It has been suggested, on the basis of hospital-based studies, that subclinical hypothyroidism and autoimmune thyroid disease are significant risk factors for coronary artery disease but this hypothesis remains to be tested in the general population.

Pituitary hypothyroidism is considered in Chapter 1. Brief reference seems appropriate here to hypopituitarism. As implied by the term pituitary myxoedema, symptoms and signs of secondary thyroid deficiency may predominate. The skin, however, tends to be finer and paler than in other forms of hypothyroidism, subcutaneous thickening is less marked, and the general aspect of the patient is accordingly somewhat different. Other endocrine deficiencies may be present; there is almost invariably amenorrhoea and pubic and axillary hair is usually absent though these features sometimes occur in primary myxoedema. The condition may be suspected when the history dates from an episode of postpartum haemorrhage followed by failure of lactation, when there is evidence of a pituitary tumour, or there is a history of previous destructive therapy to the pituitary.

HYPOTHYROIDISM IN THE CHILD

In the child, hypothyroidism may not become evident until a few weeks after birth but delayed clearance of neonatal jaundice may provide an earlier clue. The child is drowsy, sluggish in movement, fails to thrive, and there may be feeding problems. When severe hypothyroidism is present the skin is dry and puffy, the tongue protrudes, the reflexes are prolonged, and there may be an umbilical hernia. A lowered body temperature is easily produced if clothing is inadequate. While the severe cretin is easy to recognise, mild cases may present diagnostic difficulties. Growth is retarded, the child is underweight and shorter than average and with a marked delay in bone maturity. Hypothyroidism presenting later in childhood shows more of the adult features and is not usually associated with mental retardation, which depends largely on the severity of hypothyroidism and its age of onset. Complete hypothyroidism developing before birth always results in severe mental defect. Lesser degrees of hypothyroidism coming on after birth are more often the result of a partially functioning ectopic thyroid, and the prognosis is better. The date of onset of the hypothyroidism can be ascertained by X-rays, which may reveal epiphyseal dysgenesis—a misshapen fragmented epiphysis with a stippled appearance. The finding of dysgenesis in a centre indicates that hypothyroidism was present before the centre was normally due to ossify; for example, finding epiphyseal dysgenesis in the lower femoral epiphysis, which normally ossifies at thirty-six fetal weeks, implies that hypothyroidism existed before this time. Absence of an epiphyseal centre may also help to date the onset of hypothyroidism. The cuboid is known to ossify between 40 fetal weeks and one month after birth. Its absence or dysgenesis, which may only become apparent after thyroid hormone has been given, dates the cretinism to birth or earlier. Juvenile myxoedema most commonly presents as impaired linear growth. In addition to the other features of myxoedema the child is short with an impaired bone age and delayed puberty. The body proportions are often characteristic—the trunk (crown to pubis) is longer than the lower segment (pubic symphysis to ground) and the span is less than the height.

LABORATORY DIAGNOSIS

A clinical diagnosis of hypothyroidism should always be confirmed or documented by investigation. Lifelong therapy with thyroid hormone will be necessary, and subsequent physicians seeing a treated patient may, in the absence of adequate documentation, suspect the validity of the diagnosis and withdraw therapy. The diagnosis of hypothyroidism due to dyshormonogenesis and drugs has been considered earlier.

Overt hypothyroidism rarely presents any diagnostic problem since the clinical diagnosis should be obvious and conventional tests of thyroid function are almost invariably abnormal.

In a gross case of myxoedema a photograph taken before treatment compared with previous pictures of the patient and pictures taken after full response may suffice, if laboratory facilities are not available.

Thyroid hormone release tests—serum PBI, serum T4 or residual binding capacity are abnormal and can be rapidly estimated on a small volume of blood so the patient's treatment need not be delayed. The serum TSH level is usually grossly elevated. A normal TSH level excludes a diagnosis of hypothyroidism on the basis of primary thyroid disease.

Radioiodine tests may show high, low or normal values in the early stages of goitrous autoimmune thyroiditis, and even in the presence of hypothyroidism a raised level may be found. In established non-goitrous hypothyroidism a 24 hour thyroidal radioiodine uptake value is usually less than 20 per cent of the dose though the value will vary in different laboratories. Tests based on the peripheral action of thyroid hormone are cheap and sometimes helpful. Prolongation of the achilles tendon reflex, abnormalities of the electrocardiogram, and elevation of the serum creatine phosphokinase and cholesterol fall into this category. However, as mentioned earlier these tests are relatively non-specific and there is considerable overlap of values with the normal range. For example some 40 per cent of patients with hypothyroidism have an electrocardiogram which appears to be within normal limits, but *R* and *T* wave amplitude may increase with thyroid hormone. Similarly the biochemical tests can be rendered more specific by observing changes as a result of thyroid hormone treatment.

Mild hypothyroidism is often accompanied by normal routine thyroid function tests, but the diagnosis of primary thyroid failure can be confidently excluded by the finding of a normal serum TSH concentration. A raised TSH level does not necessarily indicate that the patient's symptoms are due to hypothyroidism. However, if the clinical features are suggestive and the TSH level is elevated, a therapeutic trial of thyroid hormone is justified.

Subclinical hypothyroidism is accompanied by normal routine thyroid function tests but an elevated serum TSH level.

While the thyroidal radioiodine response to TSH stimulation is almost invariably impaired or absent in patients with overt hypothyroidism, a normal response is observed in about 50 per cent of those with mild hypothyroidism and in 77 per cent of patients with subclinical hypothyroidism. The standard TSH stimulation test cannot therefore be relied upon to identify subjects with mild degrees of thyroid failure (Evered *et al.*, 1973).

The presence of thyroid antibodies in the circulation gives evidence of thyroid disease as well as indicating its nature. Low levels of thyroid antibodies may be found in thyroid carcinoma and in some multinodular goitres, but higher levels, especially a positive precipitin test, are indicative of a significant autoimmune thyroiditis. If tests are borderline and there is a clinical suspicion of mild hypothyroidism it is justifiable in some instances to give the patient a six-month trial with thyroid hormone. Where hypothyroidism is the cause of symptoms there is little doubt as to the effectiveness of therapy.

When clinical features such as loss of body hair raise the possibility of pituitary hypothyroidism it is dangerous to treat the patient with thyroid hormone without checking the plasma cortisol and if necessary correcting adrenocortical deficiency. A skull X-ray may demonstrate a pituitary lesion and a TSH test will show a rise in thyroid uptake in response to the hormone. Thyroid-stimulating hormone levels in the blood will be raised in myxoedema and lowered in hypothyroidism resulting from pituitary disease and these values may be differentiated from normal more easily by the use of TRH (*see* p. 81).

Diagnosis of hypothyroidism in infancy presents certain problems. Administration of ^{131}I is best avoided in children under the age of one year but a significant thyroid uptake of ^{132}I or ^{99m}Tc would exclude the common athyreotic variety of cretinism. Measurement of the serum TSH level is the most valuable test. Serum PBI and T4 levels are usually abnormal if there is significant thyroid failure. Estimation of the basal metabolic rate requires special apparatus in children and infants but where this is available the test can be helpful. Assessment of bone age by X-rays and the appearance of the electrocardiogram are useful indirect tests of hypothyroidism in children.

TREATMENT

Oral replacement therapy with a preparation of thyroid hormone should be started as soon as the diagnosis of hypothyroidism is established, and continued for the rest of the patient's life. In essentials, the method of treatment has not altered since Murray's day and, when properly applied and maintained, it restores the patient to complete normality.

The treatment of choice is l-thyroxine, dried thyroid extract should not be used because of its variable potency and its tendency to deteriorate in strength.

There is now considerable evidence that the previously recommended average replacement dose of 0·3 mg thyroxine daily is too high. Patients maintained on this dose have red cell sodium levels which are higher than normal and their serum TSH level does not rise in response to TRH. It is known that the range of circulating thyroid hormone levels over which a normal TSH response to TRH is obtained is very small and probably varies from patient to patient. Because of the risks of excessive thyroid hormone medication to the heart and possibly to the skeleton it is important to establish the optimal replacement dose for an individual patient. By using gradual increments of thyroxine till the patient is asymptomatic and till the serum TSH level is in the normal range, a satisfactory dose regime can be achieved. On this dose the level of circulating thyroxine and the PBI is similar to that of normal controls. There is some evidence that patients with severe hypothyroidism require a higher maintenance dose of thyroxine than those with mild hypothyroidism (Evered *et al.*, 1973).

In young patients treatment can be started with 0·1 mg thyroxine daily, the dose being increased at monthly intervals by increments of 0·05 mg daily till the patient is asymptomatic and the serum TSH level has fallen to within the normal range. The daily maintenance dose of thyroxine usually lies between 0·1 and 0·2 mg. Only a few patients require more than 0·2 mg daily. In order to minimise the risk of unmasking cardiovascular symptoms in patients over the age of 50 years, it is usual to begin with a daily dose of 0·05 mg, adding increments of 0·05 mg at four weekly intervals until the euthyroid state is achieved. In patients with ischaemic heart disease even small doses of thyroid hormone may induce angina or heart failure. Occasionally, treatment with propranolol may allow more adequate doses of thyroid hormone to be given. Thyroxine has a prolonged action, and its administration in divided dosage, though hallowed by custom is quite unnecessary: a single daily dose is preferable. Failure to respond to 0·2 mg of thyroxine daily should throw considerable doubt on the diagnosis. Some hypothyroid patients who apparently fail to respond to the usual replacement dose of thyroxine have raised TSH levels. Careful assessment reveals that they are omitting their medication, although they may deny this. It may also be noted that in euthyroid subjects, thyroactive substances in normal therapeutic dosage exert little or no physiological effect, since secretion of endogenous thyroid hormone is thereby suppressed.

Weight for weight, l-triiodothyronine is three or four times more potent than l-thyroxine, its action being shorter in duration and of more rapid onset (peak effect within twenty-four to forty-eight hours after administration). The average daily maintenance dose is in the region of 60 μg but in most circumstances there is no point in preferring it to thyroxine for routine treatment. It has a place, however, in situations in which rapid correction of hypothyroidism is desirable: e.g. preceding surgery, and in myxoedema psychosis; an intravenous preparation is available for use on these occasions. It is of value as replacement therapy following thyroid ablation for thyroid carcinoma. Because of its short half-life it only needs to be withdrawn for two weeks before scanning to detect residual thyroid tissue or tumour recurrence. The syndrome of 'non-myxoedematous hypometabolism', for which triiodothyronine was recommended is spurious.

In the child it is sometimes more difficult clinically to determine the precise dose of thyroxine since some children require the full adult dose and others need less. It is worth while checking the bone age periodically during therapy since overdosage with thyroxine will tend to increase bone maturity. Lifelong follow up is desirable to make sure treatment is conscientiously followed.

Patients with myxoedema coma are almost invariably hypothermic, but rewarming must be gradual lest ventricular fibrillation is induced. They should be placed in an unheated bed in a warm room and covered with a 'space blanket'. After removing blood for PBI and TSH to provide retrospective confirmation of the diagnosis, a stomach tube is passed and triiodothyronine is administered in low doses in suspension. A dose of 2·5–5 μg is given eight-hourly, the dose being doubled after 24 hours and again after another 48 hours. Large parenteral doses of T3 are dangerous since they may precipitate heart failure or ventricular fibrillation. It is usual to administer hydrocortisone hemisuccinate 100 mg intramuscularly at eight-hour intervals and dextrose solutions containing one fifth normal saline intravenously as required. Any infection should be vigorously treated. Once the patient regains consciousness oral thyroxine can be commenced in an initial dose of 0·025 mg daily. Myxoedema coma must be differentiated from simple hypothermia occurring in the elderly. Its mortality rate has been high probably because of over-vigorous therapy.

DE QUERVAIN'S THYROIDITIS (GRANULOMATOUS THYROIDITIS, VIRAL THYROIDITIS)

De Quervain's thyroiditis is an acute, subacute or occasionally a chronic, self-limiting inflammation of the thyroid gland which is probably viral in origin. It is commonest in the second to fourth decades and has a female to male ratio of 4:1.

Aetiology. The condition is likely to be a result of viral infection since it is often preceded by an upper respiratory infection, there is usually fever without leucocytosis and the condition may occur at the time of specific viral epidemics. Complete recovery is the rule and changing titres of viral antibodies can sometimes be demonstrated during the course of the disease. It has been reported in association with the common cold, influenza, measles, infectious mononucleosis, cat scratch fever, Coxsackie infections and mumps. Transient rises in thyroid antibody titres can often be detected over the course of the illness but they usually disappear after a few months.

Clinical Features. The disease is very variable in its severity. In some there is an acute onset of pain and tenderness in the thyroid with high fever and systemic upset. The pain may radiate to the jaws or ears and there may be pain and difficulty on swallowing. The thyroid is usually uniformly enlarged and firm. In mild cases the thyroid is only slightly enlarged and tender, there is little or no fever and few systemic symptoms. Transient hyperthyroidism can result from release of thyroglobulin and excessive amounts of thyroid hormone. The condition runs a variable course in severity and duration from a few weeks to a few months, although relapses are not uncommon. Transient hypothyroidism is not uncommon but permanent hypothyroidism is rare. Differential diagnosis is dealt with on p. 94 where pain in the thyroid is considered. The most common problem in diagnosis is that of subacute thyroiditis (subacute lymphadenoid goitre) and the differences between these two conditions are listed in Table 5.10. Where tenderness is not marked and the gland is hard, open biopsy may be required to exclude thyroid carcinoma. The follicular destruction, colloid extravasation and the round cell, polymorph and giant cell infiltration of De Quervain's thyroiditis is typical.

Treatment. Often no treatment other than mild analgesics is required. In severe cases prednisone in an initial dose of 20–30 mg daily in divided doses causes rapid symptomatic relief. Full doses should be given for one week then treatment slowly reduced over a further three weeks. If relapse occurs an increment of steroid is required for a further period and withdrawal should be made more slowly.

TABLE 5.10 *Laboratory Investigations in De Quervain's Thyroiditis and Subacute Lymphadenoid Goitre*

Test	De Quervain's thyroiditis	Subacute lymphadenoid goitre
Thyroid radioiodine uptake	Low	Normal or high
Thyroid antibodies	Low titre or absent	High titre
Plasma proteins	Raised α_2-globulin	Raised gamma globulin
ESR	Raised	Raised
White cell count	Raised or normal	Normal
PBI	Raised or normal	Raised or normal

HYPERTHYROIDISM

Classification

Graves' disease.
Neonatal Graves' disease.
Toxic multinodular goitre.
Toxic adenoma.
'Jod-Basedow phenomenon'.
Thyrotoxicosis factitia.
Struma ovarii.
Ectopic TSH syndrome.

GRAVES' DISEASE

This eponym is best retained to describe the syndrome comprising goitre, hyperthyroidism, eye signs, and rarely localised myxoedema and thyroid acropachy. All these clinical features may not occur in an individual patient. The term *ophthalmic Graves' disease* is used to describe patients with the ocular manifestations of Graves' disease in the absence of hyperthyroidism or a past history of hyperthyroidism. *Neonatal Graves' disease* is the term applied to hyperthyroid children born to mothers with Graves' disease and in whom the hyperthyroidism remits spontaneously in a few months.

Incidence. Graves' disease may affect any age group but it is uncommon in childhood and most frequent in the third and fourth decades. Females are affected six times more often than males. The incidence of Graves' disease varies in different parts of the British Isles but since diagnostic criteria are variable it is difficult to assess the significance of this finding. In a study of some general practices in England and Wales between 1955 and 1956, Logan and Cushion (1958) found hyperthyroidism had occurred in 0·3 per 1,000 men and 1·9 per thousand women. There was no relationship between the prevalence of hyperthyroidism and of 'simple goitre' but a high correlation between the occurrence of hyper- and hypothyroidism. This would be expected in view of the familial association of Graves' disease and myxoedema, both of which are now considered to be examples of autoimmune thyroid disease.

Pretibial myxoedema, a peculiar thickening of the skin and subcutaneous tissues, occurs in some five per cent of patients with Graves' disease, whereas thyroid acropachy, which resembles clubbing of the fingers, virtually never occurs in the absence of pretibial myxoedema, and is much rarer, occurring in only about 0·5 per cent of patients. There are no accurate figures for the incidence of ophthalmic Graves' disease but such patients probably comprise less than five per cent of all patients with Graves' disease. Neonatal Graves' disease is the rarest condition, though mild cases may well be overlooked.

Aetiology. Graves' disease was originally thought to result from the action of increased amounts of *thyroid-stimulating hormone*, the primary defect residing in the hypothalamus or pituitary. Evidence which renders this hypothesis untenable is summarised in Table 5.11. In very few patients with hyperthyroidism, but without

TABLE 5.11 *Evidence that TSH is Not Involved in the Pathogenesis of Graves' Disease*

1. TSH levels in the circulation are low or normal in Graves' disease (by radioimmunoassay).
2. Histology of the pituitary suggests suppression of the thyrotroph cells.
3. Graves' disease can occur after total hypophysectomy.
4. Overtreatment with antithyroid drugs in Graves' disease can cause a goitre as a result of TSH overproduction, hence the feedback mechanism is intact. Such a goitre can be reduced by thyroid hormone, which lowers TSH levels.
5. Triiodothyronine given in doses of 120 μg/day for one week fails to suppress ^{131}I uptake in patients with Graves' disease, whereas in the normal such suppression occurs. This suggests that a substance other than TSH is stimulating thyroid overactivity, since the TSH feedback mechanism is intact.

eye signs, increased levels of TSH have been found in the circulation. In some of these, pituitary tumours have been demonstrated radiologically and in one an abnormality of the hypothalamus was probably present.

When a *long-acting thyroid stimulator* (LATS) distinct from TSH was detected in the circulation of patients with Graves' disease (Fig. 5.5) it seemed that the pathogenesis had been solved.

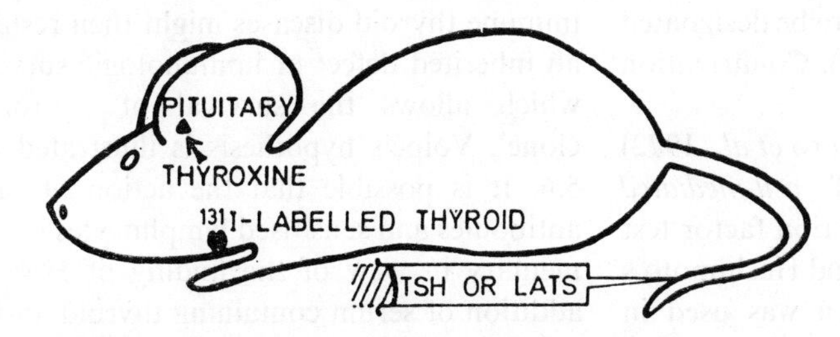

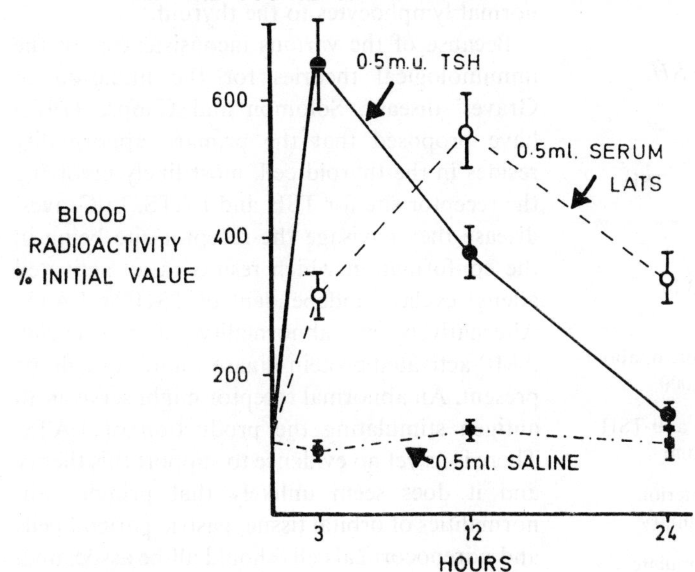

FIGURE 5.5 The contrasting 'short-acting' and 'long-acting' time courses of action of TSH and LATS in the McKenzie bioassay. (*Courtesy of* Prof. D. S. Munro)

The characteristics of LATS and a comparison of LATS with TSH is shown in Table 5.12. However, more recently evidence has accumulated which throws some doubt as to the role of LATS in the pathogenesis of Graves' disease and this is summarised in Table 5.13. Some now consider that LATS is an epiphenomenon secondary to primary events within the thyroid and may not be crucial to the initiation of the disease. Others still consider that bioassay insensitivity may contribute to the negative results observed in some patients with Graves' disease and consider that the coincidental presence of a thyroid-stimulating immunoglobulin in an immunological disease would be surprising.

Whatever the outcome of the LATS controversy, the evidence for an autoimmune basis for Graves' disease, summarised in Table 5.14 is remarkably convincing. The finding of an IgG in the serum that protects LATS from inactivation by anti-LATS in extracts of thyroid cells is still controversial. This material, designated '*LATS-protector*' or LATSP can be detected by some workers in LATS negative serum from hyperthyroid patients. It has been claimed that LATSP, like LATS and TSH causes an increase in the number of intracellular colloid droplets in human thyroid slices but unlike LATS and TSH the activity of LATSP is specific to the human thyroid and it can therefore be designated a *human thyroid-stimulator* (HTS). Confirmation of these reports is awaited.

Volpé and his co-workers (Munro *et al.*, 1972) have shown the presence of *cell-mediated immunity* by the migration inhibition factor test in patients with Graves' disease and Hashimoto's disease. A crude thyroid antigen was used in these studies. Some patients, mostly those with

TABLE 5.12 *Comparison of TSH and LATS*

	LATS	TSH
Peak of action in mouse assay	10–12 hr	2–3 hr
Structure and molecular weight	IgG, 150,000	Protein, about 28,000
Inhibition of activity	By anti-IgG serum	By anti-TSH serum
Source	Lymphocytes	Anterior pituitary
Action	Stimulates thyroid	Stimulates thyroid
Circulating level reduced by	High doses of corticosteroids	Thyroid hormone
Overproduction in	Graves' disease	Some pituitary tumours

pretibial myxoedema, showed positive results with leg skin antigen. The hypothesis has been advanced that Graves' disease may prove to be a disease of delayed hypersensitivity, induced by thymic-dependent lymphocytes situated within the thyroid gland and stimulating the thyroid cells directly. Studies of the age-specific incidence rate and observations in twins suggest that the condition may occur at random in a genetically preselected population, without the need for initiation by any thyroid antigen. The autoimmune thyroid diseases might then result from an inherited defect of immunologic surveillance which allows the survival of a 'forbidden clone'. Volpé's hypothesis is illustrated in Fig. 5.6. It is possible that the action of humoral antibodies and sensitised lymphocytes is complementary in view of the finding of Hobbs that addition of serum containing thyroid antibodies causes a marked increase in the attachment of normal lymphocytes to the thyroid.

Because of the various inconsistencies of the immunological theories for the initiation of Graves' disease, Solomon and Chopra (1972) have proposed that the primary abnormality resides in the thyroid cell, most likely involving the receptor site for TSH and LATS. In Graves' disease they envisage the receptor site being in the conformation which results in an activated adenyl cyclase, independent of TSH or LATS. Alternatively an abnormality of the cyclic-AMP-activated protein-kinase complex might be present. An abnormal receptor might serve as an antigen stimulating the production of LATS. There is as yet no evidence to support this theory and it does seem unlikely that primary abnormalities of orbital tissue, gastric parietal cells and adrenocortical cells should all be associated.

The pathogenesis of the eye signs remains uncertain, although it seems likely that parallel but distinct immunological mechanisms are involved. There is good evidence that patients with Graves' disease and active eye signs have a circulating IgG distinct from LATS which induces exophthalmos in fish. It is reasonable to designate this agent *exopthalmos-producing sub-*

stance (EPS). In addition this group of patients have *lymphocytes sensitised to retro-orbital antigens* suggesting that exophthalmos like hyperthyroidism might result from a 'forbidden clone' of cells. Winand and his colleagues have suggested that an IgG molecule from patients with exophthalmos enhances the binding of an *exophthalmogenic fragment of the TSH molecule* (which has no thyroid-stimulating activity) to orbital tissue. Similarly Hobbs has shown that

TABLE 5.13 *Evidence Against LATS Being a Major Cause of Graves' Disease*

1. LATS is not present in all patients with Graves' disease and even with concentration of IgG only between 50 and 80 per cent of patients are LATS positive.
2. LATS levels do not correlate with the presence or severity of the eye signs or of hyperthyroidism.
3. T3 treatment can cause suppression of the thyroidal radioiodine uptake in some patients with circulating LATS.
4. Previous reports of the production of an LATS-like substance by immunisation of animals with thyroid tissue have now been shown to be erroneous.
5. Immunisation of animals with thyroid tissue has not caused hyperthyroidism.

TABLE 5.14 *Evidence for Autoimmune Basis for Graves' Disease*

1. Lymphocytic and plasma cell infiltration of thyroid and retro-orbital tissues.
2. Deposition of IgG, IgM and IgE in the thyroid.
3. Enlargement and/or hyperplasia of lymph nodes, thymus and spleen and peripheral lymphocytosis.

TABLE 5.14 *Continued*

4. LATS is an IgG and possibly an antibody, LATS activity being an inherent part of the IgG molecule (Smith *et al.*, 1969); it stimulates animal and human thyroids; it binds specifically to thyroid homogenates, thyroid membranes and a 4S soluble thyroid fraction from which it can be dissociated by procedures known to separate antigen/antibody complexes; LATS may be produced by lymphocytes from patients with Graves' disease; passage of LATS across the placenta is probably responsible for neonatal Graves' disease; LATS is only found in patients with Graves' disease or their relatives and rarely in Hashimoto's disease.
5. Graves' disease, Hashimoto's disease and myxoedema occur in the same families and rarely patients may progress from one type of autoimmune thyroid disease to another.
6. Circulating thyroid and gastric antibodies are found more frequently and in higher titre in patients with Graves' disease and their families than in control subjects.
7. Other organ-specific autoimmune diseases occur more frequently in patients with Graves' disease and their families.
8. Lymphocytes from patients with Graves' disease may stimulate thyroid cells *in vitro*.
9. Lymphocytes specifically reactive to thyroid antigens are present in Graves' disease as demonstrated by the migration-inhibition factor test.
10. Patients with Graves' disease show an impaired reactivity with dinitrochlorobenzene suggesting a possible defect in immunosurveillance.
11. Corticosteroids and immunosuppressive agents may cause remission of the hyperthyroidism and eye signs in Graves' disease.

serum from patients with exophthalmos enhances the binding of lymphocytes to orbital tissue. Further studies are required to define the role of the various mechanisms which have been described so far.

Genetics. An increased prevalence of goitre, Graves' disease, and hypothyroidism is found in the relatives of patients with Graves' disease, particularly their sisters and mothers. Not infrequently several generations may be affected with autoimmune thyroid disease. It is now generally accepted that genetic factors are involved in the pathogenesis of Graves' disease; certainly the tendency to develop thyroid antibodies is so determined. Since only a proportion of the persons with the Graves' diathesis develop clinical disease, it is likely that environmental factors play some as yet unknown part.

CLINICAL FEATURES OF GRAVES' DISEASE

The clinical features of Graves' disease can be considered in three categories:

1. the thyroid
2. the effects of increased thyroid hormones
3. the extra-thyroid abnormalities:
   (*a*) the eye signs
   (*b*) localised myxoedema and thyroid acropachy
   (*c*) vitiligo
   (*d*) splenomegaly

1. *The Thyroid*

Patients with Graves' disease usually have enlarged thyroid glands but this is not invariably the case. In men, the goitre may be small and difficult to feel and is often not easily distinguished from the sides of the trachea because of its firmness. Although the thyroid is usually said

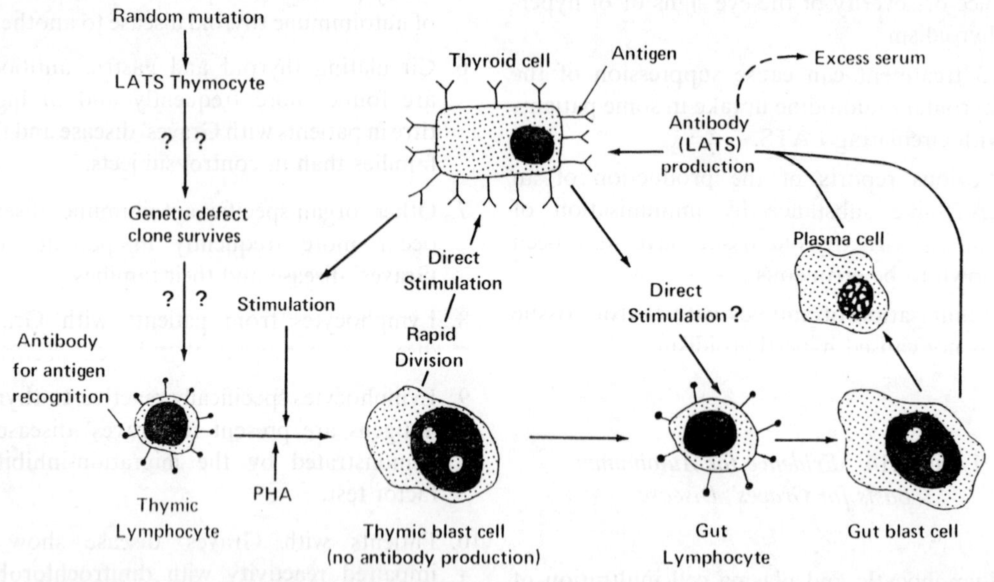

FIGURE 5.6 Delayed hypersensitivity in Graves' disease (Volpé, R., Edmonds, M. W., Clarke, P. V., *et al.*, 1970, *Acta Endocrinol. Panam.*, **1,** 155 by permission).

Graves' disease specific thymocyte (T-lymphocyte) produced normally by random mutation is allowed to survive because of a genetic defect. This cell then proliferates, possibly with thyroid antigenic stimulation. The T-lymphocyte may then stimulate the thyroid directly by cell-to-cell interaction but cannot release LATS. As well it may stimulate B-lymphocytes (bursa-equivalent or gut lymphocytes) to produce and release LATS within the thyroid gland with varying spillover of both LATS and LATS-producing lymphocytes into the circulation.

to be diffusely enlarged without palpable nodules there are many exceptions. Quite often the gland is asymmetrical with one or more nodules and except in gross cases it is sometimes difficult to make a distinction between a multinodular goitre and the type of gland felt in Graves' disease.

The goitre is variable in consistency but is not often very firm unless the patient has had recurrent hyperthyroidism. An enlarged pyramidal lobe can be felt in some instances on one or other side of the larynx. Increased vascularity of the gland is a very important physical sign—it is very rarely found in patients without hyperthyroidism unless they have recently been treated for this condition. The vascularity is sometimes indicated by a systolic thrill but is best demonstrated as a systolic bruit heard when the stethoscope is lightly placed over the isthmus; the bruit is less often heard when the gland is small and firm. It must be distinguished from murmurs conducted into the neck from the great vessels, e.g. aortic or pulmonary stenosis, from carotid stenosis which is usually asymmetrical, and from a venous hum. Occluding the jugular vein, by pressure above and lateral to the upper pole of the thyroid, eliminates venous murmurs, which in any case are more continuous, have a different high-pitched musical quality, and tend to vary in intensity with respiration. Although increased vascularity is an important sign of hyperthyroidism it is only detectable in about half the patients —mainly in those who are severely hyperthyroid. Tracheal displacement is uncommon.

2. *The Effects of Increased Thyroid Hormones*

Table 5.15 lists the main clinical features of hyperthyroidism. The effects of increased amounts of thyroid hormone must be distinguished from the physiological actions of thyroid hormone. At physiological levels thyroid hormones stimulate growth and development, increasing the synthesis of many enzymes. At pharmacological levels, catabolic effects supervene with increased heat production and oxygen consumption related in part to uncoupling of oxidative phosphorylation.

Many of the effects of excessive thyroid hormone appear to be mediated by way of the sympathetic nervous system—tachycardia, increased cardiac output, excessive sweating, and tremor, which can be largely reversed by 'sympathetic blocking agents' such as propranolol or guanethidine. The sympathetic overactivity seen in many patients with anxiety states accounts for the frequent mistakes in diagnosis.

Little difficulty in diagnosis is presented by the classical case of Graves' disease. The patient, usually a woman, complains of nervousness, irritability, palpitations, excessive sweating, and weight loss in spite of a good or increased appetite. She may be intolerant of heat and almost invariably admits to preference for cooler weather. The paradoxical association of loss of weight with normal or increased appetite is particularly suggestive, though it is sometimes encountered in diabetes mellitus and states of defective alimentary absorption. In rare instances the increase in appetite more than offsets that in metabolic rate, so that weight is actually gained. Examination reveals a nervous, sometimes agitated patient who displays exaggerated and purposeless movements—hyperkinesis. The palms are warm and moist and there is a fine tremor of the outstretched fingers often best appreciated by palpation. The pulse is full and bounding, tachycardia is almost invariable, and the systolic blood pressure is raised. The presence of eye signs and a goitre is helpful in diagnosis.

Hyperthyroidism in the elderly requires special mention. Signs and symptoms of cardiovascular strain tend to predominate over those already described or they may occur alone. Atrial fibrillation, occasionally paroxysmal, is frequent. In some instances the patient is in congestive heart failure when first seen, and evidence of the underlying thyroid disorder is scanty. Unexplained heart failure after middle age should always arouse suspicion of hyperthyroidism, especially when there are indications of a high cardiac output. Also very suggestive is failure of digitalis in normal dosage to control the rapid heart rate.

TABLE 5.15 *Clinical Features of Hyperthyroidism*

	Symptoms	Signs
Heat production increased	Feels warm, heat intolerance*, increased sweating	Warm*, moist skin*, fever, rarely hyperpyrexia
Gastro-intestinal system	Weight loss* with an increased appetite*; in older patients appetite is sometimes decreased, in young patients weight may actually increase; diarrhoea*	Loss of body fat, emaciation is rarely severe
Cardiovascular system	Palpitations and rapid heart action, shortness of breath on exertion*, angina, and symptoms of heart failure in the elderly	Tachycardia*, sleeping pulse rate over 80/minute, systolic hypertension with high pulse pressure, paroxysmal sinus tachycardia, atrial fibrillation and, in the elderly, signs of heart failure, cutaneous vasodilation*, systolic murmur due to increased blood flow
Neuromuscular system	Undue fatiguability* and muscular weakness, shaking of the hands, 'can't keep still'*	Proximal muscle weakness* (thyrotoxic myopathy) detectable in the majority of patients, reflexes hyperactive, myasthenia gravis is rare association, tremor is non-specific, hyperkinesia*, choreo-athetoid movements in children
Skeletal system and growth	Pain in the back, increased growth in some children	Thyrotoxic osteoporosis sufficient to cause kyphosis and loss of height is very rare
Integument	Loss of hair	Nails may show recession from the nail bed
Psychiatric	Irritability*, nervousness*, symptoms of an anxiety state; rarely, a psychosis may be produced; insomnia	

* Clinical features of most value.

Less common modes of presentation need to be borne in mind. One of these is muscular weakness with signs pointing to a proximal myopathy and others include diarrhoea and oligo- or amenorrhoea; very rarely myasthenia gravis is associated. Osteoporosis giving rise to back pain and even to kyphosis is another unusual presentation. Hypercalcaemia with its clinical sequelae is very rare. Glycosuria may be due to unmasking of latent diabetes, and difficulty in stabilising a diabetic patient is sometimes the first clue to the thyroid disorder. Hyperthyroidism in children can cause disorders of growth; an increase in height is usually accompanied by an advance in bone maturity. Rarely patients with hyperthyroidism present with polyuria and polydipsia, the polyuria and low serum osmolality being directly due to an increased fluid intake resulting from abnormal thirst (Evered *et al.*, 1972).

3. *The Extra-thyroid Abnormalities*

(*a*) *Eye signs.* The eye signs of Graves' disease comprise swelling of the eyelids, irritation of the conjunctivae, exophthalmos (proptosis), lid retraction, and ophthalmoplegia, and they may occur alone or in any combination. In ophthalmic Graves' disease they are found in the absence of hyperthyroidism.

Swelling of the eyelids is of two types. Firstly, swelling of the lids can occur in association with any type of exophthalmos when it is due to overfilling of the orbit. It is then a non-specific sign. Secondly, swelling of the eyelids can occur in the absence of exophthalmos when the lids appear congested and 'oedematous', often as part of the syndrome of 'congestive ophthalmopathy', a dangerous complication of Graves' disease.

Irritation of the conjunctivae causing grittiness and soreness of the eyes is a common complaint. The conjunctivae are inflamed, and sometimes there is oedema of the conjunctivae (chemosis) which may ulcerate or actually prolapse between the lids. The appearance of prominent vessels at the lateral canthi is usually a sign that the ocular manifestations are going to be troublesome.

Exophthalmos means protrusion of the eyeball. It is usually recognised by the appearance of sclera between the lower lid and the limbus of the cornea in the position of forward gaze. It can be measured by means of a Hertel exophthalmometer, an absolute reading of 18 mm or more or a difference between the eyes of 2 mm or more being taken as significant, especially if the patient complains of prominence of the eyes. In Graves' disease with hyperthyroidism the exophthalmos is usually symmetrical, whereas in ophthalmic Graves' disease asymmetry of protrusion of the eyes is common, though it rarely exceeds 5 mm. Exophthalmos in Graves' disease is caused by increased bulk of the orbital contents—the fat is increased and the muscles are enlarged, infiltrated with lymphocytes, and contain increased amounts of water and mucopolysaccharide. Exophthalmos is, however, a non-specific sign and can be caused by any space-occupying lesion in the orbit or by involvement of the orbit from outside. Orbital tumours cause progressive unilateral exophthalmos, the asymmetry usually exceeding 5 mm by the time the patient is seen. Enlargement of the globe caused by longstanding myopia should cause little difficulty in diagnosis. The exophthalmos of Graves' disease usually alters little with treatment and may be remarkably persistent. In a small proportion of patients the exophthalmos is progressive (malignant exophthalmos) and may cause loss of vision if effective treatment is not given.

Lid retraction is recognised by the appearance of sclera between the upper lid and the limbus of the cornea when the patient is looking straight ahead and is not staring. Minor degrees of asymmetrical lid retraction can be detected by comparing the amount of cornea covered by the upper lids. Normally 2 to 3 mm of cornea are covered by the upper lid in the forward position of gaze. The significance of the sign depends on the care the clinician takes to make sure the patient is relaxed. *Lid lag* is said to occur when the sclera between the upper lid and cornea becomes visible as the patient's gaze follows the examiner's finger downwards from the position of maximum elevation. It may confirm the presence of minor degrees of lid retraction but is subject to such observer error that in itself it is not a reliable eye sign of Graves' disease.

Lid retraction in Graves' disease is of two types—spastic and paralytic. Spastic lid retraction is diagnostic of Graves' disease. It is present in all positions of gaze and is one of the commonest eye signs in Graves' disease. In ophthalmic Graves' disease it is frequently unilateral. The mechanism of its production is uncertain; spasm of the striated levator palpebrae superioris and sympathetic stimulation of the superior orbital muscle of Muller have both been postulated. Paralytic lid retraction is much rarer and is not specific for Graves' disease though it may coexist with spastic lid retraction. It occurs only in the presence of limitation of upward gaze whether this is due to disorder of the muscles (Graves' disease, ocular myopathy), neuromuscular junction (myasthenia gravis), or nervous system (upper brain stem lesions, e.g. infarction). Paralytic lid retraction is thought to be caused by over-innervation of the levator palpebrae superioris when an attempt is made to look up; muscles of elevation have a common innervation with the levator palpebrae. This type of lid retraction diminishes or disappears when the gaze is directed downwards; presumably, in this position there is less stimulation of the levator palpebrae. Lid retraction is a cause of conjunctival irritation and keratitis when it prevents lid apposition during sleep. Commonly the lower limbus is affected and symptoms are worst in the morning.

Ophthalmoplegia. Paresis of one or more of the extraocular muscles usually causes diplopia. Upward gaze is reduced most often, and movement in the upwards and outwards direction is reduced four times as often as all other movements. Upwards and inwards gaze is the next most frequently affected. In some instances limitation of upward gaze may be due to tethering and adhesions of the inferior oblique and inferior rectus where they cross one another. Ophthalmoplegia is more common in ophthalmic Graves' disease. It is one of the most unpleasant ocular complications of Graves' disease and may be remarkably persistent. The patient complains of diplopia and may attempt to avoid this by extending the neck or covering one eye.

Congestive ophthalmopathy (*malignant exophthalmos*) is the term used to describe the severe and often progressive ocular changes in Graves' disease. The former term is to be preferred since exophthalmos is not invariably present. Usually the eyes are prominent, the lids and conjunctivae swollen and inflamed, and there is marked ophthalmoplegia. The patient often complains of severe pain in the eye. Retinal veins may be prominent, and papilloedema or oedema of the macula may develop, but often the fundal appearance is surprisingly normal. Ocular tensions may be high. The cornea is at risk from keratitis but this is easily recognised. Failure of vision from pressure on the optic nerve may be sudden and complete even in the presence of a normal fundus. This development is a medical emergency requiring immediate admission to a unit with experience in dealing with such cases (*see* Treatment, p. 127).

(*b*) *Localised Myxoedema and Thyroid Acropachy.* Localised myxoedema (pretibial myxoedema) occurs in about five per cent of patients with Graves' disease. As its name implies, it usually affects the front of the shins but other parts of the body may be affected, e.g. the face. The swelling often extends over the dorsum of the feet and toes where it is sometimes associated with tissue overgrowth. Biopsy scars in the area almost invariably develop keloid. The skin is coarse and purplish-red in colour, often with a peau-d'orange appearance, and hairs in the affected areas are coarse. The superficial layer of the skin is infiltrated with the mucopolysaccharide hyaluronic acid which can be demonstrated by appropriate staining techniques.

Localised myxoedema rarely occurs in the absence of ocular manifestations of Graves' disease and, as mentioned previously, there is usually a high titre of LATS in the circulation. It tends to develop after hyperthyroidism has been treated by surgery or, more particularly, with radioactive iodine. The latent interval between the treatment for hyperthyroidism and the clinical onset of pretibial myxoedema varies from 4 to 32 months with a mean time of one year in a series reported by Kriss *et al.* (1964).

Thyroid acropachy resembles hypertrophic pulmonary osteoarthropathy but the clubbing in acropachy is not usually accompanied by an increased blood flow. Radiologically the two conditions can be distinguished by the distribution of the new bone formation. In acropachy, subperiosteal new bone formation resembles soap bubbles on the surface of the bone, with coarse spicules, whereas in hypertrophic arthropathy new bone is formed in a linear distribution. Sometimes the new bone formation along the phalanges and metacarpals is both visible and palpable, but the patient is rarely concerned.

(*c*) *Vitiligo*. This is a condition in which there is patchy depigmentation of the skin surrounded by areas of increased pigmentation (*see* p. 92).

(*d*) *Splenomegaly*. This is found in five per cent of patients with Graves' disease though the degree of enlargement is only slight. The lymph nodes may be moderately enlarged and the muscles and thymus may also be involved in this lymphoid hyperplasia. Active germinal follicles are found in the thymus, which is sometimes enlarged though special techniques, e.g. pneumomediastinography may be needed to demonstrate this.

CLINICAL COURSE OF GRAVES' DISEASE

Before the advent of effective therapy Graves' disease had a mortality of about 10 per cent. About 25 per cent of patients, usually those with mild disease, remitted spontaneously within one year. A number of patients are seen who have spontaneous remissions and relapses of the disease, and antithyroid therapy must be considered against this background of a chronic remitting disease. Years after successful therapy of hyperthyroidism the patient may develop exophthalmos or ophthalmoplegia which persists or disappears in spite of therapy.

DIAGNOSIS OF GRAVES' DISEASE

Clinical. In most patients the clinical features are so obvious that there is little difficulty in diagnosis. It merely remains to document the diagnosis with one or more thyroid function tests. It might be argued that tests are unnecessary in the obvious case but, unfortunately, standards of clinical diagnosis vary and even the best clinicians are occasionally in error. Since a positive diagnosis implies treatment by potentially hazardous drugs or operation, it is necessary to be certain.

The clinical diagnosis may be made more objective and reproducible by using the diagnostic index of Gurney *et al.* (1970) shown in Table 5.16. Positive or negative scores are allocated to certain symptoms and signs to give the best discrimination between the hyperthyroid and euthyroid states. Methods of eliciting the items for use in the index require standardisation as indicated below.

USE OF THE NEWCASTLE INDEX

Psychiatric Items

In the case of the two personality traits of 'frequent checking' and 'marked anticipatory anxiety' it is important that the patient understands that these refer to their premorbid state and not to the period of illness (when they may occur as symptoms). This is a clinical index and not a questionary. However, the following general form of questioning is recommended.

Psychological Precipitant. 'We know that the symptoms you have can sometimes be brought on by shock or worry. Can you think of any strain or worry which may have played a part in causing your symptoms (e.g., worry about physical illness in yourself or someone close to you; and upset with a relative or friend; worries about work, money, moving house, etc.)?'

Frequent Checking. 'Before your illness began did you check you actions a lot? For instance, when you locked the door, switched off the gas, etc., or when you had to do your accounts, add up bills, etc., did you usually go back two or three times and check that you had done it properly?'

Severe Anticipatory Anxiety. 'Before your illness began, did you tend to worry a lot about things which were to happen in the future? For instance, if you had to do something which was a bit out of the ordinary, but not critically important (e.g. if you had to say a few words in public, have a routine interview or examination, pay a routine visit to a dentist or doctor, etc.) would you worry about it for some days before it was due to happen?'

Physical Items (Similar to those of Wayne's Index).

Increased Appetite. The question, 'How is your appetite?' should be an inquiry about whether it is regarded as less than normal, normal or excessive.

Palpable Thyroid. The gland should be significantly enlarged.

Definite Thyroid Bruit. A systolic murmur heard over the isthmus or lateral lobe of the thyroid; not obliterated by occluding the internal jugular vein, or by rotation of the head; elicited by light pressure of the stethoscope.

Exophthalmos. When sclera is visible between the limbus of the cornea and the lower lid, in the position of forward gaze.

Lid Retraction. When sclera is visible between the limbus of the cornea and the upper lid in the position of forward gaze; the gaze should be relaxed and not staring.

Hyperkinesis. The movements of removing and replacing clothing have to be unusually rapid and jerky, conveying an impression of over-reaction, wasted energy, and clumsiness. It is the combination of rapidity and inaccuracy of movement which is significant.

Fine Finger Tremor. With the patient's eyes closed, the outstretched separated fingers should show a fine tremor. Coarse tremor is ignored, but if doubt exists, the sign is regarded as present.

Pulse-rate. This is counted for one minute at the end of the examination.

Crooks (1967) has pointed out that, usually the first step in the diagnosis of hyperthyroidism is made by the general practitioner who asks the question 'is the patient hyperthyroid or not?'. In this context the finding of a goitre indicating the presence of thyroid disease is an important diagnostic clue. The diagnostic criteria are changed when the patient is referred to a hospital physician who asks the question, 'is the patient really hyperthyroid?'. In this context a goitre is less significant, but the finding of even minor eye signs is very significant since they indicate the presence of Graves' disease. In fact, some 75 per cent of patients referred to some hospital clinics with an initial diagnosis of hyperthyroidism are not hyperthyroid but are suffering from some pyschiatric disorder, usually an anxiety state or some neurotic illness. It is, therefore, important to take a psychiatic history from patients referred to hospital with suspected hyperthyroidism. Hyperthyroid patients usually have a less neurotic personality and few hysterical symptoms. The age of onset is later than in patients with anxiety states and there is less often an identifiable precipitating cause. The physical symptom of most significance in separating the two groups is increased appetite, especially if combined with weight loss.

Laboratory. In any patient with suspected hyperthyroidism it is wise to document the diagnosis with at least two tests of thyroid function. The tests chosen will depend on the preference and facilities of the individual physician. The authors routinely use the PBI and an index of residual binding capacity such as the 'Thyopac-3', calculating the free thyroxine index. The effective thyroxine ratio (ETR) can also be used to provide a similar answer.

In patients where the clinical diagnosis is difficult the limited investigations mentioned above usually settle the issue. When the initial

TABLE 5.16 *Newcastle Thyrotoxicosis Index*

Item	Grade	Score
Age of onset	15–24	0
	25–34	+4
	35–44	+8
	45–54	+12
	55 and over	+16
Psychological precipitant	Present	−5
	Absent	0
Frequent checking	Present	−3
	Absent	0
Severe anticipatory anxiety	Present	−3
	Absent	0
Increased appetite	Present	+5
	Absent	0
Goitre	Present	+3
	Absent	0
Thyroid bruit	Present	+18
	Absent	0
Exophthalmos	Present	+9
	Absent	0
Lid retraction	Present	+2
	Absent	0
Hyperkinesis	Present	+4
	Absent	0
Fine finger tremor	Present	+7
	Absent	0
Pulse-rate	Over 90 per min.	+16
	80–90 per min.	+8
	Under 80 per min.	0

Euthyroid range −11 to +23. Doubtful range +24 to +39. Toxic range +40 to +80.

tests are borderline or contradictory it is usually wise to reassess the clinical picture and to question the patient about drugs that might have modified the clinical features or the tests. Further tests are then employed to confirm the diagnosis. The *triiodothyronine suppression test* is useful in distinguishing raised thyroid radioiodine uptakes caused by iodine deficiency from those of hyperthyroidism; suppression of the thyroid radioiodine uptake by triiodothyronine excludes a diagnosis of hyperthyroidism, but failure of suppression occurs in Graves' disease without hyperthyroidism and in the presence of one or more autonomous thyroid nodules as well as in hyperthyroidism.

The thyrotrophin-releasing hormone test is valuable in the exclusion of hyperthyroidism (*see* page 81). A normal TSH response to a small (200 μg) dose of intravenous TRH excludes hyperthyroidism. An absent or impaired response is often due to hyperthyroidism but may have other explanations for example ophthalmic Graves' disease, some euthyroid patients with Graves' disease in apparent clinical remission, autonomous adenomas, multinodular goitres, pituitary disease and variety of drugs such as corticosteroids and thyroid hormones. Because of its safety, speed and convenience, the TRH test is likely to replace the T3 suppression test in clinical practice. There is a good correlation between the results of the two tests, patients with a normal TRH test show normal thyroid suppressibility and those with impaired or absent TRH responses show impaired or absent suppressibility.

Estimation of the *absolute iodine uptake* by the thyroid is occasionally of value since it allows for alterations in the plasma iodide levels. Measurements of *serum T*3 may be of value in the diagnosis of hyperthyroidism, particularly in the syndrome of T3 toxicosis (*vide infra*).

Thyroid antibody tests are useful in borderline cases since they give a clue to the presence and extent of autoimmune thyroiditis; they also have prognostic significance (*see* p. 123).

SPECIAL DIAGNOSTIC PROBLEMS

Pregnancy. The raised metabolic rate that occurs in pregnancy simulates the peripheral manifestations of hyperthyroidism, and the resemblance is increased by the thyroid enlargement that is a common sequel of pregnancy. Patients with previous Graves' disease who become pregnant are often suspected to have relapsed, especially if they have psychiatric symptoms or other complications of pregnancy such as anaemia. Radioiodine tests are best avoided in pregnant women even though the radiation dose to mother and foetus with ^{132}I is very low. The PBI is elevated because of an increase in thyroxine-binding globulin. In this situation estimation of the free thyroxine index obtained by the product of the PBI or T4 and the T3 resin uptake gives a surer indication of the level of thyroid function as does estimation of the 24 hour output of urinary free T4.

During Antithyroid Therapy. Thyroid radioiodine uptakes 2½ hours or more after the tracer dose are not helpful in assessing thyroid function during carbimazole therapy. By using early measurements, e.g. the 20-minute thyroid uptake of an intravenous dose of ^{132}I or ^{99m}Tc, a measure of thyroid trapping can be obtained independent of drug therapy. This may be useful in determining whether the thyrotoxicosis has remitted, since thyroid suppressibility with triiodothyronine returns with remission (*see* below).

Estimation of the PBI during effective antithyroid therapy may give misleadingly low values because the gland produces greater amounts of triiodothyronine during treatment. Triiodothyronine is less well bound to TBG, and the patient can be euthyroid with low or borderline levels of PBI. Estimations of plasma or urinary T3 levels will be of value in the assessment of patients receiving antithyroid drugs.

After Antithyroid Therapy. After a course of antithyroid therapy has been discontinued it is sometimes necessary to determine the level of thyroid function, e.g. if a relapse is suspected. During antithyroid therapy the thyroid becomes depleted of iodine, and after treatment is stopped the thyroid repletes its iodine stores at the expense of the other iodine in the body. The plasma inorganic iodide level falls and a greater proportion of a tracer dose of radioiodine is taken up by the thyroid. If the physician is not aware of this, the patient may be given further treatment unnecessarily. The body iodine stores can be repleted by administration of potassium iodide 2 mg daily for two weeks, carrying out a six-hour radioiodine uptake test one month after stopping the iodide. A raised value will then suggest hyperthyroidism. Alternatively, and more simply, the PBI or T4 and/or T3 resin uptake and also if possible the blood or urine T3 can be measured.

Renal failure complicates thyroid function tests, especially those employing radioiodine. Renal failure causes retention of iodine, increasing the plasma inorganic iodide which will tend to reduce the uptake of a tracer dose, whereas failure of excretion of the radioiodine will tend to increase uptake. The final result will depend on the balance of these two opposing factors. Many of the drugs employed in the treatment of renal failure may also affect the tests. Loss of TBG in the nephrotic syndrome lowers the PBI, though the thyroid status is unaffected because the free thyroxine level is normal.

Cardiac Failure. Expansion of the extracellular fluid volume will increase the volume of distribution of iodine and tend to lower the radioiodine uptake. Effects from impairment of renal function and drugs may be superimposed, e.g. organic mercurial diuretics interfere with the PBI estimation, giving falsely low values.

T3 Toxicosis. Direct measurement of circulating triiodothyronine levels has allowed recognition of the syndrome of T3 toxicosis (Hollander and Shenkman, 1972). Features of this syndrome are contrasted with those of typical hyperthyroidism in Table 5.17. The frequency of T3 toxicosis varies in different areas and true prevalence figures are not yet available. In non-iodine deficient areas perhaps about 5 per cent of patients with hyperthyroidism have this syndrome whereas in iodine deficient areas the prevalence is some three times higher. Any variety of hyperthyroidism may be associated with T3 toxicosis but it appears rather more often in patients with autonomous thyroid nodules, in recurrences in those previously subject to destructive therapy to

TABLE 5.17 *Comparison of Clinical and Biochemical Features of Typical Hyperthyroidism and T3 Toxicosis*

	Typical Hyperthyroidism	T3 Toxicosis
Cause	Any variety of hyperthyroidism	Any variety of hyperthyroidism
Clinical features	Hyperthyroidism	Hyperthyroidism
Predisposing factors		Iodine deficiency, ? early feature of typical hyper-thyroidism, ? feature of re-current hyper-thyroidism
Serum triiodo-thyronine	Raised	Raised
Urine triiodo-thyronine	Raised	Raised
Serum thyroxine	Raised	Normal
Free thyroxine	Raised	Normal
Resin uptake tests	Hyperthyroid range	Usually normal
Serum thyroxine—binding globulin	Normal or lowered	Normal
Radioiodine uptake by thyroid	Raised	Raised or normal
T3 Suppression test	Impaired or absent suppression	Impaired or absent suppression
Serum TSH response to TRH	Impaired or absent	Impaired or absent

the thyroid and as a premonitory finding early in the development of conventional hyperthyroidism. Even in untreated patients, raised levels of serum T3 do not necessarily imply clinical hyperthyroidism. Some patients with autonomous thyroid nodules or with ophthalmic Graves' disease have a relatively stable state of 'subclinical T3 toxicosis' which can persist for several years. Since conventional thyroid function tests including thyroid uptake measurements are normal in T3 toxicosis a number of patients have been erroneously diagnosed as suffering from anxiety states. If a T3 assay is not available, thyroid autonomy can be established by impaired thyroid suppressibility by T3 or an impaired or absent TSH response to TRH. Patients with clinical features suggestive of hyperthyroidism in whom thyroid autonomy is demonstrated, warrant a careful therapeutic trial of antithyroid drugs.

Hidden hyperthyroidism is not uncommon in elderly patients who present with unexplained atrial fibrillation, atrial tachycardia, palpitations, angina of effort or heart failure. Other presentations are: myopathy, weight loss, anxiety, apparent choreoathetosis in children, tremor in adults, pyrexia of unknown origin, diarrhoea, poorly controlled diabetes mellitus. Occasional patients show the reverse of the usual hyperkinetic state, the so called 'apathetic hyperthyroidism'. Such patients may have a 'bloated' or hypothyroid appearance and be depressed with an emotionally flat affect and hypokinesis. Routine tests are usually abnormal but the diagnosis is easily overlooked because of the absence of the classical features of hyperthyroidism.

TREATMENT

A. HYPERTHYROIDISM

Once a diagnosis of hyperthyroidism is established it is necessary to decide on the appropriate treatment for the particular patient. Three standard forms of therapy are available, antithyroid drugs, partial thyroidectomy and radioactive iodine. There is no general agreement as to the indications for these forms of therapy and none of them is ideal and each is associated with both short and long-term sequelae. The choice of a particular form of therapy depends on the patient's wishes and clinical state and on the preference of the physician, which, in turn, will depend in part on the facilities available to him. Only a general outline of the aims and plan of therapy can be given.

Antithyroid Drugs

All patients with hyperthyroidism can be controlled by antithyroid drugs. Some physicians regard permanent therapy with drugs as the treatment of choice for hyperthyroidism, but they are in a minority. Because of the variations in the disease, exacerbations, remissions and relapses, the dose of drugs may need to be varied and the patient needs to attend his doctor every few months. Again, the goitre may persist or increase with antithyroid drugs, particularly if too large a dose is given. Finally, a proportion of patients with hyperthyroidism remit spontaneously or during the course of therapy and it seems unnecessary to treat such patients permanently.

Indications for Antithyroid Drugs

1. *Children.* Partial thyroidectomy is more difficult in children and the complication rate is higher. Radioiodine is contra-indicated because of the possible hazard of thyroid malignancy. Children with hyperthyroidism are prone to relapse, but it is wiser to delay surgery as long as possible, giving several courses of antithyroid drugs if necessary.

2. *Pregnancy.* Operation is best avoided in the pregnant patient who can usually be easily controlled with drugs. The dose should be kept as low as possible, especially in the last two months of pregnancy, for goitre in the fetus is usually the result of overenthusiastic therapy. Radioiodine therapy is absolutely contra-indicated in pregnancy since the thyroid gland of the fetus is able to concentrate iodide from the third month onwards.

3. *Patients with Small Goitres.* Relapse after a course of antithyroid drugs is less common in patients with small glands. Patients with large glands and, possibly, those with detectable LATS on routine testing or a family history of thyroid disease are more prone to relapse.

4. *Patients in whom Surgery is Contra-indicated.* These can be treated medically. The contra-indications vary: a patient may be afraid of an operation, his job may not allow suitable time off work for the procedure, or his medical condition may be unsuitable.

5. *Thyroid Surgery.* Thyroid surgery is a specialised procedure and the complications depend largely on the skill and experience of the surgeon. It is usually best to concentrate thyroid operations in the hands of only one or two surgeons in each major hospital. If a thyroid surgeon is not available, medical therapy or radioiodine may be used more freely. This caution does not apply to surgery of the non-toxic goitre, which is less difficult.

6. *Relapse after Previous Thyroidectomy.* This is a contra-indication to further operation, distortion of the local anatomy by the first operation rendering a second operation more difficult, and repeated relapse being common. Antithyroid drugs or radioiodine are used in this group of patients.

7. *Patients with Medical Complications of Hyperthyroidism.* Heart failure or thyroid crisis require urgent therapy with antithyroid drugs, usually in combination with iodine which is used because of its speed of action.

SELECTION OF PATIENTS FOR ANTITHYROID DRUGS OR DESTRUCTIVE THERAPY

Alexander *et al.* (1973) suggest that antithyroid drugs should be the treatment of choice for the majority of patients with Graves' disease under the age of 45 years, coupled with repeated assessment of the response to therapy at six-monthly intervals. Patients are treated with carbimazole in an initial dose of 30 or 40 mg daily, reduced when they become euthyroid to a maintenance dose of 15 to 20 mg daily in divided doses. Every patient also receives 80 μg of triiodothyronine daily as four doses of 20 μg. The 20-minute ^{132}I-uptake (^{131}I or ^{99m}Tc can also be used) and free-thyroxine index are measured initially and at six-monthly intervals. Remission is assumed to occur when the 20-minute uptake falls into the normal range ($<$8 per cent). Several patterns of response may be observed and the plan of treatment in these is outlined below.

1. *Remission after Six Months of Antithyroid Therapy:* Plan: Discontinue carbimazole, continue T3 as before (optional, allows further

thyroid uptake measurements); follow free-thyroxine index at three or six month intervals for a further two or three years; if no relapse then arrange long-term follow-up by family doctor.

2. *Remission after Six Months but Subsequent Relapse:* Plan: Give second course antithyroid drugs, as before, if further relapse occurs refer for appropriate destructive therapy with subsequent long-term follow-up.

3. *No Remission after Two Years Antithyroid Therapy:* Plan: Give destructive therapy to thyroid.

This rational regime warrants further study since it avoids destructive therapy with its risk of hypothyroidism in those patients who remit spontaneously (or as a result of therapy). The proportion of patients who undergo spontaneous remission may well vary from place to place and its size is difficult to ascertain because of selection bias. It is likely that somewhere between 30 and 50 per cent of hyperthyroid patients do remit spontaneously.

Methods of Use. The antithyroid drugs in common use are shown in Table 5.18.

There is little to choose between the first three drugs shown in the table. In most clinics in the UK carbimazole is used. Toxic effects are rare,

TABLE 5.18 *Antithyroid Drugs in Common Use*

Drug	Initial dose mg/day	Minimum dose mg/day
Carbimazole	40	5
Propylthiouracil	400	25
Methylthiouracil	200	25
Potassium perchlorate	800	200

and apart from an increased tendency to aplastic anaemia—a serious and often fatal complication—and a nephrotic syndrome, both associated with potassium perchlorate, there is little difference in their incidence with the different drugs (Table 5.19).

TABLE 5.19 *Side Effects of Antithyroid Drugs*
(excluding potassium perchlorate)

Side effect	Approximate incidence %
Skin rashes (macular or papular and itchy)	5
Agranulocytosis	0·5–1·0 (neutropenia is more common)
Fever with lymphadenopathy and splenomegaly	Very rare
Arthropathy, polyarteritis nodosa, polyneuritis	Very rare
Prothrombin deficiency	Very rare (only with propylthiouracil)

Dosage. The initial dose, e.g 40 mg of carbimazole daily, is given for one to two months depending on the patient's response. It is preferable to spread the dose out, taking 2 tablets (10 mg) on rising, 2 tablets at noon, 2 tablets in late afternoon, and 2 tablets before retiring, because some patients are not so easily controlled on a twice daily regime. The patient's response can be assessed by improvement of the symptoms of hyperthyroidism and gain in weight. Tests are difficult to interpret, e.g. the PBI is lower than expected when the patient is euthyroid because the drug-blocked gland secretes more triiodothyronine. Failure to respond to antithyroid drugs means that the initial diagnosis was incorrect or the patient is not taking the medication. Very few patients require an initial dose of carbimazole in excess of 40 mg/day. Enlargement of the thyroid is usually an indication of over-treatment. If the patient becomes hypothyroid on treatment it is best to reduce the dose of carbimazole to about 15 mg/day and to add thyroxine. The patient should attend for supervision at not less than three-monthly intervals, having been warned to discontinue the drug and to report at once should any rashes, mouth ulcers or a sore throat develop. If the patient remains euthyroid on 5 to 10 mg of carbimazole daily for two months, treatment can be withdrawn and the patient observed in three months. A course of treatment is usually given for one to two years. Less than 50 per cent of patients remain in permanent remission after an 18 month course of carbimazole. Relapse after a course of antithyroid drugs may be induced in some cases by iodide administration. Conversely, a low plasma inorganic iodide after antithyroid drugs may sometimes delay relapse and it is probably worth advising such patients to avoid fish and iodised salt if this is not too great a hardship to them.

Thyroxine, 0·1 to 0·2 mg/day, is combined with antithyroid drugs as a matter of convenience in some clinics. It is not then necessary to titrate the dose of antithyroid drug so carefully and somewhat larger doses can be used without the risk of hypothyroidism. Such combined therapy does not alter the progress of the eye signs of Graves' disease except in so far as it prevents hypothyroidism which may lead to exacerbation of the eye signs.

It should be noted that potassium perchlorate, which prevents concentration of iodide by the thyroid gland, acts synergistically with the other listed drugs which interfere with the organic binding of iodine. If iodide is administered concurrently with perchlorate, the antithyroid action of the latter is overcome and this antagonism, if overlooked prior to surgery, may lead to operation being performed on a thyrotoxic patient. This means that if perchlorate is used as the antithyroid drug prior to surgery, iodine must not be given, and the advantages of preoperative iodine medication (*see* below) are lost.

Partial Thyroidectomy

Removal of part of the thyroid gland is a satisfactory method of treating hyperthyroidism and in some clinics it is the treatment of choice for most patients. The results in terms of cure of the hyperthyroidism and the incidence of complications depend to a large extent of the skill and experience of the surgeon. The patient to be treated by surgery should first be rendered euthyroid by antithyroid drugs and then treated with iodine for two weeks prior to operation (unless treatment has been with potassium perchlorate). This should preferably take place in hospital, where the patient can rest away from the cares of the home. Iodides in large doses have an antithyroid action, for they interfere with the organification of iodine and they also slow thyroid hormone secretion rate. In addition, they may reduce the size and vascularity of the gland and make the operation easier to carry out. Potassium iodide 5 mg three times daily by mouth is an adequate dose. Sensitivity and skin rashes are very rare.

The amount of gland removed bears little relation to the original gland size. Taylor and Painter (1967), who measured the size of the thyroid tissue left, considered a volume of about 8 ml to be ideal. If too much gland is left, recurrence of hyperthyroidism will be more frequent, if too little, hypothyroidism ensues.

Complications of surgery can be divided into those that occur during the operation, those following soon after, and those that tend to develop months or years after operation.

Operative complications are those of any major surgical procedure. If the patient is properly prepared the general anaesthetic should be uneventful.

Early post-operative complications are again mainly avoided by good preparation and surgical technique. Haemorrhage at the operation site may cause asphyxia, and a laryngoscope and surgical tray should always be available on the ward to allow intubation and re-opening of the wound.

Thyroid crisis consists of hyperpyrexia and

exacerbation of the features of hyperthyroidism occurring within the first day or two of operation. It may also occur during intercurrent infections in untreated hyperthyroid patients. The pulse rate is rapid, dehydration occurs, and atrial fibrillation and heart failure may develop if treatment is not vigorous. This complication was common in poorly prepared patients and is usually a sign of mismanagement. Release of hormone from the thyroid at operation and afterwards may be one factor in its causation. Treatment is given with large doses of iodide *by mouth*, 10 mg four-hourly for four doses, then six-hourly will suffice. Antithyroid drugs are given by mouth or intramuscularly in standard doses (initial dose shown in Table 5.18). Sympathetic blocking agents such as propranolol, guanethidine or reserpine are helpful in reducing sympathetic overactivity. Intravenous glucose and saline may be needed and temperature is reduced by fans and sponging if there is hyperpyrexia. Chest complications are common after thyroidectomy, and basal collapse with infection may simulate a thyroid crisis.

Tetany may start shortly after operation. The incidence will depend very much on the surgeon's technique. Hypoparathyroidism is more often caused by interference with the blood supply to the parathyroids, which are supplied by end arteries, than to their removal. Tetany begins with cramps in the hands or feet, which may take up the characteristic position, and paraesthesiae especially round the mouth can be an early sign. After taking blood for calcium and phosphate estimations (the former is low, the latter raised) treatment is initiated with intravenous calcium gluconate (20 ml of 10 per cent solution). This is then followed by oral calcium salts, about 8 g/day and calciferol 50,000 units daily or dihydrotachysterol (AT10) 1 to 3 ml/day, the aim being to restore the serum calcium to normal as soon as possible, avoiding both hypo- and hypercalcaemia. Frequent checks of the serum calcium are needed, especially in the early stages. In some patients, parathyroid function improves and therapy can be withdrawn, while in others lifelong treatment is required, the serum calcium being checked at not less than six-monthly intervals even when the dose is stabilised. All patients who have undergone partial thyroidectomy should have a serum calcium estimation three months after operation since the development of hypoparathyroidism may be delayed. If the serum calcium remains within the normal range it is unnecessary to carry out tests of parathyroid reserve, e.g. with phytate or EDTA.

Damage to the recurrent laryngeal nerves should be rare and is usually indicated by persistent hoarseness or inability to sing.

Late complications of thyroidectomy include *hypothyroidism* and *recurrent hyperthyroidism.* Recent studies suggest that the low incidence rate of hypothyroidism reported in many series is due to inadequate or short-term follow-up. The most comprehensive follow-up study by Hedley *et al.* (1970) of 146 patients treated by partial thyroidectomy for hyperthyroidism classified 55 per cent as euthyroid, 5 per cent equivocal, 36 per cent hypothyroid and 6 per cent with recurrent hyperthyroidism. The incidence of post-operative hypothyroidism is related to the amount of gland removed, possibly to the iodine intake and, also, to the extent of the lymphoid infiltration of the gland. This can be predicted by estimation of thyroid antibodies, for the titre of thyroglobulin and/or microsomal antibodies correlates with the extent of the lymphocytic infiltration. Patients with negative tests for both antibodies stand a reduced chance of becoming hypothyroid. In the presence of low titres of antibodies there is about an 8 per cent risk, whereas patients with microsomal antibody titres of 1/32 or more have almost a 25 per cent risk of hypothyroidism within the first year after operation. Thus, high titres of microsomal antibodies are a relative contra-indication to operation.

The prevalence of recurrent hyperthyroidism varies from centre to centre but probably should not exceed 6 per cent. Hedley *et al.* (1971) have shown that partial thyroidectomy is associated with a fall in circulating thyroid antibodies including LATS. Two populations of patients can be detected: those in whom thyroid suppressibility returns to normal (70 per cent) where the prevalence of thyroid cytoplasmic antibodies and LATS is lower and where recurrent hyperthyroidism is rare; those in whom lack of thyroid suppressibility persists (30 per cent), the prevalence of thyroid cytoplasmic antibodies and LATS is higher and where recurrence is common.

Assessment of Thyroid Function after Thyroidectomy. Tests of thyroid function are difficult to interpret following thyroidectomy. High radioiodine values may result from iodide depletion occurring during preoperative antithyroid therapy. High $PB^{131}I$ values at 24 or 48 hours may be due to the lowered intrathyroidal iodine pool caused by surgery. The best tests are the PBI or T4 and T3 resin uptake from which the free-thyroxine index can be calculated. Following partial thyroidectomy, serum TSH levels almost invariably rise, in response to lower than optimal circulating levels of thyroid hormones. In patients who remain euthyroid the TSH level peaks a few months after operation then falls towards the normal range, presumably as thyroid regeneration restores thyroid hormone output. In patients who become hypothyroid TSH levels remain high indicating inadequate thyroid regeneration possibly due to a small thyroid remnant, to inadequate blood supply or to the presence of thyroiditis. A raised TSH level is not in itself an indication of clinical hypothyroidism but if the value is high (e.g. >30 μU per ml) and the routine thyroid function tests borderline and the patient has symptoms compatible with early hypothyroidism then a therapeutic trial of thyroid hormone is indicated.

Indications for Partial Thyroidectomy. These vary from clinic to clinic. If the regime suggested by Alexander is substantiated it will be possible to select those patients with hyperthyroidism who are prone to relapse after antithyroid drugs and advise surgery or radioiodine on the basis of serial T3 suppression tests. It is suggested that, at present, operation might be regarded as the treatment of choice (after preoperative preparation with antithyroid drugs) in the following groups of patients:

1. Patients with large goitres, especially if they are nodular or causing pressure effects.
2. Patients who relapse after a course of antithyroid drugs. Treatment of this group of patients should be flexible. Apart from the risk of a further relapse there is no reason why a further course of drugs should not be given if the patient wishes. Older patients may be given radioiodine therapy. Children or pregnant women may be given a further course of drugs or be treated by surgery.
3. Patients who prefer surgery to a course of drugs.
4. Patients who are unable to take drugs regularly because of toxic reactions or unreliability.
5. Patients who show failure of thyroid suppression after two years drug therapy.

Radioactive Iodine

Radioiodine therapy is an effective method of controlling hyperthyroidism and it causes no discomfort to the patient. The difficulty is to calculate the dose required to render the patient euthyroid—too small a dose will not control the hyperthyroidism, too large a dose will cause hypothyroidism. The amount of radiation given to the gland depends on many factors:

1. The dose of radioiodine given—this can easily be measured;
2. the proportion of the dose taken up by the thyroid—this can be determined by previous tracer tests;
3. the length of time the radioiodine stays in the gland—this can be assessed by tracer studies;
4. the volume of the gland in which the radioiodine is distributed, (the gland size)—a big variable in calculating the dose. Wilson and his colleagues (Smith and Wilson, 1967) have carefully controlled their clinical assessment of gland size by measuring the weight of thyroid removed at thyroidectomy, adding

on the estimated weight of the thyroid remnant. Another easier method is to cut out and weigh the paper outline of a thyroid scan, obtaining the frontal area of the gland. Multiplying this value by the mean height of the thyroid lobes and a constant 0.32 gives a rough figure for thyroid weight in grammes (Myhill *et al.*, 1965);

5. the radiosensitivity of the gland is probably variable and cannot be measured.

Indications for Radioiodine Therapy. These vary from clinic to clinic and only the general principles can be given.

1. Patients who relapse after thyroidectomy.

   This group should not be subjected to a second operation. Under the age of forty years, a course of antithyroid drugs can be used, over that age radioiodine treatment is recommended.

2. Patients over the age of forty.

   The age limit for radioiodine therapy varies, and in many clinics in the USA it is as low as twenty years. Because of the possible long-term hazards it is suggested that the upper age limit is preferable.

3. Patients in any age group who have a poor prognosis because of some other disease.

   In this group, for example patients with severe heart failure, long-term antithyroid drugs or radioiodine are equally satisfactory alternatives.

Complications of Radioiodine Therapy. 1. *Malignant Disease.* In adults there is no increase in thyroid carcinoma after radioiodine therapy, in fact the risk is possibly lower than in patients with hyperthyroidism. In children, again, there is no statistically significant increase, but in view of of the well-documented increase in thyroid carcinoma in children treated with external radiation to the head and neck for other conditions it is wise to use alternative treatment. There is no increase in the incidence of leukaemia in patients treated with radioiodine. There is no increase in the incidence at other sites of radioiodine concentration viz. salivary, gastric or bronchial glands.

2. *Hypothyroidism.* This is the commonest complication of radioiodine therapy, the incidence depending on the dose given. Using doses to deliver 8–10,000 rads to the thyroid, about 10 per cent of patients are hypothyroid at one year and about 40 per cent at ten years, with subsequent yearly increments of about 3 per cent. Although hypothyroidism is easily treated, there is difficulty in ascertaining all the patients who develop hypothyroidism, and the morbidity and mortality is significant. Because of this the low dose level radioiodine regime is recommended.

3. *Radiation at Other Sites.* The radiation dose to the ovaries is small and there is no increase in the incidence of congenital abnormalities in children of parents treated with ^{131}I for hyperthyroidism during childhood or adolescence. The parathyroid glands are irradiated by radioiodine—clinical hypoparathyroidism is very rare but diminished parathyroid reserve can sometimes be detected by refined tests.

There is no evidence for reduced calcitonin levels or bone disease resulting from radiation to the parafollicular cells.

Method of Use of Radioiodine. To reduce the risk of hypothyroidism, treatment with radioiodine can be given using a low dose, controlling hyperthyroidism in the meanwhile with antithyroid drugs. A dose of 3,500 rads is given—calculated by the method of Blomfield *et al.*, 1959. The incidence of hypothyroidism with this dose is 7 per cent after five years, and 85 per cent of patients are then euthyroid and do not need any therapy. The majority of patients require additional therapy with antithyroid drugs for the first year at least.

Alternatively many groups prefer to give standard doses such as 5mCi of ^{131}I irrespective of the size of gland, repeating this after six to nine months if the patient remains hyperthyroid. In many patients no other treatment is needed but in the elderly or those with severe hyperthyroidism antithytoid drugs or propranolol (for example 40 mg t.d.s.) can be used. The advantage of the latter is that it is possible to follow the response by thyroid function tests and assess if retreatment is necessary. The advantage of the former is that it can render the patient euthyroid and can be withdrawn after an interval to determine whether relapse is going to occur. Prior treatment with antithyroid drugs appears to confer some degree of radioresistance on the gland and is best avoided unless the hyperthyroidism is severe or the patient is elderly or has some other disease making urgent therapy desirable. Rendering the patient euthyroid with antithyroid drugs does prevent the acute hyperthyroidism seen in some patients treated with radioiodine usually within the first 72 hours after the dose. Such an exacerbation may be treated with propranolol and iodides.

Elderly patients or those with concurrent disease can be rendered rapidly euthyroid and inevitably hypothyroid with a large therapy dose of radioiodine. It is mandatory that every patient treated with radioiodine (or by partial thyroidectomy) should be followed up on a long-term basis, preferably by some automated follow-up scheme involving the general practitioner. If hypothyroidism ensues the patient should be stabilised on thyroxine, the need for life-long medication stressed and follow-up continued by the general practitioner. The problem of failure of medication is a difficult one, particularly in a population which is mobile.

Use of ^{125}I for Hyperthyroidism. Because of the two major disadvantages of ^{131}I therapy viz. slow control of hyperthyroidism and the high risk of hypothyroidism, Greig and his colleagues have pioneered the use of ^{125}I therapy. Radiation effects of ^{125}I are of shorter range than ^{131}I, being concentrated on the apex of the thyroid cell adjacent to the colloid which is active in hormone synthesis and release. Radiation to the nucleus which is nearer to the base of the cell is less with ^{125}I than with ^{131}I, hence the risk of nuclear damage and reduced cell growth and hypothyroidism is less. Until the effects of ^{125}I therapy have been established in terms of the rate of control of hyperthyroidism, and the long-term incidence of hypothyroidism and thyroid neoplasia, this isotope should be regarded as an experimental form of therapy and its use restricted to special centres with facilities for meticulous follow-up.

B. TREATMENT OF THE EYE SIGNS

In most patients with Graves' disease no treatment is required for the eyes. Lid retraction tends to get better as the patient is rendered euthyroid and she is usually satisfied with the improvement in her appearance. Exophthalmos, on the other hand, shows little change with therapy. Rundle described a group of 104 patients with Graves' disease followed up for fifteen years. In 5 patients the eyes receded by more than 2 mm, in 75 the prominence of the eyes remained unchanged, and in 24 it increased by more than 2 mm. Ophthalmoplegia improved in some two-thirds of the patients, and lid retraction disappeared in a similar proportion.

The commonest complaint, that of grittiness of the eyes, can often be helped by methyl cellulose eye drops, combined with antibiotics if there is any infection. When lid retraction is pronounced, the complaint of early morning soreness of the eyes suggests corneal exposure during the night due to inadequate lid closure. Retraction can be helped by 5 per cent guanethidine eye drops—one drop inserted into each eye night and morning. Keratitis must always be looked for by slit lamp examination when the patient complains of soreness of the eyes, especially while receiving guanethidine eye drops, and antibiotic drops prescribed if it is found. Corneal exposure from lid retraction and exophthalmos may necessitate tarsorrhaphy (suture of the lids preferably only at the lateral canthi) but this should usually be a limited procedure. Patients should be advised to wipe their eyes from the outer angle inwards if necessary, for if there is significant proptosis and this advice is not heeded the globe may be caused to proptose forward with the upper lid falling behind the globe. Tarsorrhaphy helps to prevent this as well as helping lid closure and improving the appearance.

Congestive Ophthalmopathy. Early symptoms of congestion of the eyes—pain and swelling of the lids, usually associated with exophthalmos and chemosis—may respond to diuretics and elevation of the head of the bed. When these features become progressive, which is rare, high doses of steroids should be employed, starting with 60 mg of prednisone daily, and increasing the dose in a few days if there is no improvement. Deterioration in vision not due to keratitis with or without papilloedema is an indication for immediate steroid therapy, and if there is not significant improvement over a day or two surgical decompression of the orbit should be carried out. This is a major neurosurgical procedure in which, through an anterior craniotomy and extradural approach, the lateral wall and roof of the orbit are removed and the orbital fascia incised. Such decompression will reduce the raised pressure within the orbit.

Many therapeutic regimes have been advocated for the ocular complications of Graves' disease, including total thyroidectomy, retrobulbar and sub-conjunctival injections of long-acting steroid preparations, pituitary ablation by surgery or by radioactive substances, radiation to the orbit, and drugs such as reserpine or thyroxine. None of these methods of therapy is of proven value and they are not recommended till further adequately controlled trials are carried out. The only value of treatment with thyroid hormone is to correct or prevent hypothyroidism.

C. TREATMENT OF LOCALISED MYXOEDEMA

If this is localised to small areas and is asymptomatic no treatment is indicated and there is often spontaneous improvement. More extensive disease causes difficulty in walking and discomfort and requires treatment. Probably the most effective therapy is the nightly application of locally active steroid creams, e.g. betamethasone under occlusive polythene dressings. This causes marked improvement, though treatment may have to be continued up to a year, and even then the condition sometimes relapses when it is stopped. Resistant areas usually respond to local infiltration with steroids, e.g. triamcinolone. Erythema doses of ultra-violet radiation may also cause improvement in the condition. Tissue overgrowth, seen particularly on the backs of the toes, may rarely require surgical removal and skin grafting.

NEONATAL GRAVES' DISEASE

Very rarely, children born to mothers with Graves' disease are found to be hyperthyroid at birth or shortly afterwards. A goitre is usually present, and this may be vascular. The pulse rate is high, and cutaneous vasodilation may be a striking feature. Undue restlessness and failure to feed properly and gain weight may give a clue to the diagnosis. Although ocular manifestations are much less striking than in the adult, swelling of the eyelids, lid retraction and minimal exophthalmos may be seen. Treatment should not be delayed longer than is required to confirm the diagnosis by PBI, T3 resin uptake, or an early thyroid radioiodine uptake. It should be remembered that the PBI is usually raised above the accepted normal range during the first week of life. Iodides and antithyroid drugs should be used in about half the adult dose. Treatment should be adjusted according to the clinical response and can be withdrawn altogether in three of four months when a complete recovery is made.

Neonatal Graves' disease is probably due to the transplacental passage of LATS and possibly other humoral agents. In most cases LATS can be recognised in the circulation of both mother and child. It disappears from the child, having a half-life of about one month (like other IgG molecules), and this coincides with the spontaneous remission of the disease. The mother usually gives a history of hyperthyroidism but is not usually hyperthyroid at the time. The risk is highest if the mother has localised myxoedema—LATS levels are usually very high in the presence of this condition. If the mother shows neither eye signs of Graves' disease nor localised myxoedema the chance of neonatal Graves' disease is remote.

Occasional cases of neonatal hyperthyroidism have been reported where the hyperthyroidism was more prolonged than would have been expected from the rate of catabolism of IgG. These may represent early onset Graves' disease superimposed on the neonatal syndrome since they have occurred in families with a high incidence of Graves' disease.

TOXIC MULTINODULAR GOITRE

Most workers in the thyroid field are impressed by the similarities between classical Graves' disease and toxic multinodular goitre rather than by their differences. Hyperthyroidism in older patients tends to be associated with greater nodularity of the goitre, and eye signs are less common, but there are many exceptions. In a number of patients with toxic multinodular goitre the excess of thyroid hormones is derived from overactivity of the paranodular tissue rather than of the nodules themselves. These patients are likely to have Graves' disease superimposed on a longstanding nodular goitre, and the finding of LATS in a proportion of these patients supports this view. However, scanning of the thyroid has shown that occasional patients with toxic multinodular goitre have one or more active nodules (*see* Toxic Adenoma, below).

Antithyroid drugs, partial thyroidectomy, or radioiodine can be used to treat the thyroid overactivity. Surgical treatment is more commonly employed if the gland is large and multinodular, especially if there are pressure effects. Radioiodine is less satisfactory, and a larger dose is needed than in the patient with classical Graves' disease.

TOXIC ADENOMA

This term is applied to patients with hyperthyroidism resulting from one or more functioning adenomas of the thyroid. Various types of functioning adenoma, some of which do not cause thyroid overactivity, can be recognised by thyroid scans. It is not certain whether or not the categories listed below represent the stages of evolution of the autonomous nodule.

1. Thyroid nodule present, scan normal, activity over rest of gland but not over nodule suppressed by T3.
2. Thyroid nodule present, scan shows increased uptake by nodule compared with rest of gland, uptake of nodule not suppressed by T3, uptake of rest of gland increased by TSH.
3. Thyroid nodule present, scan shows activity in nodule but none in rest of gland, nodule activity unaffected by T3, activity of rest of gland restored by TSH, patient euthyroid.
4. Thyroid nodule, hyperthyroidism present, scan findings as in 3 above.

The prevalence of toxic adenoma of the thyroid varies in different parts of the world. In this country it is uncommon, only some five per cent of cases with hyperthyroidism being caused by toxic adenoma; the disorder is much commoner in women, the maximum prevalence being between forty and sixty years of age. The secretory capacity of the nodule depends on its mass and on the iodine supply in the diet. The larger the nodule the more likely is it to produce thyroid hormone in excess.

Thyroid function tests are not infrequently equivocal in patients with toxic adenoma. Overproduction of triiodothyronine but not of thyroxine is not uncommon. Some adenomas produce an iodoprotein which is measured in the PBI but not in the serum T4 estimation. It is likely that in some patients the adenoma is producing more thyroid hormone than is optimal for the patient yet not sufficient to cause clinical hyperthyroidism. Some patients pass from this state of 'sub-clinical hyperthyroidism' to one of clinical hyperthyroidism.

Treatment of the autonomous adenoma gives excellent results, since usually the rest of the gland is normal. A small proportion of the adenomas in euthyroid patients are TSH-dependent and can be reduced in size by thyroid hormone. If thyroid hormone does not reduce the adenoma in three to six months, surgical removal is carried out. If the adenoma is causing hyperthyroidism, this can be controlled with antithyroid drugs though the response is often found to be poor. Surgical removal of the nodule after the patient has been rendered euthyroid is the treatment of choice. Radioiodine can be used but large doses may be required to eliminate overactivity. The incidence of subsequent hypothyroidism is lower because ^{131}I uptake by the rest of the gland is suppressed and it thus receives only a low dose of radiation.

JOD-BASEDOW PHENOMENON

When iodine is given to goitrous patients in areas of iodine deficiency an occasional patient develops hyperthyroidism. This occurrence is referred to as the Jod-Basedow phenomenon. Two possible factors may be responsible. Firstly, the hyperplastic gland of an iodine deficient patient may continue to take up iodine even when the deficiency is corrected, and an increased hormone production results. In this situation it is difficult to understand why the thyroid overactivity should persist after correction of the iodine deficiency. Secondly, iodine deficiency may be preventing overproduction of thyroid hormone in a patient with one or more autonomous adenomas (which are common in endemic goitre regions) or Graves' disease, and correction of the deficiency unmasks the latent disease. Because of the risk of inducing hyperthyroidism (albeit a small one), patients with goitres (especially those which are nodular), should not be treated with iodine unless there is clear evidence of iodine deficiency, or the iodine is being given as treatment for pre-existing hyperthyroidism.

THYROTOXICOSIS FACTITIA

Some patients enjoy the effects of thyroid overactivity and treat themselves with thyroid hormone. They exhibit the clinical features of hyperthyroidism without the eye signs of Graves' disease. They are easily recognised by tests, which show a suppressed thyroid radioiodine uptake. The PBI may be high, normal or low, depending whether the thyroid hormone preparation used is thyroxine, thyroid extract, or triiodothyronine respectively.

STRUMA OVARII

Overproduction of thyroid hormone may very rarely develop in thyroid tissue present in a struma ovarii. Thyroid uptake will be suppressed, but a scan may indicate the ectopic thyroid tissue.

ECTOPIC TSH SYNDROME

(*see* Chapters 10 and 20)

Hyperthyroidism may be associated with malignant disease. Usually this will represent the chance coincidence of two common diseases. Rarely, hyperthyroidism with increased thyroidal radioiodine uptake is caused by a thyroid-stimulating agent produced by gastro-intestinal tumours, bronchogenic carcinomas, or trophoblastic tumours.

THYROID ADENOMA

Classification

Thyroid adenomas are classified by their histology as follows: Embryonal, fetal, follicular, Hürthle cell, and papillary. They are all benign neoplasms of thyroid tissue.

CLINICAL FEATURES

Thyroid adenomas are commoner in women and are found in about three per cent of the population. Many are asymptomatic and may be found at a routine medical examination. The patient's complaint is of a lump in the neck, which is rarely large enough to cause pressure symptoms. Sudden enlargement may be caused by haemorrhage into an adenoma.

Examination reveals a nodule in the thyroid, the rest of the gland being impalpable. A lump in the thyroid should be referred to as a *nodule* not an adenoma, which is a histological diagnosis. Thyroid nodules may represent the largest nodule of a multinodular gland, a cyst, a localised area of thyroiditis, a thyroid carcinoma, or a thyroid adenoma. Lymphadenopathy suggests that a nodule is malignant but can occur in thyroiditis. Most adenomas increase slowly in size for many years. In younger patients the nodule is more likely to be single whereas in older age groups it is more likely to be the most obvious nodule in a multinodular gland. Symptoms of hyperthyroidism may develop from a thyroid adenoma or there may be only sufficient thyroid hormone produced to suppress the rest of the gland (subclinical toxic adenoma). Toxic adenomas are dealt with in the section on 'hyperthyroidism', p. 128. The true prevalence of thyroid carcinoma in the single thyroid nodule is not known because of the variable selection methods employed before a patient comes to surgery. An overall figure of about five per cent seems reasonable if the nodule is found by chance. If the nodule is symptomatic because of increasing size, pressure effects or pain the prevalence of carcinoma will be increased.

Routine tests of thyroid function are usually normal, and a scan may show an area of increased or reduced uptake or a normal thyroid outline. Areas of reduced uptake can be due to poorly functioning adenomas, cysts, or thyroid carcinomas. The nodule is usually about 1 cm in diameter before it can be detected clinically, and the scans now available are not more discriminating. Occasional autonomous nodules show suppression with T3, in these patients circulating thyroid antibodies are often present and the treatment of choice is thyroxine.

THERAPY

If a scan shows an area of reduced uptake three courses are available:

1. *No Therapy*. This may worry the patient and may delay treatment of a carcinoma. In children, particularly, a policy of waiting is to be deprecated because of the high incidence of papillary carcinoma in single nodules. In older patients where the nodule has been found incidentally a policy of observation may be justifiable.

2. *Thyroid Hormone*. Experience varies with this line of treatment. Some workers report a reduction of size of most nodules with full replacement doses of thyroid hormone, others are less impressed. It is reasonable to try the effect of thyroxine for a few months in some small asymptomatic nodules, in adults.

3. *Surgery*. When a patient complains of a lump in the neck, and a solitary nodule is found, with reduced uptake on a scan, many physicians would recommend exploration of the neck, biopsy of the nodule, and subtotal lobectomy if the nodule is benign. The authors agree with this policy with the reservation that in some instances no therapy is indicated and in others a trial with thyroid hormone may be attempted. Occasionally, subtotal lobectomy is carried out for what is thought to be a benign adenoma and the substantive pathology report returns several days later indicating a carcinoma. In this instance, if the carcinoma was well localised, a policy of observation may be followed. If incomplete removal is indicated re-exploration of the neck may then be justified.

THYROID CARCINOMA

Classification

Malignant tumours of the thyroid can be divided into two major groups: differentiated and anaplastic.

The differentiated group includes:

(*a*) papillary;
(*b*) follicular;
(*c*) medullary;

The anaplastic group includes:

(*a*) anaplastic carcinoma in which squamous cells, spindle cells, giant cells or small round cells predominate;
(*b*) malignant lymphoma.

Secondary invasion of the thyroid by carcinomas from breast, lung and kidney and malignant melanomas is rather more frequent than primary thyroid tumours. Table 5.20 provides a simple classification and the major features of the commonest malignant tumours of the thyroid.

Incidence

Thyroid carcinomas are rare, making up about 0·2 per cent of all carcinoma deaths in men and 0·5 per cent in women in the United Kingdom. The incidence of various types of carcinoma varies in different countries and in different centres. In 1966, 122 men and 287 women died of cancer of the thyroid in England and Wales.

TABLE 5.20 *Classification and Major Features of Malignant Tumours of the Thyroid*

Type	Histology	Incidence %	Average age years	Early spread	10 year survival %	Comments	Treatment
Papillary	Fronds of cells	60	40	Lymph nodes	80	Commonest variety in children	Radical surgery and radioiodine, suppressive doses of thyroid hormone
Follicular	Resembles normal thyroid	25	50	Blood-stream	60	Often mixed with papillary	Radical surgery and radioiodine, thyroid hormone
Anaplastic	Undifferentiated, variable	10	60	Local and distant	1		Palliative DXT
Medullary	Regular cells, amyloid in stroma	5	50	Local	50	Arises from parafollicular cells, secretes calcitonin and other humoral factors causing diarrhoea, familial syndrome with phaeochromocytomas, ectopic ACTH syndrome	Radical excision, radio-resistant
Lymphoma	Variable, reticulum cell sarcoma lympho-sarcoma	1	60	Local, may be multi-focal	?10	Associated with auto-immune thyroiditis and gastro-intestinal lymphomas	Palliative DXT

Aetiology

Despite many claims to the contrary there is no good evidence that non-toxic goitre of any variety predisposes to thyroid carcinoma. Most thyroid carcinomas develop in otherwise normal glands. Of course, if nodular goitre is common in a particular area a proportion of carcinomas will be found to develop in association with the pre-existing goitre but this does not imply an aetiological relationship. Malignant change in a thyroid adenoma is very rare. Because of the extremely slow growth of some thyroid carcinomas and because of the difficulty in distinguishing histologically some benign adenomas from follicular carcinomas, it may sometimes be impossible to separate the two conditions.

There is no doubt that external irradiation applied to the head and neck in childhood increases the risk of subsequent thyroid carcinoma, usually after a latent period of several years—average nine years. After radioactive iodine therapy in children thyroid nodules have been found to develop. Very rarely, these nodules are due to low grade thyroid carcinoma and it is for this reason that radioiodine therapy should be avoided in children. In adults given external or internal radiation to the thyroid there is no convincing evidence of a significantly increased incidence of thyroid carcinoma or leukaemia.

Thyroid carcinomas have been reported to occur in certain dyshormonogenetic goitres. Although invasion of blood vessels and thyroid capsule was demonstrated, the behaviour of the neoplasms did not indicate malignancy since no local or distant metastases occurred. Judgement must be reserved on this question.

Certain workers have reported a high incidence of thyroid carcinoma in Hashimoto's disease but there is no general agreement about this association. Subclinical thyroiditis is common and it is not surprising that lymphoid infiltration of a greater or lesser estent is found in many glands containing a thyroid carcinoma. Malignant lymphoma of the thyroid may be difficult to distinguish from thyroiditis and may, in fact, be associated with it. It is sometimes difficult to separate 'true malignant lymphoma' from a small round-cell carcinoma, and indeed from an active diffuse thyroiditis. The differing prognosis reported from patients in this category may reflect the different diseases included in this grouping. Some malignant lymphomas have been reported to metastasise to the alimentary tract, but this might represent a multifocal origin.

Pathology

Papillary Carcinoma. This is the commonest type of thyroid carcinoma, particularly in children. Columnar cells are arranged around stalks containing blood vessels. Papillary carcinomas often contain psammoma bodies which are laminated calcium-containing bodies of unknown origin that tend to appear in better differentiated tumours. Metastases occur by the lymphatics both inside and outside the gland even when the primary tumour is small. The so-called lateral aberrant thyroid is now known to be a metastasis from a small thyroid carcinoma. Long-term survival rates with treatment reach 80 per cent at ten years with this type of carcinoma. Certain papillary tumours may show areas with a follicular or solid pattern.

Follicular Carcinomas. Follicular carcinomas may show a great resemblance to normal thyroid tissue. Sometimes both the primary tumour and secondary deposits are indistinguishable from the normal thyroid. Usually, the malignant nature of the tumour can be recognised by invasion of blood vessels, thyroid capsule, and lymphatics. Papillary elements may be found in some areas. Invasion occurs predominantly by the blood stream, especially to bone, brain, and lung. Long-term survivals are less than for the papillary carcinoma group.

Medullary Carcinomas. Williams (1967) has clarified our knowledge of this rare type of differentiated thyroid carcinoma. The tumour is solid with a uniform yellowish-grey surface, well demarcated from the rest of the gland. The cells, occurring in solid nests, are usually regular in size and shape with granular cytoplasm and only a few mitoses. The stroma sometimes contains amyloid which may be calcified. Females are rather more often affected than males, the highest incidence being in the fourth decade. Prognosis is similar to that of other differentiated thyroid carcinomas despite the lack of papillary or follicular pattern. Growing evidence indicates that the tumour originates from the parafollicular cell system.

The unique associations and clinical features of the medullary carcinoma certainly distinguish it from other thyroid carcinomas and will be considered at this point. The associations of medullary carcinoma can be divided into two groups, genetic and humoral.

1. *Genetic.* The familial occurrence of medullary carcinomas has been reported, and phaeochromocytomas, often bilateral, may be found in some of the affected individuals. Other unusual inherited features that may be associated are multiple mucosal neuromas, especially of the eyelids and tongue, diffuse thickening of the lips, intestinal ganglioneuromatosis, pes cavus, a high arched palate, a proximal myopathy and skin pigmentation.

2. *Humoral.* Medullary carcinomas may secrete a variety of humoral agents affecting, particularly, plain muscle. Flushing attacks may be due to secretion of 5-hydroxytryptamine, and diarrhoea to release of prostaglandins. Cushing's syndrome caused by secretion of ACTH—like peptides from the tumour has been reported. Medullary carcinomas originate from the parafollicular cells that produce calcitonin and many patients have been described whose medullary carcinomas secrete calcitonin. Serum calcium and phosphate levels are almost invariably normal because extra parathormone is secreted to maintain the calcium level, and there are no overt skeletal abnormalities. Estimations of plasma calcitonin levels are helpful in the diagnosis of medullary carcinomas and are also useful in predicting complete removal of the tumour or its recurrence. Because of the lack of sensitivity of calcitonin immunoassays it may be necessary to measure calcitonin levels during a calcium infusion a procedure which stimulates calcitonin secretion. In view of the familial occurrence of the variety of medullary carcinoma associated with thickening of the lips and Marfanoid habitus it is wise to screen first degree relatives of the propositus by calcitonin measurements.

It has recently been shown that there is a high content of the enzyme histaminase in medullary carcinomas and detection of this enzyme in the circulation is associated with extrathyroidal deposits of the tumour. The enzyme is also present in normal kidney and ileum and can be detected in the serum during pregnancy and after the administration of heparin.

Biochemistry

Many of the more differentiated thyroid carcinomas are able to concentrate iodine although less well than normal thyroid, and in a few, iodotyrosines and iodothyronines are synthesised and released. Hyperthyroidism may result from a thyroid carcinoma but is rare. More often the tumour secretes an iodoalbumin which is not calorigenically active. A similar compound is also found in the thyroid and circulation in some congenital goitres, in Hashimoto's disease, and in thyrotoxicosis.

CLINICAL FEATURES

These depend on the type of tumour, its rate of growth, and the extent of its metastases. Most patients complain of a lump in the neck that is increasing in size. On occasion, the lump may have been present for many years. The lump may be painful and tender. Invasion of local structures causes hoarseness, dysphagia, and cervical lymphadenopathy. Rarely, the presenting feature is the result of a distant metastasis, e.g. bone pain or paraplegia. Examination usually reveals a single hard nodule in the thyroid; fixation of the gland or evidence of local spread are late signs. The criteria that warrant exploration of the neck in patients with Hashimoto's disease have been dealt with. Patients presenting with a multinodular goitre are only rarely found to have a thyroid carcinoma. Solitary nodules should be scanned. 'Hot nodules' are rarely malignant, 'cold nodules' may be malignant but more often are found to be cysts or poorly functioning adenomas. Undue hardness of a goitre may also be caused by fibrosis, as in Hashimoto's disease or Riedel's thyroiditis, or by calcification in a thyroid nodule. Cervical lymphadenopathy does not always indicate malignancy since it is found occasionally in Hashimoto's disease. It may also result from spread from other tumours or be due to a coincident reticulosis.

Diagnosis of thyroid carcinoma can often be made from the clinical features, but when diagnosis is uncertain it is best to explore the neck, biopsying any suspicious areas and sending these for frozen section. Treatment can then be adapted to the particular tumour found. A drill biopsy may give misleading results as well as implanting malignant cells in the needle track. Its only justification is in the seriously ill patient, when open biopsy is less desirable.

TREATMENT

Before undertaking treatment it is important to determine the nature and extent of the tumour. Most differentiated tumours have quite a good prognosis whereas the more anaplastic carcinomas are usually rapidly fatal. Four main methods of therapy are available which may be used alone or in combination.

1. Thyroidectomy
2. External radiation
3. Radioiodine
4. Thyroid hormone.

1. *Thyroidectomy* should be considered in all cases, especially if the tumour is differentiated. Total thyroidectomy should be undertaken only by an experienced thyroid surgeon who is able to protect the parathyroids and recurrent laryngeal nerves. A compromise procedure is adopted by some surgeons who prefer a hemi-thyroidectomy on the side of the lesion. Unfortunately, the contralateral lobe is not infrequently affected, either because of multifocal origin of the tumour or intrathyroidal lymphatic spread (seen particularly in papillary carcinoma). When lymph nodes are involved lymph node dissection is carried out—the mediastinal glands are easily accessible in some cases. Fixation of the gland to the trachea or recurrent laryngeal palsy indicates the tumour to be inoperable, as do distant metastases. In these cases thyroidectomy may still be justifiable if the tumour is differentiated to facilitate subsequent radioiodine therapy. In anaplastic carcinomas surgery is rarely of much use except to confirm the diagnosis.

2. *External radiation* is the treatment of choice for anaplastic carcinomas and the malignant lymphomas. Some of these are very radiosensitive and the tumour melts away only to return locally or at distant sites after an interval. This method of therapy is also effective for metastases, especially if these are painful.

3. *Radioiodine therapy* with the isotope ^{131}I is reserved for differentiated tumours of the papillary or follicular type which cannot be completely removed surgically. As total a thyroidectomy as possible is first performed by surgery or radioiodine, giving a dose of 150 mCi. Replacement therapy with thyroid hormone is withheld until the patient becomes hypothyroid or until uptake can be demonstrated by tumour

tissue. A further therapy dose of ^{131}I is then given checking the uptake over the tumour site by scanning techniques some five days after the dose. At this time blood is taken for measurement of plasma protein-bound ^{131}I. When the $PB^{131}I$ exceeds 0·004 per cent of the dose per litre of plasma, tumour tissue (which is secreting organically-bound radioiodine) can usually be detected. Afterwards replacement treatment with 0·2–0·3 mg of T4 or 20 μg four times daily of T3 is given. Scanning of the deposits is carried out a few months later after withdrawal of T4 for four weeks or of T3 for two weeks. Administration of TSH (e.g. 10 IU of bovine TSH intramuscularly) can enhance uptake of radioiodine even when T4 and T3 are continued, but repeated injections of animal TSH may lead to allergic reactions. Secretion of endogenous TSH can be stimulated by TRH injections or infusions without the risk of sensitivity reactions. Repeated scanning and treatment of tumour deposits should be performed until there is no residual activity. Long-term survival or 'cure' can be induced by this regime in more than half of patients with metastatic differentiated tumours. Normal thyroid tissue usually takes up radioiodine more avidly than malignant thyroid, hence it is not possible to decide that a malignant thyroid metastasis has failed to take up radioiodine until all normal thyroid tissue has been ablated by surgery and/or radioiodine and the ablation confirmed by scanning after a large tracer dose. The first ablation dose of ^{131}I after a surgical diagnosis of thyroid carcinoma may merely ablate the residual normal gland preparing the field for subsequent and repeated treatment of the metastases. If a substantial amount of normal thyroid tissue has been left after surgery, this is ablated with a smaller dose of ^{131}I such as 80 mCi before administering a 150 mCi dose to the metastases. About three months are allowed to elapse between these treatments.

4. *Thyroid hormone* administration suppresses pituitary TSH output on which some tumours depend for their growth. It is well worthwhile treating most patients with thyroid carcinoma as it is difficult to predict which tumours are hormone dependent. The maximum therapeutic dose should be used (0·2 to 0·4 mg of thyroxine daily). Triiodothyronine may be useful since its effects wear off more rapidly and allow the neck and metastases to be scanned for evidence of recurrence. A full replacement dose would be 20μg three or four times daily.

REFERENCES

Laboratory Diagnosis of Thyroid Disease

Alexander, W. D., and Harden, R. McG. (1967). *Brit. med. J.*, **1**, 669.

Burke, C. W., Shakespear, R. A., and Fraser, T. R. (1972). *Lancet*, **ii**, 1177.

Chan, V., and Landon, J. (1972). *Lancet*, **i**, 4.

Chan, V., Besser, G. M., Landon, J., and Ekins, R. (1972). *Lancet*, **ii**, 253.

Clark, F. (1963). *Lancet*, **ii**, 167.

Clark, F., and Horn, D. B. (1965). *J. clin. Endocrinol.*, **25**, 39.

Crooks, J., Murray, I. P. C., and Wayne, E. J. (1958). *Lancet*, **i**, 604.

Ekins, R. P., Williams, E. S., and Ellis, S. (1969). *Clinical Biochemistry*, **2**, 252.

Goolden, A. W. G., Bateman, D., and Torr, S. (1971). *Brit. med. J.*, **2**, 552.

Hall, R., Ormston, B. J., Besser, G. M., Cryer, R. J., and McKendrick, M. (1972). *Lancet*, **i**, 759.

Hall, R. (1972). *Clin. Endocr.*, **1**, 115.

Hesch, R. D., and Evered, D. C. (1973). *Brit. med. J.*, **1**, 645.

Larsen, P. R. (1972). *Metabolism*, **21**, 1073.

McGowan, G. K., and Sandler, M. (Eds) (1967). 'Symposium on the thyroid gland,' *J. clin. Path. Suppl.*

Ormston, B. J., Garry, R., Cryer, R. J., Besser, G. M., and Hall, R. (1971). *Lancet*, **ii**, 10.

Refetoff, S., Robin, N. I., and Alper, C. A. (1972). *J. clin. Invest.*, **51**, 848.

Sandler, G. (1959). *Brit. Heart J.*, **21**, 111.

Thorson, S. C., Mincey, E. K., McIntosh, H. W., and Morrison, R. T. (1972). *Brit. med. J.*, **2**, 67.

Van't Hoff, W., Pover, G. G., and Eiser, N. M. (1972). *Brit. med. J.*, **4**, 203.

Wayne, E. J. (1960). *Brit. med. J.*, **1**, 1478.

Wayne, E. J., Koutras, D. A., and Alexander, W. D. (1964). *Clinical Aspects of Iodine Metabolism*. Oxford: Blackwell.

Non-toxic Goitre and Hypothyroidism

Calder, E. A., McLeman, D., Barnes, E. W., and Irvine, W. J. (1972). *Clin. exp. Immunol.*, **12**, 429.

Evered, D., and Hall, R. (1972). *Brit. med. J.*, **1**, 290.

Fagge, C. H. (1871). *Med.-Chir. Trans. Lond.*, **54**, 155.

Gull, W. W. (1874). *Trans. clin. Soc. Lond.*, **7**, 180.

Hall, R., Dingle, P. R., and Roberts, D. F. (1972). *Clinical Genetics*, **3**, 319.

Halliburton, W. D. (1893). *J. Path. Bact.*, **1**, 90.

Kilpatrick, R., Milne, J. S., Rushbrooke, M., Wilson E. S. B., and Wilson, G. M. (1963). *Brit. med. J.*, **1**, 29.

Means, J. H. (1948). *The Thyroid and its Diseases*, 2nd Edition. Philadelphia: Lippincott.

Murray, G. R. (1891*a*). *Proc. Northumberland and Durham med. Soc.*, p. 91.

Murray, G. R. (1891*b*). *Brit. med. J.*, **2**, 796.

Ord, W. M. (1878). *Med.-Chir. Trans. Lond.*, **61**, 57.

Osler, W. (1898). *Principles and Practice of Medicine*, 3rd Edition. New York: Appleton.

Semon, F. (1883). *Brit. med. J.*, **2**, 1073.

Wayne, E. J. (1960). Ibid., **i**, 1.

Hyperthyroidism

Adams, D. D. (1965). *Brit. med. J.*, **1**, 1015.

Adams, D. D., and Kennedy, T. H. (1967). *J. clin. Endocrinol.*, **27**, 173.

Alexander, W. D., Harden, R. M., Skimmins, J., McLarty, D., and McGill, P. (1967). *Lancet*, **ii**, 681.

Blomfield, G. W., Eckert, H., Fisher, M., Miller, H., Munro, D. S., and Wilson, G. M. (1959). *Brit. med. J.*, **1**, 63.

Cassano, C., and Andreoli, M. (Eds) (1965). *Current Topics in Thyroid Research*. London: Academic Press.

Crooks, J. (1967). 'The diagnosis of hyperthyroidism,' in 'Symposium on the Thyroid Gland' (G. K. McGowan and M. Sandler, Eds), *J. clin. Path., Suppl.*, 373.

Crooks, J., Murray, I. P. C., and Wayne, E. J. (1959). *Quart. J. Med.* (N.S.), **28**, 211.

Evered, D. C., Hayter, C. J., and Surveyor, I. (1972). *Metabolism*, **21**, 393.

Hedley, A. J., Flemming, C. J., Chesters, M. I., Michie, W., and Crooks, J. (1970). *Brit. med. J.*, **1**, 519.

Hedley, A. J., Ross, I. P., Beck, J. S., Donald, D., Albert-Recht, F., Michie, W., and Crooks, J. (1971). *Brit. med. J.*, **4**, 258.

Hollander, C. S., Shenkman, L. (1972). *Brit. J. Hosp. Med.*, Oct., 393.

Irvine, W. J. (Ed.) (1967). *Thyrotoxicosis. Proc. Edinburgh Symposium*. Edinburgh: E. S. Livingstone.

Kriss, J. P., Pleshakov, V., and Chien, J. R. (1964). *J. clin. Endocrinol.*, **24**, 1005.

Logan, W. P. D., and Cushion, A. A. (1958). *Morbidity Statistics from General Practice*, Vol. 1 (General). London: HMSO.

McGowan, G. K., and Sandler, M. (Eds) (1967). 'Symposium on the thyroid gland,' *J. clin. Path., Suppl.*

Morris, C. J. (1962). *Proc. roy. Soc. Med.*, **55**, 540.

Myhill, J., Reeve, T. S., and Figgis, P. M. (1965). *Amer. J. Roentgenol.*, **94**, 828.

Pitt-Rivers, R., and Trotter, W. R. (Eds) (1964). *The Thyroid Gland*, Vol. 2. London: Butterworth.

Smith, B. R., Dorrington, K. J., and Munro, D. S. (1969). *Biochim. Biophys. Acta*, **192**, 277.

Smith, R. N., and Wilson, G. M. (1967). *Brit. med. J.*, **1**, 129.

Taylor, G. W., and Painter, N. S. (1962). *Lancet*, **i**, 287.

Werner, S. C., and Platman, S. R. (1966). *Lancet*, **ii**, 751.

Thyroid Carcinoma

Doniach, I. (1963). 'Aetiological considerations in thyroid carcinoma,' in *The Thyroid and Its Diseases* (A. S. Mason, Ed.). London: *Pitman Medical*, p. 106.

Halmar, K. E. (1963). 'Choice of treatment for thyroid carcinoma,' in *The Thyroid and Its Diseases* (A. S. Mason, Ed.). London: *Pitman Medical*, p. 112.

Lindsay, S. (1964). 'Pathology of the thyroid gland,' in *The Thyroid Gland*, Vol. 2 (R. Pitts-Rivers and W. R. Trotter, Eds). London: *Butterworth*, p. 223.

Tata, J. R., and Pochin, E. E. (1964). 'Thyroid cancer,' in *The Thyroid Gland*, Vol. 2 (R. Pitt-Rivers and W. R. Trotter, Eds). London: *Butterworth*, p. 208.

Williams, E. D. (1967). 'Medullary carcinoma of the thyroid,' in 'Symposium on the Thyroid Gland' (G. K. McGowan and M. Sandler, Eds), *J. clin. Path., Suppl.*, p. 395.

6

ADRENAL

ANATOMY AND EMBRYOLOGY

The adrenal cortex and medulla have separate embryological origins, the cortex being derived from mesoderm, and the medulla from ectoderm. In mammals, the cortex encloses the medulla, but in fish the cortex and medulla exist as distinct entities. At about the fifth week of fetal life, mesodermal cells near the base of the dorsal mesentery migrate dorsally to form the fetal adrenal cortex. These cells are soon invested by a further layer of cells, from the same origin, which form the permanent cortex. By the eighth week the adrenal is larger than the kidney, its main bulk being derived from the fetal cortex which begins to atrophy at birth and disappears by the end of the first year of life. The fetal cortex depends on ACTH stimulation, as it is absent in the anencephalic fetus, but can be restored by administration of ACTH. By the third week of life the adrenal weight is half that at birth, but it is not until the third year of life that the permanent cortex is fully differentiated into its three zones (*see* below).

The adrenal medulla is, like the sympathetic neurones, derived from ectodermal cells of the neural crest. These chromaffin cells, so called because they stain brown with chromium salts, invade the medial side of the cortex at about the seventh week of intrauterine life to take up their central position within the gland.

Accessory adrenal glands made up of cortex and medulla are occasionally found in adult life in the cortex of the kidney or in the region of the coeliac plexus. Separate cortical or medullary components occur more frequently in various sites on the posterior abdominal wall and in the pelvis. Cortical tissue may be found in close relationship to the testis or ovary, reflecting their similar embryological origin.

There are two adrenal glands, lying retroperitoneally, one at the upper pole of each kidney. The right gland is triangular in shape and is related posteriorly to the right crus of the diaphragm, anteriorly and above to the right lobe of the liver, and is bounded laterally by the kidney and medially by the inferior vena cava. The left gland is more semilunar in shape and is related posteriorly to the diaphragm and splanchnic nerves, anteriorly in its upper two-thirds to the lesser sac and below to the pancreas and splenic vessels, medially to the aorta and laterally to the kidney.

In normal children up to twelve years, each adrenal weighs 1·5 to 3 g. In adults the average weight of the normal gland is 4 g with an absolute range in both sexes of 2 to 6 g, but at autopsy the weight varies depending on the cause of death. The lower part of each adrenal contains more medulla than the upper, the cortex-medullary ratios being 5:1 and 18:1 respectively.

HORMONES OF THE ADRENAL CORTEX AND THEIR MEASUREMENT

Although more than 40 steroids have been isolated from the human adrenal cortex, the main ones found in adrenal vein blood are cortisol, corticosterone, aldosterone, dehydroepiandrosterone (DHA), androstenedione, and 11-hydroxyandrostenedione. The human adrenal secretes each day about 25 mg of cortisol, 2 mg of corticosterone, 200 μg of aldosterone and 25 mg of DHA.

These hormones can be grouped into three types according to their main metabolic activities:

1. Glucocorticoids, principally cortisol and small amounts of corticosterone.
2. Mineralocorticoids, principally aldosterone and small amounts of desoxycorticosterone.
3. Androgens, e.g. dehydroepiandrosterone (DHA), androsterone and testosterone.

In addition, small amounts of oestrogens and progesterone are produced.

STRUCTURE OF STEROID HORMONES

Natural and synthetic steroids contain three 6-carbon rings labelled A, B, and C, one 5-carbon ring labelled D, and certain side chains. The carbon atoms are numbered as shown in Fig. 6.1. The simplest method of classifying natural steroids is by the number of carbon atoms in the molecule. (Note that C_{21} means a molecule with 21 carbon atoms, but C-3 refers to carbon atom number three.) Corticosteroids, a term which includes glucocorticoids and mineralocorticoids, are C_{21} compounds; androgens are C_{19} compounds, and oestrogens C_{18} derivatives (Fig. 6.2).

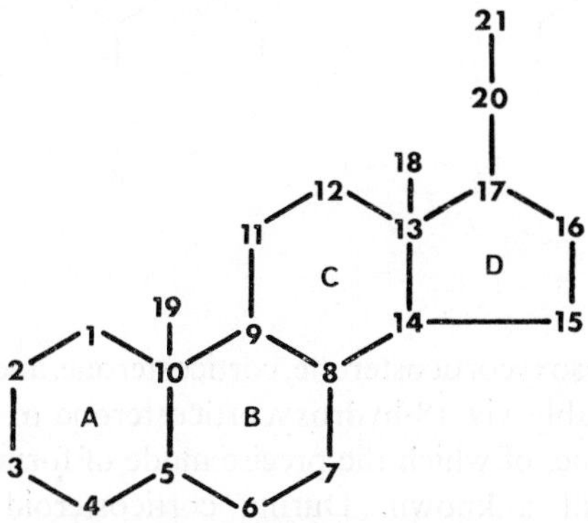

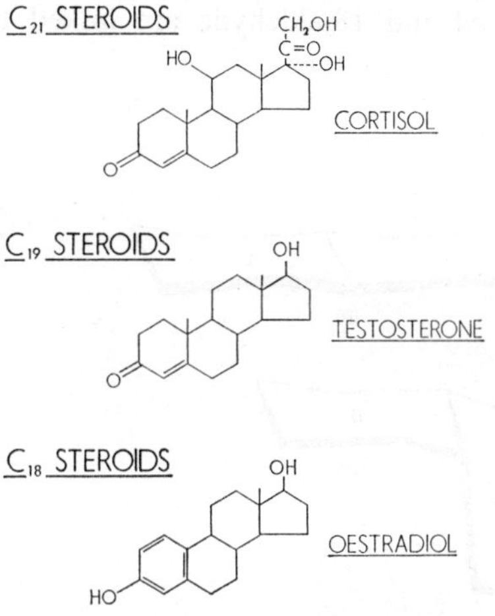

21
20
18
12 17
11 13 16
C D
19
9 14 15
1
2 10 8
A B
3 5 7
4 6

FIGURE 6.1 Corticosteroid structure showing numbering of carbon atoms and lettering of rings

C_{21} STEROIDS
CH_2OH
C=O
HO
OH
O
CORTISOL

C_{19} STEROIDS
OH
O
TESTOSTERONE

C_{18} STEROIDS
OH
HO
OESTRADIOL

FIGURE 6.2 Types of steroid produced by the adrenal cortex

Stereoisomerism related to rings A and B is termed 'cis' and 'trans', rings C and D always being in the 'trans' position in biological compounds (Fig. 6.3). Any substitution in rings A and B is related to the methyl group at C-10, which is considered to be above the plane of the ring. Alpha groups lie below the plane and are linked by a dotted line; beta groups lie above the plane and are linked by a solid line. All active corticosteroids have a 17α-hydroxyl group and a 21'β'-alpha ketol grouping

CH_2—C—
| ‖
OH O

at carbon 17. The 11-hydroxyl group of the natural corticosteroids is in the β-position. Desoxycorticosterone which lacks a hydroxyl group at C-11 is only a very weak glucocorticoid. All active steroids (except DHA) have a double bond between carbon atoms four and five (Δ^4) and an oxygen atom attached to C-3. *Aldosterone* has an aldehyde group (—CHO) attached to C-18 and is capable of existing in two forms, in one of which the 11-hydroxyl and 18-aldehyde are linked to form the hemiacetal. The natural hormone is d-aldosterone. The *androgens*, which contain 19 carbon atoms, have an oxygen atom at C-17, hence their designation 17-oxosteroids (also called 17-ketosteroids).

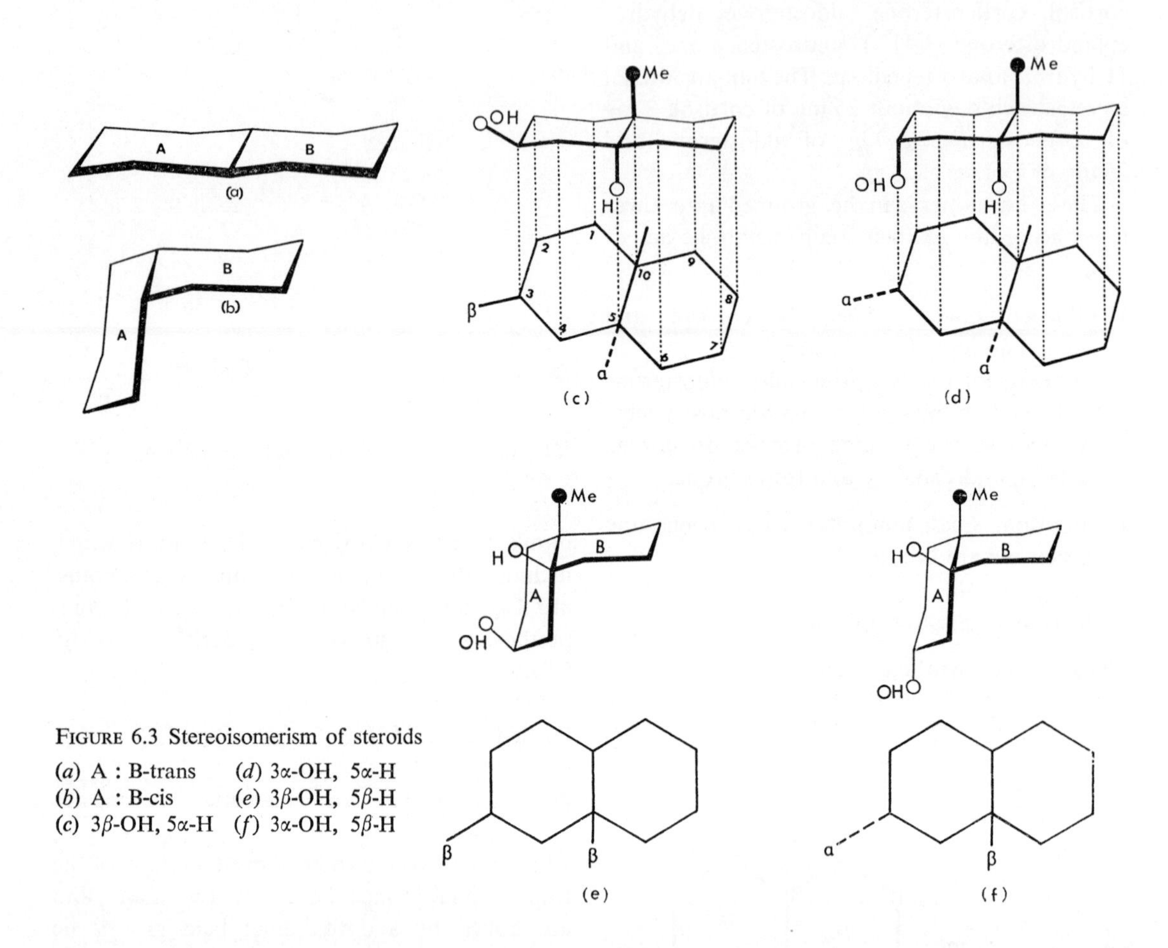

FIGURE 6.3 Stereoisomerism of steroids

(*a*) A : B-trans (*d*) 3α-OH, 5α-H
(*b*) A : B-cis (*e*) 3β-OH, 5β-H
(*c*) 3β-OH, 5α-H (*f*) 3α-OH, 5β-H

BIOSYNTHESIS OF STEROIDS (Fig. 6.4)

Cholesterol and its esters are largely derived from acetate and are stored in the lipid-rich cells of the zona fasciculata. Δ^5-pregnenolone is then formed and is a precursor of all types of adrenal corticosteroids. Individual enzyme steps via progesterone, 17α-hydroxyprogesterone, and 11-desoxycortisol lead to cortisol production. Alternatively, progesterone may be converted to 11-desoxycorticosterone, corticosterone, and then probably via 18-hydroxycorticosterone to aldosterone, of which the precise mode of formation is still unknown. During corticosteroid biosynthesis hydroxyl groups are introduced at positions 11β, 17α, and 21β of the steroid nucleus. The various enzymes involved in steroid biosynthesis can be isolated from different cell fractions, e.g. 11β-hydroxylase is largely in mitochondria, 3β-dehydrogenase is in the so-called microsomal fraction, while both the 17- and 21-hydroxylating systems are in the soluble fraction of the cell. This distribution may not, however, represent the true location of the enzymes *in vivo*. During androgen biosynthesis, 17α-hydroxy-pregnenolone is converted into DHA and, hence, into the other androgens. DHA has an androgenic potency somewhere between 3 and 20 per cent that of testosterone. Small amounts of testosterone are normally synthesised by the adrenal, though larger quantities are produced in some patients with hirsutism. Like testosterone, oestrogens are normally produced in very small quantities by the adrenal and it is only in certain rare adrenal tumours that significant amounts of oestrogens are released.

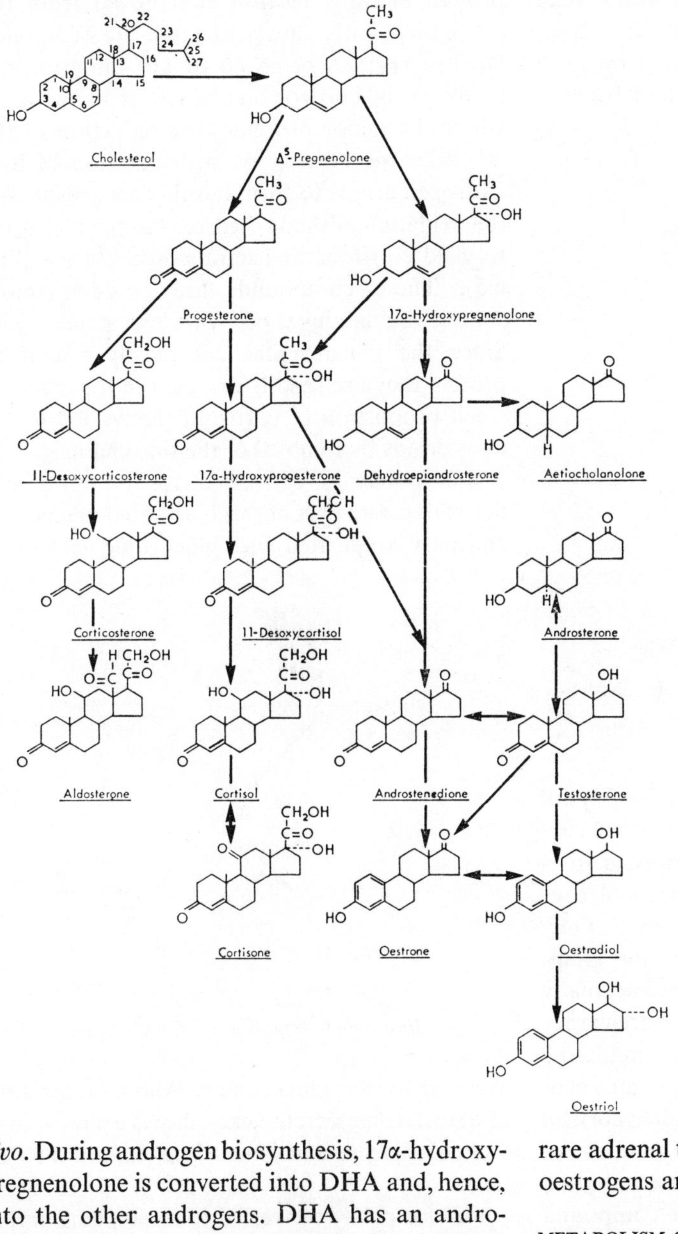

FIGURE 6.4 Biosynthesis of steroids in the adrenal

METABOLISM OF CORTICOSTEROIDS

(*a*) *Protein Binding*. Most of the cortisol entering the bloodstream is bound to protein, especially to an α-globulin termed transcortin. This protein has a much higher affinity for cortisol than has albumin though the total capacity of albumin for cortisol is much greater because it is present in much larger amounts. Usually, more than 95 per cent of the cortisol present in the circulation is bound to protein, this portion being in equilibrium with the free or unbound fraction

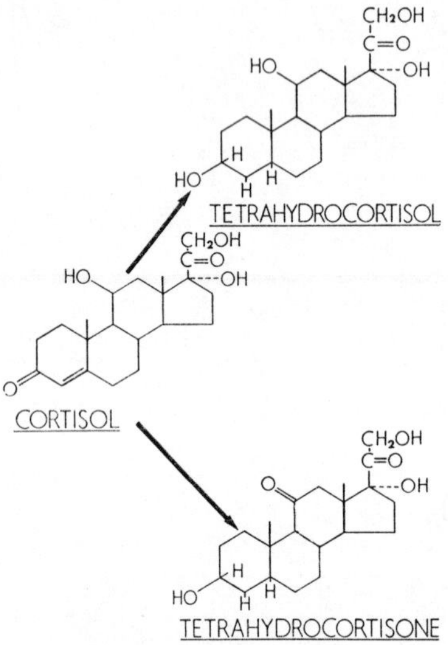

FIGURE 6.5 Conversion of cortisol to tetrahydrocortisol and tetrahydrocortisone

that is able to enter cells and exert its physiological effect. As the blood levels of cortisol rise, the cortisol binding capacity of transcortin is exceeded and the amount of free cortisol rises and may exceed 25 per cent of the total. Only the free hormone can be filtered by the glomerulus, so that the amount of cortisol normally found in urine is very small. During pregnancy or after oestrogen administration circulating levels of transcortin rise, increasing the amount of bound cortisol, but since the level of free cortisol is normal there are no clinical features of cortisol excess. Because of the increase in bound cortisol the rate of destruction of the compound is reduced during pregnancy. In cirrhosis and certain dysproteinaemias, there is a decrease in cortisol binding power. Normally, about 60 per cent of aldosterone is bound to albumin but this fraction is reduced when albumin levels fall, e.g. in the nephrotic syndrome.

(*b*) *Degradation.* Because of the high degree of protein binding, *cortisol* is removed from the circulation fairly slowly, the half-life of injected labelled cortisol being 80 to 110 minutes. The main site of cortisol breakdown is in the liver, where the major processes are reduction of the Δ^4, 3-ketone of ring A, with addition of four hydrogen atoms to form tetrahydrocortisol, and the oxidation of the 11-hydroxyl to the 11-ketone to yield cortisone and tetrahydrocortisone (Fig. 6.5). These compounds are rendered more soluble by conjugation with glucuronic acid. Since the glucuronides are poorly bound to protein they are readily excreted in the urine. A small proportion of cortisol is converted to 17-oxosteroids by removal of the side chain.

Aldosterone is converted to its tetrahydro derivative, and part of this is excreted unchanged and part conjugated with glucuronic acid to be excreted as the glucuronide. About 5 per cent of aldosterone secreted each day is excreted as a 3-oxo-conjugate and only 0·5 per cent in the free form.

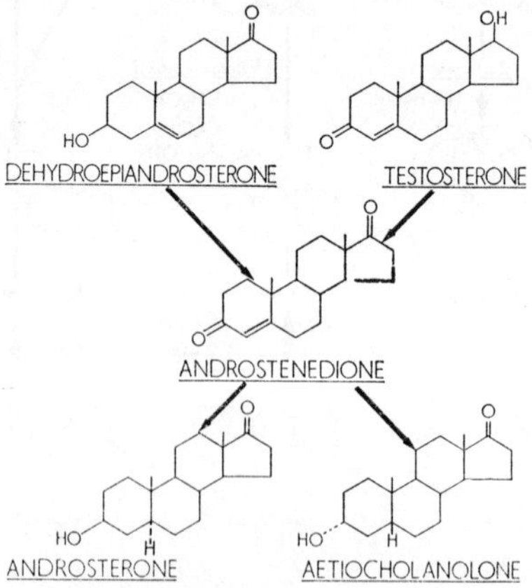

FIGURE 6.6 Metabolism of androgens

DHA is partly converted to its sulphate and is also metabolised to aetiocholanolone and androsterone. Androstenedione is similarly converted to these two compounds (Fig. 6.6).

(*c*) *Renal Excretion.* The kidney excretes steroids and their metabolites, the amounts excreted depending on the extent of protein binding, which largely determines the amount filtered, and the tubular reabsorption. Only 10 per cent of filtered cortisol is excreted because of tubular reabsorption. Less than 80 μg of cortisol are found in the urine each day and about 60 μg of cortisone.

DETERMINATION OF THE RATE OF SECRETION OF CORTICOSTEROIDS

The rate of secretion of corticosteroids can be determined by measurements of:

1. Gland steroid content.
2. Adrenal vein steroid output.
3. Blood concentration of steroids.
4. Renal excretion of steroids.

Only methods (3) and (4) are routinely possible in man. Blood estimations have the disadvantage that they represent only one point in time, and it is known that the adrenal output of steroids is variable and, in addition, usually only microgram amounts are measured. Urinary measurements are prone to all the risks of incomplete collection but do give a measure of steroid output over a longer time and, therefore, much larger amounts are involved. Traditionally assessment of adrenocortical activity in health and disease has depended on estimation of the corticosteroid metabolites in urine, but these only indirectly relate to true cortisol secretion or excretion, and may often be misleading. Since the introduction by Mattingly in 1962 of a rapid and reliable plasma corticosteroid assay, assessment of adrenocortical activity has switched more and more to plasma measurements since the ease of their assay has made frequent sampling during dynamic test procedures a practical proposition. Diagnostic reliability has greatly improved as a result.

CORTISOL AND ITS METABOLITES

Compounds having a 17-hydroxyl group and a 'dihydroxyacetone' type of side chain react with the Porter-Silber reagent (phenylhydrazine and strong sulphuric acid) to give a yellow colour, and are referred to as 17-hydroxycorticosteroids (17-OHCS). These compounds include cortisol, cortisone, and their tetrahydro metabolites, as well as other interfering chromogens, but not pregnanetriol. The method is more widely used in the USA than in the United Kingdom and is usually applied to urine corticosteroid estimations. It has in the past also been used for blood corticosteroid measurements but is tedious to perform and has a low capacity. It has now been replaced by fluorescence or protein binding techniques.

The urinary corticosteroid method most favoured in Europe depends on the destruction of existing 17-oxosteroids (17-OS) in the urine by sodium borohydride and the subsequent oxidation of the side chain on C-17 by sodium bismuthate. The 17-oxosteroids produced are derived from 17α-hydroxyprogesterone, pregnanetriol, 11-desoxycortisol, cortisol, cortisone, and their tetrahydro compounds cortol and cortolone. Various substances such as glucose and meprobamate interfere with the reaction but the method is simple, rapid, and reproducible. Normal values for men and women at different ages are shown in Fig. 6.7. The term 17-oxogenic steroids is used to signify the group of steroids measured by the sodium bismuthate reaction without destroying the existing 17-oxosteroids which are allowed for by a separate estimation.

Routine estimation of corticosteroids in blood and urine have been greatly facilitated by the method of Mattingly, which measures the total (protein bound and free) cortisol concentration together with the small amount of corticosterone present. The technique involves extraction of plasma or urine with methylene chloride and measurement of fluorescence in the presence of concentrated sulphuric acid and ethanol. There is a small amount of non-steroid fluorescence amounting to about 2 to 4 μg/100 ml equivalent of cortisol. Plasma fluorogenic corticosteroids (often inaccurately but more simply called 'plasma cortisol') vary with the time of day, the 9.30 a.m. values range from 8 to 26 μg/100 ml in adults. Levels are lowest at midnight and maximal between 6 and 8 a.m. Plasma cortisol can also be measured by 'protein-binding' methods, in which radioactively labelled cortisol competes with the unlabelled cortisol extracted from the plasma, for the binding sites on transcortin. The source of the transcortin is plasma obtained from oestrogen-treated or pregnant patients in whom transcortin levels are high. The more cortisol there is in the original blood sample, the less labelled cortisol will bind and by comparing the amounts bound with those obtained when standard solutions of cortisol are assayed, the original concentrations can be calculated. This method is no more specific than the fluorimetric assay since it also measures corticosterone, and it is rather less convenient, but the non-steroid background is less. Both the fluorimetric and protein binding methods of cortisol assay may be used to measure the amount of free corticosteroids excreted in the urine and this is a sensitive index of the amount of cortisol excreted per day (*see* Appendix).

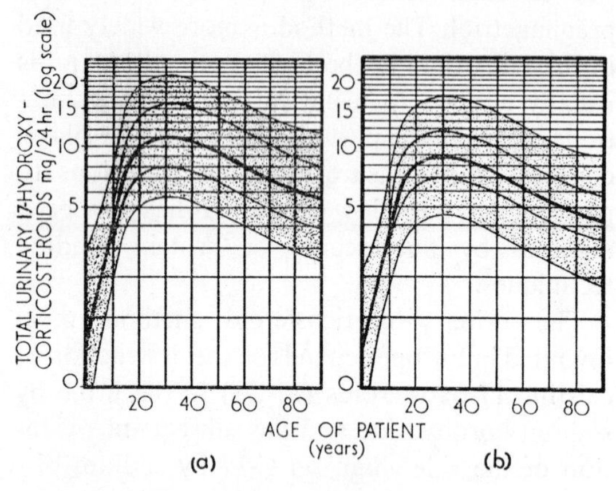

FIGURE 6.7 Urinary 17-hydroxycorticosteroid excretion (*a*) men, (*b*) women. (Linder, A., and Riondel, A. (1957), *Acta Endocr. Kbh.*, **25**, 33)

The secretion rate of cortisol can be determined by an isotope dilution method. Isotopically labelled cortisol (usually ^{14}C-cortisol) is administered, and the secretion rate of naturally produced cortisol calculated from the formula—

$$\frac{\text{administered steroid} \times \text{specific activity of administered steroid}}{\text{specific activity of unique urinary metabolite}}$$

A unique metabolite is one derived solely from the steroid hormone being investigated, e.g. tetrahydrocortisol or tetrahydrocortisone in the case of cortisol. Cortisol secretion rates in normal subjects range from 5 to 28 mg/day with a mean of 16 mg/day. The test is time-consuming and requires considerable technical skill as well as requiring the administration of a radioisotope to a patient (though only a small amount of radiation is involved).

During pregnancy, the plasma levels of corticosteroids rise, reaching a peak at the ninth month, normal values being restored by the sixth day after delivery. The rise in cortisol is due to increase in hepatic production of transcortin, so that most of the circulating corticosteroid is protein bound and metabolically unavailable. The free hormone concentration only rises slightly. After the first week children have plasma steroid levels similar to those of adults, although no circadian rhythm for several months.

ALDOSTERONE AND ITS METABOLITES

Aldosterone estimations in urine are not readily available for routine use since methods are tedious and require high technical skill. Satisfactory techniques for determining plasma levels have only recently been developed, but again are technically very difficult. A mean urinary excretion in normal subjects of 10·5 μg/24 hr has been reported (range 4·6–18·9 μg). Output is lowest at night and shows a peak at noon. No sex difference has been demonstrated. Potassium administration, sodium restriction, or a decrease in extracellular fluid volume can stimulate aldosterone output. During pregnancy, the urinary output of aldosterone increases six-fold.

Plasma aldosterone levels are extremely low—mean 6 μg/100 ml (range 2 to 15 μg). Only 65 per cent of aldosterone in the plasma is bound to protein. Most of the aldosterone is removed from the blood during passage through the liver, which is its major site of degradation. Secretion rates can be determined by isotope dilution methods, the mean figure being about 130 μg/24 hr (range 50 to 200 μg).

ANDROGENS AND THEIR METABOLITES

The adrenal androgens are largely excreted as 17-oxosteroids in the urine. In the male, only 24 per cent of testosterone from the testis is converted to 17-oxosteroids, mainly androstenedione and, hence, to androsterone and aetiocholanolone, which are measured as 17-oxosteroids in the urine. The 5-hydrogen atom of aetiocholanolone lies above the plane of the molecule, which is therefore called a 5β-compound. In androsterone, which has the same formula, the 5-hydrogen atom lies below and the compound is said to have the 5α-configuration. Most of the 17-oxosteroids in the urine are rendered more soluble by conjugation with glucuronic and sulphuric acids. Measurement of 17-oxosteroids depends on the colour produced by their reaction with m-dinitrobenzene in the presence of alcoholic potassium hydroxide, the so-called Zimmerman reaction. The effect of other compounds in the urine that produce a colour in this reaction can be eliminated by readings at several wavelengths, and the application of a correction factor. Some drugs, such as meprobamate, can interfere with the reaction.

DHA can be separated from most of the other oxosteroids because of its 3β-hydroxyl grouping, which allows its precipitation by digitonin. It is found in large amounts in the urine of some patients with adrenal carcinoma and was formerly thought to be derived only from the adrenal but it is now known to be produced in the ovary and testis in addition. Much of the DHA present in blood is in the form of sulphate ester though the role of this ester has not been defined.

Androsterone is derived from DHA, testosterone, and androstenedione. Aetiocholanolone has a similar origin but can also be produced from 17-hydroxyprogesterone. 11-oxygenated oxosteroids are mainly formed from cortisol and its metabolites though this forms only a minor pathway of cortisol degradation. During pregnancy, metabolites of progesterone may be estimated along with 17-oxosteroids but refined techniques indicate that there is no elevation of true 17-oxosteroid output. The urinary 17-oxosteroid levels are low in children, rising at puberty. Adult levels are somewhat higher in the male, largely because of the greater contribution of the testis than the ovary. The highest values are found in early adult life and decline with age (Fig. 6.8). Since so little testosterone is converted to 17-oxosteroids, and it is a very potent androgen, marked virilisation can occur due to over-secretion of testosterone, yet there may be no change in 17-oxosteroid excretion.

PHYSIOLOGY OF CORTISOL

The factors which regulate cortisol secretion, via ACTH, are:

1. the circadian rhythm,
2. the negative feedback and
3. stress mechanisms.

The latter is the most powerful of the three.

Plasma cortisol concentrations are not normally constant throughout the day, being highest just before waking, then under quiet conditions gradually falling throughout the day to reach their lowest values at about the time of retiring, only to begin rising again some four hours before waking. This circadian rhythm is maintained by pituitary ACTH secretion and is controlled by an intrinsic 'biological clock' mechanism within the midbrain, and is mediated by variations in corticotrophin-releasing factor (CRF) secretion from the median eminence of the hypothalamus. CRF passes down the capillary plexus of the pituitary stalk to act on the basophil cells of the anterior pituitary causing them to synthesise and release ACTH and also β-MSH. Unlike lower species, there is very little α-MSH in the human pituitary gland which contains no intermediate lobe cells, and only β-MSH appears to be secreted in man, and then apparently always with ACTH. In addition to the circadian rhythm, there is another control mechanism 'feedback'. Thus the stress mechanism is much more powerful than the others, and very high levels of plasma cortisol may be achieved during physical or psychological stress, higher than those ever seen under basal conditions. If this stress response fails due to adrenocortical insufficiency resulting from adrenal gland disease (primary adrenocortical failure), pituitary (secondary) or hypothalamic (tertiary) disease, then

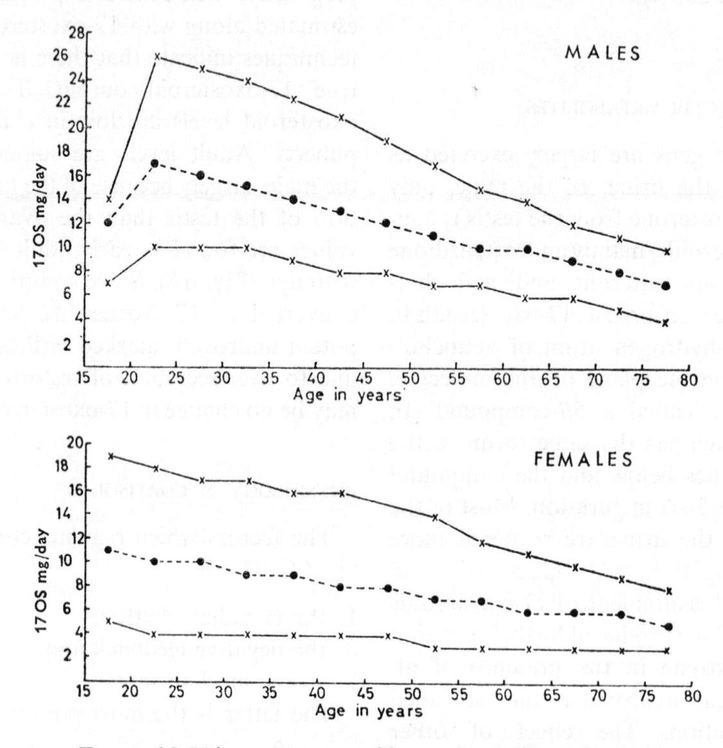

FIGURE 6.8 Urinary 17-oxosteroid excretion (Mills, I. H., 1964)

which operates under basal conditions, the negative feedback, whereby CRF, ACTH and therefore cortisol secretion are reduced or inhibited when plasma corticosteroid levels are too high, and increased when corticosteroid levels are inappropriately low. Finally the third control system is that which operates during stress. Under stressful conditions CRF, ACTH and cortisol secretion are promptly increased, irrespective of the time of day or operation of the the patient is likely to collapse in circulatory failure, although the mechanisms whereby cortisol allows the body to cope with stress are unknown. The control of ACTH secretion is further discussed in Chapter 1.

Some of the *main actions* of cortisol and other glucocorticoids are listed in Table 6.1. The relationships between the biochemical and physiological properties of the corticosteroids are uncertain. Deamination of amino-acids is increased because of enhanced activity of enzymes involved in deamination and transamination. Cortisol is known to enhance the activity of many enzymes by a process of enzyme induction, particularly in the liver. It is also able to stabilise the membranes of the lysosomes that contain many proteolytic enzymes. Though the physiological significance of this action is unknown it may be responsible for the anti-inflammatory action of cortisol.

TABLE 6.1 *Main Actions of Cortisol*

Carbohydrate, protein and fat metabolism:	Enhances gluconeogenesis; peripheral antagonism to insulin along with growth hormone causes hyperglycaemia and may lead to permanent diabetes mellitus; causes centripetal distribution of fat, hyperlipaemia and hypercholesterolaemia.
Anti-inflammatory:	Decreases all components of inflammatory response, reduces passage of fluid and cells out of capillaries, reduces fibrous tissue formation.
Immunological:	In large doses causes lysis of lymphocytes and plasma cells with release of antibody; subsequently, antibody levels are lowered.
Water metabolism:	Enhances water diuresis, prevents shift of water into cells, maintains extracellular fluid volume, antagonises vasopressin action on renal tubule, increases vasopressin destruction by liver, and may suppress vasopressin output from posterior pituitary.
Haemopoiesis and haemostasis:	Lowers eosinophil and lymphocyte counts, increases neutrophil leucocytes, red cells and platelets, increases clotting tendency.
Gastro-intestinal:	Increases gastric acid and pepsin production, reduces gastric mucus; in excess, may cause peptic ulceration.
Cardiovascular:	Sensitisation of arterioles to the action of noradrenaline, thereby maintaining blood pressure; enhances production of angiotensinogen which can then increase angiotensin level which, in turn, stimulates aldosterone output; in excess causes atherosclerosis.
Skeletal:	Impairs both growth hormone secretion from the pituitary and also its actions on the tissues; impaired formation of cartilage, decreased bone formation and osteoporosis, decreased absorption of calcium from the gut (where cortisol antagonises action of vitamin D), increased renal excretion of calcium.
Neuromuscular:	Increased slow wave activity on EEG, lowers threshold for electrical excitation of brain; both deficiency and excess cause psychiatric disturbances and muscular weakness.

CLINICAL EFFECTS OF CORTISOL

OVERPRODUCTION OF CORTISOL (Cushing's syndrome)

The term Cushing's syndrome is used to describe the clinical disorder that results from supraphysiological levels of corticosteroids in the circulation whether this is endogenously produced or administered to the patient. Certain patients with Cushing's syndrome may also show features of androgen excess, especially if the disorder is due to an adrenal adenoma or carcinoma. Like many endocrine diseases, Cushing's syndrome may vary in severity in an individual patient, and spontaneous remissions have occasionally been reported.

AETIOLOGY (*see also* Chapter 1)

The syndrome may be divided into two main groups depending on whether or not the condition derives from exposure to excess ACTH:

ACTH Dependent Causes:

1. Pituitary-dependent bilateral adrenocortical hyperplasia, conventionally called Cushing's disease, due to increased pituitary ACTH secretion.
2. The ectopic ACTH syndrome—secretion of ACTH by malignant or benign tumours of non-endocrine origin.
3. Iatrogenic—resulting from treatment with ACTH or its synthetic analogues.

Non-ACTH Dependent Causes:

1. Adenomas or carcinomas of the adrenal cortex.
2. Iatrogenic—resulting from treatment with supraphysiological doses of corticosteroids.

Clearly the feature distinguishing the two main groups is that there is detectable ACTH in the circulation in the first, whereas in the second group circulating ACTH levels will be very low or undetectable.

When the iatrogenic and ectopic groups are excluded, pituitary-dependent Cushing's disease comprises 80 per cent of the cases, whereas adenomas and carcinomas each make up about 10 per cent.

In *Cushing's disease* although there is increased ACTH secretion, the abnormality probably lies at the hypothalamic level resulting in excessive CRF secretion. Instead of a normal circadian rhythm of ACTH and cortisol secretion, a continuous secretion is found. Although the blood corticosteroid levels may not be elevated outside the normal morning range in early cases, they remain at these levels all the time and are thus too high throughout the second half of the day and early night. The excess exposure of the adrenal cortex to ACTH results in hyperplasia so that glands above the normal maximal size (6 g each) are found. About 20 per cent of patients with Cushing's disease have an enlarged pituitary fossa when they are first seen, due to the presence of an expanding pituitary tumour. A higher proportion have tiny microadenomas. The tumours are usually basophilic but only rarely are large enough to compress the visual pathways. Very rarely they may be locally invasive.

Adrenocortical tumours, either adenomas or carcinomas, may secrete very large amounts of cortisol, often with various androgens, especially DHA and, occasionally, aldosterone. Atrophy of the contralateral adrenal is caused by suppression of ACTH production by the steroids produced by the adrenal tumour although occasionally they are bilateral. Adrenal rests in spleen and ovary or other sites may be the site of tumours or may rarely lead to a recurrence of

Cushing's disease after bilateral adrenalectomy. Extra-adrenal carcinomas, especially of lung, may secrete ACTH-like peptides in very large amount, stimulating the adrenals to produce extremely high quantities of cortisol. This is the so called ectopic ACTH syndrome and is dealt with in Chapter 20. Adrenocortical carcinomas are the commonest cause of Cushing's syndrome in childhood.

CLINICAL FEATURES

Cushing's syndrome is a disease affecting women four times more commonly than men and has a peak age incidence between 35 and 50 years. The major clinical signs are obesity, purple striae, excessive bruising, hypertension, hirsutism, osteoporosis, and spontaneous fractures.

Obesity is mainly of proximal distribution and is responsible for the characteristic appearance of the patients. The reason for this unusual localisation of fat is unknown, the face, supraclavicular fossae, the area over the seventh cervical vertebra, and the abdomen are particularly affected. Cortisol stimulates appetite, liberates glucose from gluconeogenesis, which is available for fat synthesis, and reduces peripheral glucose utilisation.

Hypertension is one of the contributors to death in patients with Cushing's syndrome. Salt retention, induced by cortisol, may be one factor causing the hypertension but cortisol probably also has a direct action on the peripheral vessels synergistic with the catecholamines. Associated with the hypertension, oedema, heart failure and cardiac arrhythmias may be found.

Purple striae may be found on the arms, breasts, abdomen or thighs even in patients who have not become unduly obese. They must be distinguished from the paler pink striae often seen in obese patients, particularly in girls, or pregnant women, and which result from stretching of the skin by the increased fat. In Cushing's syndrome, loss of protein from the skin renders it unduly fragile and thin, and this is a useful clinical sign. The *polycythaemia* often found in Cushing's syndrome is possibly a minor factor in determining the colour of the striae but, associated with the thinning of the skin, it is largely responsible for the facial plethora. *Excessive bruising* is common, especially on the legs, and may be due to capillary weakness, possibly resulting from loss of protein from the vessel wall. *Osteoporosis* of the spine and *spontaneous fractures*, which typically occur in the ribs, femora and feet, are said to be due to loss of the protein matrix of bone. They heal badly and are often accompanied by excessive callus formation. *Hirsutism* is not usually associated with clitoral hypertrophy except in occasional adrenal tumours. The fine downy overgrowth of hair produced by cortisol can sometimes be distinguished from the coarser androgen-determined hairs associated with the high androgen levels produced by some adrenal tumours. *Muscular weakness* of proximal distribution, so-called Cushing's myopathy, may be prominent in some cases, where the loss of muscle mass may cause the limbs to appear unduly thin. Few patients with significant Cushing's syndrome can rise from the squatting position without assistance. *Menstrual disturbances* are common, either amenorrhoea or irregular menstruation may occur and impotence is common in men. *Psychoses*, irritability or emotional instability are frequent and do not always revert with treatment of the disease. *Polyuria* and *nocturia*, with undue *thirst* may occur without glycosuria although the cause is unknown. *Hyperglycaemia* and *glycosuria* develop in some patients because cortisol interferes with the action of insulin and this is usually reversible with correction of the hypercortisolaemia. *Skin pigmentation* of Addisonian type is found in some patients with Cushing's disease who may mention that they tan more easily or that scars have become pigmented. Such pigmentation is found when both ACTH and β-MSH levels are high, and indicates that there is likely to be bilateral adrenal hyperplasia which may be due to a pituitary tumour or to a malignant tumour, usually of the lung. It is most common after total adrenalectomy for

Cushing's disease (*see* later), but is not seen with adrenocortical adenomas or carcinomas.

DIAGNOSIS

In most patients with Cushing's syndrome the diagnosis is obvious and tests are required merely to document the raised cortisol production, determine its cause, and to look for complications. Occasionally, the disease may be so early, so mild, or so fluctuant in its course that diagnosis is impossible and the clinician must be content to observe the patient over a longer period of time.

Investigations are required to *confirm the overproduction of cortisol* and then to *determine the cause* of this abnormality. The excess of cortisol may be determined indirectly by certain metabolic effects of cortisol or directly by measurement of corticosteroid production.

Direct evidence of cortisol overproduction can be made by measurement of the *cortisol production rate* by the technique of isotope dilution. This is the absolute test for Cushing's syndrome against which all other tests must be compared, but because the method is difficult less direct estimations must suffice.

Plasma cortisol levels can be used to demonstrate cortisol overproduction. The earliest sign may be loss of the normal circadian rhythm, and a *raised midnight cortisol* level is of much value in diagnosis; less often the morning levels are raised. In normal patients the midnight plasma cortisol rarely exceeds 8 μg/100 ml (Fig. 6.9). When taking blood for this estimation, care must be taken not to alarm the patient as even minimal stress may cause a rise in cortisol production and it is best taken when the patient has been asleep, as soon as possible after waking.

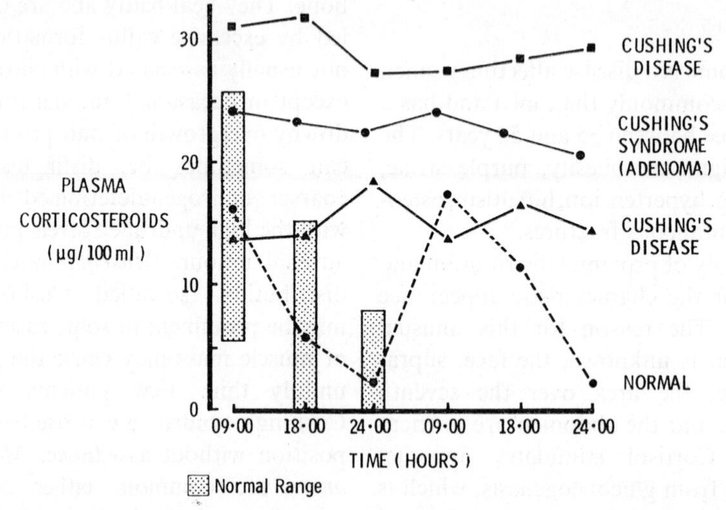

FIGURE 6.9 Circadian rhythm of plasma fluorogenic corticosteroids in one normal subject, two patients with Cushing's disease and one with an adrenal adenoma and Cushing's syndrome (from Besser and Edwards, *Clinics in Endocrinology*, Vol. 1, No. 2, 1972, by permission of the Editor).

Estimation of the *urinary 17-hydroxycorticosteroids* (17-OHCS) or *oxogenic steroids* (17-OGS) is useful in severe cases of Cushing's syndrome but when cortisol over-production is moderate, urinary tests often show values within the normal range. At higher levels of cortisol production the 24-hour urinary 17-OHCS output is approximately half the cortisol production rate. 17-*oxosteroid* (17-OS) *output* in the urine is even less helpful in the diagnosis of Cushing's syndrome except in those cases due to adrenal tumours where androgen output is often high. Much of the raised 17-oxosteroid output in Cushing's syndrome is due to 11-oxygenated oxosteroid products of cortisol metabolism, but, since only a small fraction of cortisol is metabolised by this route, only minimal increases in 17-OS output are to be expected. In some patients there is also a minor qualitative alteration in the pattern of 17-OS excretion, the reason for which is unknown. By far the most useful urinary excretion test for routine use involves measurement of the *urinary fluorogenic corticosteroids* (*see* Appendix) by the method of Mattingly. Most patients with Cushing's syndrome show a raised 24-hour excretion, which correlates surprisingly closely with the cortisol production rate. Values over 320 μg/24 hr are usually obtained in Cushing's syndrome but because of the fluctuations in steroid output from day to day, several estimations should be carried out. Determination of the true urinary free cortisol output by protein binding is also very helpful, though the estimation is more time-consuming. Both these tests are based on the fact that small elevations of the plasma cortisol increase the percentage of free cortisol in the plasma and, hence, its excretion in the urine.

The tests described so far for the confirmation of a suspected diagnosis of Cushing's syndrome allow estimation of adrenocortical function under basal conditions. They are not entirely satisfactory since complete urine collections are not always easy to obtain especially in outpatients, and both these and plasma cortisol levels may be altered by stressful situations such as infection, pain, anxiety or depression. Under these conditions the increased adrenocortical activity is appropriate to the stressed condition of the patient and a Cushingoid state does not develop even though there is an increased cortisol production rate.

To differentiate these situations from Cushing's syndrome two dynamic test procedures may be used. Since for ACTH the feedback control mechanism is set to a supranormal level in Cushing's disease, or the condition is not dependent on pituitary ACTH in patients with the ectopic ACTH syndrome or adrenal tumours, adrenal corticoid production will not be switched off by doses of dexamethasone which suppress the adrenals of normal patients. Plasma or urinary cortisol or 17-OHCS, or 17-OGS may be measured. Endocrinologically normal patients, but not those with any cause of Cushing's syndrome, will suppress adrenocorticoid output when given 2 mg *dexamethasone* daily for two days (as 0·5 mg four times a day). Dexamethasone does not interfere with the estimations of the corticosteroids and adequate suppression has occurred if the morning plasma fluorogenic corticosteroids have fallen to 6 μg/100 ml or less, urinary fluorogenic corticosteroids to 60 μg/day or less or urine 17-OHCS or 17-OGS to less than 5 mg/day, on the second day of dexamethasone. An overnight dexamethasone suppression test has been described (1·5 mg given on retiring, plasma cortisol taken on waking should be less than 7 μg/100 ml) but is less reliable. The 2 mg per day or 'low dose' dexamethasone suppression test is reliable for screening patients suspected of having Cushing's syndrome, and is particularly valuable in differentiating the obese patient. However, inadequate dexamethasone suppression may still be found in a stressed patient without Cushing's syndrome. A very reliable test in the diagnosis of Cushing's syndrome is the *insulin tolerance test* since patients who have Cushing's syndrome do not increase their plasma cortisol levels despite a fall in blood sugar below 40 mg/100 ml and sweating (*see* Appendix and Chapter 1). This is because the inappropriately elevated cortisol levels have suppressed the hypothalamic response to stress. It is sometimes necessary to give larger doses of insulin than usual (0·3 to 0·5 units/kg body weight, instead of 0·15 units/kg) to obtain adequate hypoglycaemia since cortisol has anti-insulin actions. The test should not be performed if there is myocardial ischaemia. A rise of plasma cortisol of at least 8 μg/100 ml excludes Cushing's syndrome, and such increments are retained in stressed patients without Cushing's syndrome, even if they have elevated plasma or urinary cortisol levels. A further feature of Cushing's syndrome is an impaired growth hormone response to hypoglycaemia.

Thus the following tests are useful for *establishing a diagnosis* of Cushing's syndrome irrespective of the precise cause:

1. Abolition of the circadian rhythm of plasma cortisol,
2. Raised urinary corticosteroids,
3. Resistance to suppression of blood or urine corticosteroids on dexamethasone 2 mg daily for 2 days.
4. Failure of plasma cortisol to rise during adequate insulin-induced hypoglycaemia.

Tests 2 to 4 may be used as screening tests in outpatients.

Once overproduction of cortisol is confirmed and a diagnosis of Cushing's syndrome established, it is necessary to determine which of the various causes is present (*see* p. 148). Undoubtedly *plasma ACTH* measurements by radioimmunoassay offer the quickest and most reliable means of making this differential diagnosis (Fig. 6.10).

If ACTH is detectable in the plasma the cause of the Cushing's syndrome is Cushing's disease

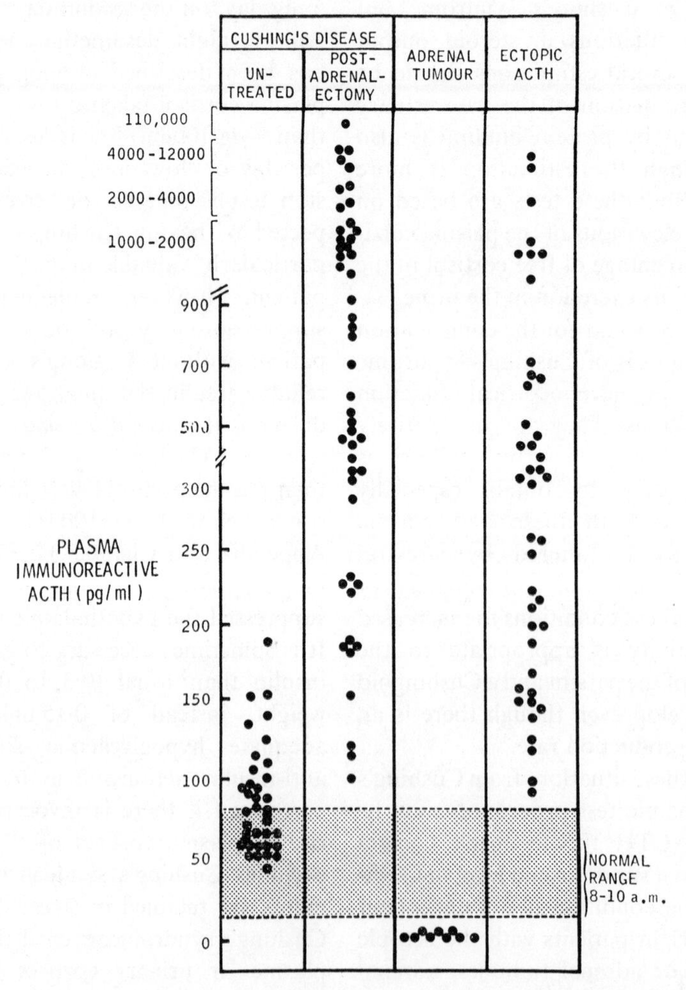

FIGURE 6.10 Plasma immunoreactive ACTH levels in 137 cases of Cushing's syndrome (from Besser and Edwards, *Clinics in Endocrinology*, Vol. 1, No. 2, 1972, by permission of the Editor).

(pituitary-dependent adrenocortical hyperplasia) or the ectopic ACTH syndrome, the latter being favoured if the levels are very high (over 200 pg/ml). If ACTH is undetectable then the patient has an adenoma or carcinoma of the gland. Unfortunately plasma ACTH assays are not widely available so less reliable differential tests have sometimes to be used.

Of the remainder the *metyrapone* test is the best. This drug blocks 11-hydroxylation of corticosteroids (the last step in cortisol synthesis) so that plasma cortisol falls, ACTH secretion increases and pre-cortisol metabolites accumulate and are excreted as 17-OHCS or 17-OGS in urine. When the hypothalamic-pituitary output of ACTH is suppressed as in patients with adrenocortical tumours producing Cushing's syndrome or in the ectopic ACTH syndrome, there will be little or no increase in ACTH, pre-cortisol metabolites or urinary 17-OHCS or 17-OGS. However in pituitary ACTH dependent Cushing's disease there will be a very great ACTH increase and an exaggerated urinary corticosteroid response, thus differentiating the causes. Details of the test procedure is given in the Appendix.

A *high dose dexamethasone* suppression test is often recommended to differentiate Cushing's disease from adrenal adenomas or ectopic ACTH production. When 8 mg per day of dexamethasone is given (2 mg four times daily) to patients with Cushing's disease, most will show at least 50 per cent suppression of plasma or urinary corticosteroids since the negative feedback control of ACTH production is still operating in this condition but at a higher level than normal. No suppression is seen with other causes of Cushing's syndrome. However negative suppression or even a paradoxical rise in corticosteroids is not infrequently seen in Cushing's disease and the test is therefore not reliable.

In summary the following tests may be used to *differentiate between the different causes* of Cushing's syndrome:

1. Plasma ACTH assay—present or elevated in Cushing's disease and ectopic ACTH syndrome, absent in adrenal tumours.
2. Metyrapone test—excessive responses in Cushing's disease, absent or impaired in adrenal tumours or ectopic ACTH syndrome.
3. Suppression with high dose (8 mg/day) dexamethasone given for 2 days in Cushing's disease, not in adrenocortical tumours or ectopic ACTH syndrome.

Indirect evidence of cortisol excess can be obtained by haematological and radiological investigations and by estimation of the electrolytes. Cortisol stimulates red cell and polymorph production, causing polycythaemia and a polymorph neutrophil leucocytosis with a low eosinophil count. The plasma sodium level is often at the upper end of the normal range, and hypokalaemia is especially marked in patients whose Cushing's syndrome results from a bronchogenic carcinoma, when it is usually accompanied by an elevated plasma bicarbonate, indicating an extracellular alkalosis. Cortisol, like aldosterone, facilitates the exchange of potassium for hydrogen ions at the distal renal tubule. This is thought to cause an intracellular acidosis which is compensated by the loss of hydrogen ions in the urine producing the extracellular alkalosis. X-rays of the bones may show osteoporosis and pathological fractures; chest X-rays a bronchogenic carcinoma; and skull X-ray an enlarged pituitary fossa. If the latter is enlarged, examination of the visual fields is mandatory. A glucose tolerance test may indicate diabetes mellitus.

Further information about the site of the underlying lesions may be obtained before proceeding to therapy. This may have been demonstrated by the initial X-rays, e.g. a pituitary tumour or a bronchogenic carcinoma secreting ACTH. Pelvic examination should always be carried out in women to exclude an ovarian tumour producing cortisol. A plain X-ray of the abdomen may show calcification in an adrenal tumour, usually a carcinoma. An intravenous pyelogram may indicate downward displacement of the kidney or distortion of the calyces by an adrenal tumour. Perirenal air or oxygen insufflation is rarely performed these days to determine adrenal size. Both adrenals may appear normal or enlarged if there is bilateral adrenal hyperplasia, or one enlarged and one small if there is an adrenal tumour, though false positive and negative results are not infrequent. Aortography can be modified to render the adrenals visible in some cases, and the increased vascularity of a tumour may be a helpful finding. Retrograde injection of dye up the adrenal veins may outline a tumour. Renal or adrenal vein catheterisation may also be performed to obtain blood samples to lateralise an adrenal tumour by differential cortisol assay. However the tumours may be bilateral and catheterisation of adrenal veins is difficult.

DIAGNOSTIC DIFFICULTIES

Most patients suspected of Cushing's syndrome referred to an endocrinologist are obvious examples of obesity due to over-eating. Striae, when present, are pale or pink; there is no thinning of the skin, and muscle-wasting and weakness are absent. Many obese females have rather more body hair than the average female but it is not usually of the same pattern or type as that produced by cortisol. Obese patients share some of the abnormalities of cortisol metabolism seen in Cushing's syndrome. They may have a slightly raised cortisol production rate, even when this is corrected for weight or surface area, and this abnormality returns to normal after weight loss. Their urinary cortisol output falls in the upper normal range. They retain the normal hypothalamic control of ACTH production and unlike patients with Cushing's syndrome show a normal circadian pattern of plasma cortisol levels. This test is most helpful in difficult cases as it is usually abnormal in even the mildest cases of Cushing's syndrome and the corticosteroids in blood and urine usually suppress normally during a low dose dexamethasone suppression test.

Another diagnostic problem is the woman with the polycystic ovary syndrome. Such patients frequently have obesity, hirsuties, menstrual irregularity, and infertility. Corticosteroid output from the adrenal is normal though the urinary 17-OS output is often slightly elevated. Urinary cortisol output is normal and so is the circadian rhythm of plasma cortisol. Ovarian enlargement can be demonstrated by pelvic examination, by peritoneal air insufflation, by culdoscopy, or by laparoscopy.

TREATMENT

If a diagnosis of Cushing's syndrome can be established, efforts should be made to treat the condition. In children, the cortisol excess interferes with growth hormone action and permanent stunting of growth may ensue. In adults, the most serious complication is hypertension with the enhanced risk of renal, cardiovascular, and cerebral sequelae; osteoporosis and diabetes mellitus are further hazards. Treatment will obviously depend on the cause of the Cushing's syndrome.

Adrenal adenoma and carcinoma should have been diagnosed from the criteria mentioned previously. Treatment involves removal of the affected adrenal. If the site of the tumour has not been determined before laparotomy, the surgeon using an anterior approach will note the atrophy of the unaffected adrenal. After removal of an adrenal tumour the residual atrophic adrenal can be revived by a course of ACTH but, as in the case of long-term steroid therapy, the major hazard lies in failure of the hypothalamic ACTH releasing mechanism, which may remain impaired for many months.

Metastatic adrenal carcinoma can be treated with o,p'D.D.D., an amphenone-like substance that has a direct toxic action on adrenocortical tissue (Hutter and Kayhoe, 1966). Unfortunately, the drug may cause intractable nausea and anorexia in therapeutic doses and usually has only a transient effect on the tumour.

Extra-adrenal carcinoma causing Cushing's syndrome can easily be missed since the wasted pigmented patient is not always suspected of having an endocrine disorder (*see* Chapter 20). However, cortisol production is usually greatly increased, causing the serum potassium to be lower than in most other patients with Cushing's syndrome. Removal of the carcinoma or radiotherapy only rarely leads to remission as these tumours are often highly malignant and metastasise early. Adrenalectomy can cause remission of the complication but is only justified if metastases cannot be detected or the clinical course is prolonged. Drugs affecting the adrenal, e.g. metyrapone or o-p'D.D.D., have little to offer.

Bilateral adrenal hyperplasia can be treated at the pituitary or at the adrenal level. Very good results can be obtained by bilateral adrenalectomy, which cures the overproduction of cortisol except in the rare cases with accessory adrenal tissue. Cortisol cover is needed over the operation, which can be carried out in one or two stages. Permanent replacement therapy with cortisol and a mineralocorticoid is then needed in similar dosage to that described for Addison's disease. Unilateral adrenalectomy with subtotal (usually nine-tenths) adrenalectomy on the opposite side has been performed in the past but has now been abandoned in view of the high incidence of either infarction of the remnant or recurrence of the disease. After adrenalectomy some 20 per cent of patients might be expected to develop the 'post-adrenalectomy syndrome' when the persisting disease process with high plasma ACTH and β-MSH levels (*see* Fig. 6.10) leads to pigmentation of the skin and enlargement of the pituitary fossa. This condition, described by Nelson, may respond to full external pituitary irradiation or internal irradiation using yttrium-90. Irradiation of the pituitary at the time of the adrenalectomy should prevent the development of Nelson's syndrome, and should be considered especially if plasma ACTH rises markedly after adrenalectomy.

Pituitary irradiation using 4,500 rads externally applied from the cobalt unit or linear accelerator, or more effectively using a proton beam, cures Cushing's disease in about 40 per cent of patients although about half of these may require supplementary treatment with some adrenocortical inhibiting drug such as metyrapone (250 to 750 mg, 2 or 3 times daily) and/or aminoglutethimide (250 mg, 3 times daily). Some advocate the use of intrapituitary implants of yttrium-90 as the source of the irradiation. Pituitary irradiation with administration of adrenal inhibitors should be considered in all mild or moderately severe cases of Cushing's disease as primary treatment. If the high blood cortisol levels do not respond adequately over the next 18 months, adrenalectomy should be carried out. If the patient's Cushing's disease is severe, and adrenalectomy is to be carried out as the primary treatment, patients may benefit from administration of adrenal enzyme inhibitors for a while preoperatively, to lower the cortisol levels. Surgical attack to the pituitary is less effective in Cushing's disease than the other methods of treatment indicated above and should not be used unless visual field involvement from a large expanding pituitary tumour is present. This is very unusual and the simple presence of an abnormal fossa should not alter the plan of treatment except that Nelson's syndrome is more likely to occur and the pituitary should be irradiated.

ADRENOCORTICAL INSUFFICIENCY

Adrenocortical insufficiency may be primary, that is due to destruction of the adrenal glands themselves, secondary, due to pituitary, or tertiary due to hypothalamic disease resulting in impaired ACTH secretion and consequent adrenocortical atrophy.

Hypoadrenalism may be acute or chronic. Chronic primary adrenocortical insufficiency was first described by Thomas Addison in 1855, and the term Addison's disease is used to refer to the form of chronic hypoadrenalism which results from destruction of the adrenal glands from a variety of pathological processes.

ADDISON'S DISEASE

AETIOLOGY

In the United Kingdom, the two most frequent causes of *chronic hypoadrenalism* are probably *autoimmune adrenalitis* and *tuberculous disease* of the adrenals. *Autoimmune adrenalitis* is likely to include most cases previously referred to as idiopathic adrenocortical insufficiency. In this group of patients antibodies to adrenal cortex can be detected by immunofluorescence and by complement fixation in 80 per cent of females and in 10 per cent of males (Irvine *et al.*, 1967). Titres of antibodies are usually low and there is no correlation between the duration of the illness and the presence or absence of antibodies. There is a clinical and immunological overlap between idiopathic Addison's disease and autoimmune thyroid, gastric, ovarian and parathyroid failure. Histology of the adrenal gland shows loss of glandular cells with lymphocytic infiltration and fibrous tissue, the appearance resembling that seen in Hashimoto's disease of the thyroid. The disease process is mainly confined to the adrenal cortex, unlike tuberculous adrenalitis which affects both cortex and medulla. Rarer causes of hypoadrenalism are secondary metastatic deposits, especially from bronchogenic carcinoma, other granulomas (except for sarcoidosis, which almost never involves the adrenals), amyloidosis, haemochromatosis, and some fungal diseases.

Congenital adrenal hyperplasia, due to deficiency of one or other of a number of specific enzymes in the adrenal cortex, may present with symptoms of hypoadrenalism and pigmentation of the skin, but most often the relative adrenocortical insufficiency is well compensated for by adrenal hyperplasia (*see* Chapter 13).

Acute hypoadrenalism may occur in any patient in the later stages of chronic hypoadrenalism or may be precipitated in these patients by any form of stress, e.g. infections or operations. Surgical removal of the adrenals in the treatment of metastatic breast carcinoma or other malignant disease or for Cushing's syndrome is a not infrequent cause of hypoadrenalism. Fulminating infections such as meningococcal septicaemia associated with subcutaneous ecchymoses may lead to adrenal haemorrhage and acute adrenal failure. Adrenal haemorrhage may occur in the newborn, especially if the labour is prolonged or difficult; sometimes breech presentation may also be a factor. Adrenal vein thrombosis and infarction of the gland are very rare sequelae of trauma to the back.

CLINICAL FEATURES

The clinical features depend on the nature of the underlying disease process, especially its chronicity and severity, and on the pattern of deficiency of the different types of adrenocortical hormones —glucocorticoids, mineralocorticoids, and androgens.

Chronic hypoadrenalism is not an all-or-none phenomenon but varies from complete failure of hormone production to minor impairment of adrenal reserve capacity. Basal hormone secretion may be normal and the diagnosis can be established only by tests determining the impaired reserve capacity of the gland.

Pigmentation of the skin is often the feature that raises the suspicion of hypoadrenalism.

It is due to increased melanin in the skin and is most obvious in exposed areas. Pigmentation may be more marked in the nipples, in the buccal mucosa, in scars made after the onset of the hypoadrenalism, and in areas subject to pressure, sunlight or irritation. Pigmentation of the skin is caused by the raised levels of β-MSH which accompany the elevated ACTH levels resulting from the low plasma cortisol. In some patients, pigmentation may precede other features of hypoadrenalism by many years, probably due to a very slowly progressive destructive lesion. Before effective therapy was available it was noted that patients in whom pigmentation was a prominent feature tended to live longer.

Vitiligo, patchy areas of depigmentation of the skin surrounded by increased pigmentation, occurs in some 15 per cent of patients with idiopathic Addison's disease. It is of interest that vitiligo is also associated with other organ-specific autoimmune diseases (Cunliffe *et al.*, 1968).

Tiredness is a common but rather non-specific complaint. It rapidly improves with cortisol therapy, unlike the fatigue that accompanies various psychiatric disorders. Profound lassitude in a patient with a possible cause of hypodrenalism, e.g. a pituitary tumour, should be an indication for immediate investigation and cortisol therapy.

Gastro-intestinal complaints are also non-specific but may occur early—anorexia, nausea, vomiting, weight loss, and occasionally diarrhoea. Faecal fat excretion may be increased in the absence of diarrhoea, normal fat output being restored by cortisol therapy. Vague abdominal pain may also lead to difficulties in diagnosis.

Hypotension particularly when the patient is erect can be caused by cortisol deficiency alone, and the blood pressure can usually be restored by cortisol though the large doses usually used will have a significant sodium-retaining action. Cortisol, as mentioned previously, acts synergistically with noradrenaline to maintain vascular tone. Normal reflex maintenance of the blood pressure is also impaired and there is a failure of peripheral vasoconstriction in the presence of hypotension; hence, dizziness and syncopal attacks may result from postural hypotension. Chronic sodium depletion with loss of water will also reduce the extracellular fluid volume and it is certainly a factor in causing the lowered blood pressure.

Hypoglycaemia occurs in some patients with hypoadrenalism because of the lack of cortisol which is one of the physiological antagonists of insulin. Reactive hypoglycaemia several hours after a carbohydrate meal is another complaint.

Loss of body hair is more prominent in women than in men, who have an alternative source of androgens from the testes. Sexual functions are usually well maintained and amenorrhoea is unusual (antibodies to ovary may be found in some patients with amenorrhoea).

Depression, psychoses, and other mental disturbances are not uncommon and respond well to cortisol medication.

Acute Hypoadrenalism. The patient with acute hypoadrenalism is gravely ill, and treatment should not be delayed to carry out investigations. Nausea, vomiting, diarrhoea, profound muscular weakness, and hypotension are the salient features. Without treatment such patients become comatose and die. However before starting emergency treatment in such a patient it is wise to obtain a blood sample for subsequent cortisol assay so that the diagnosis can be substantiated in retrospect.

DIAGNOSIS

Diagnosis depends on demonstrating impaired production of adrenal hormones, usually of cortisol, and if possible in determining the underlying cause of the disease.

Direct evidence of hormonal deficiencies should be demonstrated before making a diagnosis of hypoadrenalism. *Cortisol production rate* is usually reduced but may be just within the normal range under basal conditions but will not increase if the patient is stressed, i.e. the adrenocortical reserve is reduced. This can be demonstrated by administration of exogenous ACTH and showing an impaired response. However production rate measurements are not generally available for clinical use and are unnecessarily complex.

Like cortisol production rates plasma or urinary corticosteroids may either be reduced or be within the normal range under resting conditions, but show impairment of reserve and cannot increase under stress or ACTH administration. The change in plasma cortisol, measured fluorimetrically or by protein-binding methods, in response to exogenous ACTH is the most useful diagnostic procedure when seeking to confirm a diagnosis of Addison's disease. As a screening test, 250 μg of tetracosactrin (Synacthen) is given intramuscularly and blood obtained before and at 30 and 60 minutes afterwards for corticosteroid assay (the 'short' tetracosactrin or Synacthen test, *see* Appendix). Tetracosactrin is a synthetic polypeptide identical with the first 24 amino-acids of ACTH which are responsible for steroidogenesis. The test is best carried out at about 9 a.m. and can easily be performed on ambulant outpatients. If the plasma corticosteroids rise by more than 7 μg/100 ml to a level over 20 μg/100 ml a diagnosis of Addison's disease can be confidently excluded. If the results are impaired (Fig. 6.11) then the diagnosis probably lies between primary adrenocortical failure (Addison's disease) and adrenal atrophy secondary to either pituitary or hypo thalamic disease and consequent ACTH deficiency, or to corticosteroid therapy. The patient should then be given a long acting form of tetracosactrin (Synacthen-depot) 2 mg i.m. daily for 3 days, and the short tetracosactrin test repeated. This is the 'long' tetracosactrin or Synacthen test (*see* Appendix). In Addison's disease there will still be little or no corticosteroid response, but if the glands are merely atrophic the cortisol will rise above 20 μg/100 ml. Primary disease and secondary adrenal atrophy can thus be differentiated. Alternatively the two parts to the test can be combined; if 2 mg of tetracosactrin depot is given and samples taken

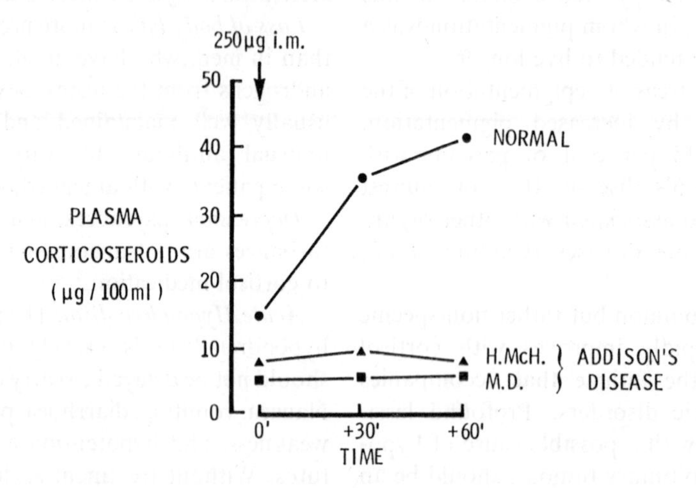

FIGURE 6.11 Short tetracosactrin (Synacthen) test in two patients with Addison's disease compared with a normal control.

0, 1, 4, 8 and 24 hours later for corticosteroid measurement, in Addison's disease there will be a markedly impaired response throughout, whereas in secondary adrenal atrophy the initial response will be impaired but later the levels will rise. It is quite unnecessary to withhold treatment from patients with suspected adrenocortical insufficiency, since a synthetic corticosteroid such as prednisolone (in a dose of 5 mg twice daily) can be given and this will not interfere with the plasma corticosteroid measurements. It is best to start treatment while awaiting the results once the short tetracosactrin test has been completed if clinical suspicion is strong. If an adrenocortical crisis is suspected under stressed conditions, plasma should be obtained for subsequent cortisol assay and treatment initiated immediately with 20 mg prednisolone intravenously and also intramuscularly; proper investigation under prednisolone cover can be deferred until later.

Cortisol deficiency can be demonstrated indirectly by the failure of excretion of a water load although the mechanism by which cortisol influences renal water excretion is not well understood. Cortisol deficiency may also lead to *electrocardiographic abnormalities* with lowered amplitude of T waves and, occasionally, prolongation of the PR and QT intervals and low voltage complexes. These revert to normal shortly after cortisol administration. Tests involving eosinophil counts before and after ACTH are of historical interest only.

Aldosterone deficiency is indicated in some cases by abnormalities of plasma electrolytes and urea but, again, normal levels are often found. The plasma sodium and chloride levels are low in some patients but the sodium levels are rarely less than 120 mEq/litre. The low sodium is due partly to renal loss because of aldosterone deficiency and partly to water retention, since plasma vasopressin levels are raised secondary to the reduced plasma volume. The plasma potassium is elevated due to lack of aldosterone and blood urea levels may be raised because of hypotension and lowering of the glomerular filtration rate. In some patients treated with cortisol alone the blood urea remains elevated until a mineralocorticoid preparation is given.

A plain X-ray of the abdomen may show suprarenal calcification caused by tuberculosis. Chest X-ray may also show evidence of tuberculosis but healed pulmonary lesions are so common that this finding is not very helpful in determining the cause of hypoadrenalism. Evidence of a bronchogenic carcinoma or bronchiectasis (causing amyloidosis) will rarely help in the diagnosis of hypoadrenalism. It may be possible to distinguish Addison's disease caused by tuberculosis or other destructive lesions from that due to autoimmune processes by demonstrating the presence of anti-adrenocortical antibodies in the latter group. In response to stress (e.g. hypoglycaemia) in normal persons, and in those with idiopathic Addison's disease, there is a rise in plasma or urinary adrenaline output whereas in patients with destructive lesions that also involve the adrenal medulla there is a poor or absent catecholamine response.

DIFFERENTIAL DIAGNOSIS

Many patients have rather brown skin and feel tired but only a very small minority of these are found to have hypoadrenalism. Pigmentation of the skin may be racial or constitutional or due to a wide variety of diseases. A history of recent increase in pigmentation is of greater significance than pigmentation of long standing. Pigmentation is usually due to increased melanin in the skin but may occasionally be caused by iron (as well as melanin) in haemochromatosis, or by other metals. Melanin pigmentation may be local or generalised. *Local pigmentation*, especially of the buccal mucosa, may raise the suspicion of hypoadrenalism but it is more often an incidental finding. Rarely, it may be due to the Peutz-Jegher's syndrome where small intestinal polyposis is accompanied by freckles and melanosis of the lips and buccal mucosa. Local pigmentation may also be seen in regional ileitis, ulcerative colitis, cirrhosis of the liver, melanosarcoma, acanthosis nigricans, neurofibromatosis, and polyostotic fibrous dysplasia. Many chronic disorders, especially malignant disease, are associated with a *general increase in pigmentation*. Lassitude and weight loss occur commonly in these diseases and the picture may closely resemble hypoadrenalism. Malabsorption syndromes, chronic infections, especially tuberculosis, malignant disease, including the reticuloses, leukaemia and salt-losing renal disease all fall into this category. Urinary 17-OHCS and 17-OS may be normal or lowered in many of these non-endocrine diseases associated with malnutrition but plasma cortisol levels are normal and the response to ACTH unimpaired. Pigmentation may occur in other endocrine diseases such as thyrotoxicosis, as well as in Cushing's disease. Only in the latter condition is there a raised level of ACTH and β-MSH.

TREATMENT

(*a*) *Chronic Adrenocortical Insufficiency*. All patients with hypoadrenalism require permanent maintenance therapy with a glucocorticoid. Since the physiological hormone is available it is best to use this in a schedule that mimics the normal circadian variation of cortisol output from the adrenal, and most patients are well controlled on cortisol 20 mg each morning and 10 mg each evening. The morning tablet should be taken on waking, since it is at this time that the plasma cortisol levels should be at their highest. Occasional patients have difficulty in sleeping if the evening dose is given too late. Cortisol levels should be checked (*see* p. 31). Patients should be given a steroid card giving details of their therapy and asked to carry this with them always and it is also wise to suggest they wear a MedicAlert bracelet or necklace (*see* Appendix); they should be warned to increase the dose if they develop an infection, or if an operation is to be carried out. Routine corticosteroid maintenance therapy will not reduce resistance to infection. Cortisone acetate in a dose of 25 mg each morning and 12·5 mg each evening is a reasonable alternative to cortisol but it is sometimes poorly absorbed and it has to be converted to cortisol before it is effective and has any physiological action. Other synthetic glucocorticoids such as prednisone, triamcinolone, or dexamethasone are less suitable for long term replacement treatment because of their weak salt-retaining action.

Deficient aldosterone production may be expected in patients with primary hypoadrenalism. Orthostatic hypotension or a rather low blood pressure while the patient is receiving maintenance cortisol therapy indicates a need for mineralocorticoid therapy. Some patients maintained only on cortisol show an elevation of the blood urea and serum potassium levels which fall to normal only with mineralocorticoid treatment. Often, however, there will be no clear indication that the patient requires such therapy and it is probably best to administer a mineralocorticoid to all patients with more than the most trivial hypoadrenalism. The mineralocorticoid of choice is at present fludrocortisone, starting with a daily dose of 0·05 mg and increasing if necessary to 0·1 to 0·2 mg/day. Most patients can be controlled on a dose of 0·05 mg/day. Signs of overdosage are those of sodium retention—hypertension, oedema, headaches, and arthralgia—and of potassium depletion—hypokalaemic alkalosis and muscular weakness.

It is unnecessary to see well-controlled Addisonian patients more often than six monthly.

(*b*) *Acute Hypoadrenalism*. This is a major medical emergency that requires immediate intravenous injection of 100 mg of hydrocortisone hemisuccinate. If there is difficulty in entering a vein because of the circulatory collapse, an intramuscular injection should be given while a drip is being erected, by cut-down if necessary. One litre of normal saline (preferably containing 5 per cent dextrose to correct hypoglycaemia) should be given within half to one hour. Subsequent infusion will depend on the patient's condition—if there is severe sodium and water depletion 3–4 litres of saline may be required. A total of 200–300 mg of hydrocortisone may be given intravenously in the first 24 hours though, very rarely, massive doses are required to restore the blood pressure, but when this occurs alternative causes of hypotension should obviously be sought. The following day, if the patient has improved, 20 mg of hydrocortisone can be given by mouth 6 to 8 hourly. On subsequent days the dose may be reduced till a maintenace level is reached. When the oral dose is greater than 60 mg daily there should be sufficient mineralocorticoid action but at dose levels less than this mineralocorticoids will often be required. Infections that may have triggered off the acute hypoadrenalism must be looked for and treated vigorously with antibiotics.

It is sometimes possible to distinguish whether the acute hypoadrenalism is mainly due to aldosterone or to cortisol lack though often the two deficiencies go hand in hand. Aldosterone deficiency may be precipitated by sodium loss and presents with dehydration and hypotension and the blood urea is usually raised. Cortisol deficiency may be precipitated by any stress, and causes nausea, vomiting, profound weakness, fever, hypotension and coma, and dehydration may even be absent. The hypotension of adrenocortical insufficiency responds very poorly to noradrenaline infusion and this should be avoided.

(*c*) *Pregnancy and Hypoadrenalism.* Pregnancy is an additional stress to the patient with hypoadrenalism but, with care, complications can be avoided. Maintenance therapy with cortisol and a mineralocorticoid should be continued throughout. Vomiting or toxaemia is an indication for an increase in cortisol dosage (and mineralocorticoid if necessary) sometimes by the intramuscular or intravenous routes. A slight increase in cortisol dosage, e.g. by 10 mg/day may be desirable because of the increase in binding protein concentration during pregnancy which will tend to reduce the level of free cortisol. Anaesthetics or Caesarian section will be an indication for increased cortisol dosage. Labour should be covered with an increase in cortisol, as for a major surgical procedure see (*e*).

(*d*) *Hypoparathyroidism and Hypoadrenalism.* Hypoparathyroidism is occasionally associated with hypoadrenalism, and, like idiopathic Addison's disease, hypoparathyroidism may sometimes result from an organ-specific autoimmune disease. The antagonism that occurs between cortisol and vitamin D in the absorption of calcium from the gut may lead to difficulties when both drugs are required. Increased doses of cortisol may necessitate an increase in dose of vitamin D, which will need to be reduced along with the subsequent reduction in cortisol therapy.

(*e*) *Operations and Hypoadrenalism.* Any patient with adrenocortical insufficiency, whether due to adrenal disease, previous steroid therapy, adrenalectomy or hypopituitarism, will require careful regulation or corticosteroid dosage over the period of an operation. The regime suggested by Plumpton *et al.* (1969) is satisfactory:

1. *Major surgery* (e.g. laparotomy, hip osteotomy, etc.)
   100 mg hydorcortisone hemisuccinate is given intramuscularly each six hours, starting with the premedication and is continued for 72 hours or until the patient is taking food orally; after this the dose is given orally and is reduced over the next 5 days to the normal replacement dose of hydrocortisone and fludrocortisone. If complications occur, the full parenteral dose should be continued; if the patient is well but merely not taking food by mouth (e.g. after gastrectomy) the dose should be continued as 50 mg hydrocortisone hemisuccinate 8 hourly intramuscularly.

2. *Minor surgery* (e.g. herniorrhaphy)
   100 mg hydrocortisone hemisuccinate is given i.m. each 6 hours for 24 hours, starting with the premedication. Thereafter in the absence of complications the normal oral replacement is given.

3. *Minimal procedures* (e.g. endoscopy)
   A single i.m. injection of 100 mg hydrocortisone hemisuccinate is all that is required.

(*f*) *Withdrawal of Corticosteroid Medication.*

Any patient not suffering from Addison's disease who has received therapeutic doses of glucocorticoids for long periods will present the clinician with two major problems. First, is it possible to withdraw the steroids safely; and secondly, if steroids have already been satisfactorily withdrawn and the patient is required to undergo an operation, has been involved in an accident, or has acquired a major infection, should a 'covering' course of steroids be given?

The ease with which steroids can be withdrawn depends on the dose and duration of therapy. There is not usually any problem if the dose of steroids has been small and the duration of treatment less than one year. Prolonged steroid therapy suppresses the output of ACTH from the pituitary and the pituitary ACTH-releasing mechanism may become permanently impaired. Secondary adrenal atrophy occurs but this can almost always be reversed by a course of ACTH. Adrenal responsiveness can easily be confirmed by changing the steroid medication to a synthetic analogue, e.g. prednisolone or dexamethasone, and following the response in plasma corticosteroids to ACTH over several days. After withdrawal of all medication the plasma cortisol is initially low but if the ACTH-releasing mechanism is intact there is a gradual rise in plasma cortisol to normal levels within 72 hours. If, after this interval, the plasma cortisol remains less than 6 μg/100 ml at 9 a.m. profound damage has occurred and prolonged steroid therapy may be needed but this is very rare. Maintenance therapy with prednisolone 7·5 mg per day may be continued and attempts to remove this should be made every few months. Restoration of plasma cortisol to normal levels does not necessarily indicate that the patient will be able to respond to stress with a rise in plasma cortisol. To test the stress response an insulin tolerance test (*see* Appendix) must be carried out to confirm the rise in plasma cortisol caused by hypoglycaemia. A normal response to this test appears to correlate well with the ability to respond to other stresses, e.g. surgical operations. The stress response can also be tested by bacterial pyrogen. The problem of cortisol cover for operations is such a common one that it is not practicable to investigate all patients in the thorough manner indicated above and it is routine practice to give cortisol cover for an operation to any patient who has received corticosteroid medication within the last two months. In patients who have not received steroids so recently, cover is not normally necessary, but any unaccounted fall in blood pressure should be treated as hypoadrenalism with cortisol (Plumpton *et al.*, 1969).

SECONDARY ADRENOCORTICAL INSUFFICIENCY

This has also been discussed in Chapter 1. ACTH deficiency due to pituitary or hypothalamic disease causes atrophy of both adrenal glands. It is not always complete, and may only become apparent when a patient collapses with low plasma cortisol levels under stressful conditions. Since gonadotrophins, prolactin and growth hormone secretion are usually impaired well before ACTH in patients with progressive pituitary or hypothalamic disease, ACTH deficiency under these circumstances occurs as part of a general picture of hypopituitarism. However very rarely 'isolated ACTH deficiency' has been described. Chronic high dose corticosteroid therapy suppresses hypothalamic CRF and pituitary ACTH secretion both under basal conditions and under stress and adrenocortical atrophy ensues. Should corticosteroid therapy be inadvertently stopped or reduced suddenly, particularly if the patient is severely stressed, he is likely to go into adrenocortical failure.

Since basal aldosterone secretion does not depend on ACTH, secondary adrenocortical failure is not associated with mineralocorticoid deficiency. The clinical picture is similar to that of Addison's disease except that pigmentation is not present (blood ACTH and MSH levels are low not high) and there will usually be signs of deficiency of other pituitary hormones. The treatment is the same as for Addison's disease except that fludrocortisone is not required. The diagnostic tests for ACTH deficiency are discussed in Chapter 1 and in the earlier section of this chapter.

ALDOSTERONE

PHYSIOLOGY

The overall effect of aldosterone is to increase the amount of sodium in the body, its main action being to increase sodium absorption from the distal renal tubule and, also, from the ascending limb of the loop of Henle and the collecting ducts by exchange for potassium and hydrogen ions. Potassium excretion is dependent on aldosterone action and, also, on the availability of sodium ions at the distal tubule which, in turn, depends on the amount of sodium that leaves the proximal tubule. Sodium retention resulting from aldosterone is accompanied by water retention produced by the release of vasopressin in response to the increase in plasma osmolality. This limits the extent of the rise in serum sodium concentration.

When aldosterone is administered continuously, to a normal person for more than about two weeks, the induced sodium and water retention ceases, by an escape mechanism thought to be mediated by a natriuretic hormone which has not yet been isolated. This hormone appears to have a molecular weight of between 800 and 1000, possibly originates in the brain and is released in response to an increase in central blood volume. Potassium excretion which is increased both by way of the gut and the kidney in response to aldosterone does not show this escape phenomenon, nor does the sodium excreted by the sweat glands.

The absence of oedema in the majority of patients with aldosterone-producing tumours is explained by this escape mechanism. In oedematous states such as the nephrotic syndrome, cirrhosis and congestive cardiac failure, plasma aldosterone levels are usually high but hyperaldosteronism is not the primary cause of the oedema although it may tend to make fluid retention worse.

CONTROL OF ALDOSTERONE SECRETION

The rate of aldosterone production is influenced by many different factors. Increased secretion results from sodium restriction, increased sodium loss caused by diuretics, potassium administration, haemorrhage and dehydration, reduction in plasma volume, injection of angiotensin (*see* below), and assumption of the upright position. Decreased secretion follows potassium depletion, sodium administration, and any increase in plasma volume, as well as assumption of the horizontal position.

It is now well established that changes in aldosterone secretion in response to these various stimuli are mediated predominantly by the renin-angiotensin system. Although ACTH infusion induces a transient increase in aldosterone secretion, and a pituitary factor is necessary to maintain the adrenal in a condition in which it can respond normally to stimuli to aldosterone production, aldosterone levels are dissociated from cortisol levels in many physiological situations, indicating that ACTH is not the major factor controlling aldosterone. Similarly hyperkalaemia and hyponatraemia in the blood perfusing the adrenal, are known to stimulate aldosterone secretion but cannot account for changes in aldosterone levels observed under various conditions of diet and posture. By contrast in normal animals and man changes in plasma aldosterone are almost invariably associated with parallel changes in plasma renin concentration or angiotensin II levels, indicating the overriding importance of renin in the control of aldosterone.

The exact mechanisms by which the various stimuli to aldosterone secretion trigger renin release are not finally established. The most likely main stimulus to aldosterone secretion is a tendency to a reduction in central blood volume brought about by blood or salt and water loss or by pooling of blood in the legs with assumption of the erect posture; this then stimulates the sympathetic nervous system via the carotid sinus and beta adrenergic stimuli pass via the renal nerves to the kidney and lead to renin release. This would be brought about either by stimulation of the renin producing cells directly, or possibly by inducing arteriolar constriction proximal to baroreceptors in the afferent arterioles thus lowering the pressure at the receptor. An alternative more direct mechanism has also been postulated, namely that the sodium reaching the distal tubule is reduced as the filtration pressure falls, leading to reduced sodium concentration at the macula densa part of the juxtaglomerular apparatus. Renin is produced by cells of the juxtaglomerular apparatus in the wall of the afferent arteriole and is released into the circulation where it acts enzymatically on angiotensinogen, derived from the liver, to form a decapeptide angiotensin I. This is converted to the octapeptide angiotensin II by 'converting enzyme' which is present in the circulation and in high concentration in the lungs. The octapeptide is a potent vasopressor agent as well as the major factor stimulating the secretion of aldosterone (Fig. 6.12).

ALDOSTERONE ANTAGONISM

Spironolactones are synthetic steroids that are competitive inhibitors of aldosterone action on the renal tubules. Aldosterone causes a rise in urinary potassium and magnesium excretion and both effects can be blocked by spironolactone. Sodium loss by the kidney is influenced only in so far as the exchange of sodium with potassium is concerned. Thus, the spironolactones are effective only when a condition of aldosteronism exists, be it primary or secondary.

The newer potassium sparing diuretics triampterene and amiloride have direct actions on the distal tubules blocking sodium reabsorption and potassium excretion independently of the presence or absence of aldosterone. They may be useful in the treatment of patients with primary aldosteronism who are unable to tolerate large doses of spironolactone, although they are more commonly used for their potassium sparing effect.

CLINICAL EFFECTS OF ALDOSTERONE

OVERPRODUCTION OF ALDOSTERONE

Aldosteronism is the condition produced by an excess of aldosterone. This is said to be primary when it is due to disease of the adrenal gland itself, usually a single adrenal adenoma (approximately 60 per cent of cases), or bilateral micronodular hyperplasia with or without multiple adenomata (approximately 40 per cent). Adrenal carcinoma is an exceedingly rare cause of aldosteronism. Secondary aldosteronism results when overproduction of aldosterone is due to excessive stimulation of normal adrenals as a result of extra-adrenal disease. Conditions which lead to reduction in blood volume such as the nephrotic syndrome, cirrhosis and sodium-losing nephritis, or to ischaemia of the kidney as in renal artery stenosis and most cases of malignant hypertension, result in a compensatory mechanism involving release of renin. This increases secretion of aldosterone tending to cause sodium retention and an increased blood volume thus offseting the initial stimulus. A rare cause of secondary aldosteronism is hyperplasia of the juxtaglomerular apparatus with overproduction of renin.

Primary and secondary aldosteronism can be readily differentiated by measurement of the plasma renin or angiotensin II level, low levels indicating primary and high levels secondary aldosteronism.

PRIMARY ALDOSTERONISM

Conn (1964) reviewed experience of this condition over the ten years that elapsed from his first description, analysing the clinical features of 145 cases. Primary aldosteronism is usually the result of small aldosterone-producing adrenocortical adenomas. In 91 per cent of Conn's cases a small adenoma was present; 68 per cent of the tumours weighed less than 6 g; 73 per cent measured less than 3 cm in diameter. Females were affected some two and a half times more often than males, and 72 per cent of cases were between the ages of thirty and fifty years, though any age group can be affected. Subsequent experience has confirmed these observations although it now seems that only about 60 per cent of patients have a single adenoma, the remainder have bilateral adrenal hyperplasia. Adrenal carcinomas may secrete aldosterone along with cortisol, adrenal androgens, oestrogens, and other non-hormonally active steroids but they will not be considered further.

Clinical Features

The symptoms and signs of primary aldosteronism can be classified into three main groups as shown in Table 6.2.

1. Those related to the abnormal renal function.
2. Those due to neuromuscular abnormalities.
3. Those associated with hypertensive-vascular disease.

The renal features are mainly due to potassium depletion, as are the muscular ones of weakness and paralysis and impaired carbohydrate tolerance. Tetany and paraesthesiae are probably related to magnesium depletion. The biochemical and functional alterations observed in aldosteronism are summarised in Table 6.3, and the classification of coexisting hypertension and hypokalaemia in Table 6.4.

Diagnosis of Primary Aldosteronism

Primary aldosteronism is usually suspected when a patient with hypertension is found to have a low serum potassium, though recent studies by Conn suggest that hypokalaemia is not invariably present (*see* below). The problem then is to decide which patients with this combination have primary aldosteronism and which have aldosteronism associated with malignant hypertension and/or renal artery stenosis or renal ischaemia, or as a result of diuretic therapy. For hypertensive patients with borderline serum potassium levels a simple screening procedure is to give 200 mEq of sodium a day for a week, on the last three days estimating the serum potassium level. In a normal person, sodium loading reduces aldosterone secretion but in a patient with primary aldosteronism this reduction does not occur and the greater amounts of sodium presented to the distal tubule are exchanged for potassium under the influence of aldosterone, causing an increase in urine potassium excretion and a resultant fall in the serum potassium level.

Although low serum potassium levels can result from diuretic therapy, particularly with the thiazide group of drugs, severe hypokalaemia and muscle weakness presenting early after the initiation of diuretic therapy may give a clue to the presence of an aldosterone-secreting tumour.

Again, the finding of a low serum potassium in a hypertensive patient may not necessarily indicate overproduction of aldosterone; nor does the demonstration of increased aldosterone production or reversal of hypokalaemia by aldosterone antagonists confirm a diagnosis of primary aldosteronism if malignant hypertension or renal disease is present, for in either of these conditions there may be secondary aldosteronism. It is helpful, but again not diagnostic, to know that the hypokalaemia is due to renal loss,

TABLE 6.2 *Symptoms and Signs of Primary Aldosteronism*

Renal:	Polydipsia, polyuria, and nocturia.
Neuromuscular:	Weakness, usually episodic, flaccid paralysis, latent or overt tetany, paraesthesiae.
Hypertensive:	Hypertension of any grade, headache, cardiomegaly, and retinopathy slight in relation to blood pressure elevation.
Negative features:	Oedema, usually absent or minimal, and papilloedema is very rare.

TABLE 6.3 *Primary Aldosteronism (Tumour): Biochemical and Functional Alterations*

(With acknowledgements to J. W. Conn *et al.* (1964), by permission of the Editor, *American Journal of Surgery*.)

Location	Alteration
Blood	Hypokalaemia*
	Hypernatraemia
	Hypochloraemia
	Hypomagnesaemia
Urine	Increased aldosterone excretion and/or secretion*
	Normal 17-OS and 17-OHCS*
	Decreased concentrating ability on:
	water restriction
	vasopressin administration
	Decreased ability to acidify:
	neutral or alkaline urine
	decreased H^+ and increased NH_4^+
	Decreased renal conservation of K^+
Na, K and body fluids	Increased body exchangeable Na* } high
	Decreased body exchangeable K* } Na/K
	Low Na/K of saliva
	Increased plasma volume†
	decreased hematocrit
Electrocardiogram	Changes compatible with hypokalaemia*

* Most common. † Not invariable.

TABLE 6.4 *Aetiological Classification of Coexisting Hypertension and Hypokalaemia*

(With acknowledgements to J. W. Conn *et al.* (1964), by permission of the Editor, *American Journal of Surgery*.)

Category	Condition
I	Primary aldosteronism (tumour)
II	Congenital aldosteronism (bilateral hyperplasia)
III	Diuretic therapy in hypertensive patients
IV	Accelerated (malignant) hypertension: renal ischaemia (unilateral or bilateral)
V	Potassium-wasting renal disease: Fanconi syndrome renal tubular acidosis advanced chronic nephritis chronic pyelonephritis
VI	Conditions associated with large production of hydrocortisone: Cushing's syndrome: adrenal hyperplasia or tumour, ACTH-producing pituitary tumour, neoplasms producing ACTH-like compounds: lung, thymus, pancreas, and gall-bladder
VII	Miscellaneous: a few benign hypertensives with all the characteristics of primary aldosteronism but no tumour aberrant aldosteronoma a familial renal disorder with hypokalaemia factitious (pseudoprimary aldosteronism) chronic ingestion of liquorice subnormal aldosterone excretion and secretion

and repeated daily urinary potassium excretion >20–30 mEq, when the serum potassium is less than 3·5 mEq/litre, support this. Patients with primary aldosteronism tend to show hypokalaemia resistant to oral potassium administration, more and more potassium being lost in the urine. The so-called hypokalaemic alkalosis with raised serum bicarbonate levels is merely a reflection of the severity of potassium depletion.

How then can we distinguish between the groups of hypertensive patients with primary and secondary aldosteronism? Most patients with primary aldosteronism tend to have serum sodium levels greater than 140 mEq/litre whereas secondary aldosteronism is very often provoked by sodium depletion, and serum sodium levels are often less than 135 mEq/litre. Indeterminate values are often found and more precise differentiation is necessary. Secondary aldosteronism may have an obvious cause in hypertensives, such as renal disease, but this is often not the case.

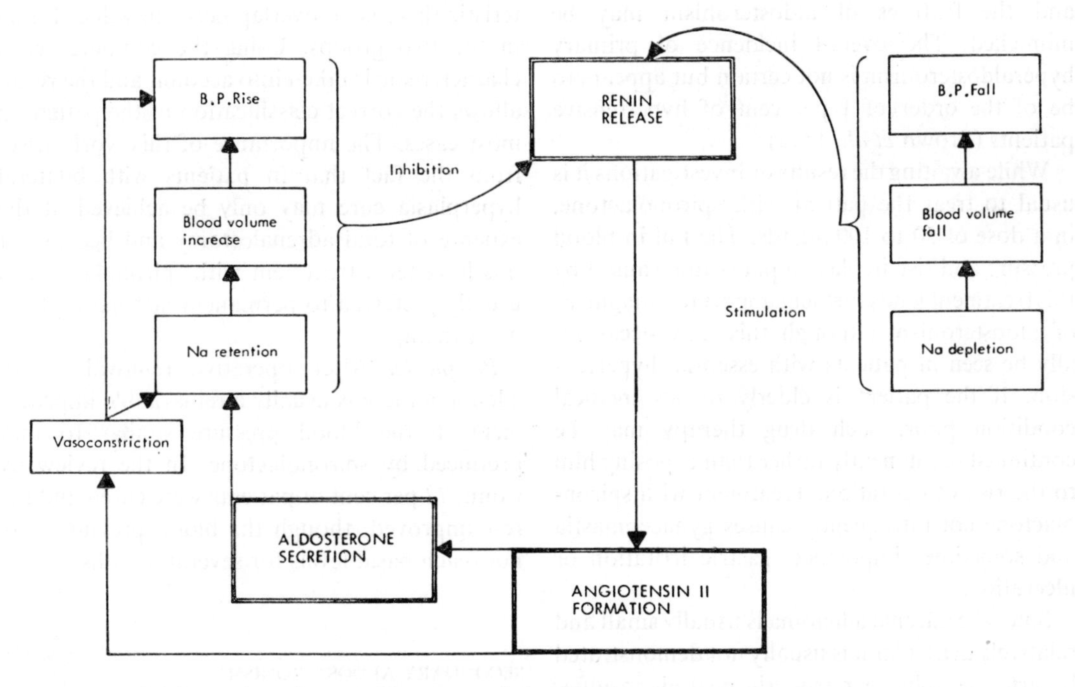

FIGURE 6.12 Renin, angiotensin, and aldosterone relationships

The only means by which primary and secondary aldosteronism can be reliably differentiated is by measurement of plasma renin levels. In primary aldosteronism high plasma and urinary aldosterone levels are associated with sodium retention and increased intravascular volume and renin levels are low; in secondary aldosteronism renin is the initiator of the increased aldosterone secretion and plasma levels are elevated.

Methods of estimating plasma renin are difficult but are now more readily available and such measurements should be obtained in hypertensive patients with unprovoked hypokalaemia. Even after sodium restriction to 10 mEq/day for 3 days and maintenance of the upright position, plasma renin levels tend to remain low in patients with primary aldosteronism and it has been shown that they exhibit an approximate inverse relationship to the serum sodium concentration. A clinical clue to the finding of a low plasma renin is a raised plasma sodium level in a hypokalaemic patient with hypertension. It must be remembered that hypokalaemia may be intermittent in primary hyperaldosteronism.

Before diagnosing aldosteronism as a cause of hypertension and hypokalaemia it is essential to rule out cortisol overproduction since high levels of cortisol have a mineralocorticoid action and the features of aldosteronism may be mimicked. The overall incidence of primary hyperaldosteronism is not certain but appears to be of the order of 1 per cent of hypertensive patients (Brown *et al.*, 1972).

While awaiting the results of investigations it is usual to treat the patient with spironolactone, in a dose of 50 to 100 mg tds. The fall in blood pressure and rise in plasma potassium caused by this treatment lends further support to a diagnosis of aldosteronism although this may occasionally be seen in patients with essential hypertension. If the patient is elderly or his medical condition poor, such drug therapy may be continued permanently rather than exposing him to the risk of operation. Treatment with spironolactone not infrequently causes gynaecomastia and sometimes impotence, gastric irritation or ulceration.

Since the adrenal adenoma is usually small and relatively avascular it is usually not demonstrated by arteriography or retroperitoneal air insufflation. The investigation of choice to locate the adenoma is adrenal vein catheterisation via the femoral vein with venography to demonstrate distortion of the veins by the relatively avascular tumour and collection of blood samples for determination of aldosterone levels, high levels being found on the side containing the tumour. Unfortunately the procedure is technically difficult and injection of contrast medium carries the risk of adrenal infarction. Adenomata are more common on the left and are rarely bilateral.

Preoperative distinction between single adenoma and bilateral hyperplasia may now be possible without resorting to adrenal vein catheterisation. Ferris *et al.* (1970) have used a computer to analyse the data from patients with primary aldosteronism in order to categorise them into the two groups. The analysis is based on the observation that all the biochemical features of primary aldosteronism, i.e. hypernatraemia, hypokalaemia, alkalosis, hyporeninaemia, and increased plasma aldosterone are in general more marked in the tumour than the hyperplasia group although for any one characteristic there is an overlap between values found in the two groups. Using the computer each characteristic is taken into account and the result allows the correct classification of the patient in most cases. The importance of this work arises from the fact that in patients with bilateral hyperplasia cure may only be achieved at the expense of total adrenalectomy and because of this long term treatment with spironolactone is usually preferred to permanent adrenal replacement therapy.

Prognosis. After operative removal of an adenoma there is usually a remarkable improvement in the blood pressure similar to that produced by spironolactone. In the review by Conn, 72 per cent of patients were cured and the rest improved, though the blood pressure may not reach basal levels for several months.

SECONDARY ALDOSTERONISM

Secondary aldosteronism can be classified into the following categories:

1. *With fluid retention*—there is not usually hypokalaemia or hypertension, unless the latter is the underlying cause for cardiac failure. In this category we include some cases of cardiac and 'idiopathic' oedema, cirrhosis of the liver with ascites, and the nephrotic syndrome.
2. *Without fluid retention*, but associated with hypertension and hypokalaemia. Here are included renal ischaemia (usually renal artery stenosis), malignant hypertension, and sodium-losing nephritis.
3. Due to liquorice, carbenoxolone, or other drugs.

Cardiac Oedema

Despite numerous studies the pathogenesis of cardiac oedema is poorly understood. When urinary aldosterone excretion is raised in some patients with congestive cardiac failure there does seem to be an increase in aldosterone production, but reduced aldosterone destruction in the liver is sometimes a factor. A low salt diet and diuretic therapy are also potent factors in causing increased aldosterone production. However, of 15 cases with resistant cardiac oedema studied by Cope only 3 had aldosterone secretion outside the normal range, despite intensive diuretic therapy. The stimulus to increased aldosterone production in heart failure is unlikely to be stretching of the right atrium (which in any case tends to reduce aldosterone production) since patients with raised venous pressure due to tricuspid incompetence do not always have a raised aldosterone output. Nor does a fall in pulse pressure on the arterial side of the circulation seem to be a major stimulus since aldosterone output is not usually raised in left ventricular failure or in aortic stenosis. The most likely stimulus is probably a leak of fluid and sodium out of the vascular compartment, which increases aldosterone production and causes sodium retention, but this is not usually sufficient to raise the plasma sodium level to normal.

Idiopathic Oedema

Persistent oedema without any of the usual causes is referred to as 'idiopathic' oedema. In some of these patients aldosterone production is normal, and in others it is raised. Atypical primary aldosteronism may occasionally present in this manner despite the fact that oedema is extremely rare in this condition. The defect in most cases, however, is unknown but a change in capillary permeability has been postulated, and in one case the protein content of the oedema fluid was high. Patients with this syndrome show much greater fluid retention in the upright position than occurs in normal persons. Loss of fluid from the vascular compartment into the interstitial fluid would, by reducing intravascular volume, tend to stimulate aldosterone production causing sodium retention and aggravation of the oedema. The condition can sometimes be improved by aldosterone antagonists.

Cirrhosis of the Liver with Ascites and the Nephrotic Syndrome

In both these groups of diseases there is loss of fluid from the plasma into the extravascular compartment, and aldosterone production is frequently raised, despite an increased body sodium content. Treatment with aldosterone antagonists may, especially in the former group, be a useful adjunct to diuretic therapy.

Renal Ischaemia

Narrowing of a renal artery leads to ischaemia and increased production of renin, thence of angiotensin and aldosterone. Angiotensin is responsible for hypertension, which may be associated with papilloedema, and aldosterone for hypokalaemia. Renin levels are raised in contrast to primary aldosteronism where renin levels are low. It is particularly helpful to catheterise both renal veins and obtain blood for renin assay. Demonstration of an elevated renin concentration in blood from the kidney suspected of having a stenosed renal artery, compared with the other side, confirms the clinical diagnosis. Clinical evidence of renal artery obstruction may be indicated by the presence of a bruit on auscultation of the upper abdomen. Radiological evidence is obtained by the delayed excretion of contrast media on the affected side in films a few minutes after injection. There may be an increased concentration of dye on the side of the lesion and the kidney may be smaller. Renal arteriograms are helpful in diagnosis, but before operating on the blocked segment it is best to demonstrate a pressure gradient across the block at operation. Vascular reconstruction on the affected side may allow conservation of the less damaged kidney. If this is not possible nephrectomy may be indicated. A significant proportion of cases so treated show improvement or cure of their hypertension.

Malignant Hypertension

In malignant hypertension there is often hypokalaemia and secondary aldosteronism although papilloedema may rarely occur in primary hyperaldosteronism. Presumably the mechanism of production of the secondary aldosteronism is renal arteriolar spasm, ischaemia and therefore increased renin and angiotensin formation. Treatment of the hypertension may improve the renal damage and is often able to reverse the malignant phase that may be superimposed on any type of hypertension.

Sodium-losing Nephritis

Some patients with chronic renal disease, usually chronic pyelonephritis, have excessive renal loss of sodium which stimulates aldosterone production and results in hypokalaemia. An elevated plasma renin level helps to distinguish this variety of secondary aldosteronism from primary aldosteronism. If renin assays are not available, the effect of a low sodium diet on the hypokalaemia may help in the differential diagnosis. In primary aldosteronism lowered sodium intake reduces the amount of sodium presented to the distal tubule which is available for exchange with potassium, and the hypokalaemia improves. In secondary aldosteronism, sodium restriction aggravates the condition, renal sodium loss continues, the hypokalaemia is not corrected and, in addition, the blood urea rises. Some of these patients are hypotensive or normotensive but as renal disease progresses the blood pressure tends to rise.

Juxtaglomerular Hyperplasia

Patients with this rare syndrome, first characterised by Bartter, present with clinical sequelae of aldosteronism, particularly hypokalaemia, but are normotensive. They have increased production of renin, angiotensin, and aldosterone, and renal biopsy shows hyperplasia of the juxtaglomerular apparatus. They are resistant to the pressor action of angiotensin though the nature of this defect is not understood. Treatment with aldosterone antagonists is effective though occasionally sodium restriction may also be needed.

Renin Secreting Renal Tumours—primary reninism

Rarely patients may be found who have high blood renin and aldosterone levels with hypertension and hypokalaemia. They are initially suspected of having renal artery stenosis but this is excluded by arteriography and there is no evidence of chronic renal disease. Such patients may have a renin secreting tumour of the juxtaglomerular cells of the kidney—a haemangiopericytoma, and the plasma renin level in the renal vein blood is higher on the side of the lesion. These lesions are usually too small to show up on renal arteriography, but can be found if the kidney is laid open at surgery. Removal cures the condition.

UNDERPRODUCTION OF ALDOSTERONE

Underproduction of aldosterone most commonly occurs as part of the syndrome of Addison's disease. Selective failure of aldosterone production in the presence of normal cortisol production and responsiveness to ACTH is very rare. A few patients have been described, usually with hyperkalaemia, and the cardiac complications of this such as complete heart block. Salt retention may be poor and muscle weakness and postural hypotension may also occur. After removal of an aldosterone-producing tumour, hypoaldosteronism may be present for a while.

Some patients with Addison's disease and those who have had bilateral adrenalectomy may show evidence of aldosterone deficiency if their mineralocorticoid replacement therapy is inadequate—the blood urea and serum potassium levels are raised but rapidly respond to corrective therapy with fludrocortisone.

Recently a hypotensive patient has been described with low renin and aldosterone levels, who responded to infusion of angiotensin. Deficient renin production appeared to be present, and the patient did well with fludrocortisone replacement alone.

OVERPRODUCTION OF ADRENAL ANDROGENS

This is dealt with in Chapters 8 and 13.

ADRENAL MEDULLA

The adrenal medulla is derived from the ectoderm of the neural crest and secretes the hormones adrenaline and noradrenaline into the circulation. Noradrenaline is also a neurotransmitter, being secreted locally by sympathetic nerve endings.

THE CATECHOLAMINES

Catecholamines are low molecular weight compounds which contain a catechol nucleus and an amine group. Noradrenaline, adrenaline, and their precursor dopamine are the most important catecholamines in man. They are synthesised from the amino-acids phenylalanine and tyrosine in the brain, in chromaffin tissue (mainly in the adrenal medulla), and in the sympathetic nerve endings of most tissues (Fig. 6.13). The enzymes responsible for the synthesis of the catecholamines from tyrosine have been identified and their intracellular localisation and action is shown in Fig. 6.14. Adrenaline (epinephrine) is formed from noradrenaline (norepinephrine) by action of the enzyme phenylethanolamine N-methyl transferase which is largely confined to the adrenal medulla. In this chromaffin tissue noradrenaline migrates from the chromaffin granules, where it is stored, to the cytoplasm, to be converted to adrenaline which re-enters the chromaffin granule. It is likely that glucocorticoids from the adrenal cortex are involved in this transformation of noradrenaline to adrenaline. Most of the noradrenaline and adrenaline in tissues is localised within storage granules that also contain adenosine triphosphate (ATP). The chromaffin granules are large, measuring 500–4,000 Å in diameter, whereas the granules in sympathetic terminals are only about 500 Å in width. Certain specific functions may be attributed to the storage granules:

(*a*) uptake of dopamine (a precursor of noradrenaline);
(*b*) conversion of dopamine to noradrenaline;
(*c*) storage of noradrenaline and adrenaline;
(*d*) uptake of noradrenaline and adrenaline from the circulation;
(*e*) protection of noradrenaline and adrenaline from degradation by monoamine oxidase present in the tissue;
(*f*) release of noradrenaline or adrenaline in response to nervous stimulation;
(*g*) recapture of part of the released noradrenaline.

The granules act as a tissue buffer for catecholamines which can be compared with the tissue or serum binding proteins that react with other hormones.

Release of Catecholamines

Most of the adrenaline in the circulation is derived from the adrenal medulla. Bilateral adrenalectomy causes the urinary adrenaline output to fall by over 80 per cent but noradrenaline excretion remains unchanged. After several years urinary adrenaline excretion approaches the original level, suggesting that extra-adrenal chromaffin tissue has taken over the role of the adrenal medulla in synthesising this hormone. The adrenal medulla releases adrenaline in response to stress of various sorts, e.g. fear, hypoglycaemia, or surgical trauma. Usually both catecholamines are released, but it is not known whether separate chromaffin cells are responsible for the release of each hormone.

Noradrenaline is secreted into the circulation both by the adrenal medulla and by sympathetic nerve endings, the latter being the main source. Much of the noradrenaline in the blood is derived from sympathetic nerves in the heart, where the large blood flow washes out the hormone.

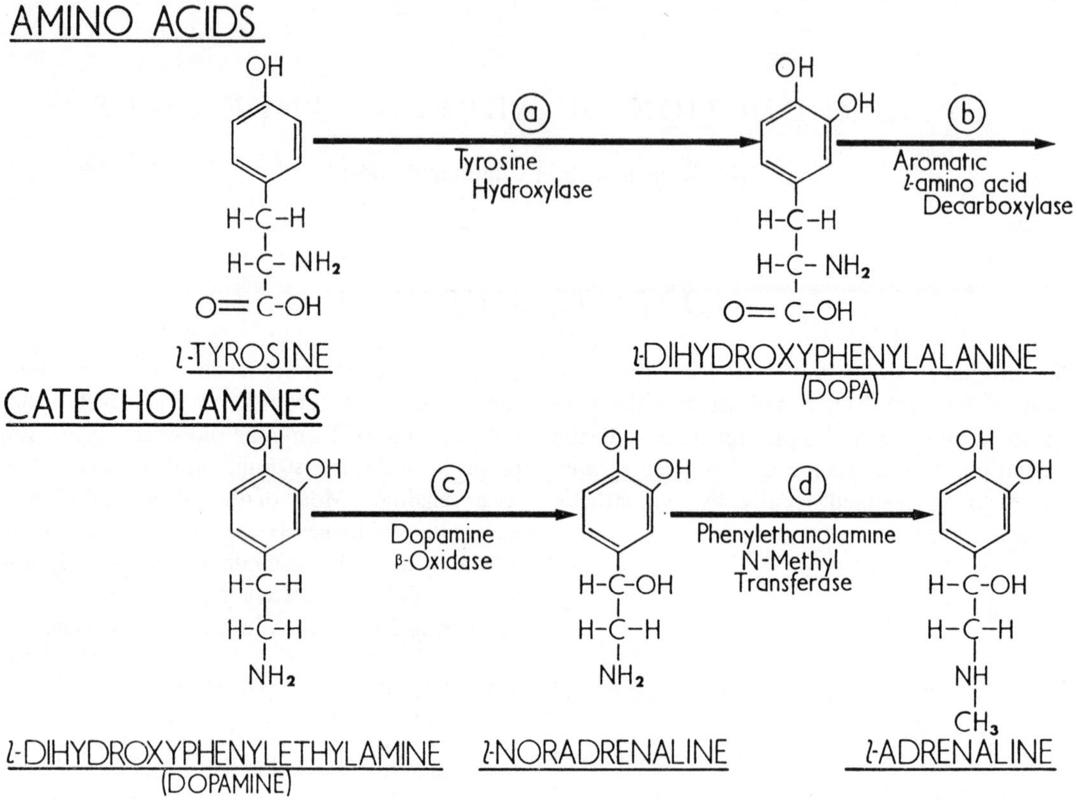

AMINO ACIDS

(a) Tyrosine Hydroxylase

(b) Aromatic *l*-amino acid Decarboxylase

l-TYROSINE

l-DIHYDROXYPHENYLALANINE (DOPA)

CATECHOLAMINES

(c) Dopamine β-Oxidase

(d) Phenylethanolamine N-Methyl Transferase

l-DIHYDROXYPHENYLETHYLAMINE (DOPAMINE)

l-NORADRENALINE

l-ADRENALINE

FIGURE 6.13 Biosynthesis of catecholamines

Fate of Catecholamines

The circulating catecholamines are either taken up by tissues to be stored or degraded, or are excreted in the urine. Tissue uptake of catecholamines depends on the blood supply of the tissue and the extent of its sympathetic innervation. When the sympathetic innervation is rich, the catecholamines are taken up and bound in the storage granules. Brain tissue takes up very little circulating catecholamine and its content is largely derived from endogenous synthesis. Sympathetic denervation abolishes the ability of a tissue to concentrate catecholamines.

pool, which is degraded mainly by monoamine oxidase.

Tissues such as liver and kidney which are rich in catechol-o-methyl transferase convert most of the catecholamines to normetadrenaline and

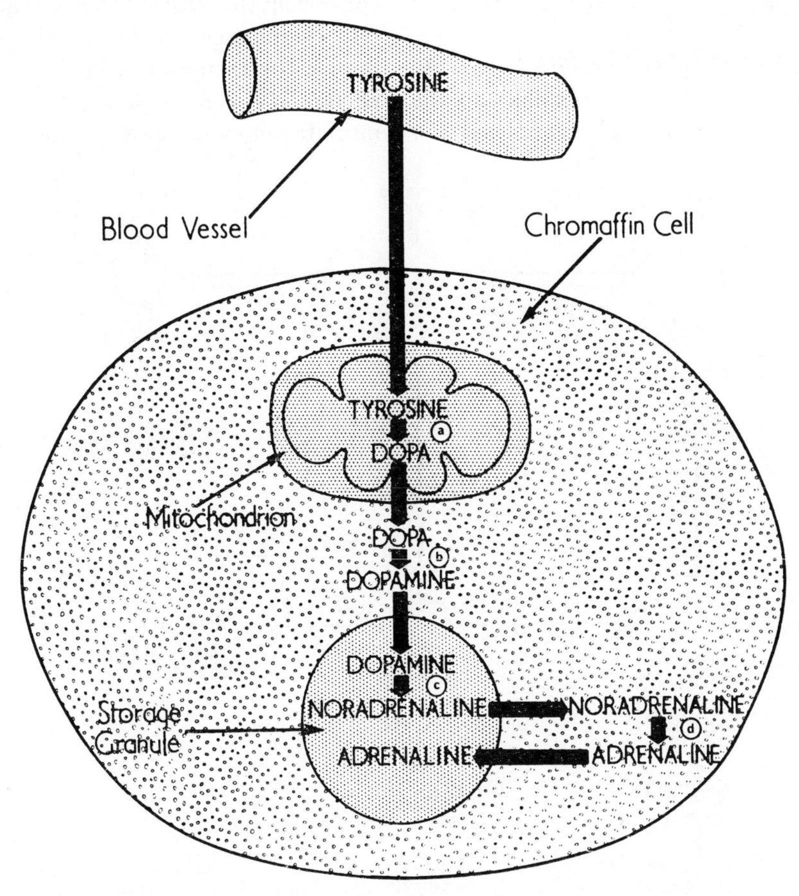

FIGURE 6.14 Intracellular localisation of enzymes and subtrates involved in catecholamine biosynthesis. (a, b, c, and d refer to enzymes labelled in Fig. 6.13)

Tissue catecholamines are derived from endogenous synthesis and from the circulation. At least two pools of catecholamines can be detected: pool 1 is an active pool that turns over rapidly, and can be released by tyramine or by sympathetic nerve activity, when it is destroyed in the circulation or taken up again into nerve endings to be stored or to be o-methylated. Pool 2 is relatively inactive and acts as a store of catecholamines. Tyramine has little effect on this

metadrenaline which, in turn, are acted on by monoamine oxidase to yield 4-hydroxy-3-methoxymandelic acid (HMMA), which is also known as vanillyl-mandelic acid (VMA) though the former is the more correct designation (Fig. 6.15). HMMA is the major degradation product of the catecholamines, largely originating from pool 2. HMMA excretion is more closely related to catecholamine synthesis than to the activity of the sympathetic nervous system.

Dopamine, a better substrate for monoamine oxidase than either adrenaline or noradrenaline, tends to be oxidatively deaminated before it is o-methylated to homovanillic acid (HVA). This compound can then be converted to HMMA and other metabolites.

Biological Activity of Catecholamines

The biological effect of catecholamines in the circulation will depend on the amount fixed in the tissue which, as mentioned previously, is related to its blood supply and sympathetic innervation, and also to the sensitivity of the binding sites of tissue receptors. The tissue receptors have not been isolated and are largely a convenient theoretical concept. They are divided into α-adrenergic receptors which cause smooth muscle contraction, e.g. in skin and the dilator of the iris, and β-adrenergic receptors which mediate smooth muscle relaxation, e.g. in the

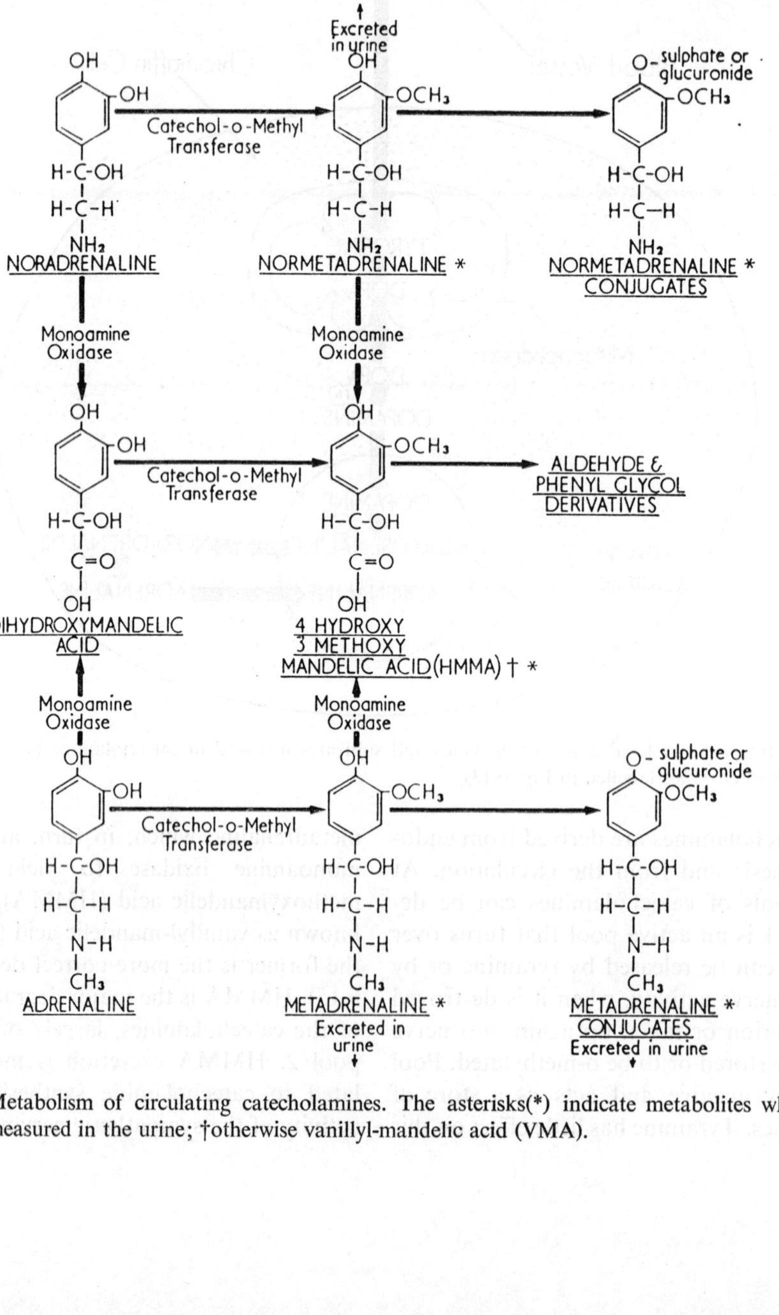

FIGURE 6.15 Metabolism of circulating catecholamines. The asterisks(*) indicate metabolites which may be conveniently measured in the urine; †otherwise vanillyl-mandelic acid (VMA).

bronchi. Adrenaline is thought to act on both α- and β-receptors, causing smooth muscle contraction in certain sites and relaxation in others. Adrenaline mobilises fatty acid by a mechanism mediated through β-adrenergic receptors. The synthetic adrenergic agent isoprenaline acts almost exclusively on β-receptors in the heart, smooth muscle of bronchi, skeletal muscle, blood vessels, and the gut. Noradrenaline acts mainly on α-receptors and has little action on β-receptors except in the heart. The main actions of adrenaline and noradrenaline are shown in Table 6.5. The receptors responsible for some of the metabolic actions of catecholamines cannot be readily fitted into the α-, β-receptor theory. Certain drugs interfere with the actions of catecholamines at one or other type of receptor. Propranolol and practolol act largely as β-adrenergic blockers although the action of the latter is more or less restricted to the heart; thymoxamine, phentolamine and phenoxybenzamine are α-adrenergic inhibitors, although with the exception of thymoxamine the actions of these compounds are not pure in that under many circumstances they show α-agonist activities before their blockade is apparent. The use of these drugs in the diagnosis and management of phaeochromocytoma will be discussed later.

TABLE 6.5 *Effects of Adrenaline and Noradrenaline*

(After Goldenberg, Aranow, Smith, and Faber, 1950, by permission of the editor, *Archives of Internal Medicine*.)

Action	Adrenaline	Noradrenaline
Cardiac:		
Heart rate	+	−*
Stroke volume	++	++
Cardiac output	+++	0, −
Arrhythmias	++++	++++
Coronary blood flow	++	+++
Blood pressure:		
Systolic arterial	+++	+++
Mean arterial	+	++
Diastolic arterial	+, 0, −	++
Mean pulmonary	++	++
Peripheral circulation:		
Total peripheral resistance	−	++
Cerebral blood flow	+	0, −
Muscle blood flow	++	0, −
Cutaneous blood flow	−	+, 0, −
Renal blood flow	−	−
Splanchnic blood flow	++	0, +
Metabolic effects:		
Oxygen consumption	++	0, +
Blood sugar	+++	0, +
Blood lactic acid	+++	0, +
Eosinopenic response	+	0
CNS:		
Respiration	+	+
Subjective sensations	+	0, +

+ = increase; − = decrease; 0 = no change; * = after atropine

Mechanism of Action of Catecholamines

The action of adrenaline on carbohydrate metabolism is thought to be mediated by stimulation of the formation of cyclic 3′, 5′-adenosine monophosphate from ATP. Cyclic AMP causes activation of phosphorylase which breaks down glycogen to form glucose-1-phosphate which is then converted to glucose-6-phosphate. Glucose-6-phosphate is available for the formation of free glucose or to enter the hexose monophosphate or Embden-Meyerhof pathways.

Effect of Drugs on Catecholamine Metabolism

Many drugs exert their clinical effects by interfering with catecholamine metabolism, and a brief outline of some of these actions will be given. Some drugs have more than one action.

1. *Drugs interfering with catecholamine uptake by sympathetic nerve endings*—cocaine, imipramine, ephedrine and amphetamine. These

drugs potentiate catecholamine action since uptake of the hormones by nervous tissue is one of the chief methods by which they are removed from the circulation.

2. *Drugs causing release of bound catecholamines*—phenylephrine, epinine, tyramine, ephedrine, amphetamine and reserpine. Some of these agents also elevate the blood pressure by a direct action on α-receptors. Reserpine usually causes a fall in blood pressure because the catecholamines it releases are broken down by monoamine oxidase, and its central hypotensive action is unopposed.
3. *Drugs blocking release of catecholamines*—bethanidine, guanethidine, ganglion blocking agents and inhibitors of monoamine oxidase. Bethanidine and guanethidine first discharge catecholamines and then block any further release from tissues. Ganglion blocking drugs which interfere with preganglionic sympathetic nerve impulses prevent the release of catecholamines by the post-ganglionic terminals. Monoamine oxidase inhibitors break down catecholamines within the nerve terminal, particularly from the second storage pool.
4. *False transmitters* are formed as the result of the presence of α-methyldopa and are taken up by the storage granules in competition with catecholamines. They therefore lower tissue catecholamine content and sympathetic activity.
5. *Drugs interfering with the peripheral action of catecholamines* include α-adrenergic blockers (thymoxamine, phenoxybenzamine or phentolamine) and β-adrenergic blockers (propranolol, practolol).

DISORDERS OF THE ADRENAL MEDULLA

Total removal of both adrenal glands can be corrected by administration of adrenocortical hormones alone and there is no evidence that adrenal medullary deficiency has any clinical sequelae. As mentioned previously, after adrenalectomy extra-medullary chromaffin tissue gradually takes over the role of the adrenal medulla in secreting adrenaline.

OVERPRODUCTION OF ADRENAL MEDULLARY HORMONES

This is caused by tumours of the adrenal medulla or of accessory chromaffin tissue. Tumours that arise from tissues having their origin in the neural crest are sympathoblastomas, neuroblastomas, ganglioneuromas, phaeochromocytomas, neurofibromas, melanomas, neurilemmomas, and argentaffinomas. The first four tumours in this list are derived from sympathetic nervous tissue, the first two of them being embryonic in type, and the second two mature. Recently some patients with retinoblastomas, which are also of sympathetic origin, have been shown to excrete an excess of catecholamine metabolites in the urine. Very rarely, secretion of catecholamines can be demonstrated by carotid body (glomus jugulare) and melanotic neuroectodermal tumours.

Cell	*Tumour*
1. Sympathogone	Sympathoblastoma
2. Sympathoblast	Neuroblastoma
3. Ganglion cells	Ganglioneuroma
4. Chromaffin cells	Phaeochromocytoma

1. SYMPATHOBLASTOMA (sympathogonioma)

These highly malignant tumours occur during intrauterine life or during the first year. They show a fibrillary stroma and small cells arranged irregularly or in clusters.

2. NEUROBLASTOMA (sympathoblastoma, neurocytoma)

Neuroblastomas are, again, highly malignant and are one of the most common neoplasms in childhood. Most cases occur before the age of five years but no age group is exempt. Neuroblastomas usually arise along the line of migration of sympathoblasts from the neural crest to the adrenal medulla. About one-third occur in the adrenal medulla but it is sometimes difficult to be sure of the site from which a retroperitoneal neuroblastoma has arisen. Some 25 per cent of tumours arise in the thorax. Metastases by the blood and lymphatics reach the liver, bones, and lymph nodes. When metastases have occurred, the prognosis is virtually hopeless. Microscopically, the tumours show fibrillary fibrous septa and there is a tendency for the tumour cells to be arranged in whorls or rosettes. Occasionally, mature ganglion cells are interspersed and, very rarely, in patients who survive, the neuroblastoma cells may mature to form ganglion cells. Calcification is not infrequent and may be sufficient to be visible on X-ray.

The *clinical features* of the tumour are usually the result of local or distant spread, and less commonly due to catecholamines which the neoplasm may produce. Malaise, vomiting, abdominal pain or difficulty in walking are the commonest presenting features. The incidence of symptoms and signs caused by overproduction of catecholamines and possibly other humoral factors is not well known but a proportion of cases have hypertension, sweating attacks, pallor, and diarrhoea. There is a possible association between neuroblastomas and adrenocortical hyperplasia.

Diagnosis may be suggested by calcification shown on X-rays of thorax or abdomen. In about half the cases in most series, marrow examination reveals malignant cells which should not be mistaken for reticulum cells. Ewing's tumour may occasionally cause difficulty in diagnosis. In most cases, even in those without features of catecholamine excess, catecholamines or their degradation products can be detected in the urine in increased amounts. Dopamine, HVA, adrenaline, noradrenaline, and HMMA (VMA) may be found. In practice, HMMA or HVA screening is usually carried out. If this is positive, the diagnosis is confirmed. Occasionally, tests for total catecholamines are positive when HMMA is negative and, rarely, no catecholamines or their metabolities can be found.

Treatment when possible is usually by surgery followed by radiotherapy, though the 'cure' rate is only about 10 per cent at present. Response to therapy can sometimes be assessed by changes in catecholamine excretion.

3. GANGLIONEUROMA

Ganglioneuromas are rare tumours occurring in young adults. They may be benign or malignant and are often an incidental finding at autopsy. Occasionally, malignant neuroblastomas have been found to mature to benign ganglioneuromas.

4. PHAECHROMOCYTOMA (chromaffinoma)

Phaeochromocytomas (PCC) occur in either sex, usually in adults aged from 25–55 years. They are rare in children but when they do occur they affect boys more commonly. Familial cases occur, and these are more often associated with neurofibromatosis or, more rarely, medullary carcinoma of the thyroid or other endocrine adenomas. Some 90 per cent of all PCC originate in the adrenal medulla, 10 per cent being malignant, when they are usually bilateral. Extra-adrenal PCC may develop anywhere along the course of the sympathetic chain from neck to pelvis and even in the bladder wall, but often the paired para-aortic bodies of Zuckerkandl are affected. Children are more prone than adults to develop extra-adrenal, multiple PCC.

Pathology. PCC are variable in size, usually well encapsulated, vascular and, on sectioning, they may show areas of haemorrhage and necrosis in a grey-brown surface. Histologically the tumours resemble adrenal medullary tissue, and like normal adrenal medulla, they stain brown with dichromate, hence their designation chromaffin. The brown staining results from oxidation products of the catecholamines present in granules within the cell.

Clinical Features

These are typically the result of increased catecholamine production by the tumour. The PCC is a great mimic, simulating anxiety, hysteria, hyperthyroidism, spontaneous hypoglycaemia, diabetes mellitus, renal disease and, most importantly, essential hypertension. Its clinical features will be considered under the headings hypertension, hypermetabolism, and hyperglycaemia.

Hypertension. About 0·5 per cent of all cases of hypertension are due to PCC, but because PCC are usually benign they represent an important curable group of the hypertensive population. Hypertension may be paroxysmal, or persistent, when essential hypertension is simulated. Paroxysmal hypertension is accompanied by headaches, nausea and vomiting, precordial or abdominal pain, pallor and sweating. The attacks last anything from a few minutes to a few hours and usually terminate spontaneously. They may cause death from intracranial haemorrhage, ventricular fibrillation, or acute heart failure. They are due to the intermittent release of catecholamines from the tumour which occurs spontaneously, from emotional upsets, from changes in posture, from exertion, from massage of the tumour or operative handling, and from drugs such as histamine or certain anaesthetics. The pattern of attacks varies with the amount and type of catecholamine released. Rarely, the paroxysms are associated with hypotension and diarrhoea. Renal damage may result from the hypertension, acute renal failure following some severe paroxysms of hypertension, and chronic renal failure resulting from sustained hypertension. In children and less commonly in some adults PCC may be present with sustained hypertension. During pregnancy PCC may simulate pre-eclamptic toxaemia. Pressor attacks similar to those occurring in PCC are seen in some patients receiving monoamine-oxidase inhibitors. These occur after the ingestion of cheese, game, some wines, broad beans, and yeast extracts, when the catecholamines, such as tyramine, which they contain, remain unoxidised and lead to massive noradrenaline release.

Hypermetabolism and hyperglycaemia, due largely to adrenaline, may be paroxysmal or persistent. The raised metabolic rate suggests hyperthyroidism and this resemblance is increased by the tachycardia, tremor, excessive sweating, diarrhoea, and weight loss which accompany it, but tests of thyroid function are normal. Abnormalities of carbohydrate metabolism result from overproduction of catecholamines—hyperglycaemia, abnormal glucose tolerance, and glycosuria. Removal of the PCC corrects these abnormalities in some patients but not in others. Presumably, patients constituted as diabetics are more susceptible.

There is in addition a reduced blood volume in patients with PCC possibly due to vasoconstriction particularly in the venous circulation. This may give rise to problems when the tumour is removed (*see* below).

Diagnosis

The history of intermittent headache and sweating, especially in a hypertensive patient, should always raise the possibility of PCC. All hypertensive patients should be screened for the presence of PCC. Three main groups of tests are applied to patients with possible PCC:

1. Direct estimation of catecholamines or their degradation products in blood and urine.
2. Blocking tests with phentolamine.
3. Provocative tests with histamine or tyramine.

Once overproduction of catecholamines has been confirmed tests should be used to determine the site of the tumour.

1. *Direct Estimation of Catecholamines and Metabolites.* Plasma levels of total catecholamines are normally less than 1·0 μg per litre and daily urine excretion less than 20 μg of adrenaline and 70 μg of noradrenaline. Much higher amounts are found in most patients with phaeochromocytomas. It is sometimes important to know the type of catecholamine the tumour is secreting—extra-adrenal PCC secrete largely noradrenaline, as do metastases from adrenal tumours. If adrenaline is secreted in excess it is likely that the tumour arises in the adrenal medulla. Malignant PCC have a tendency to secrete large amounts of the catecholamine dopamine, but not all tumours secreting dopamine and its metabolites are malignant. Since only a small part of the catecholamines secreted each day are excreted unchanged in the urine, and since the plasma levels of catecholamines are low, the urinary excretion of their metabolites should be assayed.

The routine procedure of choice in most laboratories is estimation of the daily urine output of HMMA (VMA). Figures vary from different laboratories but, normally, less than about 8 mg of HMMA are excreted each day. To prevent false positive results the patient should avoid coffee, tea, chocolate, ice cream and bananas, and all drugs for 48 hours before the start of the urine collection. Measurement of the excretion of metadrenaline and normetadrenaline must also be performed since not only may they be helpful in determining the type of catecholamine the tumour is producing and hence suggesting whether the tumour is intra- or extra-adrenal, but also some patients with PCC have elevated metadrenaline output with normal HMMA excretion. A few patients show normal basal urinary catecholamines with a rise only after an episode of hypertension.

Occasionally, PCC secrete hydroxytyramine which has less of a pressor action than noradrenaline. Another rare variant is the patient with PCC who is normotensive or hypotensive and has flushing of the skin. It is possible that 'inert' catecholamine precursors are secreted by their tumours and taken up by the storage granules, to interfere with catecholamine release and action. Other humoral agents may cause the polycythaemia or diarrhoea seen very occasionally in patients with PCC.

2. *Blocking Tests.* In past years reliance has been placed on the blood pressure response to the α-adrenergic blocking drug phentolamine. The blood pressure is taken each 30 seconds during a 10 minute control period and then one or two control saline injections are given, by a separate observer through an indwelling needle, while the blood pressure record continues. Then 5 mg of phentolamine is given intravenously, and the test is considered to be significant if the blood pressure falls by more than 35/25 within 3 minutes, the effects passing off within 15 minutes. Unfortunately false negatives may occur in patients with PCC who only rarely have sustained hypertension anyway; also false positives may be seen in patients with essential hypertension without PCC. There seems to be little place now for the phentolamine test.

3. *Provocative Tests.* These may be dangerous and should no longer be performed now that urinary catecholamine excretion can be measured reliably and with relative ease. In the past intravenous tyramine or histamine was given and an excessive rise in blood pressure suggested the presence of PCC.

When overproduction of catecholamines has been confirmed an attempt is made to determine the site of the tumour. As mentioned previously, the type of catecholamine secreted may be helpful. A plain X-ray of abdomen may show displacement of the renal outline or, rarely, calcification. An intravenous pyelogram is useful if there is downward displacement of the kidney. Selective adrenal arteriography or aortography is helpful if the tumour is more than 1 cm in diameter. Such procedures may provoke hypertensive attacks and patients should be prepared as for surgery (see below). Perirenal air insufflation is of little value. If the tumour cannot be located by these techniques, catheterisation of the inferior vena cava, taking serial blood samples for catecholamines as the catheter is withdrawn, can sometimes indicate the level of the tumour.

Treatment

It is essential that the surgeon examines both adrenals since PCC may be multiple, and therefore an anterior approach is to be preferred. During such manipulations there may be transient but marked elevations of blood pressure due to release of catecholamines, and these can be treated by the anaesthetist by administration of intravenous phentolamine. Following removal of the tumour there is often a profound fall in blood pressure due to sudden relaxation of the tone of the vascular bed and an insufficiency of blood to fill the vascular volume. This must be treated with blood transfusion, often with large volumes of blood.

These complications may largely be avoided by intensive preoperative (or pre-aortogram) preparation of the patient for at least 3 days. Intravenous phenoxybenzamine infusions are given (0·5 mg per kg body weight in 250 ml of 5 per cent dextrose over 2 hours) each day. After the first phenoxybenzamine infusion, propranolol is started (40 mg each 8 hours by mouth). This regime, described by Ross *et al.* (1967) allows the increased vascular tone to relax so that the plasma volume becomes normal, and also prevents hypertensive episodes. If for any reason operation has to be delayed, some measure of protection can be afforded by adminstering phenoxybenzamine by mouth (10 mg, 8 hourly) with propranolol (40 mg, 8 hourly). Patients with PCC who experience hypotensive episodes should not be treated with phenoxybenzamine.

REFERENCES

General

Cope, C. L. (1972). *Adrenal Steroids and Disease.* 2nd Edition. London: Pitman Medical.

Adrenal Cortex

Addison, T. (1855). *On the Constitutional and Local Effects of Disease of the Suprarenal Capsules.* London: D. Highley.

Besser, G. M., and Edwards, C. R. W. (1972). '*Cushing's Syndrome*,' in *Clinics in Endocrinology and Metabolism*, Vol. 1 (2), p. 451 (Mason, A. S., Ed). London: Saunders.

Bartter, F. C., Pronove, P., Jillo, J. R., and MacCardle, R. C. (1962). *Amer. J. Med.*, **33**, 811.

Brown, J. J., Fraser, R., Lever, A. F., and Robertson, J. I. S. (1972). 'Aldosterone: Physiological and Pathophysiological Variations in Man', in *Clinics in Endocrinology and Metabolism*, Vol. 1 (2), p. 397 (Mason, A. S., Ed). London: Saunders.

Conn, J. W., Knopf, R. F., and Nesbit, R. M. (1964). *Amer. J. Surg.*, **107**, 159.

Cope, C. L. (1966). *Brit. med. J.*, **ii**, 847.

Ferris, J. B., Brown, J. J., Fraser, R., Kay, A. W., Neville, A. M., Robertson, J. I. S., Symington, T., Lever, A. F., and D'Muircheartigh, I. G. (1970). *Lancet*, **2**, 995.

Hutter, A. M., Jr., and Kayhoe, D. E. (1966). *Amer. J. Med.*, **41**, 581.

Irvine, W. J., Stewart, A. G., and Scarth, L. (1967). *Clin. exp. Immunol.*, **2**, 31.

Irvine, W. J., and Barnes, E. W. (1972). 'Adrenocortical Insufficiency', in *Clinics in Endocrinology and Metabolism*, Vol. 1 (2), p. 549 (Mason, A. S., Ed). London: Saunders.

Neville, A. M., and Mackay, A. M. (1972). 'The Structure of the Human Adrenal Cortex in Health and Disease', in *Clinics in Endocrinology and Metabolism*, Vol. 1 (2), p. 361 (Mason, A. S., Ed). London: Saunders.

Orth, D. N., and Liddle, G. W. (1971). *New England Journal of Medicine*, **285**, 243.

Plumpton, F. S., Besser, G. M., and Cole, P. V. (1969). *Anaesthesia*, **24**, 3 and 12.

Adrenal Medulla

Goodman, L. S., and Gilman, A. (Eds) (1970). *The Pharmacological Basis of Therapeutics*, 4th Edition. New York: Macmillan Co.

Ross, E. J., Prichard, B. N. C., Kaufman, L., Robertson, A. I. G., Harries, B. J. (1967). *Brit. Med. J.*, **1**, 191.

Varley, H., and Gowenlock, A. H. (Eds) (1963). 'The clinical chemistry of mono-amines,' *Proc. Symp. Clin. Chem. of Mono-amines*, Manchester, 1962. London: Elsevier Publishing Co.

7

OVARY

The ovaries secrete oestrogens and progesterone, which cause maturation and maintenance of the female genitalia and secondary sex characteristics, as well as affecting the metabolism of other body tissues. The ovaries also produce ova capable of fertilisation, implantation, and development into a fetus. The endometrium is prepared for implantation of the fertilised ovum by secretion of progesterone from the corpus luteum, which is formed from the ruptured Graafian follicle, and which subsequently maintains the endometrium in a state capable of supporting the fertilised ovum. These ovarian functions are controlled by the gonadotrophins secreted by the anterior pituitary (*see* Chapter 1).

EMBRYOLOGY

The primordial sex cells are differentiated at an early stage in the development of the embryo. Initially, they are situated in the wall of the yolk sac, from where they migrate to the root of the mesentery and thence to the genital ridge. The cells in the genital ridge induce the formation of the fetal ovary and act as stem cells for the primordial ova present at birth. In the gonad destined to become an ovary there are initially two layers of cells—the cortex and the medulla. The medulla soon becomes atrophic, although it can, in the adult, be the site of androgen-producing adenomas or hyperplasia. The medulla of the ovary is analogous to the testis. In the cortex of the ovary are situated the germ cells and other cells that will assume an endocrine function. The secondary reproductive structures are derived from the Wolffian ridges. In the female, the Müllerian ducts grow out of these ridges and give rise to the uterus, Fallopian tubes, and part of the vagina. In the normal female, only vestigial remnants of the Wolffian ducts are present. Fuller details on the embryology of the ovary are considered in Chapter 13.

ANATOMY AND HISTOLOGY

The ovaries are situated one on each side of the uterus in relation to the lateral wall of the pelvis, and attached to the posterior or upper layer of the broad ligament, behind and below the uterine tubes. They are greyish pink in colour, and with advancing age show an increasing degree of puckering and unevenness of the surface. Each ovary is about 3 cm long, 1·5 cm wide, and 1 cm thick. The arterial blood supply to the ovaries arises from the aorta. The venous drainage leaves the ovarian hilum in a plexus, the pampiniform plexus, from which the ovarian veins are formed. The right ovarian vein drains to the inferior vena cava, and the left to the left renal vein.

The surface of the ovary is covered with a layer of cuboidal cells, the germinal epithelium, which gives the ovary its typical colour. Immediately beneath the germinal epithelium is a condensed layer of connective tissue—the tunica albuginea. The ovarian follicles are embedded in the stroma of the cortex, which surrounds a richly vascular central area where the vestigial remnant of the primitive medulla is situated. The stroma consists of reticular connective tissue

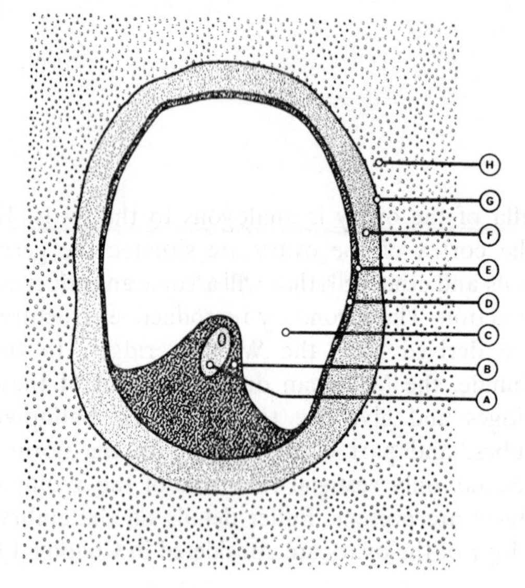

FIGURE 7.1 The Graafian follicle (diagrammatic)

A ovum
B discus proligerus
C antrum filled with follicular fluid
D stratum granulosum
E membrana granulosa
F theca interna and externa
G theca folliculi
H stroma of ovary

fibres and spindle-shaped cells. During prenatal life the stroma of the cortex of the ovary contains groups of interstitial cells; after puberty these are only present in the theca of atretic follicles.

The cortex at birth contains numerous *primary ovarian follicles*, consisting of a large central cell, the öogonium, surrounded by a single layer of small cuboidal cells—the follicular cells. It was previously thought that most primary follicles degenerated during childhood, a few remaining dormant until puberty, when some would develop each month to form the vesicular Graafian follicles, of which one would mature and rupture. However, there is now evidence that suggests that all of the primary follicles degenerate during childhood, and that each month new follicles form as ingrowths of the germinal epithelium. During the childbearing years, the cortex of the ovary contains follicles and corpora lutea in various stages of development.

The fully developed Graafian follicle is 10 mm or more in diameter and is surrounded by a capsule, the theca folliculi, derived from the ovarian stroma. Internal to this are the theca externa and theca interna, the latter being separated from the stratum granulosum by a thin basement membrane. The centre of the follicle is vesicular and filled with the liquor folliculi, and the ovum surrounded by the discus proligerus (derived from the stratum granulosum) is attached peripherally (Fig. 7.1). As a rule, only one follicle reaches full maturity and ruptures, although occasionally several ova may be released. Several follicles also develop partially each month and then undergo degeneration; these are the atretic follicles. The cells of the theca interna of these atretic follicles form the interstitial cells, which are the equivalent of the interstitial cells of the testes. Cycles in the months following the menarche are often anovulatory.

Ovulation. The mechanism by which one particular follicle is selected for full development is not known. The primordial germ cell migrates towards the centre of the ovary and is surrounded by other cells. As the cell mass reaches its final position, it develops a small cleft, called the antrum. This process takes place in several primitive follicles simultaneously. Up to this stage, development of the follicle may occur independently of FSH. However, FSH is necessary for follicular ripening and causes accumulation of fluid within the antrum as the cell mass moves peripherally. With further secretion of liquor folliculi and cell growth, the follicle reaches maturity. The events leading to ovulation are not fully understood. The follicle now forms a bulge on the surface of the ovary, the area from which ovulation will occur being termed the stigma. A ring of blood vessels which surround the stigma constrict and produce necrosis of the follicular wall. It seems that at the time of ovulation, when LH levels rise sharply, the cell wall becomes sufficiently weakened to rupture and the follicular fluid is released, carrying with it the ovum and its surrounding cumulus. The ovum passes along the Fallopian tubes, where it may be fertilised. The walls of the ruptured ovarian follicle collapse and become folded. Cells of the stratum granulosum increase in size and a yellowish carotenoid pigment (lutein) is formed in their cytoplasm. These are the lutein cells; they form the major part of the corpus luteum which, unless fertilisation of the ovum occurs, functions for 12 to 14 days after ovulation and then degenerates. The hormonal control of follicle development and ovulation is further discussed later.

THE OVARIAN HORMONES

The ovarian hormones are steroids and may be considered in three groups:

1. oestrogens
2. progesterone
3. androgens.

The biosynthesis of the ovarian steroids is dependent on the pituitary gonadotrophins, and is normally cyclical, unless fertilisation of an ovum occurs, in which case ovarian secretion becomes continuous. The major precursor of the ovarian hormones is cholesterol. The biosynthetic pathways involved are shown in Fig. 7.2.

1. OESTROGENS

The ovarian oestrogens are secreted by cells of the theca interna and the stratum granulosum. The oestrogens are characterised by the presence of a benzene ring and a phenolic hydroxyl group (Fig. 7.3). 17β-oestradiol and oestrone are the primary oestrogens produced in the ovary, the former being the most potent. They are inter-convertible, and the enzymes responsible for the conversion are found in many tissues, hence the active circulatory oestrogen in non-pregnant women is probably an equilibrium mixture of the two. Oestriol is an irreversible metabolite of oestradiol and is much less potent in terms of its effect on the endometrium. However it does have marked effects on the cervix and vagina which may be regarded as its target organs. All three oestrogens circulate in the blood bound to protein and are excreted in the bile and in the urine mainly in the form of conjugates with glucuronic and sulphuric acids. Conjugation of the oestrogens is carried out in the liver, and renders the compounds more soluble. A number of other oestrogenic metabolites have been identified in small quantities in human urine.

Actions of Oestrogens. Oestrogens are responsible for initiating and maintaining maturity of the female genitalia and the secondary sex characteristics. These will be discussed in the section on puberty in the female. The oestrogens, together with progesterone, are responsible for the maintenance and control of normal menstruation. Although oestrogens stimulate growth, excessive levels may in fact lead to short stature due to premature fusion of the epiphyses. Oestrogens tend to antagonise the effects of androgens on the skin, thus reducing sebaceous gland activity. They cause deposition of subcutaneous adipose tissue, and are responsible for the characteristic distribution of fat in the mature female. This action of oestrogen is made use of by farmers and others concerned with food production who add oestrogens to the feed of livestock to increase carcase fat and produce more tender meat. Oestrogens inhibit the secretion of FSH. In large doses they also cause sodium and water retention, which may lead to oedema, or, rarely, precipitate heart failure in a susceptible individual. In pharmacological amounts, oestrogens may induce painful swelling of the breasts, dysfunctional uterine bleeding, nausea, and vomiting. Venous thrombosis is a proven complication of oestrogen therapy (*see* p. 206). The administration of oestrogens in early pregnancy is a possible cause of vaginal adenosis and adenocarcinoma in female offspring with a latent period of up to two decades. (Herbst *et al.*, 1970).

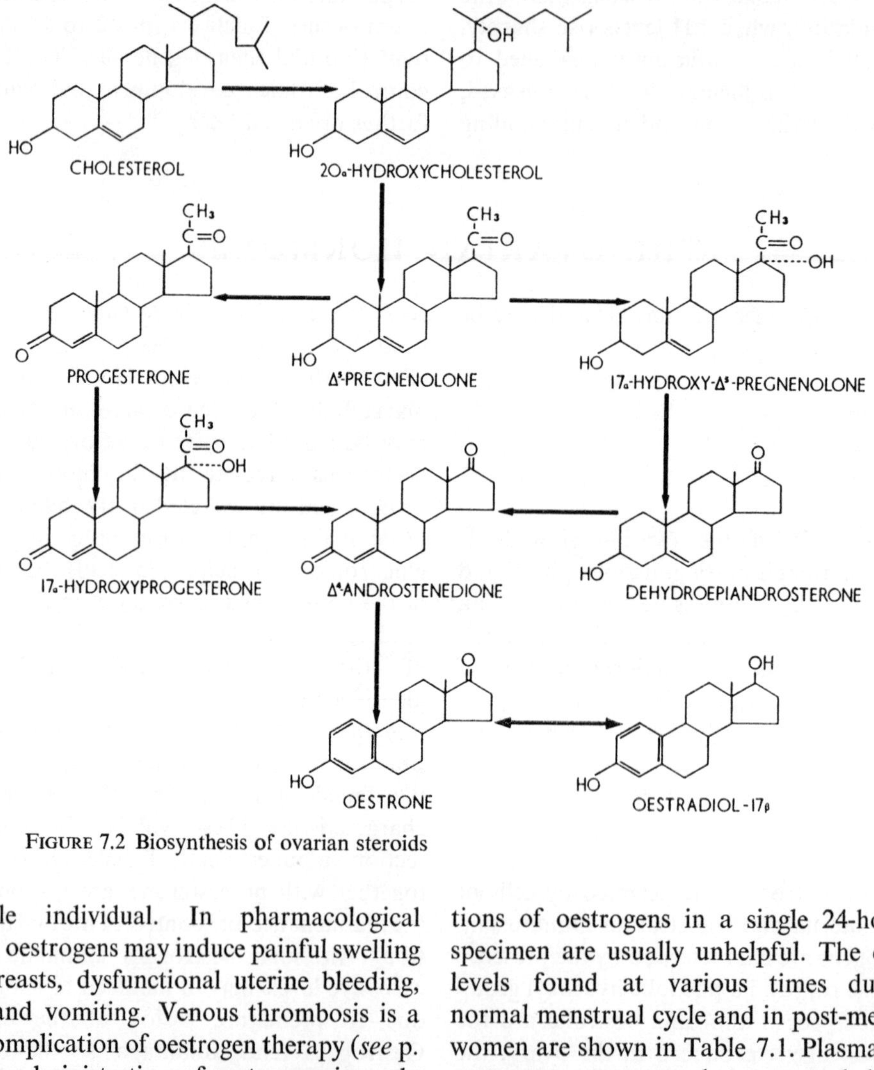

FIGURE 7.2 Biosynthesis of ovarian steroids

Assay of Oestrogens. Chemical and biological methods are available for the quantitation of urinary oestrogens. The normal range for urinary oestrogen excretion in the female is wide and fluctuates in a cyclical fashion, depending on the stage of the monthly cycle at which the specimen is collected. For this reason, estimations of oestrogens in a single 24-hour urine specimen are usually unhelpful. The oestrogen levels found at various times during the normal menstrual cycle and in post-menopausal women are shown in Table 7.1. Plasma levels of oestrogens can now be measured by radio-immunoassay. Levels of 17β-oestradiol vary during the menstrual cycle from a mean level of about 50 pg/ml during the early follicular phase.

TABLE 7.1 *Oestrogen Levels during the Menstrual Cycle and After the Menopause*
(from Brown, J. B., 1955a, b)

Time in cycle	Urinary excretion (mg/24 hr), mean and range		
	oestriol	oestrone	oestradiol
Onset of menstruation	6 (0–15)	5 (4–7)	2 (0–3)
Ovulation peak	27 (13–54)	20 (11–31)	9 (4–14)
Luteal maximum	22 (8–72)	14 (10–23)	7 (4–10)
Post-menopausal	3·3 (0·6–8·6)	2·5 (0·8–7·1)	0·6 (0–3·9)

Indirect estimates of oestrogen secretion may be obtained from examination of vaginal or cervical secretions. The absence of cornification in the vaginal epithelial cells indicates a marked reduction in oestrogen secretion. In the fern test, a sample of cervical secretion is spread on a glass slide and dried. A fern-like configuration indicates the presence of adequate oestrogen concentrations.

Indications for Oestrogen Therapy. Oestrogens have been used in the treatment of a wide variety of disorders and only some of the commoner uses will be considered here. They are effective in controlling many of the complications of the menopause (*see* p. 188). In high dosage they are capable of stopping the prolonged phase of bleeding seen in metropathia haemorrhagica, but oral contraceptive regimes using combined oestrogen-progesterone preparations are now preferable. Similarly combined regimes are effective in the treatment of endometriosis. So long as a uterus is present it is possible to induce withdrawal bleeding with cyclical oestrogen regimes, preferably in combination with a progestogen. Oestrogens may be used to accelerate epiphyseal fusion in tall girls from tall families but treatment must be started before the age of 12 years. Lactation may be suppressed by a high dosage of oestrogens but this treatment may induce venous thrombosis and is best avoided. Secondary sexual characteristics can be induced or restored with oestrogens in females with ovarian failure. Osteoporosis can probably be avoided in women subjected to early oophorectomy if they are treated with oestrogens and they may also prevent the complication of premature coronary atheroma which follows this procedure. In men oestrogens in high doses can cause temporary remission of metastatic prostatic carinoma. Habitual male sexual offenders may obtain a reduction in libido by periodic oestrogen implants. Oestrogens may also be used to treat slight elevations of the serum calcium level in post-menopausal women with primary hyperparathyroidism (*see* p. 405).

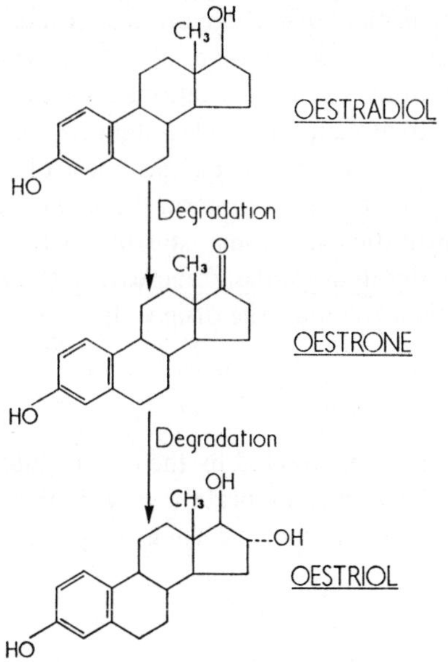

FIGURE 7.3 The oestrogens

Oestrogen Preparations. Ethinyl oestradiol is the most potent oestrogen preparation and is the drug of first choice. It can be used in a dose of 0·01 mg once or twice daily to induce withdrawal bleeding or to control menopausal symptoms. It is usual to give courses of three weeks duration with one week off the drug. For severe menorrhagia larger doses are required, e.g. ethinyl oestradiol 0·05 mg four times daily for two or three days until the bleeding has stopped and the dose is then gradually reduced over a week. Stilboestrol is not used routinely in females as it tends to cause pigmentation of the nipples. The conjugated equine oestrogens such as Premarin are also effective in cyclical regimes and in the control of menopausal symptoms and there is some evidence suggesting that they cause less impairment of carbohydrate tolerance in pre- and latent diabetics than do other oestrogen preparations. Local applications may be of value in the treatment of senile vaginitis, either as creams or as pessaries. Stilboestrol is still widely used for the long-term therapy of metastatic prostatic carcinoma starting with 0·5 mg twice daily and gradually increasing the dose if the patient tolerates the drug well.

2. PROGESTERONE

This hormone, secreted by the corpus luteum, is a steroid with a configuration very similar to that of the adrenocortical steroids (Fig. 7.4). Progesterone is also synthesised in the adrenal cortex and testes, where its main function is to serve as a precursor in the steroid biosynthetic pathways. Progesterone is thought to circulate in a form bound to protein. It is largely degraded in the liver, and a small fraction appears in the urine as the inactive conjugate pregnanediol glucuronide.

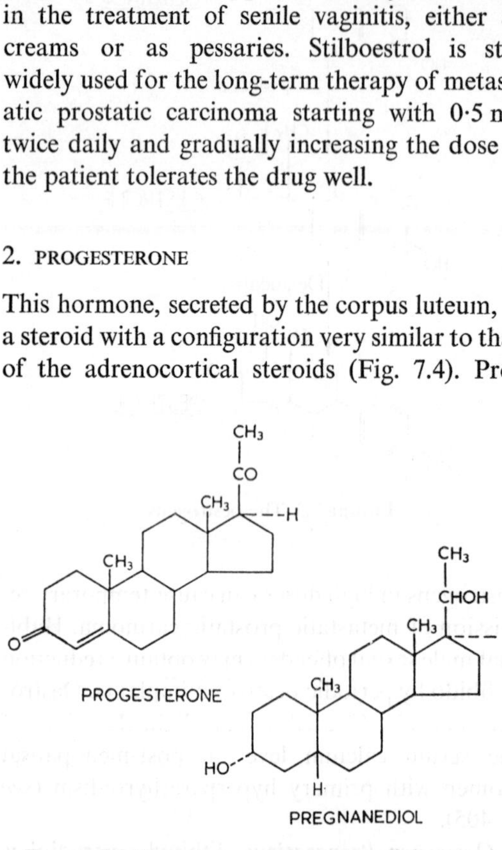

FIGURE 7.4 Progesterone and pregnanediol

Actions of Progesterone. The main action of progesterone is concerned with the preparation of the endometrium for implantation and the maintenance of pregnancy. It causes the secretory changes in the endometrium necessary for implantation of the fertilised ovum and it suppresses uterine mobility. During pregnancy it is at least in part responsible for inhibition of ovulation and for further development of the breasts. Its systemic effects are less well defined than those of oestradiol. Progesterone is pyrogenic, and a daily basal temperature recording that reveals an abrupt rise of about 1°F in the middle of the cycle maintained until menstruation suggests the presence of a functioning corpus luteum and hence, that ovulation has occurred. Side-effects of progestogens include acne, breast tenderness, reduced menstrual loss, cholestatic jaundice and virilisation of a female fetus.

Assay of Progesterone. Progesterone secretion is routinely assessed by the estimation of its breakdown product pregnanediol in a 24-hour urine specimen. In the follicular phase of the cycle the excretion of pregnanediol is less than 1 mg in 24 hours and in the luteal phase this rises to 2 to 5 mg in 24 hours. A further indication of progesterone production is the finding of secretory changes in an endometrial biopsy. Plasma progesterone levels can now be measured by radioimmunoassay. During the follicular and mid-luteal phases of the menstrual cycle mean reported levels are, respectively: 545 pg per ml and 8561 pg per ml.

Indications for Progesterone Therapy. Progestogens are used in the treatment of dysfunctional uterine bleeding. They may be of value in the treatment of premenstrual swelling and tenderness of the breasts. They have been used in the treatment of habitual abortion but are now considered to be of doubtful value. Some women with metastatic breast cancer show improvement with progestogens. Progestogens may be used alone or in combination with oestrogens as oral contraceptives.

Progesterone Preparations. Progesterone itself must be given by intramuscular injection in a dose of 20 to 60 mg daily. Preparations which are active by mouth are now preferred to progesterone. Of these the drug of choice is norethisterone given in daily doses of 5 to 20 mg.

3. ANDROGENS

Recently, attention has been drawn to a possible endocrine role played by the stroma cells of the ovary, which show cyclical histological changes during the monthly cycle. The stroma is able to synthesise different steroids from those produced by the ovarian follicle and the corpus luteum, and these steroids appear to be mainly androgens. Under normal circumstances, androgens, particularly androstenedione, are secreted in very small amounts by the ovary (Fig. 7.2). The physiological significance of these ovarian androgens is uncertain, although the adrenal androgens are involved in bringing about the pubertal growth spurt.

Androgen secretion by the ovaries is greatly increased in some pathological conditions in which there is abnormal steroidogenesis (as in the Stein-Leventhal syndrome) or tumour formation (such as arrhenoblastoma).

THE HORMONAL CONTROL OF THE MENSTRUAL CYCLE

The secretion of oestrogens and progesterone is under the control of the pituitary gonadotrophins. During the first half of the cycle the Graafian follicle develops under the influence of the low tonic secretion of FSH and LH. There is a gradual increase in the secretion of 17β-oestradiol which eventually triggers off a reflex discharge of LH/FSH-RH from the hypothalamus which in turn causes a surge of LH and FSH secretion from the anterior pituitary. Both oestrogen and 17α-hydroxyprogesterone are secreted by the theca interna cells of the developing Graafian follicle whose activity begins to decline prior to ovulation.

The surge of LH causes rupture of the follicle and release of an ovum, probably after a time interval of about 24 hours. The granulosa cells then undergo hypertrophy and hyperplasia to form the corpus luteum whose principal product is progesterone. Theca interna cells also invade the corpus luteum and are probably responsible for

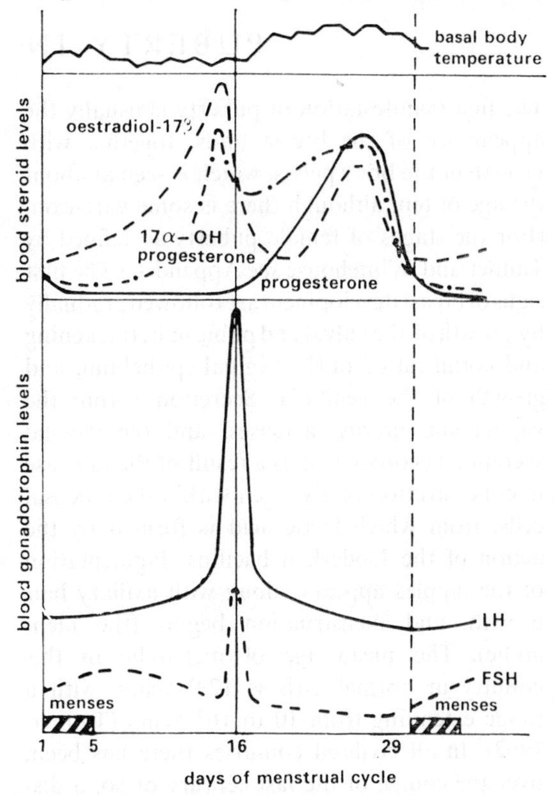

FIGURE 7.5 Hormone changes in the menstrual cycle (by permission of Dr R. Short)

the rise in 17β-oestradiol and its precursor 17α-hydroxyprogesterone in the second half of the cycle. After about two weeks the corpus luteum regresses, levels of oestrogen and progesterone decline and menstruation ensues.

The endometrium undergoes proliferative changes during the first half of the cycle in response to the oestrogens whereas in the second half of the cycle progesterone induces secretory changes in the endometrium. In animals prostaglandin $F_{2}\alpha$ is secreted by the endometrium and this factor is responsible for regression of the corpus luteum. In man the factors responsible for corpus luteum regression are unknown.

Clinical tests for the occurrence of ovulation are still inadequate. The rise in body temperature resulting from the action of progesterone is a useful guide as is measurement of urinary pregnanediol excretion. The increased progesterone production which follows normal ovulation can be measured by radioimmunoassay of plasma progesterone and this method should soon be generally available.

PUBERTY IN THE FEMALE

The first manifestation of puberty is usually the appearance of the breast buds, together with growth of the bony pelvis, which is seen at about the age of ten, although there is some variation. (For the stages of female puberty as defined by Tanner and Whitehouse *see* Appendix.) The first signs of breast development are followed gradually by growth of the vulval and pubic hair, thickening and cornification of the vaginal epithelium, and growth of the genitalia. Secretion within the vagina and uterus increases, and the vaginal secretion becomes acid as a result of the increase in concentration of glycogen within the mocosal cells, from which lactic acid is formed by the action of the Doderlein bacillus. Pigmentation of the nipples appears, along with axillary hair growth, and menstruation begins (the menarche). The mean age of menarche in this country in normal girls is 12·9 years, with a range extending from 10 to 16½ years (Tanner, 1962). In all civilised countries there has been, over the course of the last century or so, a distinct and often marked tendency for the menarche to occur at a progressively earlier age. The age at which the menarche occurs is at least partly determined by genetic factors. At the time of puberty, growth is stimulated by oestrogens and by androgens, the latter arising mainly from the adrenal cortex in females, the growth spurt often preceding the onset of menstruation. As ovarian oestrogen secretion increases, the rate of growth slows, and fusion of the epiphyses occurs. Plasma 17β-oestradiol levels correlate with bone age, chronological age, and with the clinical evaluation of sexual development. It is presumed that decreased sensitivity of the hypothalamus to the negative feedback of the gonadal hormones is responsible for the development of puberty. Thus, the levels of steroid secreted by the immature gonads become incapable of inhibiting the production of the pituitary gonadotrophins, and puberty begins. Sexual maturation is accompanied by a marked increase in the secretion of FSH which plateaus after mid-puberty while LH, like 17β-oestradiol slowly increases with advancing sexual maturation.

Menstruation (which occurs only in primates) consists of breakdown of the endometrium as a result of withdrawal of oestrogens and progesterone. The menstrual loss is composed of endometrial cells, secretions, and blood. It normally occurs in a regular cyclical fashion from the menarche to the menopause, being interrupted only by pregnancy. The duration of menstrual loss is 3 to 7 days, and the cycle occurs approximately every four weeks.

THE MENOPAUSE

At some time, usually in the late forties, the secretion of oestrogens and progesterone is diminished and ovulation ceases. Commonly, the periods become progressively more irregular, infrequent and scanty, and eventually stop, but in some individuals the cessation of menstruation may be sudden. The term menopause refers only to cessation of menstruation but this is only one feature of a complex of changes which extend over a much longer period (Williams, 1971). To these, which include vasomotor symptoms and signs of oestrogen deficiency, the term climacteric is applied. Cycles at the time of the menopause may be anovulatory, but, on the other hand, ovulation may occur in a few women after menstruation has ceased. Persistent menorrhagia, or uterine bleeding after a period of more than six months amenorrhoea, is *not* a normal feature of the menopause, and requires investigation.

Since the menopause is a type of primary ovarian insufficiency, the urinary gonadotrophin excretion is found to be high.

Hormonal Changes. In women approaching the menopause, LH levels rise to values seven times higher than in normal young women, whereas FSH levels are only three-fold elevated. The increase in urinary LH occurs before the onset of vasomotor symptoms. After the menopause there is a 15-fold increase in the production rate of FSH and a five-fold increase in LH while the metabolic clearance rates are unchanged; so there is an early increase in LH production and excretion which is later exceeded by that of FSH. Oestrogen secretion by the ovaries falls after the menopause and eventually ceases, when excreted oestrogens are derived from peripheral conversion of androgens.

Physical and Psychological Changes. After the cessation of menstruation the ovaries become smaller and sclerotic and appear white and wrinkled, the uterus is reduced in size and the cervix tends to become flush with the vault, the endometrium is thin and atrophic and the vagina narrows and becomes smaller and the labia regress. There is a tendency to vaginal infections as the vaginal pH rises and the cervical and vaginal secretions decrease. The pubic hair becomes sparse, the skin thinner and the breasts become smaller. Muscles, ligaments and fascia of the pelvic floor lose their flexibility and prolapse is commoner.

After the menopause there is a progressive diminution in bone mass which is a feature of osteoporosis (*see* Chapter 18). This is largely due to oestrogen deficiency and it can be halted and possibly improved, in some instances at least, by the administration of oestrogens. Bilateral oophorectomy causes a more rapid bone loss than after a normal menopause but the final level reached is usually no lower than that found in normal women one year after the menopause. A number of vasomotor changes which take the form of periodic feelings of warmth in the face neck, and upper chest, associated with flushing, and often with severe sweating (hot flushes and flashes) may also occur at this time. These symptoms result from the low oestrogen levels which occur at this time. Cholesterol, triglyceride and phospholipid levels rise and this is associated with a greater incidence of cardiovascular disease. Women castrated ten or more years before the age of 50 years have a greater prevalence of coronary artery disease. Lipid levels can be lowered towards normal by oestrogen administration and there is a good case for administering oestrogens to all women subjected to oophorectomy at an early age. Nervousness, irritability, and lassitude may also occur, and depressive illnesses are not uncommon. Although there may be an endocrine basis for these symptoms, psychological factors contribute to a large extent. Women at this age often feel unwanted and unloved as their sexual attractiveness wanes and their children present adolescent problems or are leaving home. Outlets for their energies diminish and over-eating and obesity may be expressions of emotional tensions.

Treatment

If menorrhagia should occur at this time, if there is marked irregularity of menstruation or if bleeding recurs after a six-month interval of amenorrhoea, examination under anaesthesia is required with dilatation and curettage to exclude local pathology. Treatment for iron deficiency anaemia may be needed. If no local pathology is found it is wise to wait for three months to see if the periods will become regular or cease. If they do not become regular a combined oestrogen-progesterone contraceptive pill should be given for several cycles and then withdrawn. If the periods still remain irregular and/or heavy, a further course of hormone treatment may be attempted which, if unsuccessful, is followed by a hysterectomy. Hormone treatment should not be continued for more than a year without a repeat pelvic examination and curettage.

Hot flushes and other vasomotor symptoms usually disappear in a year or two without any treatment. If they are only occurring once or twice a day, no treatment is required whereas frequent flushes causing disability warrant treatment with small doses of oestrogens administered cyclically. Suggested regimes are ethinyl oestradiol 0·01 to 0·05 mg b.d. for three weeks in every month; or chlorotrianisene ('TACE') 24 to 48 mg daily for 30 days. The dose should be kept as low as possible to avoid endometrial bleeding which often has to be investigated to exclude uterine pathology.

A reduction of vaginal secretion which often causes dyspareunia will respond to cyclical oestrogen therapy but if this is not indicated to treat vasomotor symptoms, local oestrogen creams or pessaries often suffice.

Psychological upsets can often be alleviated by kindness and understanding from the husband and doctor. The transient nature of many of the symptoms should be emphasized. Other outlets for her energies should be sought, part-time employment can often provide a useful boost to her morale. Depressive illness should be treated promptly with specific anti-depressant drugs.

Avoidance of the menopause has been advocated using long-term administration of oestrogens or oestrogen-progesterone combinations taken cyclically in low doses. It has been suggested that such therapy avoids or reduces the prevalence of osteoporosis, cardiovascular disease and other psycho-sexual menopausal problems. Further data on the benefits and possible complications of such long-term hormone medication are required before it can be generally recommended.

HYPOGONADISM IN THE FEMALE

A suggested classification of hypogonadism in the female is given in Table 7.2. This classification is not meant to be completely inclusive, and broad headings, rather than specific causes are given.

The following conditions are not included in this table:

1. Failure of menarche with normal ovarian function due to imperforate hymen or congenital defects of the vagina or uterus. Such patients usually have good secondary sexual characteristics.
2. Pregnancy, which although the commonest cause of secondary amenorrhoea during the childbearing years, cannot be considered to be a failure of sexual function.
3. Conditions such as testicular feminisation where the chromosome pattern is male. Here breast development is good but there is absence of pubic and axillary hair.

FAILURE OF SEXUAL MATURATION

As mentioned previously, there is considerable variation in the age when sexual maturation occurs, due to acceleration or delay in the normal functioning or co-ordination of the delicately balanced hypothalamico-pituitary-ovarian mechanisms. Genetic factors play a part in determining the time of onset of puberty, and a history of late puberty in the mother or sisters should always be sought. Many such patients will be referred because of the combination of obesity

TABLE 7.2 *Hypogonadism in the Female*

Failure of Sexual Maturation (*'Primary amenorrhoea'*)	*Failure of Established Sexual Function* (*'Secondary amenorrhoea'*)
1. *Due to ovarian causes*	1. *Due to ovarian causes*
(*a*) *ovarian failure*	(*a*) *ovarian failure*
congenital hypoplasia	menopause
'castration'	'castration'
radiation damage	radiation damage
chromosomal abnormalities	chromosomal abnormalities (rare)
non-masculinising tumours	non-masculinising tumours
(*b*) *excess androgen production*	(*b*) *excess androgen production*
masculinising tumours	masculinising tumours
	Stein–Leventhal syndrome
2. *Due to hypothalamico-pituitary causes*	2. *Due to hypothalamico-pituitary causes*
neoplasm	neoplasm
vascular	vascular
trauma	trauma
infection	infection
granulomas	granulomas
'functional'	'functional', includes depression, anorexia nervosa and other varieties of psychogenic anorexia, post-oral contraceptives
	iatrogenic (including pituitary ablation)

3. *Associated with other endocrine and metabolic disturbances**
   congenital adrenal hyperplasia
   Cushing's syndrome
   Addison's disease
   obesity
   undernutrition (including anorexia nervosa)
   malabsorption syndromes
   hyperthyroidism, hypothyroidism
   administration of androgens or anabolic steroids

4. *Associated with chronic debilitating disease**
   e.g. renal failure, diabetes, tuberculosis, connective tissue disorders

* The hypogonadism is assumed in most cases to be mediated through the hypothalamico-pituitary centres.

and failure to develop sexually, and the overwhelming majority can be reassured that there is no organic defect, that there is merely a physiological delay in the onset of puberty which will usually begin and proceed normally if weight is lost. However, if by the age of fifteen to sixteen definite signs of sexual maturation have not begun to appear, more investigation is necessary to exclude any organic abnormality.

1. *Due to Ovarian Causes.* In such cases the uterus does not enlarge, there is no breast development or growth of pubic and axillary hair, and menstruation does not begin. The patient may be excessively tall because of failure of epiphyseal closure, and the proportions may be eunuchoid in that the arm span exceeds the height by more than 5 cm and the pubis to floor measurement is considerably in excess of half the total body height. Such proportions are, however, not always seen in patients with hypogonadism due to ovarian abnormalities, and short stature is invariable in Turner's syndrome. Apart from those patients with a chromosomal abnormality, discussed in Chapter 13, primary ovarian insufficiency may result from congenital hypoplasia or absence of ovaries, or from 'castration' due to ovarian disease, surgery, or radiation. Rarely, ovarian tumours may present with failure of sexual maturation, but other signs and symptoms are usually more prominent. When the child with primary ovarian insufficiency reaches the age at which puberty would be expected to occur, pituitary gonadotrophins are released, but there is no response from ovarian tissue. Thus, the urinary excretion of oestrogens and pregnanediol is low or absent, whilst the urinary gonadotrophin excretion is considerably elevated.

2. *Due to Hypothalamico-pituitary Causes.* Here the primary cause is a failure of gonadotrophin secretion, which may be the result of destructive lesions of the hypothalamus or the pituitary. Lesions responsible include tumours such as craniopharyngiomas or chromophobe adenomas, vascular causes such as haemorrhage, or trauma to the base of the skull; rarer causes include basal meningitis, granulomatous conditions such as Hand-Schuller-Christian disease, or the Laurence-Moon-Biedl syndrome. The syndromes produced by these lesion vary according to the nature of the lesions, its size, and its location but in most cases there will be evidence of hypopituitarism, and many will present with visual failure or evidence of increased intracranial pressure. Failure of sexual maturation is often an incidental finding, the patient showing more striking or disturbing features that draw attention to her condition. Hypogonadism is common in gigantism and acromegaly. Isolated gonadotrophin deficiency may precede by many years other signs of pituitary disease.

In the majority of patients with gonadotrophin deficiency there is no evidence of organic hypothalamic or pituitary disease, and it is presumed that there is a 'functional' defect resulting in a failure of gonadotrophin-releasing hormone secretion. In the mildest cases there may simply be a delay in the onset of normal puberty, while in more severe cases there is complete failure of sexual maturation.

In all patients grouped under this heading the urinary gonadotrophin excretion would be expected to be low, and the finding of a high value would virtually exclude hypothalamic or pituitary disease or dysfunction as a cause of hypogonadism. If urinary gonadotrophins are normal, it is difficult to be certain whether the cause is primarily of pituitary or ovarian origin.

3. *Associated with Other Endocrine and Metabolic Disturbances*, and

4. *Associated with Chronic Debilitating Disease.* Congenital adrenal hyperplasia leads to increased androgen secretion and virilisation. Ovarian insufficiency occurs and is believed to be due to the inhibitory effect of adrenal androgens on gonadotrophin secretion. Therapy with cortisol usually leads to normal sexual maturation. In the rare condition of juvenile Cushing's syndrome there is ovarian hypofunction, although breast development and growth of body hair may occur. Failure of sexual maturation may also

result from the administration of androgens or anabolic steroids.

In the other conditions listed, e.g. obesity, thyrotoxicosis, undernutrition, and chronic diseases such as diabetes and renal failure, hypogonadism and delayed puberty are not uncommon. It is presumed that this is due to a functional disturbance of pituitary gonadotrophin secretion. Puberty may be expected to occur normally and sexual maturation to proceed when the primary condition is effectively treated. In all of these cases failure of sexual maturation is usually an incidental finding.

FAILURE OF ESTABLISHED SEXUAL FUNCTION

Failure of sexual function in the adult woman is usually indicated by secondary amenorrhoea or oligomenorrhoea. The causes are similar to those discussed in the previous section on primary amenorrhoea but the emphasis is altered. Physiological causes of secondary amenorrhoea such as pregnancy or the menopause should always be excluded. The amenorrhoea is sometimes preceded by a variable period of infrequent and scanty menstruation. If the ovarian insufficiency is permanent or protracted a variable degree of hypo-oestrogenism will occur.

1. *Due to Ovarian Causes.* The menopause is a manifestation of primary ovarian failure. There is a considerable variation in the age at which it may occur. Amenorrhoea occurring earlier than the age of forty is unusual and should arouse suspicion of pregnancy or of organic disease. Patients with an early menopause often give a history of a late menarche, of irregular or scanty periods and impaired fertility, and may mention a similar occurrence in other members of the family. The periods may cease suddenly or gradually, menopausal symptoms such as hot flushes are frequent, and the urinary gonadotrophin excretion is elevated. While chromosomal abnormalities typically cause a failure of sexual maturation, menstruation may be established in some patients with the triple-X and isochromosome-X abnormalities. Secondary amenorrhoea may subsequently occur. Sexual maturation is always impaired in Turner's syndrome. The Stein-Leventhal syndrome is a common cause of failure of normally established sexual function and is discussed in Chapter 8. A number of ovarian tumours may be responsible for hypogonadism in the adult, sometimes with the development of features of virilisation.

2. *Due to Hypothalamico-pituitary Causes.* The causes of failure of established sexual function listed under this heading are similar to those causing failure of sexual maturation. The most important additional abnormality is panhypopituitarism due to post-partum infarction of the pituitary, though this is much less frequent than in previous years due to improved obstetric facilities.

Perhaps the most common cause of secondary amenorrhoea in the adult is a functional disturbance of the normal hypothalamico-pituitary-ovarian axis. Amenorrhoea frequently occurs in patients without demonstrable organic disease in any system. In many cases the menarche, sexual maturation, and sexual function in adult life have been quite normal, and commonly a history of acute psychological stress is obtained preceding the amenorrhoea, which may occur suddenly or be preceded by oligomenorrhoea or other menstrual disturbances. Some patients show evidence of oestrogen deficiency on examination. Menstrual function may return to normal after a variable period, but in others cyclical hormone therapy may be needed.

The syndrome of amenorrhoea and galactorrhoea occurring post-partum or after withdrawal of oral contraceptives is another example of a functional disturbance of gonadotrophin secretion, in which the normal cyclical secretion of FSH and LH is lost, while prolactin is secreted in large quantities. This syndrome may be an early manifestation of a tumour of the pituitary or hypothalamus.

3. *Associated with Other Endocrine or Metabolic Abnormalities;* and

4. *Associated with Chronic Debilitating Disease.* Those abnormalities discussed in the section on

failure of sexual maturation may also be responsible for failure of established sexual function. Very rarely, in congenital adrenal hyperplasia the manifestations of virilisation may be delayed until adolescence or later. As in the child, the administration of androgens or anabolic steroids may result in hypogonadism with virilisation. Anorexia nervosa is discussed elsewhere (*see* Chapter 1). It is important to remember that in some patients amenorrhoea precedes the onset of anorexia and weight loss, pointing to a primary disturbance of the hypothalamic centres. In anorexia nervosa, although amenorrhoea is almost invariable, there is usually no loss of body hair, and although fatty tissue is lost from the breast there is little atrophy of the glandular tissue. In some successfully treated patients with anorexia nervosa, there may be prolonged delay in the establishment of normal menstruation, and in these hormonal therapy may be necessary. Mild forms of psychogenic anorexia are not uncommon, and in these patients menstrual irregularities often improve when weight is gained. Many chronic diseases may be associated with secondary amenorrhoea, presumably as a result of functional disturbances in gonadotrophin secretion. Treatment of the primary condition will usually result in the return of normal ovarian function. Primary ovarian failure may also develop in patients with Addison's disease, when antibodies to ovarian tissue may sometimes be detected in the serum.

INVESTIGATION

1. *Failure of Sexual Maturation.* In any girl referred because of suspected failure of sexual maturation a full history must be taken and physical examination carried out, particular attention being paid to the height and skeletal proportions. Stigmata of Turner's syndrome must be looked for, such as webbing of the neck and cubitus valgus. In the majority of such patients referred to the endocrinologist, no physical abnormality is present and they are merely normal girls in whom there is a physiological delay in the onset of puberty, commonly associated with simple obesity. In some, a family history will be of value. The time of puberty is at least partially genetically determined, and a family history of delayed onset of puberty in the mother may be of significance.

The decision to be made is when to undertake investigation in such patients. In some patients with Turner's syndrome, congenital adrenal hyperplasia or pituitary tumour it will be immediately apparent that investivation is needed. In others, who have an associated endocrine or metabolic disturbance such as hyperthyroidism or diabetes, investigation will initially be directed towards the primary condition. Patients first seen at the age of twelve or thirteen who show no physical abnormalities, merely require a skull X-ray to exclude an obvious intracranial lesion, and a buccal smear should be examined at this stage if the patient is of short stature. The further investigations considered below may be postponed until the age of sixteen to seventeen, when they will be justified if there is no evidence of sexual maturation.

Suggested Investigations in Primary Amenorrhoea

1. height, span, and pubis-to-floor measurement;
2. chest and skull X-ray;
3. buccal smear and karyotype by white cell culture;
4. X-ray of hands and wrists for bone age, and of knees for state of epiphyseal development;
5. 24 hour urinary 17-oxosteroids, 17-hydroxycorticosteroids and urinary 'free cortisol';
6. plasma and urinary gonadotrophins:
   (*a*) *If gonadotrophins are low:*
   Continue investigation to exclude an organic intracranial lesion.
   Investigate for other systemic disease such as diabetes, renal failure, chronic infection, thyroid disease.
   (*b*) *If gonadotrophins are high:*
   Direct investigation towards an ovarian cause. Pelvic examination, culdoscopy laparoscopy or laparotomy and on occasion gonadal biopsy may be required, (Black and Govan, 1972).

(*c*) *If gonadotrophins are normal:*
Investigation of both the hypothalamic-pituitary axis and the ovaries should be carried out.

In patients with primary amenorrhoea without obvious cause laparoscopy with gonadal biopsy may provide useful information. Dysgenetic gonads and gonadal tumours can be recognised; the presence or absence of ovarian follicles can be ascertained; anatomical abnormalities such as absence or maldevelopment of the uterus and tubes can be defined.

In many cases no abnormality will be found as a result of these tests. If low gonadotrophins are the only abnormal finding, it is presumed that there is likely to be a functional disturbance of gonadotrophin secretion. Under these conditions a further period of observation may be decided upon before cyclical hormone therapy is prescribed, lest the patient is at the extreme range of normal as regards pubertal development. Normal gonadotrophin levels in the absence of any other abnormality suggest that puberty may be imminent and that the patient should be observed. If ovarian hypoplasia or absence is demonstrated, cyclical hormone therapy will be indicated.

2. *Failure of Established Sexual Function.* The general scheme of investigation is the same as in primary amenorrhoea. The history and examination alone may provide a strong clue to the cause; thus, generalised hirsutes will suggest an abnormal source of androgens such as occurs in the Stein-Leventhal syndrome, in certain masculinising tumours of the ovary, or in the rare cases of late onset congenital adrenal hyperplasia. A history of failure of lactation and amenorrhoea following an obstretic haemorrhage, coupled with loss of pubic and axillary hair, will suggest post-partum hypopituitarism.

Estimation of the plasma and urinary gonadotrophin levels differentiate those cases with hypothalamico-pituitary defects from those with ovarian disease. The finding of increased gonadotrophins will, in general, point towards primary ovarian failure, although when there is an abnormal source of androgens, gonadotrophin excretion is usually diminished. In all patients with failure of established sexual function a vaginal examination carried out by a gynaecologist is mandatory, if necessary with the patient under an anaesthetic.

Investigation will usually be negative, and in the older patient (forty years onwards) an early menopause is likely if the gonadotrophin levels are high. In others with normal or low gonadotrophins and no evidence of pituitary or ovarian disease, it is usually assumed that the cause of the failure of established sexual function is either functional failure of gonadotrophin secretion or loss of the normal cyclical pattern of gonadotrophin release. In the younger single woman early anorexia nervosa must always be considered.

Whenever obvious hypothalamico-pituitary or ovarian disease is excluded it is necessary to search for some other endocrine or metabolic disorder or chronic debilitating disease.

TREATMENT OF FAILURE OF SEXUAL MATURATION

Therapy should first be directed towards the causative condition, where this is possible (Table 7.2). Successful therapy along these lines may by itself result in the rapid onset of maturation. Sometimes this may not occur, even though the primary cause is dealt with. In other cases the primary cause is not amenable to treatment, e.g. 'castration', ovarian hypoplasia or aplasia, and chromosomal abnormalities. In these patients, and in the vast majority where no organic lesion can be detected, treatment must be directed towards producing regular menstrual cycles together with normal feminisation and growth. Oestrogens, while causing a temporary growth spurt, will ultimately retard growth by bringing about fusion of the epiphyses. When the child is tall and of eunuchoid proportions, early fusion of the epiphyses will probably be desired, and thus fairly large doses of oestrogens may be given. Similar doses may be used in patients who have little or no potential for further growth, as indicated by premature fusion of the epiphyses.

The aim of cyclical hormone therapy is to produce normal feminisation and the psychological benefits of regular menstruation, even though ovulation will not be possible and the menstrual bleeding is simply due to oestrogen withdrawal. Regular withdrawal bleeding is more easily achieved if a progestational compound is given towards the end of the cyclical course of oestrogen. The authors usually give an initial dose of 0·01 mg of ethinyloestradiol twice daily for 24 days, with the addition of norethisterone (Primolut N) 5 mg daily for the last 10 days of the course. Withdrawal of therapy is usually followed by bleeding, and if so, the cycle is restarted at the end of menstruation. Bleeding may not occur for the first one or two cycles, in which case the therapy is begun again after a pause of 4 to 5 days. It may sometimes be necessary to increase the dose of ethinyloestradiol up to 0·2 mg daily, in order to produce withdrawal bleeding. The dose needed to produce regular withdrawal bleeding should be determined individually for each patient, and once adequate feminisation has been achieved, the smallest dose of oestrogen that will produce regular bleeding should be used, treatment being withdrawn at intervals to see if spontaneous menstruation will ensue. Where skeletal X-rays show no evidence of epiphyseal maturation, and when the child is small, greater caution must be exercised to avoid premature fusion of the epiphyses and, thus, cessation of growth. It is usually best to delay cyclical hormone therapy for as long as possible in these patients in the hope that additional growth will be obtained.

As an alternative to the regime outlined above, oral contraceptives may be used in the same cyclical manner in order to produce menstrual cycles and feminisation. However, the cyclical regime utilising ethinyloestradiol and norethisterone will usually suffice and allows much more latitude in dosage.

TREATMENT OF FAILURE OF ESTABLISHED SEXUAL FUNCTION

In general, the principles of treatment of failure of established sexual function in the adult are the same as those pertaining in the child with primary amenorrhoea, though it will not always be necessary to give replacement therapy to an older woman.

Recently there have been considerable advances in the therapy of secondary amenorrhoea and infertility resulting from hypothalamico-pituitary dysfunction. In certain patients, treatment with the drug clomiphene is effective; others benefit from human gonadotrophins, though these should be used only in centres where facilities are available for the biochemical estimations mandatory for their control. By the use of test-dosage schemes, the lowest effective amount of FSH may be selected, thereby reducing the risk of multiple pregnancies and of the rare but serious hyperstimulation syndrome. Clomiphene may be used in similar situations, though it is somewhat less effective (*see* Chapter 1).

OVARIAN TUMOURS

A classification of the ovarian tumours that secrete hormones is given in Table 7.3. Non-functional tumours, such as the various types of cystadenoma, are much more common than those listed here.

The clinical syndromes produced by these functional tumours are:

Virilisation:

- arrhenoblastoma
- hilus cell tumour
- adrenal-cell tumour (often with features of Cushing's syndrome)
- very rarely, granulosa or theca cell tumour.

Precocious puberty (pseudo-precocity):

granulosa cell tumour
theca cell tumour
luteoma
teratoma and chorionepithelioma.

Thyrotoxicosis (very rare):

struma ovarii

These syndromes are discussed under the appropriate headings in other chapters.

TABLE 7.3 *Functional Ovarian Tumours*

Source and type	Hormone secretion	Malignancy	Comments
Arising from primitive mesenchyme			
Arrhenoblastoma	Androgens	Rare	Solid, usually unilateral
Granulosa cell	Oestrogens (occasionally progesterone; rarely androgens)	Not common	Often cystic, usually unilateral
Theca cell	As for granulosa cell	Rare	Usually solid, unilateral
Luteoma	Oestrogens and progesterone	Rare	Represent luteinisation in a granulosa or theca cell tumour
Hilus cell (Leydig cell)	Androgens	Rare	May be hyperplasia (bilateral) or adenoma (unilateral
Arising from ova			
Teratoma, chorionepithelioma	Chorionic gonadotrophin, oestrogens, and progesterone	Highly malignant	Principally in prepubertal female
Struma ovarii	Thyroid hormones	Rare	Very rare. Teratoma in which predominant tissue is thyroid. Unilateral
Arising from cell rests			
Adrenal cell	Androgens, cortisol, rarely oestrogens	Not common	A number of tumours described under this heading. Confusion regarding cellular origin exists since proliferating adrenocortical cells closely resemble luteal cells
Complex origin			
Gonadoblastoma	Androgens	Doubtful	

Gonadal Neoplasms in Dysgenetic Gonads
The prevalence of gonadal neoplasms is greatly increased in patients with various types of dysgenetic gonads; dysgerminomas, seminomas, teratomas and gonadoblastomas have all been described. The risk of malignancy in a dysgenetic gonad is highest in patients with XO/XY or XO/XX forms of mosaicism, whatever the phenotype, and in those with 'pure gonadal dysgenesis' whether they have a normal XX or XY karyotype or a sex chromosome anomaly. Often the tumours are 'silent' but they may secrete androgens or oestrogens and they can sometimes be recognised by the radiological demonstration of calcification. Laparotomy and prophylactic gonadectomy is advisable in patients with XO/XY mosaicism and in those with pure gonadal dysgenesis, particularly if the karyotype is XY. Such patients are usually reared as females and appropriate substitution therapy is required at the normal time of puberty. It is usually best not to divulge the nature of the chromosomal anomaly to the patient because of the psychological implications.

EXCESSIVE GROWTH DURING PUBERTY

Excessive linear growth during puberty is usually a familial condition which, nevertheless, causes concern and embarrassment to the patient and her relatives. Organic disease is very rarely present, but it is wise to carry out a skull X-ray in such cases. If menstruation is established and sexual maturation is proceeding normally, it is hardly ever necessary to carry out any more detailed investigations. An X-ray of the knees should be taken to determine the extent of epiphyseal fusion so that the patient may be given a prognosis as regards the likelihood of further growth. Treatment may be considered in a girl whose predicted adult height is 178 cm (5 ft 10 in) or more. It should be started when the patient's height is approaching 167·5 cm and preferably before the menarche. A cyclical regime of oestrogens should be prescribed, for example ethinyl oestradiol 0·05 to 0·1 mg daily for 24 days, with norethisterone 5 mg twice a day for the last ten days. A period will begin on withdrawal, and the cycle restarts on its completion. The patient should be seen at regular intervals for assessment of height and of the radiological appearance of the epiphyses around the knee, the regime being discontinued when fusion has occurred. The results of therapy are difficult to assess, particularly if treatment is begun after the age of twelve.

INFERTILITY IN THE FEMALE

Inability to conceive is one of the commonest of problems presented to the endocrinologist or the gynaecologist. It is generally considered that a marriage should not be regarded as infertile until a year of normal coitus without contraception of any sort has passed.

CAUSES

In some patients the reason for infertility will be apparent after a full physical examination at the first visit, but such patients are in the minority. It is always necessary to remember that the husband is at fault as frequently as the wife when infertility is present, and that factors on the male side are primarily and solely responsible in about 33 per cent of cases. In about the same number, both partners contribute towards the inability to conceive, and the causation of infertility is often multifactorial. Thus, a female with a comparatively minor genital abnormality which predisposes to subfertility may have the misfortune to be married to a male whose potential is also below average. Neither partner is completely infertile, but the combination of subfertility on each side is sufficient to render the marriage barren. Infertility in the male is dealt with in Chapter 11, and the remainder of this section will be confined to the causation, investigation, and treatment of the subfertile or infertile female.

Fertility in women depends upon the normal production, fertilisation, and tubal transport of ova, as well as the uterine entry, development, implantation, and maintenance of the fertilised ovum. Defects of fertility in the female are related to the production of ova and interference in their union with spermatozoa, and of their implantation in the endometrium. A failure of maintenance of the implanted and fertilised ovum will, of course, lead to recurrent abortion rather than to infertility, but this may be difficult to differentiate from inability to conceive when the cycles are irregular and miscarriage takes place at an early stage. It is obvious that pregnancy will not occur unless ovulation takes place, and the problems and causes of amenorrhoea, irregular menstruation, and lack of ovulation have previously been discussed. Such a state of affairs may arise because of ovarian disease (e.g. Stein-Leventhal syndrome), more generalised pelvic disease (e.g. tuberculosis), abnormality of other endocrine glands (e.g. Cushing's syndrome), systemic disease (e.g. chronic infections or connective tissue diseases), or to disturbance of normal hypothalamico-pituitary-ovarian function.

In the presence of ovulation, infertility in the female is usually due to interference with the ascent of the spermatozoa and to factors which prevent their union with the ovum. Such causes may be located in the vagina, the cervix and uterus, or the Fallopian tubes.

Vaginal Causes. Congenital malformation or infection may interfere with fertilisation by preventing normal coitus, and dyspareunia (often due to some deep-seated emotional cause) may have a similar effect.

Cervix and Uterus. The spermatozoa may be prevented from ascending higher because of chronic cervicitis or oestrogen deficiency, both of which cause qualitative or quantitative disturbances in cervical mucus production during the preovulatory phase of the cycle—the 'hostile cervix'. The mid-cycle increase in mucus volume is usually accompanied by a significant decrease in viscosity, and these variations in physical state are also associated with chemical changes which have as yet not been fully delineated in the human. The viscosity is reflected in the 'spinnbarkeit' or ability to form a thread of mucus when it is stretched between a slide and coverslip. The clear leucocyte free secretion is most penetrable to spermatozoa when there is minimal viscosity and maximal threadability, which occurs around the time of ovulation.

Abnormalities in the uterus itself may contribute to infertility. Sometimes, retroversion prevents adequate contact of the external os with the seminal pool, though it is by no means always associated with subfertility or infertility. Malformations of the uterus and uterine tumours such as fibroids may also contribute to infertility although they more commonly lead to recurrent abortion. Endometritis and functional progesterone deficiency have similar effects.

Fallopian Tubes. The tubes may be obstructed partially or completely by congenital narrowing, inflammation or tumours arising in the adnexae. Adhesions due to endometriosis or inflammation may prevent the ovum from reaching the Fallopian tube.

Emotional Factors. The role of emotional factors in the aetiology of infertility is still poorly defined. As in the male, they may interfere with normal coitus and, hence, contribute to infertility. They may also affect fertility by interfering with normal hormonal balance, causing failure of ovulation. It has been postulated that psychogenic factors may cause tubal spasm, and interfere in other undefined ways with the normal transport of the ovum or ascent of the sperm.

INVESTIGATION

When infertility is a problem in a marriage, it is almost invariably the female who first seeks advice. However, it will be apparent that adequate diagnosis and prognosis can be made only when both partners are present for examination and investigation. A complete history should be obtained, and examination of husband and wife should be carried out at an early opportunity. It may be that some obvious abnormality of coital technique will immediately come to light which may be corrected by suitable advice, and some indication of sexual maladjustment or other emotional conflict may be apparent. Routine laboratory procedures to exclude systemic disease should be performed when indicated. A series of more specific tests should then be carried out. Those relevant to the male are discussed elsewhere, but it must be stressed that the investigation of infertility is incomplete without a seminal analysis. The initial history may immediately point to an abnormality in the female, and such symptoms as hirsuties, amenorrhoea, oligomenorrhoea, and irregular menstruation will direct investigation towards the possibility of an ovarian or pituitary abnormality. It is suggested that the line of investigation outlined below should be followed in the female who has normal and regular menstrual cycles, and whose sole complaint is inability to conceive.

1. *Routine Vaginal Examination, including the use of a Vaginal Speculum to inspect the Cervix.* A sample of pre-ovulatory cervical mucus should be obtained for examination of clarity, cell content, threadability (normally a thread of 5 to 15 cm in length can be obtained in the immediate pre-ovulatory phase) and ferning, as a crude indication of oestrogen concentration.

2. *Evaluation of Ovulation.* Basal body temperature should be measured throughout the menstrual cycle; characteristically, a sustained rise is seen after ovulation. Urinary pregnanediol levels during the second half of the cycle may be used as an indication of ovulation, but this estimation is not readily available and no more reliable than the recording of daily basal temperature. The most reliable method for confirming that ovulation has occurred is examination of an endometrical biopsy (*see* below).

3. *Post-coital Test.* The cervical mucus should be examined some 8 to 12 hours after coitus for the number of viable spermatozoa. The test should be arranged during the ovulatory phase of the cycle, i.e. 14 to 16 days before the next period is due. The contents of the cervical canal are aspirated and examined immediately under the microscope; an even distribution of at least five motile spermatozoa per high power field indicates a satisfactory test. In combination with the examination of cervical mucus, this test can be of great value. A poor post-coital test in the presence of good preovulatory mucus suggests deficiency of spermatozoa, deficiency of coital technique, or malposition of the cervix. If both test results are poor and there is normal semen analysis in the male, then it is strongly suggestive of either inflammatory disease of the cervix or some endocrine change resulting in impaired mucus formation.

4. *Tests for Tubal Patency.* This will be carried out under anaesthetic by insufflation of carbon dioxide, with recording of pressure tracings. If the test is abnormal, hysterosalpingography will usually be performed, and the latter investigation may also be carried out in patients with a normal carbon dioxide insufflation test and no other detectable abnormalities, who fail to become pregnant after an adequate period of time.

5. *Examination under Anaesthetic, Endometrial Biopsy, Culdoscopy and Laparoscopy.* These are performed to demonstrate the presence of secretory changes in the endometrium which indicate that ovulation has occurred, and to exclude any organic endometrial or ovarian disease.

TREATMENT OF INFERTILITY

Patients who demonstrate incomplete sexual maturation and hypogonadism will be treated as outlined in a previous section. Many couples conceive after their initial interview, or after preliminary investigations have been carried out and before any treatment is advised, but this may be fortuitous. It is of vital importance that the physician should prevent, by his handling of the patients and his discussion of the problem, any feelings of guilt or accusation on either side. When emotional factors are a problem, more detailed psychotherapy is sometimes needed. The couple should also be advised on the most suitable time to have intercourse, based on temperature charts recorded throughout the cycle. In general, the therapy of the infertile couple will be determined in a large part by the findings on physical examination and as a result of investigation. Any defects, either major or minor, detected in either the husband or wife should be treated so far as possible, in order that the total potential of the couple may be increased to its maximum level. Specific therapy for the male partner is discussed in Chapter 11. In the female, any vaginal or cervical infection should be treated appropriately by systemic or local antibiotics. Cauterisation of the chronically infected cervix may be necessary, and cervical dilation under anaesthetic should be performed in patients who have cervical stenosis. The retroverted uterus may be corrected by insertion of a pessary, or, if necessary, by operation. In patients who have occluded Fallopian tubes, attempts to restore patency by repeated insufflation may be carried out, and are sometimes successful. Often, however, the presence of endometriosis or chronic pelvic inflammatory disease indicates the need for surgery. The plastic repair of uterine tubes or cornual reimplantation may be of help in some cases, but surgery is much more effective when the ovaries are fixed by adhesions or endometriosis and are still ovulating, and when the uterine tubes are uninvolved in the process and are relatively normal. Myomectomy may be necessary if fibroids are found, and appropriate treatment (surgical or otherwise) may be given for ovarian cysts or tumours or the Stein-Leventhal syndrome.

Hormonal therapy may sometimes be of value. The use of clomiphene, FSH, and HCG and LH/FSH-RH is considered in Chapter 1. The patient who ovulates but has inadequate progesterone release from the corpus luteum, as shown by a poor secretory response in the endometrium during the luteal phase of the cycle, may be given small doses of progestational compounds such as norethisterone 2·5 to 5 mg daily during the last seven to ten days of the cycle, beginning four to five days after the midcycle rise in body temperature.

Despite all endeavours, a proportion of couples fail to conceive. In the authors' experience, some 50 to 60 per cent of couples who attend remain infertile. Artificial insemination, preferably by the husband, may be considered in appropriate patients, though the problem is usually resolved by adoption.

ORAL CONTRACEPTIVES

The use of oral contraceptives has increased steadily in Britain since their introduction in the early 1960s and it is estimated that at present at least 10 to 15 per cent of married women regularly use this method of birth control. The compounds in general use fall broadly into three groups. Those in the first contain an oestrogen and a progestogen in combination, and the preparation is given for cycles of 20 to 22 days. In the second group, the oestrogen is given alone for the first 15 or 16 days after cessation of menstruation, to be followed by a combination tablet containing an oestrogen and a progestogen given for a week to complete the course. In all the preparations used in the United Kingdom the oestrogenic component is either mestranol or ethinyloestradiol. A number of different progestogens are used, and recently a third regime of oral contraception has been described in which a progestogen is given alone. Here the progestogen is taken daily without interruption, usually from the first day of the cycle. Since 'progestogen only' tablets do not always inhibit ovulation, they depend for their contraceptive action on their effect on the cervical mucus and the endometrium. They have a small failure rate, rather less than one per cent. They do not inhibit lactation and they can be given safely to women who wish to breast feed. Cycle control in the first few months is poor, and even in later months is rarely as good as with combined tablets. Other unpleasant side-effects are few. Although they are simpler to use, missed tablets are more likely to lead to failure. Theoretically they have fewer health hazards. Details of the compounds in common use are given in Table 7.4.

If taken regularly and according to instructions, oral contraceptives are the most effective form of birth control, with a pregnancy rate of 0·1 to 1·0 per 100 woman years. They may be of particular use in patients in whom pregnancy is contra-indicated on medical grounds and when other forms of contraception are not possible. The combined preparations are more effective than the sequential regimes.

The mode of action of the oral contraceptives has not been fully elucidated, although it is assumed that their effect in preventing ovulation, which is brought about mainly by the oestrogenic component, is due to suppression of formation or release of LH/FSH-RH and possibly to a direct action on the anterior pituitary, inhibiting release of the gonadotrophins. The combined preparations suppress the release of LH at mid-cycle, and the sequential regimes cause a decrease in FSH secretion, although there is decreased release of both gonadotrophins if therapy is

TABLE 7.4 *Oral Contraceptive Preparations*

PRODUCT	PROGESTOGEN	OESTROGEN
	The Combined Preparations	
Anovlar 21	Norethisterone Acetate 4 mg	Ethinyloestradiol 0·05 mg
Gynovlar 21 (*Controvlar*)	Norethisterone Acetate 3 mg	Ethinyloestradiol 0·05 mg
Minovlar	Norethisterone Acetate 1 mg	Ethinyloestradiol 0·05 mg
Minovlar ED	Norethisterone Acetate 1 mg	Ethinyloestradiol 0·05 mg
Orlest 28	Norethisterone Acetate 1 mg	Ethinyloestradiol 0·05 mg
Norlestrin 21	Norethisterone Acetate 2·5 mg	Ethinyloestradiol 0·05 mg
Demulen 50	Ethynodiol Diacetate 0·5 mg	Ethinyloestradiol 0·05 mg
Ovulen 50	Ethynodiol Diacetate 1 mg	Ethinyloestradiol 0·05 mg
Minilyn	Lynestrenol 2·5 mg	Ethinyloestradiol 0·05 mg
Volidan 21	Megestrol Acetate 4 mg	Ethinyloestradiol 0·05 mg
Ortho-Novin 1·50	Norethisterone 1 mg	Mestranol 0·05 mg
Norinyl-1	Norethisterone 1 mg	Mestranol 0·05 mg

	The Sequential Preparations	
Feminor Sequential	15 × Mestranol 0·1 mg: 5 × Norethynodrel 5 mg and Mestranol 0·075 mg	
Sequens	15 × Mestranol 0·08 mg: 5 × Chlormadinone acetate 2 mg and Mestranol 0·08 mg	
C-Quens 21	14 × Mestranol 0·1 mg: 7 × Chlormadinone acetate 1·5 mg and Mestranol 0·1 mg	Strongly oestrogenic
Ortho-Norvin S.Q.	14 × Mestranol 0·1 mg: 7 × Norethisterone 2 mg and Mestranol 0·1 mg	
Serial 28	16 × Ethinyloestradiol 0·1 mg: 5 × Megestrol acetate 1 mg and Ethinyloestradiol 0·1 mg	

continued for long periods. Additional peripheral effects on the cervical mucus and the endometrium also occur. There is usually a prompt return of normal pituitary function following withdrawal of the drugs, although amenorrhoea may sometimes develop at this time (*see* below).

CHOICE OF PREPARATION

Combined (*recommended dose containing 0·05 mg of oestrogen*). This group is by far the most widely used at present. The dose of *oestrogen* is the same in all but there may be minor differences in effect between the two types, ethinyl oestradiol and mestranol, the latter being a slightly stronger oestrogen. *Progestogens* vary in potency, and also in dosage. Strong progestogens include norethisterone and its acetate, and ethynodiol diacetate. Lynestrenol, while being a strongly potent progestogen appears in addition to have some 'clinically oestrogenic' effects. Megestrol acetate and norethynodrel are relatively weaker. The dosage varies from 0·5 mg to 4 mg and the aim should be to prescribe the smallest amount of progestogen which will give reasonable cycle control. This will vary with each individual patient but some assessment can be made by the amount and frequency of menstrual loss, those with heavier and more frequent periods requiring a greater amount of progestogen. Weaker or smaller doses of progestogen are indicated for women with a tendency to obesity or greasy skins. Packs containing placebo tablets may assist in tablet taking routine but can also lead to confusion resulting in pregnancy.

Combined (*containing more than 0·05 mg oestrogen*). These are usually prescribed only when hormone therapy is needed for purposes other than contraception. High dose tablets, particularly of progestogen, are indicated in menorrhagia, functional uterine bleeding, endometriosis, and also in cases of dysmenorrhoea unresponsive to lower dose products. Higher dose oestrogen tablets sometimes benefit certain skin conditions, such as acne.

Sequential. These all contain higher amounts of oestrogen and should only be given in special cases. They carry a very small failure rate. They may be a first choice in cases of acne and premenstrual tension. Occasionally they are the only type of oral contraceptive that a patient can tolerate and may justifiably be prescribed provided that the patient is warned of the 'increased health risk'.

Management. Before a patient is prescribed an oral contraceptive, the following procedures should be completed:

1. Full medical and gynaecological history paying particular attention to hypertension, any thrombotic tendency and menstrual irregularities.

2. Examination, including—
   (*a*) weight;
   (*b*) blood pressure;
   (*c*) breast palpation;
   (*d*) pelvic examination, including cervical smear.

3. Instruction in tablet taking routine with explanation of mode of action. Reassurance of availability of medical supervision as necessary. Advice as to the need for extra contraceptive cover during first cycle.

Follow-up care should include an interview, with examination if indicated, during the second and third cycle and following this, six-monthly appointments. Although it may be considered wise to withdraw oral contraception for a few months every few years, there is no firm scientific evidence that this confers benefit.

Change of Preparation. This can be made at the first follow-up appointment if necessary although side-effects, in particular nausea and breakthrough bleeding, may well disappear after the first few cycles.

Side-effects commonly encountered can be attributed to one or other hormone component but may be due to both.

OESTROGEN EFFECTS	PROGESTOGEN EFFECTS
Fluid retention	Premenstrual depression
Premenstrual tension	Leucorrhoea
Nausea, vomiting	Dry vagina
Headache	Acne
Mucorrhoea	Greasy hair
Cervical erosion	Appetite increase—weight gain
Menorrhagia	Breast discomfort
Excessive tiredness	Reduced menstrual loss
Irritability	Leg and abdominal cramps
Vein complaints	Decrease in libido

Progestogenic effects may be alleviated by lowering the dose or a change to a different progestogen, either to one which is weaker or to one which is more 'oestrogenic' in its clinical effects. Oestrogenic side-effects may be lessened if an alteration is made to a product incorporating a weaker type of oestrogen. Alternatively the oestrogen may be totally withdrawn and a 'progestogen only' pill substituted. In some cases, however, these advised changes may well conflict with the need to maintain reasonable cycle control. When a change is made from a high dose to a low dose tablet it is rare but possible for pregnancy to occur during the first cycle of the new preparation, and patients need to be warned accordingly. Although changes in preparation can sometimes give relief from undesirable side-effects, this is by no means certain and some patients will not tolerate any form of oral contraceptive tablet.

The Menopause. Oral contraception does not interfere with the timing of the natural menopause, although it may camouflage the usual signs. Withdrawal bleeding will, in most cases, continue to occur at the end of each course of tablets but decreased loss or amenorrhoea can be due to the climacteric, but may also be due to long-term administration of the pill. An assessment should be made as to the likely age of cessation of menstruation on every woman on the pill at, or over, the age of 40. Some pointers which are helpful are, the age of menarche, and the family history of menopausal age. Nationality and nutrition may also be an influence. In the case of women approaching the age of the expected menopause who have been taking oral contraceptives for upwards of two years, it is wise to discontinue medication in order to determine whether spontaneous menstruation will occur. If no period occurs within the following three months, oral contraception should be discontinued permanently. If, however, there is a return to a normal menstrual cycle within this time, oral contraception can again be given but a similar break after a further two years is advised. A discussion about alternative methods of contraception during the interval is necessary. After the age of 48 when the chance of pregnancy is remote, it may well be unnecessary to give further contraceptive advice but this must depend on the individual feelings of the particular patient.

Contra-indications. The preparations should not be used in patients with biliary cirrhosis or congenital defects of hepatic excretory function, nor in those with recent liver disease. They are contra-indicated in those with breast or cervical carcinoma, and these lesions should be excluded by appropriate examinations before the drugs are prescribed. Patients who have a history of thromboembolic phenomena should not be given oral contraceptives, and care must be exercised when they are used in the presence of epilepsy, hypertension, advanced cardiac or renal disease with oedema, and diabetes.

Uterine fibroids may increase in size under the oestrogenic stimulus, although high progestational steroid content pills may produce a reduction in size. There is no evidence of any danger to the fetus associated with oral contraceptives in early pregnancy.

METABOLIC EFFECTS OF ORAL CONTRACEPTIVES

Abnormalities of carbohydrate and fat metabolism have been reported during the use of these preparations. Impairment of oral carbohydrate tolerance has been reported to occur in 20 per cent of patients, and in a similar number an increased maximum pyruvate increment after glucose has been observed. As many as 85 per cent of patients may develop abnormal cortisone-stressed glucose tolerance tests (Javier *et al.*, 1968). Overt diabetes mellitus is often aggravated, and diabetes or glycosuria may be precipitated in pre- or latent diabetics. The abnormalities noted are similar to those found in steroid diabetes (Wynn and Doar, 1966).

The fasting plasma free fatty acid level is often elevated, and the normal fall after glucose administration may be delayed. Thirty per cent of a group of patients receiving cyclical oral contraceptives have shown elevation of the serum triglyceride level, and blood cholesterol tends to be raised (Wynn *et al.*, 1966).

Many liver function tests are affected including bromsulphthalein retention and an increase in the serum concentration of a number of enzymes. A variety of changes have been noted in regard to plasma proteins and on occasion jaundice has been produced. Oestrogens have an effect on tryptophan metabolism, since the oestrogen component enhances the capacity for the conversion of tryptophan to nicotinic acid ribonucleotide. Possibly because this pathway is stimulated there is depression of the alternative metabolic pathway which produces 5-hydroxytryptamine (serotonin). This could account for the depression occasionally associated with oral contraceptives.

ENDOCRINE EFFECTS OF ORAL CONTRACEPTIVES

Hypertension. Hypertension occurs in a variable proportion of normotensive women receiving any variety of oral contraceptive. Prospective studies are of most value in defining the problem and indicate a significant although minor rise in mean systolic but not in diastolic blood pressure (Weir *et al.*, 1971). Women with pre-existing hypertension may be more susceptible to a further rise in their blood pressure. The mechanism of the hypertension is not fully understood but it is probably due to a rise in renin-activity consequent upon an effect of oestrogens upon hepatic production of renin-substrate. Increased angiotensin activity could then lead to a form of secondary aldosteronism. The practical implications of these findings are:

1. Avoid oral contraceptives in women with pre-existing hypertension, or, if they are used, check the blood pressure at frequent intervals afterwards.
2. Check the blood pressure of all women to be given oral contraceptives and repeat the reading at six months and one year. If no hypertension has appeared at these times all is likely to remain well.
3. Always enquire for a drug history of oral contraceptives in any young woman with hypertension.

Amenorrhoea. Amenorrhoea may follow withdrawal of any variety of oral contraceptive (Shearman, 1971). Occasionally the amenorrhoea may be due to a premature menopause. The condition is more frequent in women with a previous history of amenorrhoea or menstrual irregularity, but may also occur in those with previously regular cycles. Spontaneous remission probably occurs in about half of the cases within one year and in another quarter as a result of therapy. The mechanism is probably mediated by an action of oestrogens on the hypothalamus, which by suppressing the release or formation of LH/FSH-RH causes low LH levels and a reduction in ovarian oestrogen production. Hypothalamic dysfunction is supported by the occurrence of galactorrhoea, not always recognised by the patient, in about one-third of those with amenorrhoea. The practical implication of these findings are:

1. Avoid oral contraceptives in women with a history of menstrual irregularity whenever possible.

2. If amenorrhoea persists for six months following withdrawal of the drugs refer the patient for endocrine assessment. This should include measurement of plasma LH and FSH and urinary oestrogens and an X-ray of the skull to exclude pituitary fossa enlargement. Those with normal gonadotrophins and oestrogen excretion can be followed without therapy till one year and, if amenorrhoea persists, treated with clomiphene. Those with low hormone levels should be treated with clomiphene at once. Galactorrhoea may respond to clomiphene and remits with restoration of menstruation. Alternatively the ergot alkaloid described in Chapter 1 (p. 12) can be used. Amenorrhoea may persist for longer periods in up to a quarter of women with the syndrome and if fertility is a problem, gonadotrophins should be considered.

Pigmentation. Chloasma-like pigmentation similar to that occurring in pregnancy is a frequent feature of treatment with the pill. Recognition of the complication prevents a misdiagnosis of Addison's disease. If the woman is distressed by the pigmentation, withdrawal of the drug is usually followed by a slow regression of the pigmentation. The mechanism of its occurrence is not well understood but it is most likely to be due to a local action of oestrogens on melanocytes.

Thyroid and Adrenal Function Tests. Oral contraceptives affect the levels of many plasma proteins largely due to an effect on hepatic protein synthesis. Increased levels of thyroxine-binding globulin (TBG) and of transcortin lead to an elevation of the serum PBI, serum thyroxine and plasma cortisol levels. This may lead to erroneous diagnoses of hyperthyroidism or Cushing's syndrome. The free level of the hormones which is metabolically active is little altered and hence clinical features of hormone excess do not occur. The elevation of the PBI can be allowed for by measurement of some form of resin uptake test which will show 'hypothyroid' values to calculate a free-thyroxine index which is normal in pregnant women and in those receiving oral contraceptives.

THROMBOEMBOLIC EFFECTS OF ORAL CONTRACEPTIVES

There is an increased incidence of thrombophlebitis during pregnancy and the puerperium, and a rise in the level of certain clotting factors after administered oestrogen. During pregnancy there is an increase of Factors I, V, VII, VIII and X and oestrogens have been found to raise the level of Factor VIII in women with von Willebrand's disease and in carriers of haemophilia. Oestrogens have also been shown to increase platelet adhesiveness by enhancing their sensitivity to ADP. Superficial thrombophlebitis occurs three times more commonly in women taking oral contraceptives. There is now good evidence that there is a significant increase in venous thrombosis and pulmonary embolism in such women and an increased hazard of cerebral thrombosis although so far no definite increase in the incidence of coronary thrombosis has been demonstrated. Certain measures can be adopted to minimise the hazard. The tendency to thromboembolism depends upon the oestrogen content of the pill and preparations with an oestrogen content of >50 μg should not normally be used. In view of the increased thrombotic tendency which follows surgical operations, oral contraceptives should be withdrawn four weeks before a planned operation. Other possible conditions which may predispose to arterial thrombosis are obesity, hypertension, hypercholesterolaemia, diabetes mellitus and possibly worsening migraine.

GYNAECOLOGICAL EFFECTS OF ORAL CONTRACEPTIVES

Cervical Changes. Changes in appearance of the cervix may be difficult to interpret and florid cervical erosions which bleed on pressure are sometimes found in patients on oral contraceptive therapy. The cytological findings are usually negative in spite of the rather bizarre clinical appearance, although on occasions biopsy may show histological evidence of carcinoma in situ. There is no direct evidence linking administration of the pill with the development of carcinoma of the cervix or with malignant lesions in any site. However, cancer of the cervix occurs naturally in women of the reproductive age group and therefore occasional spontaneous occurrence of malignant change can be expected. Regular cytological examination of patients on the 'pill' should be performed.

Breast Changes. In some women cyclical engorgement and fullness occur premenstrually; enlargement of the breast may also be noted. Some women develop diffuse nodularity in the breast which subsides when therapy is discontinued. Low dosage oral contraceptive agents have no effect on the maintenance of lactation, and can be given safely to lactating women.

Vaginal Candidiasis. Oral contraceptives may precipitate or aggravate candida infection of the vagina, the oestrogen component causing changes in the acidity of the vagina which allows 'thrush' to become established. This must be distinguished from simple increased vaginal transudate. The patient complains of pruritus vulvae and a discharge and the appearances of the vagina are usually characteristic. The diagnosis should be confirmed by culture and treatment given at once with local pessaries and an oral anti-fungal preparation.

REFERENCES

Black, W. P., and Govan, E. D. T. (1972). *Brit. med. J.*, **1**, 672.

Brown, J. B. (1955a). *Lancet*, **i**, 320.

Brown, J. B. (1955b). *Mem. Soc. Endocrinol.*, **3**, 1.

Herbst, A. L., Ulfelder, H., and Poskanzer, D. C. (1971). *New Engl. J. Med.*, **284**, 878.

Javier, Z., Gershberg, H., and Hulse, M. (1968). *Metabolism*, **17**, 443.

Rifkind, A. B., Kulin, H. E., and Ross, G. T. (1967). *J. clin. Invest.*, **46**, 1925.

Shearman, R. P. (1971). *Lancet*, **2**, 64.

Tanner, J. M. (1962). In *Growth at Adolescence*, 2nd Edition. Oxford: Blackwell Scientific.

Weir, R. J., Briggs, E., Mack, A., Taylor, L., Browning, J., Naismith, L., and Wilson, E. (1971). *Lancet*, **1**, 467.

Williams, D. (1971). *Brit. med. J.*, **2**, 208.

Wynn, V., and Doar, J. W. H. (1966). *Lancet*, **ii**, 715.

Wynn, V., Doar, J. W. H., and Mills, G. L. (1966). *Lancet*, **ii**, 720.

8

HIRSUTISM AND VIRILISM

The effects of overproduction of androgen vary with the age and sex of the individual. In adult men there is little obvious effect, whereas in boys, pseudo-precocious puberty may occur with development of the secondary sexual characteristics although the testes remain small. In females, the commonest action of excess androgens is to produce an increase in body hair, which is referred to as *hirsutism*. The excess hair growth is usually noticed on the sides of the face, chin and upper lip areas, between the breasts, around the areolae, on the limbs and on the abdomen as an extension upwards towards the umbilicus of the horizontal upper limit of the normal female pubic hair. This 'male escutcheon' is, however, often seen in normal women as is a small amount of hair around the nipples or on the face. When the hair growth is mild a decision as to whether a patient has significant hirsuties is often arbitrary and the family history and constitutional origin of the patient are of particular relevance. Evidence of significant *virilism*, such as temporal hair recession with scalp hair thinning, deepening of the voice, skeletal muscle hypertrophy, acne, clitoromegaly, oligomenorrhoea or amenorrhoea indicates that a definite source of abnormal androgen production is likely to be found.

Androgens are derived from the adrenal cortex, the testis, and the ovary and are excreted in the urine as 17-oxosteroids. In the male, two-thirds of the 17-oxosteroids are derived from the adrenal cortex. The 11-oxygenated oxosteroids are mainly of adrenocortical origin and comprise some 23 per cent of the total 17-oxosteroids in the urine, the rest consisting mainly of androsterone, aetiocholanolone, and dehydroepiandrosterone. By far the most powerful androgen is testosterone, which is secreted largely from the testis; small amounts also arise in the adrenal cortex and ovary. In the normal female most of the testosterone is derived from conversion of androstenedione to testosterone in the tissues. Metabolites of testosterone itself contribute little to the total urinary 17-oxosteroids since only about 24 per cent of testosterone is converted to 17-oxosteroids. Since testosterone is such a potent androgen, slight elevation in its production rate can result in marked hirsuties without producing an elevation of the urinary 17-oxosteroids; it is evident that estimation of urinary 17-oxosteroids is rarely helpful. Even elaborate fractionations of 17-oxosteroids are of little diagnostic importance in most cases of hirsuties.

The production rate of testosterone in normal men is about 7 mg/day, and in women about 1·5 mg/day. In men the production rate correlates well with plasma testosterone levels but this is not so in women, probably due to interconversions. The plasma testosterone level in men lies between 3 and 11 ng/ml, and in women 0·2 to 0·8 ng/ml. Levels rise sharply at puberty in boys and decline in old age, whereas in females there is little variation with age or during the menstrual cycle. Urinary testosterone excretion is unaffected by ACTH in men but is increased in women. Dexamethasone causes a reduction in testosterone excretion in women. Chorionic gonadotrophin increases testosterone excretion in males but has no consistent effect in females. Testosterone production has been studied in various endocrine diseases. It is decreased in hypopituitarism, primary testicular disease and some cases of Klinefelter's syndrome and increased in Cushing's syndrome and congenital adrenal hyperplasia.

In most women with hirsutism plasma testosterone levels are raised, the extent of the elevation depending on the underlying disease process. In those patients in whom the absolute plasma testosterone levels are not raised, the concentration of the specific sex hormone-binding-globulin, to which testosterone is normally bound, is reduced. As a result the non-protein bound testosterone level, i.e. that fraction which is metabolically active and available to the tissues, is increased. The problem is usually to determine whether the testosterone is arising from the ovary or the adrenal. Estimations of adrenal or ovarian vein blood are not readily applicable in clinical practice and an indirect approach to the problem is used. Adrenocortical hormone output can usually be suppressed by dexamethasone and stimulated by ACTH, whereas ovarian or testicular stimulation may be attempted by chorionic gonadotrophin and suppression by a potent oestrogen or androgen. However, the problem is complex since in some circumstances a combined ovarian and adrenocortical abnormality appears to be present. For example elevated adrenal androgens, urinary 17-oxosteroids and testosterone levels may all occur in patients with the polycystic ovary syndrome, yet all may be suppressed with dexamethasone.

AETIOLOGY

Hirsutism is one of the commonest and least rewarding problems that presents to an endocrinologist and there is often no detectable ovarian or adrenal abnormality. The common causes of hirsutism in order of diminishing frequency are: 'idiopathic'—cause unknown, polycystic ovary syndrome, Cushing's syndrome, ovarian tumours, congenital adrenal hyperplasia, and adrenal tumours. All these diseases, apart from the first two listed, are rare. There is a wide range of body hair growth in normal women which varies with different racial groups, e.g. the Mediterranean races have more body hair than Nordic women. Many normal women, especially those with dark hair, have more hair on the upper lip than they deem ideal. A few coarse hairs on the chin, around the nipples or even extension of pubic hair to the umbilicus are frequent normal findings. All that is required in these patients is firm reassurance that they are normal and that they are not about to change sex. The major causes of hirsuties and virilism in women are shown in Table 8.1 together with the appropriate changes in androgen levels.

CLINICAL FEATURES

A number of features in the *history* are important in determining the cause of hirsutism. The age of onset of the hirsutism should first be elicited. Patients with idiopathic hirsuties and with the polycystic ovary syndrome often notice the worrying increase in body hair during the teens. An increase in hair on the face is not uncommon in elderly women. A family history of increased hair in siblings or parents is often found in idiopathic hirsuties. Enquiry should be made about the ingestion of any androgenic compounds, including anabolic steroids and hormonal compounds given for menopausal symptoms, some of which contain testosterone. *A menstrual history is vital.* Patients with idiopathic hirsuties usually have regular, normal periods, whereas those with the polycystic ovary syndrome have irregular periods, or prolonged secondary amenorrhoea. Ovarian or adrenal tumours causing hirsuties often cause amenorrhoea. Most women with hirsutism are otherwise well and attend for advice because they are embarrassed about their appearance or worried

TABLE 8.1 *Major Causes of Hirsuties and Virilism in Women* (from Besser and Edwards, *Clinics in Endocrinology and Metabolism*, (1972), W. B. Saunders, by permission of the Editor).

Cause	Plasma* Testosterone	Urinary 17-oxosteroids*	17-oxogenic steroids*
Constitutional			
familial	N	N	N
idiopathic	N	N	N
Physiological			
menopause	N	N	N
Iatrogenic			
androgens	N ↓ or ↑ †	N	N
progestogens	N ↓ or ↑	N	N
ACTH	↑	↑	↑
corticosteroids	↓ or N	↓	↓ or ↑ †
Ovarian			
polycystic ovaries	↑ or N	↑ or N	N
arrhenoblastoma or hilus cell tumour	↑	N or ↑	N
hilus cell hyperplasia	↑	N or ↑	N
Adrenocortical			
Cushing's syndrome	N or ↑	N or ↑	↑ or N
congenital adrenal hyperplasia	↑	↑	↑
virilising adenoma or carcinoma	↑	↑	N or ↑
Pituitary tumours: acromegaly	N or ↓	N or ↑	N
Gonadal maldevelopment, e.g. ovarian agenesis, intersexual states	N or ↓	N	N
Miscellaneous			
anorexia nervosa	N or ↓	↓	↓
porphyria	N	N	N

* where alternatives are given the most common finding is quoted first.
† raised if natural hormone given, usually suppressed if synthetic compound used.
N = normal
↑ = increased ↓ = decreased

about its possible implications fearing that they are undergoing a 'change' of sex.

On examination, the extent of the hirsuties should be defined and other evidence of virilisation or endocrinopathy should be sought. The more severe the virilisation the more likely is the chance of finding some treatable cause. Obesity is so common in women attending endocrine clinics that it has little discriminatory value as a sign of the polycystic ovary syndrome.

Investigations are usually unrewarding in the absence of clinical evidence of clear endocrine disease but must be carried out to detect the patients with curable conditions. In patients with the two commonest conditions, idiopathic hirsuties and the polycystic ovary syndrome, urinary 17-oxosteroids are often in the upper normal female range or just above it, especially if they are also obese. Patients with ovarian tumours causing hirsuties may have raised 17-oxosteroid output since they may be found in association with polycystic ovaries, but occasionally reduced excretion is found. Significant elevation of 17-oxosteroid excretion usually indicates an adrenal tumour. If there is any question of Cushing's syndrome, the urinary free cortisol should be estimated as this is the best single test to exclude or confirm this condition. It is usual to estimate the 24-hour excretion of pregnanetriol to exclude the very rare patients with congenital adrenal hyperplasia who present at or after puberty with hirsuties. A raised pregnanetriol excretion in the urine suggests an adrenal defect affecting the 21-hydroxylase enzyme, the commonest variant of congenital adrenal hyperplasia. Whenever possible plasma testosterone and also sex-hormone binding-globulin levels should be assayed.

The *dexamethasone suppression test* is often helpful in the differential diagnosis of patients with hirsuties and virilism. The plasma testosterone and urinary 17-oxosteroids normally suppress by more than 50 per cent during administration of dexamethasone 2 mg per day (as 0·5 mg four times a day). It must be given for at least 3 days, as the urinary androgenic metabolites are cleared relatively slowly from the body. Normal suppression will be seen in idiopathic hirsuties, the polycystic ovary syndrome and congenital adrenal hyperplasia. In patients with virilising ovarian tumours the circulating testosterone will not suppress but the 17-oxosteroids will; in Cushing's disease and adrenocortical tumours neither will suppress; in Cushing's disease suppression will be seen if 8 mg per day of dexamethasone is given.

Pelvic examination by an experienced gynaecologist may reveal bilateral ovarian enlargement suggestive of the polycystic ovary syndrome, but even experienced clinical evaluation may often not pick up the abnormality. Unilateral ovarian enlargement may still be due to the syndrome but also raises the possibility of an ovarian tumour. Since routine pelvic examination is an uncertain method of assessing ovarian size, culdoscopy or laparoscopy and examination under anaesthetic may be required. Alternatively a gynaecogram or pelvic pneumoperitoneum may be used, when gas is introduced into the pelvic cavity to outline the ovaries and uterus on X-ray.

The investigations required must be decided for the individual patient. For example, if the hirsuties is mild, menstruation regular, routine pelvic examination is normal, and the plasma testosterone and urinary 17-oxosteroids are normal, it is not usually necessary to proceed with further investigations and the patient can usually be assumed to belong to the category of idiopathic hirsuties.

IDIOPATHIC HIRSUTIES

This is the commonest category into which women with hirsuties are placed. As mentioned previously, it is a diagnosis arrived at by exclusion of other possibilities; the hirsuties is not usually severe, menstruation is normal, the ovaries are not enlarged, and the urinary 17-oxosteroids are normal.

The underlying pathogenesis of the condition is still unknown. Three possible causes have been suggested: (1) these patients tend to overreact to ACTH administration; the 17-oxosteroid rise produced by 20 IU of ACTH given twice daily for four days relative to the 17-hydroxycorticosteroid rise is much greater than normal. There may therefore be an abnormal metabolic pathway in the adrenal cortex resulting in excess androgen production. Urinary 17-oxosteroid excretion is easily suppressed with dexamethasone. (2) Some patients with idiopathic hirsuties may have minor ovarian abnormalities of androgen production. (3) Hypersensitivity of hair follicles to normal circulating amounts of androgen has been suggested, but there is no good evidence for this theory.

Plasma testosterone concentrations are often increased and if normal are associated with lowered sex hormone binding globulin levels and therefore increased free testosterone concentrations. Although rises in plasma testosterone can be produced by ACTH, and decreases follow dexamethasone therapy, some patients show a rise in level with administration of HCG during dexamethasone suppression of the adrenals. These dynamic tests therefore give equivocal results suggesting the possibility of combined adrenal and ovarian abnormalities in some cases. It is known that polycystic ovaries similar to those of the polycystic ovary syndrome can be found in patients with an androgen producing tumour of the adrenal or ovary, and possibly minor ovarian abnormalities may occur as secondary phenomena in the presence of other sources of increased androgen production, e.g. the adrenal.

TREATMENT

This may be directed at suppression of adrenocortical or ovarian androgen production, alone or in combination, or be purely palliative. If palliative it is rather unsatisfactory. Depilatory waxes and creams benefit some. Coarse facial hairs can be removed by electrolysis though this is time consuming and expensive, and occasionally causes some scarring. Shaving is often the most effective remedy and, contrary to popular belief, does not increase the rate of hair growth or cause the hairs to become coarser.

Adrenocortical suppression may usually be effected by administration of prednisolone in a dose of 7·5 mg per day although 10 mg per day may be initially required. A large proportion of the total dose (e.g. 5 mg) should be given at night on retiring, with the remainder being taken in the morning, since this produces the most effective suppression of ACTH secretion. With this treatment the hirsuties at best improves but this happens only in the minority of patients; more often the progressive worsening of the hair growth is arrested. Many patients fail to improve but at least 6 to 9 months should be allowed to elapse before the treatment is abandoned since the cycles in hair growth are slow, and this should be explained to the patients. If the periods are irregular they usually become normal and fertility is restored during corticosteroid therapy.

Ovarian suppression may be achieved using one of the oral contraceptives. Contraceptives should not be used if the patient has oligo- or amenorrhoea as they may result in prolonged amenorrhoea, with or without galactorrhoea. However if regular menstruation is restored with prednisolone, but the hirsuties is still not adequately controlled, it is then safe to add the oral contraceptive, and this combined therapy probably offers the best chance of improving the hair growth. Unfortunately some patients still may not respond.

THE POLYCYSTIC OVARY SYNDROME

This is the commonest ovarian abnormality associated with significant hirsuties and is often accompanied by mild virilism. The eponym 'the Stein–Leventhal syndrome' is confusing and uninformative since any combination of the clinical features of the condition (Table 8.2) may be present. The name should be discarded and instead the term 'the polycystic ovary syndrome' used since it is the common feature.

TABLE 8.2 *Clinical Features of Polycystic Ovary Syndrome*
(from Prunty, 1967)

Clinical features	Incidence (%)
Amenorrhoea—primary or secondary	55
Dysfunctional uterine bleeding	28
Infertility—primary or secondary	75
Evidence of ovulation	20
Hirsutism	95
Enlarged ovaries	95
Obesity	40

On reviewing the menstrual history prior to diagnosis it is sometimes found that the menarche was later than average. Often the menses were never normal or showed intervals of normality interspersed with amenorrhoea which may be prolonged. Dysfunctional bleeding may occasionally be severe. Rarely, the patient presents with primary amenorrhoea. Ovulation is absent or intermittent, and primary or secondary infertility is a common complaint. Hirsutism is usually the main problem, virilism is uncommon, but does occur. There are no specific features of the hirsutism that make it possible to arrive at a clinical diagnosis. Usually, the hirsuties is more marked than in the idiopathic variety. The breasts may show signs of activity in the nipples similar to that seen in early pregnancy and there may be galactorrhoea. Ovarian enlargement can usually be demonstrated by pelvic examination, examination under anaesthetic, culdoscopy, laparoscopy or gynaecography, depending on the obesity of the patient and on the preference of the gynaecologist concerned.

Pathology. The ovaries are usually enlarged and pearly white in appearance. The ovarian capsule is thickened due to an increased amount of collagen (normal capsular thickness 0·1 mm, polycystic ovaries 1 mm or more). Beneath the capsule there are numerous small follicles or cysts, lined with a thin layer of granulosa cells. Corpora lutea and corpora albicans occur in about 22 per cent of ovaries indicating previous ovulation. The theca interna is often thickened and shows signs of hyperactivity, and the ovarian stroma is increased in amount.

Ovarian Steroid Content. The ovarian cystic follicles contain a completely different group of steroids to normal follicles and other varieties of ovarian cysts (Fig. 8.1). Usually, in this disease the cyst fluid shows a very high concentration of androstenedione, and unlike the normal follicle, little or no oestradiol-17β or oestrone, and only small amounts of progesterone. By incubating ovaries with various radioactive substrates it has been shown that there may be an enzymatic defect in the conversion of androstenedione to oestradiol. Prior treatment with FSH and HCG reverses the abnormal steroid pattern in the ovaries though after a time the original abnormality tends to recur. A few patients with the polycystic ovary syndrome show a different steroid pattern in cyst fluid with large amounts of dehydroepiandrosterone (DHA). Ovaries from these patients are unable to convert DHA to androstenedione because of deficiency of 3β-hydroxydehydrogenase; but they easily convert androstenedione to oestradiol.

Blood and Urinary Steroids and Gonadotrophins. Ideally, ovarian vein steroids should be analysed but these samples contain a contribution from the uterus. The samples can, of course, be obtained at laparotomy or by selective venous catheterisation. Oestrogen secretion from the ovary, blood oestrogen levels, and urinary excretion are within the normal range or slightly reduced. Androstenedione and/or dehydroepiandrosterone and testosterone levels are raised in ovarian vein in some patients, in adrenal venous blood in others and in peripheral blood in most. Testosterone production rate is often raised but, when normal, it is found that the testosterone in the circulation is mainly derived from androstenedione. Plasma testosterone levels are usually higher than in the idiopathic hirsuties group but like those patients

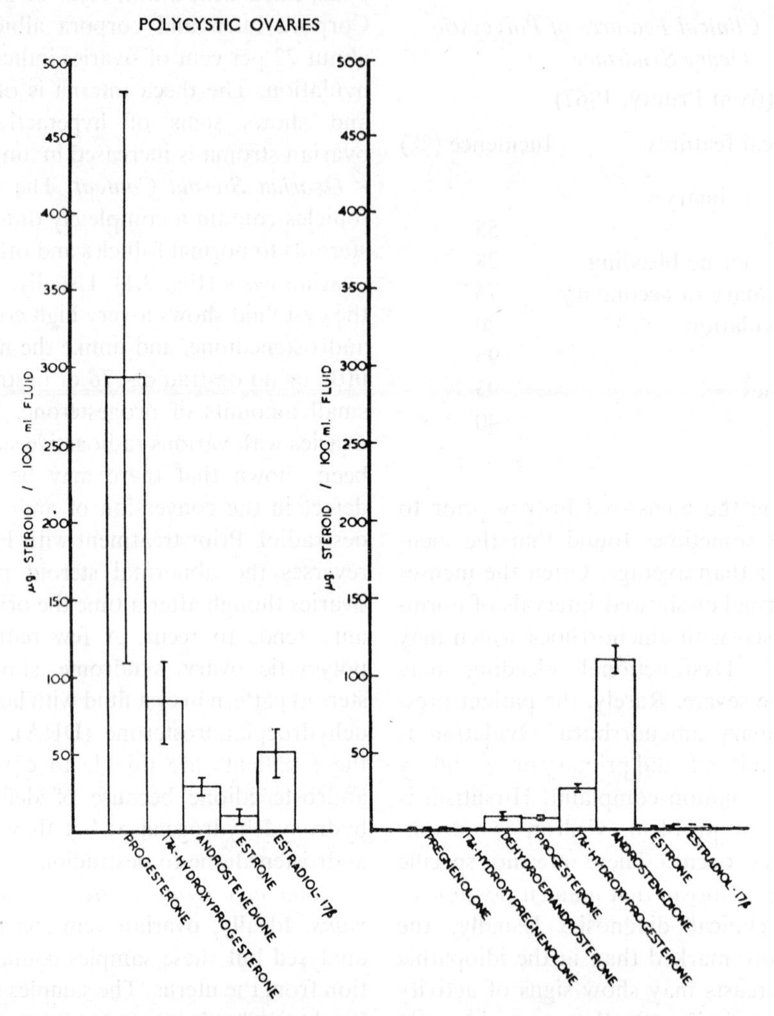

FIGURE 8.1 Steroids contained in various cystic follicles and in the polycystic ovary syndrome (from Short, R. V. (1964), in *Proc. Second Internat. Cong. Endocrin.*, London, by permission of Excerpta Medica Foundation)

there is an increase in free testosterone levels as the sex hormone binding globulin concentration is reduced. The urinary 17-oxosteroid excretion is raised in about a third of these patients though it does not exceed 30 mg/24 hours. These 17-oxosteroids comprise 11-oxy compounds of adrenal origin and 11-deoxy compounds from adrenal or ovarian sources. On the basis that dexamethasone suppresses the adrenal contribution of 17-oxosteroids, some workers describe two groups of patients; those showing good suppression of 11-deoxy 17-oxosteroids suggesting an adrenal origin, and those showing poor suppression of 11-deoxy 17-oxosteroids suggesting an ovarian origin. Stilboestrol causes reduction of 11-deoxy 17-oxosteroids in the latter group, again suggesting an ovarian origin.

However, others find that both the urinary 17-oxosteroids and plasma testosterone always suppress in this condition providing that dexamethasone is given for long enough (3 to 5 days) since the steroids may be cleared from the body only slowly. Non-suppression should suggest the presence of an antonomous ovarian or adreno-cortical tumour. Stimulation tests using FSH or HCG are of little value in diagnosis or in understanding the basic pathology of the disease. There is considerable evidence that in many patients the serum LH levels are raised and fluctuant although they do not cycle normally; the FSH levels are low. It is possible that these changes could be secondary to a primary hypothalamic, ovarian or adreno-cortical abnormality. Indeed, the whole polycystic ovary phenomenon may represent a non-specific target organ response to a variety a different abnormal stimuli since they may be associated with other causes of abnormal androgen production, e.g. ovarian or adrenal tumours and Cushing's disease.

TREATMENT

Conservative management with weight reduction and reassurence should be adopted unless the hirsuties, menstrual abnormalities or infertility are problems. Spontaneous recovery may sometimes occur.

The *hirsuties* should be managed as for a case of idiopathic hirsuties (*see* p. 212) if this is the predominant problem. If primary or secondary infertility is the principal problem then ovulation induction with clomiphene or gonadotrophins, or wedge resection of the ovaries should be considered.

Wedge Resection of the Ovaries. This used to be practised more frequently in the past than at present. Usually about one third of each ovary is removed. This results in a fall in 17-oxosteroid excretion, particularly of the 11-deoxy fraction, and testosterone formation is also reduced. In about two-thirds of patients ovulation occurs after operation and regular ovulatory cycles are restored. Fertility is highest in the earlier months but often relapses occur and infertility and oligo- or amenorrhoea return. The mechanism by which wedge resection restores normal ovarian function is unknown, though by reducing the mass of ovarian tissue, particularly the stroma responsible for androgen secretion, it may allow a normal gonadotrophin cycle to be re-established. Wedge resection rarely improves the hirsuties and since the infertility can be treated medically with ovulation induction, surgery is not as often performed as previously.

Ovulation Induction. Providing that the Fallopian tubes are patent, the uterus normal, and the partner's seminal analysis normal, the infertility associated with the polycystic ovary syndrome usually responds to clomiphene therapy. Clomiphene is an anti-oestrogen which acts on the hypothalamus to cause gonadotrophin release, although it may also have an action on the ovary. An oral dose of clomiphene, 100 to 150 mg daily for 5 days, is given each month and followed by 4,500 units intramuscularly of HCG given once, on day 14. The patient's response may be monitored by measuring the basal body temperature but this may be confused in the early phases of the cycle since clomiphene itself may elevate the temperature. It is better to follow the urinary oestrogen excretion as an index of ovarian follicle stimulation by FSH during the first half of the cycle, and pregnanediol excretion in the second half since an elevation of the urinary levels of this metabolite of progesterone indicates corpus luteum formation and therefore of anteceding ovulation. Ovulation usually occurs during the 48 hours after the HCG. Unless conception occurs menstruation follows. After two or three months of clomiphene administration the patient may continue to cycle spontaneously, unless pregnant, but the periods and fertility in most cases eventually disappear. A regime of 3 months of clomiphene administration followed by 3 months off the drug, should be followed for at least a year before the alternative gonadotrophin therapy is considered, since this is associated with a much higher incidence of multiple births or the 'hyperstimulation' syndrome with shock and great ovarian enlargement, and is much more difficult to manage. Clomiphene occasionally results in twin or triplet births, but is free of side effects in the dosage given, apart from occasional visual effects (haloes and flickering lights) and reversible minor depression.

Gonadotrophin therapy using human menopausal urinary gonadotrophin (HMG, containing FSH and LH) and HCG is also effective. In the polycystic ovary syndrome it is used in the same way as in hypopituitary patients and some details are given in Chapter 1. However, it must be remembered that polycystic ovary patients are usually much more sensitive to HMG than other infertile women and dosage should be started with not more than 3 ampoules on days 1, 3 and 5 (each ampoule of 'Pergonal' contains 75 units of FSH and 75 units of LH), followed by HCG given once on day 8 in a dose of 4,500 units.

Unfortunately, none of the lines of therapy mentioned above has much effect on hirsuties, which should be managed as previously described. Furthermore following pregnancy, the menstrual disorder and infertility often return.

OVARIAN TUMOURS

Ovarian tumours causing hirsutism and virilisation are very rare. The tumours usually secrete testosterone and can cause rapid virilisation and amenorrhoea. The tumour may be palpable on abdominal or pelvic examination but its presence can be excluded only by inspection and section of the ovaries. In patients with virilisation in whom the 17-oxosteroid excretion is normal (or occasionally lowered), laparotomy is justified to ensure that an ovarian tumour is not overlooked particularly if testosterone levels are elevated and do not suppress with dexamethasone. The nature of the hormone secreted by an ovarian tumour is not closely correlated with its histological type; e.g. granulosa cell tumours may secrete oestrogens causing pseudo-precocious puberty in girls, or androgens causing virilisation. Successful removal of an ovarian tumour is usually followed by return of normal menstruation, and hirsuties may regress. Deepening of the voice is usually permanent, though slight improvement can occur. Whatever the type of tumour the hirsutism and virilisation are usually the result of excessive formation of testosterone.

Arrhenoblastomas usually affect young women and are the commonest virilising tumours of the ovary, probably arising from the ovarian stroma. They may be of low grade malignancy but metastasise late. The whole ovary should be removed.

Hilus cell tumours (Leydig cell tumours) are very rare, usually small and benign, occurring at or after the menopause, when they may cause post-menopausal bleeding. They may develop in some patients with Turner's syndrome. They are thought to arise from ovarian hilar cells which are probably of similar origin to the Leydig cells of the testis. Occasionally hilus cell hyperplasia rather than a tumour is seen in these virilised women.

Adrenal rest tumours may cause features of Cushing's syndrome as well as virilisation. They usually appear in women under forty years of age, are unilateral, and non-malignant. It is very likely they arise from adrenal rests in the ovary. They sometimes secrete oestrogens and progesterone as well as testosterone and cortisol.

Granulosa-theca-cell tumours are usually feminising, but occasionally they cause virilisation. They are of variable malignancy.

Gonandroblastomas are of complex cellular origin and of doubtful malignancy. They tend to occur in pseudo-hermaphrodites and should be suspected if virilisation develops in such patients.

CONGENITAL ADRENAL HYPERPLASIA (CAH)

This group of diseases will be dealt with in Chapter 13. As mentioned previously, congenital adrenal hyperplasia, may not, for unknown reasons, become manifest till after puberty, when it can cause masculinisation in girls. The condition may be suspected if the urinary 17-oxosteroids are raised and are easily suppressed by dexamethasone, and if there is excess of pregnanetriol in the urine. Treatment consists of giving cortisol or prednisolone to suppress ACTH and the adrenocortical steroid production.

ADRENAL TUMOURS

Adrenal adenomas or carcinomas secreting androgens are very rare causes of hirsutism or virilism. They can be detected much more easily in women than in men. Adenomas usually secrete either androgens or cortisol, whereas carcinomas may secrete any group of steroids, including oestrogens. Usually, an adrenal tumour is suspected by the raised excretion of 17-oxosteroids in the urine, very high values sometimes being seen. The 17-oxosteroid excretion is usually fixed and unresponsive to stimulation with ACTH or suppression with dexamethasone. Some tumours secrete very large amounts of dehydroepiandrosterone, though this is not a unique metabolite of the adrenal. Adrenal calcification can sometimes be detected on X-rays and is usually indicative of a carcinoma. Localisation may be confirmed by intravenous pyelography but both glands should be inspected at operation since such tumours may be bilateral. Lateralisation preoperatively is sometimes possible if differential venous blood samples are obtained for testosterone assay from both adrenal veins and from different levels along the inferior vena cava. When the adenoma secretes only androgens, the contralateral adrenal is not atrophic. Regression of some of the masculinising features occurs after removal of the tumour, when menstruation and fertility may be restored.

REFERENCES

Besser, G. M., and Edwards, C. R. W. (1972). *Clinics in Endocrinology and Metabolism*, **1**, 491.

Jenkins, J. S. (1966). *Brit. J. Hosp. Med.*, **1**, 37.

Prunty, F. T. G. (1967). *J. Endocrinol.*, **38**, 85, 203.

9

BREAST

In the male, breast tissue is rudimentary throughout life, although a mild degree of transient physiological gynaecomastia commonly occurs at puberty (*see* below). In the female, the breasts remain rudimentary until the changes of puberty occur. Further breast development takes place during pregnancy and lactation, when the mammary glands achieve their secretory function. There is some atrophy of breast tissue after the menopause.

ANATOMY

The normal adult female breast consists of glandular, fibrous, and adipose tissue. The gland tissue is a lobulated flattened mass, consisting of some fifteen to twenty lobes, each composed of a group of lobules. Between lobules are the areolar tissue, blood vessels, and the duct system. The terminal lobules are composed of a cluster of rounded alveoli which open into the smallest branches of the lactiferous ducts. Each duct drains a lobe, the ducts converging beneath the nipple to open on to the surface. Below the nipple, the lactiferous ducts dilate, forming the lactiferous sinuses, which act as reservoirs for the secreted milk. At birth, the female breast consists almost entirely of lactiferous ducts without alveoli. At puberty there is growth of the ducts and connecting fibrous tissue, increased deposition of fat, and development of the alveoli. The alveoli are the site of milk production, but lactation does not normally begin until after parturition has occurred.

PHYSIOLOGY

Oestrogen stimulates the development of the duct system by causing elongation and thickening of the lactiferous ducts. Progesterone stimulates alveolar growth and leads to the appearance of 'buds' at the distal ends of the ducts which differentiate into the alveoli. However, while oestrogen and progesterone have a direct effect in producing breast growth and development, optimal growth of breast tissue depends also on the presence of a number of anterior pituitary mammogenic substances, and the ovarian steroids are much less effective in the absence of these hormones.

The pituitary mammogenic factors necessary for normal breast development are prolactin, possibly growth hormone, and the pituitary gonadotrophins, and these factors may have direct effects on breast growth even in the absence of oestrogen and progesterone. Prolactin has now been isolated from the human pituitary, and is the major lactogenic factor in man (*see* Chapter 1). Like growth hormone it originates from the acidophil cells. The following account of the control of lactation is based largely on animal work, and its application to human physiology should be interpreted with caution. When the breast is fully developed mainly under the influence of the oestrogens, prolactin results in further alveolar formation and the secretion of milk. Hypophysectomy is rapidly followed by the cessation of milk secretion, and failure of lactation is a well recognised feature of post-partum hypopituitarism. In addition to the hormones already mentioned, the adrenocortical steroids, thyroid hormones, and insulin also have an indirect role to play in the development of the normal breast.

LACTATION

During pregnancy, the breasts enlarge and develop further mainly in response to the placental hormones present in the circulation in very great concentration—oestrogen, progesterone, and placental lactogen. The onset and maintenance of lactation is immediately due to increased secretion of prolactin. However, a small amount of pituitary prolactin is secreted in the middle trimester of pregnancy, and this then increases progressively towards term. The mean serum immunoreactive prolactin levels in the non-pregnant woman (and in men) is 10 ng/ml and this rises to 207 ng/ml at term (Hwang *et al.*, 1971). Post-partum, the prolactin levels rise further as long as breast feeding continues. There is a marked further temporary rise during the actual period of suckling. In women who are not breast feeding, prolactin levels fall after parturition to reach non-pregnant levels by 4 to 6 weeks post-partum. The factors that initiate lactation are not yet fully understood, but it is presumed that the humoral changes that occur at the time of parturition play a major part in this process in addition to the act of suckling. It appears that modification of the secretion of prolactin depends on hypothalamic mechanisms which alter the secretion into the portal capillary circulation in the pituitary stalk of prolactin inhibiting factor (PIF). The pathway involved in secretion of PIF is dopaminergic.

Maintenance of Lactation

Lactation does not continue for long, unless the milk produced is removed, even in the presence of normal hormonal secretion. Lactation ceases after weaning but may be prolonged for considerable periods if breast feeding is continued. The maintenace of lactation depends principally upon the continued secretion of prolactin for the stimulus of suckling has been shown to produce release of pituitary prolactin, and this effect may become conditioned. Thus, the physical and emotional stimuli associated with suckling help to maintain the secretion of prolactin.

Milk secreted into the alveoli is largely unavailable to the child until the alveoli contract and milk is passed through the duct system to the lactiferous sinuses. Oxytocin causes contraction of the myoepithelial cells which partially surround the alveoli and is clearly important in many animals producing milk 'let-down', but its importance in man in this respect is far from established. This hormone is released as a result of sensory nerve stimuli from the nipple during suckling which pass to the hypothalamus. Oxytocin does not appear to be involved directly in the control of prolactin secretion.

Suppression of Lactation

When it is necessary to suppress lactation, suckling and expression of milk from the breasts should be avoided. In some cases no specific therapy is indicated. In others, however, there is severe engorgement of the breasts, with discomfort to the patient and the risk of a breast abscess. In these cases manual expression of milk may be necessary for a short period to make the patient more comfortable, and suppression of lactation has in the past been brought about by giving synthetic oestrogens in high dosage, such as chlorotrianisene, hexoestrol or stilboestrol. Recently the ergot alkaloid 2-brom-α-ergocryptine has been shown to suppress prolactin secretion from the pituitary in lactating mothers as well as in patients with pathological lactation. It is very effective in suppressing puerperal lactation, and so far no significant side effects have been reported.

Persistent Lactation

Prolactin will be released as long as suckling continues but sometimes secretion of milk continues after suckling has ceased. This is commonly associated with a delay in the return of normal menstruation and is presumably due to a failure in re-establishing normal cyclical secretion of FSH and LH. Persistent lactation and amenorrhoea is frequently termed the Chiari-Frommel syndrome when it follows pregnancy, the Argonz-del Castillo syndrome when it occurs in women who have not been pregnant, and the Forbes–Albright syndrome if an obvious pituitary tumour is present. Galactorrhoea may be the first indication of a pituitary or hypothalamic tumour but often no underlying abnormality can be detected. The eponyms should not however be used now since the conditions listed are in effect all the same condition due to hyperprolactinaemia and merge into one another. The galactorrhoea syndromes are dealt with in more detail in Chapter 1. Galactorrhoea may be diminished by cyclical oestrogen/progesterone therapy, and in some cases the regime may be discontinued after a few months with return of normal function. Clomiphene is often effective in the treatment of galactorrhoea, whatever the cause. Bromergocryptine is a most effective suppressor of both prolactin secretion and galactorrhoea and also usually results in disappearance of the amenorrhoea.

DISORDERS OF THE BREASTS

Aberrant breast tissue or accessory nipples are not uncommon, and may occur anywhere in the breast-line, which extends from mid-clavicle to the inguinal ligament. Treatment is not usually required.

SMALL BREASTS

Small breasts are a physiological variant in patients who otherwise show normal sexual maturation with regular ovulatory menstrual cycles, and little can be done by drug therapy to increase their size, although pregnancy may occasionally result in a permanent increase in the size of the breasts. Reduction in the size of the breasts may occur after a period of weight loss. Failure of development of one breast is presumed to be due to end-organ failure and in some cases other congenital defects are also present. In patients who complain of small breasts in association with other signs of delayed maturation, cyclical hormone therapy may be of help, but relatively large doses of oestrogens may need to be given. Recently, encouraging results have been obtained by the insertion of synthetic prostheses and this procedure should be considered in patients who are psychiatrically disturbed because of their small breasts.

LARGE BREASTS

Over development of the breasts is less frequently seen than is under development. It may be bilateral or unilateral. The cause is unknown, though overdevelopment may sometimes begin during pregnancy. Progesterone preparations may be helpful in reducing the breast size, due to their anti-oestrogenic action, but in severe cases plastic surgery may give a satisfactory cosmetic result.

CYSTIC MASTITIS

During each menstrual cycle there is stimulation of duct tissue by oestrogens, and of alveolar secretory activity by progesterone. This is followed by a period of involution as oestrogen and progesterone levels fall and menstruation begins. Most women experience slight tenderness of the breasts, with a feeling of heaviness, during the premenstrual period of the cycle. In some, however, these symptoms are more marked, and there may be severe tenderness and distension, associated with increased nodularity. These changes may be due to a relative deficiency in progesterone and an increase in oestrogen during the luteal phase of the cycle. If diuretics are not of help, progesterone compounds may be given during the last few days of the cycle; e.g. norethisterone, 5 mg daily or twice daily. The recurring cycle of stimulation and involution may result in later life in the development of small cysts affecting the ducts, together with nodular fibrosis. In some cases localised cysts may raise the possibility of a neoplasm. The tenderness of the cysts during the latter half of the menstrual cycle is suggestive of chronic cystic mastitis rather than of neoplasm, but any suspicious areas should be biopsied. When pain is a prominent feature, cyclical oestrogen-progesterone therapy should be given, and if this is ineffective simple mastectomy should be considered.

TUMOURS OF THE BREAST

BENIGN

Fibroadenoma. This tumour is commoner in females under the age of thirty, and may arise in a breast that already shows the changes of cystic mastitis. The tumours are rounded, well defined and mobile, with no attachment to skin or underlying structures. Excision-biopsy is mandatory, with examination of a frozen section at the time of operation.

Benign Intraduct Papilloma. This tumour may give rise to a serous or sometimes a sanguinous discharge from the nipple. It may be palpable as a small nodule, but is sometimes difficult to locate. Systematic palpation of the breast is necessary to define the lobe that gives rise to the discharge. Excision and examination of a frozen section is essential.

Other tumours such as lipomas, fibromas, and neurofibromas may occur in the breast; in many cases excision will be necessary to establish the diagnosis.

MALIGNANT

Sarcomas, of various types, are rare.

Intraduct carcinoma typically gives rise to a blood-stained discharge from the nipple. It may be impossible to distinguish this clinically from the benign papilloma.

CARCINOMA

Carcinoma is the commonest malignant tumour of the breast, and is the most frequent carcinoma in the female. It occurs with increasing frequency after the age of twenty-five until the menopause, when the incidence levels out, to rise to a second peak after the age of sixty-five.

AETIOLOGY

The cause of breast carcinoma is unknown, but both genetic and hormonal factors are presumed to play a part. There are obvious similarities between the breast carcinoma that may be produced in animals and those occurring naturally in the female, though as yet there is no evidence that viruses are involved in the development of human breast carcinoma. The incidence of breast carcinoma appears to be inversely related to the number of children suckled. It is a common belief that single women are more liable to breast cancer than are married women, but this seems to be true only in women over the age of forty-seven. Below this age, proportionately fewer nulliparous women die of breast cancer. Although the tumour does not appear to be caused primarily by oestrogens, there is no doubt that oestrogens may accelerate the growth of an existing breast cancer. Other tumours appear to be dependent on prolactin. Acceleration of growth may sometimes occur during pregnancy, though a subsequent pregnancy does not adversely affect the prognosis. It has recently been reported that about one-third of women with breast cancer have lowered plasma levels of the cortisol-binding protein transcortin. There is also evidence that abnormalities in the excretion of corticosteroid and androgen metabolites are found in women with breast cancer.

CLINICAL FEATURES

Patients with breast cancer usually present with a hard painless lump which may be fixed to skin or underlying tissues. Fixation to the skin may give the classical 'peau d'orange' appearance or dimpling. Tumours may arise in the axillary tail of Spence. During pregnancy, breast carcinomas may progress rapidly, giving the appearance of diffuse inflammation in the breast. The primary site of the neoplasm is usually in the ducts, less often the alveoli. All degrees of differentiation may occur and there is commonly dense connective tissue intermingled in the tumour, giving the typical hard scirrhous carcinoma which on incision has the feel of cutting into a unripe pear. Metastases to lymph nodes tend to occur early. Lateral lesions metastasise to the axillary or supraclavicular nodes, while medial lesions metastasise to the internal mammary chain. Metastases to distant sites occur frequently. Breast carcinoma may be classified clinically by the TNM (tumour node metastasis) method of staging.

Mammography can detect small breast cancers but the incidence is too low to justify extensive screening programmes. The technique may prove valuable in high-risk groups, e.g. those with a family history or who have had a contralateral carcinoma. It is less useful once a lump is apparent since routine practice is excision biopsy. Thermography is a sensitive though, as yet, unproven method of diagnosing breast carcinoma.

TREATMENT

The basis of treatment is surgical, although not all tumours are operable. The larger the tumour, the poorer is the prognosis. Any suspicious lesion in the breast must be biopsied and a frozen-section examined, with the surgeon prepared to continue the operation if necessary. It is not yet agreed whether radical mastectomy, 'conservative' radical mastectomy (where the pectoralis major muscle is preserved) or simple mastectomy (perhaps followed by radiotherapy) is more effective for the lesion that appears to be confined to the breast. When there are obvious lymph node secondaries in the axilla many surgeons perform a radical mastectomy with block dissection of the axilla followed by X-ray therapy, though not all agree that radiation is indicated. Patients who present with advanced metastases may sometimes be subjected to simple mastectomy or local excision (if the lesion is operable), followed by hormonal therapy of the type described below. Metastases at distant sites and local recurrences are still depressingly common, even after radical surgery and X-ray therapy.

Many breast cancers are hormone dependent, and most of the regimes recommended for the treatment of disseminated breast cancer are based on this observation. In premenopausal patients and in those who have reached the menopause within the previous five years, bilateral oophorectomy is first recommended, and results in remissions of variable duration in 30 to 40 per cent of patients. Adrenocortical steroids may be given post operatively and may prolong remission, possibly by suppressing the adrenal oestrogens. Androgens may also be used in the premenopausal patient prior to oophorectomy or as a supplement to this procedure. It has been reported that patients who have low levels of androgen in the urine have a poor prognosis and fail to respond to pituitary or adrenal ablation.

In patients who relapse or fail to show a remission after oophorectomy, and in postmenopausal women who develop disseminated malignancy after surgery, a direct surgical attack on the adrenals or the pituitary is usually indicated. It is not yet agreed whether oestrogen therapy should be used initially in postmenopausal patients, with adrenalectomy or hypophysectomy reserved for a further relapse, or whether the more radical approach should be used as the treatment of choice in this group. The protagonists of the radical approach point out that adequate time must be allowed for the response to oestrogens to be assessed, and that if such therapy is unsuccessful there may be such physical deterioration that a more radical approach cannot be employed. On the other hand, there is no good evidence that the initial form of treatment alters the ultimate prognosis for survival (Atkins *et al.*, 1966). There is evidence, however, that more patients obtain a good response from a hormone ablation operation when it is performed early rather than late.

The operations available are bilateral adrenalectomy and the various techniques of pituitary ablation. Disseminated breast cancer appears to be the only cancer (apart possibly from rare patients with prostatic tumours) in which good results may be obtained by the use of yttrium-90 pituitary ablation. There is probably little to choose between bilateral adrenalectomy, surgical hypophysectomy and yttrium implant, although the originator of the technique of yttrium implantation now considers that a greater degree of benefit may be obtained from bilateral adrenalectomy (Forrest and Stewart, 1967). Unless *complete* ablation of the pituitary is achieved, the results are disappointing.

A suggested approach for the treatment of disseminated breast carcinoma is:

1. In premenopausal patients: bilateral oophorectomy with or without subsequent prednisolone therapy. If relapse occurs, pituitary ablation should be performed where available —failing this bilateral adrenalectomy.
2. In postmenopausal patients: pituitary ablation (or bilateral adrenalectomy) is the treatment of choice.

Joplin (1965) has found that 25 per cent of women have clear objective remission as well as a striking subjective improvement after yttrium implantation. These patients survive an average of about two years after implantation, but much longer survivals are sometimes seen. Fifty per cent of cases show some objective remission.

PROGNOSIS

It is hoped that new methods for testing the *in vitro* hormone dependance of breast carcinoma may lead to more rational selection of endocrine suppressive or ablative therapy (Salih *et al.*, 1972). However, until the initial encouraging results are confirmed other indirect indicators of potential responsiveness have to be considered.

It would obviously be of value to forecast which patients are likely to respond to adrenalectomy or hypophysectomy. A good initial response to oophorectomy indicates the likelihood of a response to pituitary ablation, but this indication will not always be available. A recurrence less than two years after mastectomy indicates a poor prognosis.

Bulbrooke and his colleagues (1962) have suggested that the majority of women with advanced breast cancer who excrete normal amounts of 11-deoxy-17-oxosteroids in the urine and who show a high excretion of aetiocholanolone relative to 17-hydroxycorticosteroids are responsive to hypophysectomy or bilateral adrenalectomy, whereas those with low 11-deoxy-17-oxosteroids and a lower relative excretion of aetiocholanolone usually fail to respond to these procedures. Bulbrooke and Hayward (1967) have also suggested that the urinary excretion pattern of androgen metabolites might form the basis of a screening test for breast cancer. If these results are confirmed they will obviously be of great significance in the early diagnosis and in the management of breast carcinoma, although at present the observations seem to be mainly of theoretical interest, and not all workers have found them to give useful prognostic information (Ahlquist *et al.*, 1968).

GYNAECOMASTIA

A concentric increase in the glandular and stromal tissue of the male breast that results in enlargement of the gland is termed gynaecomastia. The condition may be unilateral or bilateral. Before the diagnosis of gynaecomastia is made, other causes of breast enlargement must be excluded. Carcinoma of the male breast and neurofibromatosis may both present as enlargement of one or other breast, but the commonest condition that may be mistaken for true gynaecomastia is the deposition of adipose tissue in the breast area. To diagnose true gynaecomastia, it must be ascertained that glandular tissue is palpable. The degree of gynaecomastia may vary from a small sub-areolar button of tissue to enlargement indistinguishable from the normal adult female breast.

Histology. The normal male breast consists of a few scattered ducts with dense surrounding connective tissue and a variable amount of adipose tissue.

Two histological patterns of gynaecomastia are seen:

1. A predominant increase in the parenchymatous elements—the ducts and lobules.
2. A predominant increase in the interlobular and periductal tissue, although an increase in duct formation is also seen.

It has been suggested that the first pattern is seen when the gynaecomastia is due primarily to the effects of oestrogens, androgens or adrenal steroids, and that the second pattern is largely due to the action of the anterior pituitary mammogenic hormones. Clinically, in the oestrogen stimulated male breast there is a firm cone of glandular tissue with no development of the areola itself, although there is often some swelling of the subareolar tissues. When stimulated by prolactin, however, there may be only a small amount of glandular tissue despite the lactation, and often there is considerable fatty deposition. In addition there is usually thickening of the areola with hypertrophy of Montgomery's tubercles giving an appearance similar to that seen in pregnancy.

AETIOLOGY

The factors that may produce gynaecomastia in the male are the same as those that are responsible for the normal development of the breast in the female; e.g. oestrogens, prolactin, growth hormone, and pituitary gonadotrophins. In the male, androgenic compounds may in certain instances also produce enlargement of the breast. A list of the main causes of gynaecomastia is given in Table 9.1 but this classification is based on clinical associations rather than aetiology. Many of the associations listed may be fortuitous, and often the pathogenesis of the gynaecomastia is quite unknown. In those cases in which there is increased secretion of oestrogens or in those resulting from exogenous oestrogen therapy there is an obvious causal relationship, but, in many cases occurring in association with systemic disease, no abnormality of circulating oestrogens, or indeed, of any other hormones can be detected.

Gynaecomastia of puberty. Visible enlargement of the breast is evident in 50 per cent of pubertal boys, and breast tissue may be palpable in most of the remainder. Occasionally it is severe enough to cause embarrassment, and tenderness of the breasts may be present. Physiological gynaecomastia of puberty is unlikely to be due to increased circulating levels of oestrogen or of testosterone. It is more likely to be caused by increased secretion of pituitary hormones but there may also be increased sensitivity to normal circulating levels of adrenal and testicular steroids.

Refeeding gynaecomastia follows refeeding after long periods of starvation and inanition, and was frequently seen in prisoners of war after their release. During the period of subnutrition there is suppression of gonadotrophin secretion. On refeeding there is increased secretion of pituitary gonadotrophins, and the individual again experiences many of the changes of puberty, with the development of gynaecomastia, and sometimes testicular tenderness. The gynaecomastia is usually only short lived. The same mechanism may also play a part in the development of gynaecomastia during the successful treatment of a number of chronic diseases in which inanition is a feature. In such cases gynaecomastia is usually associated with a period of increased appetite, physical well-being and gain in weight ('refeeding') as the condition primarily responsible for the sub-nutrition is removed or treated. While an increase in subcutaneous fat in such cases may contribute to the breast enlargement, there is no doubt that true gynaecomastia with hypertrophy of the glandular or periglandular tissue also occurs.

Gynaecomastia may be seen in most varieties of primary testicular failure and the association of gynaecomastia, pea-sized testes, and eunuchoid proportions will immediately suggest the diagnosis of *Klinefelter's syndrome.* Klinefelter's syndrome, and other causes of primary hypogonadism that may be associated with gynaecomastia are discussed in Chapters 11 and 13. It is not yet certain whether the cause of the gynaecomastia in such cases is related to increased pituitary gonadotrophin secretion, to increased tissue sensitivity to androgens secreted by the Leydig cells or to excessive oestrogen production relative to androgens by the abnormal gonads. Patients with the testicular feminisation syndrome, who have a male chromosome pattern, often have well-developed breasts. This syndrome is considered in Chapter 13.

Although gynaecomastia is frequently seen in association with *seminoma* and *teratoma* of the testis, it may occur in association with any type of testicular tumour, not only those that produce large quantities of HCG or oestrogens.

Oestrogen secreting adrenal tumours are very rare.

Exogenous oestrogens are an important cause of gynaecomastia, and the condition is well recognised in patients treated with oestrogens

TABLE 9.1 *Causes and Associations of Gynaecomastia*

Cause	Associations
1. *Physiological*—gynaecomastia of puberty	
2. '*Refeeding*' *gynaecomastia*	(*a*) Post-inanition (*b*) Treated congestive heart failure (*c*) Treated pulmonary tuberculosis (*d*) Chronic renal failure on intermittent dialysis†
3. *Primary testicular failure*	(*a*) Testicular agenesis (*b*) Bilateral torsion (*c*) Severe bilateral orchitis (*d*) Bilateral cryptorchidism (*e*) Chromosomal abnormalities
4. *Testicular tumours*	(*a*) Seminoma (*b*) Teratoma
5. *Excessive oestrogens* (*nontesticular*)	(*a*) Adrenal carcinoma (*b*) Exogenous
6. *Liver disease*	
7. *Drugs**	(*a*) Isoniazid† (*b*) Spironolactone (*c*) Digitalis (*d*) Phenothiazines† (*e*) Amphetamines (*f*) Reserpine† (*g*) Androgens and anabolic steroids (*h*) Adrenocortical steroids
8. *Non-endocrine neoplasms*	(*a*) Bronchogenic carcinoma† (*b*) Renal carcinoma (*c*) Hodgkin's disease
9. *Endocrine disorders*	(*a*) Hyper and hypothyroidism† (*b*) Acromegaly† (*c*) Diabetes mellitus* (*d*) Addison's disease (*e*) Hypothalamic and 'pineal' tumours† (*f*) Pituitary tumours†
10. *Generalised skin disease**	
11. *Miscellaneous*	(*a*) Rheumatoid arthritis (*b*) Paraplegia (*c*) Leprosy (*d*) Ulcerative colitis* (*e*) Trauma to the chest wall†
12. '*Idiopathic*' (no cause discovered)	

* In some of these cases, the mechanisms postulated under the heading of 'refeeding gynaecomastia' (*see* below) are presumed to play a part.
† May be associated with hyperprolactinaemia and galactorrhoea.

for prostatic carcinoma. Rarely, gynaecomastia may occur after prostatectomy without subsequent oestrogen therapy. The synthetic oestrogen stilboestrol more commonly gives rise to thickening and blackening of the nipples (Dodd's nipples) than to any severe degree of gynaecomastia. The so-called 'non-feminising' oestrogens such as Honvan (stilboestrol diphosphate) can also cause gynaecomastia, particularly in younger men. In some patients the source of the oestrogens may not be immediately apparent —inunction of oestrogen creams, inhalation (as in a factory where oestrogenic compounds are manufactured) or accidental contamination of other drugs during their preparation may all give rise to tenderness of the breasts and/or gynaecomastia. The possibility of self-administration of oestrogens by transexualists and homosexuals should always be borne in mind.

Liver Disease. Several mechanisms may play a part in the gynaecomastia that is not infrequently observed in association with cirrhosis of any type. The 'refeeding' phenomenon may be a factor in some cases, during the treatment of cirrhosis with a high-calorie high-protein diet. In alcoholic cirrhosis this mechanism may also be responsible for gynaecomastia in the rare patient who reforms and, at the same time, improves the quality and quantity of his diet. However, in many cases of cirrhosis the gynaecomastia seems largely to be due to hyperoestrogenism, and in these, testicular atrophy, spider naevi, and palmar erythema may also be present. It is usually postulated that in advanced liver disease there is a disturbance of the normal hepatic degradation of androgens, with consequent increased conversion to oestrogen. Gynaecomastia is relatively common in *hyperthyroidism* due to the increase in sex hormone binding globulin levels induced by the thyroid hormones. This protein binds testosterone more avidly than oestrogen, shifting the balance of available free sex hormones in favour of the oestrogens and resulting in gynaecomastia. SHBG is made in the liver.

Gynaecomastia is a rare complication of *drug therapy* except in the case of spironolactone where long-term treatment is very often complicated by breast enlargement. The pathogenesis of the gynaecomastia that occurs in association with drugs other than oestrogens is far from clear in most cases. In some instances breast enlargement may simply result from the 'refeeding' phenomenon, when administration of a drug results in increased food intake, gain in weight, and an overall improvement in physical state. In other cases accidental contamination of the drugs with oestrogenic compounds has been shown to be the causative factor. Some drugs such as phenothiazines, reserpine and antidepressants cause prolactin secretion by suppressing secretion of PIF, prolactin inhibiting factor.

Gynaecomastia is occasionally seen in association with *non-endocrine neoplasms*, particularly bronchogenic carcinoma (*see* Chapter 20). A number of patients with bronchogenic carcinoma and gynaecomastia have been shown to have elevated gonadotrophin or prolactin levels in the tumour tissue or in the urine.

Gynaecomastia, like galactorrhoea in the female, may be the first indication of a *pituitary* or *hypothalamic tumour*. It may also be associated with acromegaly, and occurs presumably, as a result of growth hormone oversecretion. Gynaecomastia has also been reported to occur in association with a number of other *endocrine disorders* and with various *non-endocrine systemic diseases*. In some cases 'refeeding' may play a part, in others the association may be fortuitous, and although urinary oestrogens may be increased there is usually no well-defined abnormality of hormonal production or metabolism.

DIAGNOSIS

The patient and his practitioner must be questioned in detail about recent drug therapy. Attention must be given to examination of the genitalia, looking in particular for evidence of hypogonadism or testicular enlargement. The presence of one small soft testis and the other normal in size or large and firm, in a patient with gynaecomastia, suggests the presence of an interstitial tumour of the testis in the normal sized gonad secreting oestrogen, suppressing the gonadotrophins and causing atrophy of the contralateral testis. Liver disease will usually be apparent on examination.

Biochemical investigation of gynaecomastia is commonly unrewarding, presumably due to the relative insensitivity of the assay techniques used. Urinary oestrogen levels are normal in the physiological gynaecomastia of puberty. Urinary and plasma gonadotrophins are usually elevated in Klinefelter's syndrome and other primary hypogonadal states. Urinary oestrogen levels are elevated only in a proportion of patients with gynaecomastia due to liver disease or systemic disease. Jull *et al.* (1964) studied the urinary steroid excretion in normal males and in fifteen men whose only complaint was of gynaecomastia. Three patients showed a reduced oestrogen excretion. In five patients urinary oestrogens were high; one of these had a chorioncarcinoma of the testis but the others showed no evidence of adrenal or testicular abnormality. In two patients, regression of the gynaecomastia was associated with a reduction of previously high urinary oestrogens, and in one, regression was accompanied by an increase in oestrogen excretion from subnormal to normal levels. There is, therefore, no consistent pattern of oestrogen excretion in patients with gynaecomastia, using present techniques. There is, however, a marked increase in urinary oestrogens in the presence of oestrogen-secreting tumours.

The following scheme may be useful in the investigation of gynaecomastia:

1. Careful drug and alcohol intake assessment.
2. Buccal smear and karyotype (unnecessary if the patient has given evidence of fertility).
3. X-ray of skull and chest.
4. Urinary oestrogen, blood gonadotrophin and testosterone estimations.
5. Liver and thyroid function tests.

Further investigations will be ordered according to the abnormalities detected as a result of these screening tests, or as seems appropriate after physical examination. Commonly, no abnormalities are detected.

TREATMENT

Physiological gynaecomastia of puberty usually regresses spontaneously and completely and no treatment is necessary other than firm reassurance, particularly when normal genital development is present. In severe cases, surgical excision may be necessary for cosmetic reasons and to prevent adverse effects on the personality. In other cases removal or treatment of the cause, when possible, may be followed by a variable degree of regression of the gynaecomastia, though mastectomy may still be needed. External radiation of the breasts prevents the development of gynaecomastia which normally follows the use of oestrogens for prostatic carcinoma. Such therapy must be given before oestrogens are started, and radiation is ineffective when gynaecomastia is already present.

CARCINOMA OF THE MALE BREAST

Carcinoma of the breast in the male is about one hundred times less frequent than in the female. The lesion presents and behaves in the same manner. Therapy is the same as in the female, except that orchidectomy instead of oophorectomy is performed. There is a highly significant association between cancer of the male breast and Klinefelter's syndrome, and the latter should be excluded in any male patient presenting with a breast carcinoma.

REFERENCES

Ahlquist, K. A., Jackson, A. W., and Stewart, J. G. (1968). *Brit. med. J.*, **i**, 217.

Atkins, H., Falconer, M. A., Hayward, J. L., MacLean, K. S., and Schurr, P. H. (1966). *Lancet*, **i**, 827.

Besser, G. M., Parke, L., Edwards, C. R. W., Forsyth, I. A., and McNeilly, A. S. (1972). *Brit. med. J.*, **iii**, 669.

Bulbrooke, R. D., and Hayward, J. L. (1967). *Lancet*, **i**, 519.

Forrest, A. P. M., and Stewart, H. J. (1967). In *Major Endocrine Surgery for the Treatment of Cancer of the Breast in Advanced Stages* (Eds M. Dargent and Cl. Romieu). Lyons: Simep Editions.

Forsythe, I. A., and Edwards, C. R. W. (1972). *Clinical Endocrinology*, **1**, 293.

Frantz, A. G., Kleinberg, D. L., and Noel, G. I. (1972). *Recent Progress in Hormone Research*, **28**, 527.

Joplin, G. F. (1965). 'Therapeutic pituitary ablation by needle implantation.' Thesis submitted for degree of PhD, University of London.

Turkington, R. W. (1972). *Am. J. Med.*, **53**, 389.

Jull, J. W., Bonser, G. M., and Dossett, J. A. (1964). *Lancet*, **ii**, 797.

Salih, H., Flax, H., Brander, W., and Hobbs, J. R. (1972). *Lancet*, **ii**, 1103.

10

HORMONAL CHANGES DURING PREGNANCY

Certain hormones such as the sex steroids, chorionic gonadotrophin (HCG), and some pituitary hormones play a specific role in pregnancy, while the secretion of other hormones from the thyroid, pancreas, adrenal, and pituitary appears to be modified by the changing conditions of pregnancy. As well as changes in the maternal hormone production in pregnancy there are major hormonal contributions from the placenta and the endocrine glands of the fetus. The placenta produces progesterone, a variety of oestrogens, HCG, placental lactogen (HPL), human chorionic thyrotrophin (HCT), human molar thyrotrophin (HMT), possibly relaxin and a variety of prostaglandins. The concept of the feto-placental unit was first introduced by Diczfalusy. According to this concept, the bulk of steroid hormones elaborated during pregnancy is formed by the complementary activity of the fetus and of the placenta, since both are deficient in certain essential steroidogenic enzyme systems. The feto-placental unit is capable of synthesizing most if not all of the biologically active steroid hormones required during pregnancy. More recently it has been shown that there is an abundant synthesis of sterols and steroids in the mid-gestation fetus, whereas little if any sterol or steroid synthesis occurs in the plancenta at this time (Diczfalusy, 1970).

The placenta also acts as a source of pituitary-like hormones which have structural and biological similarities with the hormones of the anterior lobe. HPL shares similarities with growth hormone and prolactin, HCG with LH and FSH, and HCT and HMT with TSH. The production of these protein hormones reflects the tendency of the feto-placental unit to 'complete endocrinological self-sufficiency'.

The hormones playing a specific role in pregnancy will be dealt with first, outlining their sites of production, the amounts produced, their sites of action, physiological effects, and any clinical significance. Secondly, the changes in adrenal, thyroid, and pituitary function will be considered. No attempt will be made to discuss alterations in insulin secretion, or the problem of diabetes in pregnancy.

I. *SPECIFIC HORMONAL CHANGES*

(*a*) PROGESTERONE

Progesterone is produced in the luteinised granulosa cells of the ovarian corpus luteum in each menstrual cycle. After conception, ovarian progesterone is essential for the maintenance of pregnancy. After a few weeks, however, the placenta becomes the main site of progesterone production, and pregnancy can be maintained in the absence of the ovaries. Progesterone is not produced *de nova* by the mid-term placenta since this lacks the enzyme systems necessary to convert acetate into cholesterol. The mid-term fetus on the other hand is easily able to produce cholesterol from its precursors and this fetal cholesterol is then converted in the placenta to

Most knowledge of progesterone production has been derived from measurements of the output of its physiologically inert end-product, pregnanediol, in the urine. Because of the variable conversion of progesterone to pregnanediol and alternative routes of excretion, e.g. in the faeces, urinary pregnanediol gives at best only a crude

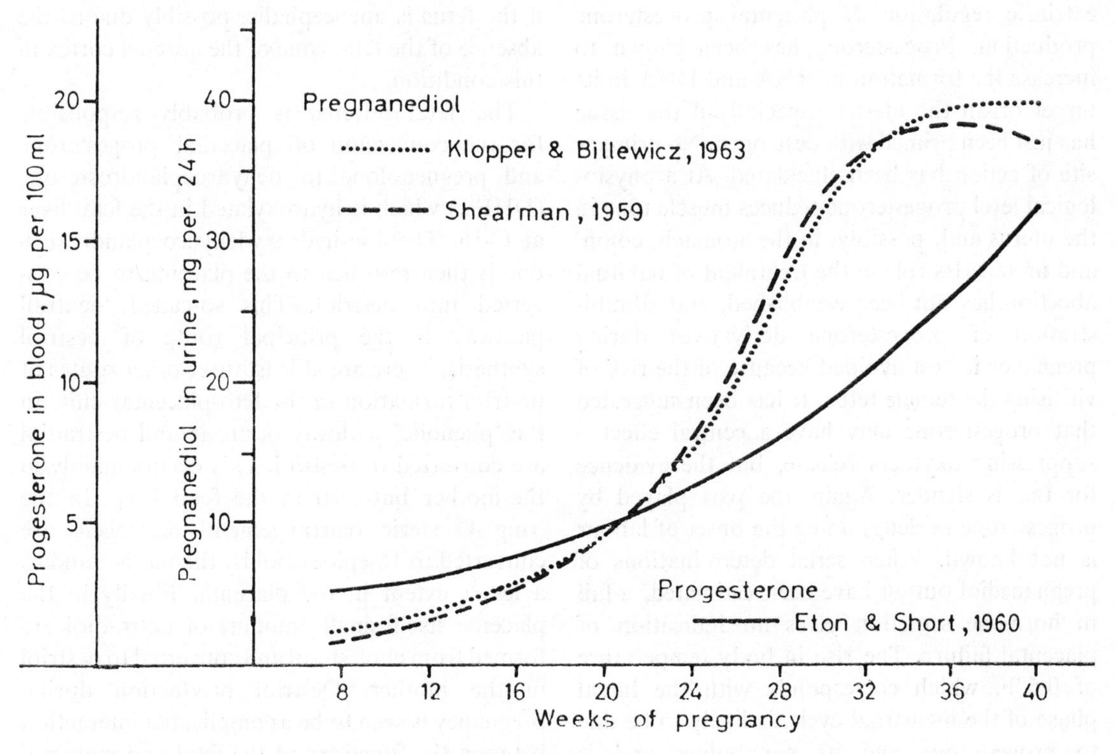

FIGURE 10.1 Excretion of pregnanediol in urine during pregnancy compared with the concentration of progesterone in the blood (from Hytten and Leitch, 1964)

a variety of steroids especially pregnenolone and progesterone and also 17α-hydroxypregnenolone, dehydroepiandrosterone, 17β-oestradiol, 20α-dihydroprogesterone and 20β-dihydroprogesterone. The adrenal glands of the mother and fetus also make a small contribution to progesterone formation. Progesterone synthesised in the placenta serves as a substrate for cortisol and other steroids formed in the fetal adrenal. As much as 50 per cent of progesterone elaborated by the placenta reaches the fetus.

reflection of progesterone production. Isotope dilution methods using tritium or carbon-labelled progesterone are prone to error since placental progesterone is released both to the maternal and fetal circulations and the labelled material cannot be assumed to be distributed in the same way. Progesterone output rises during pregnancy (Fig. 10.1), levelling off a few weeks from term, when the production rate is probably of the order of 300 mg/day, of which no more than 25 mg arises from the ovaries. Progesterone is transported in the circulation both by albumin and by corticosterone-binding globulin and less than 10 per cent is in the free form. There is an almost linear increase in plasma progesterone during pregnancy to a level of about 14 μg per 100 ml at term.

Progesterone is not taken up specifically by any tissue and there is no evidence for any extrinsic regulation of placental progesterone production. Progesterone has been shown to increase the formation of RNA and DNA in its target organ the uterus, especially if the tissue has just been primed with oestrogen. No primary site of action has been elucidated. At a physiological level progesterone reduces muscle tone in the uterus and, possibly, in the stomach, colon, and ureters. Its role in the treatment of habitual abortion has not been established, and administration of progesterone derivatives during pregnancy is best avoided because of the risk of virilising the female fetus. It has been suggested that progesterone may have a central effect—suppressing oxytocin release, but the evidence for this is slender. Again, the part played by progesterone in determining the onset of labour is not known. When serial determinations of pregnanediol output have been estimated, a fall in hormone secretion gives an indication of placental failure. The rise in body temperature of 0·5°F, which corresponds with the luteal phase of the menstrual cycle, is likely to be due to progesterone and its metabolites and is continued after conception till about mid-pregnancy. In the presence of oestrogen, progesterone increases alveolar tissue growth in the breast. The extensive storage of depot fat during pregnancy may be determined by progesterone, but firm proof of this is still lacking. The reduction in alveolar and arterial pCO_2 which is seen during pregnancy is likely to be due to a central stimulatory action of progesterone.

(*b*) OESTROGENS

At least 27 different oestrogens have been isolated from the urine in pregnancy. It is likely that the true ovarian hormone in the human is 17β-oestradiol which is readily converted to oestrone and oestriol. By the second to third months of pregnancy the placenta has taken over from the ovary as the main site of oestrogen production. Small amounts of oestrogens also arise from the adrenal cortex and from the fetus. Specific deficiency of the fetal contribution occurs if the fetus is anencephalic, possibly due to the absence of the fetal zone of the adrenal cortex in this condition.

The fetal adrenal is probably responsible for the conversion of placental progesterone and pregnenolone to dehydroepiandrosterone (DHEA) which is hydroxylated in the fetal liver at C-16. The 16α-hydroxydehydroepiandrosterone is then returned to the placenta to be converted into oestriol. This so-called 'neutral' pathway is the principal route of oestriol synthesis. There are at least three other routes of oestriol formation in the feto-placental unit. In the 'phenolic' pathway oestrone and oestradiol are converted to oestriol. This occurs mainly in the mother but also in the fetal liver. In the 'ring D steric rearrangement' androgens are converted to 16-epioestriol by the mother and to a lesser extent in the placenta. Finally in the placenta itself small amounts of oestradiol are formed from cholesterol and converted to oestriol in the mother. Oestriol production during pregnancy is seen to be a complicated interaction between the functions of the fetal and maternal adrenals and livers and those of the placenta. The clinical value of urinary oestriol assays in monitoring the condition of the fetus will thus depend on the relative contributions of the four pathways. The 'neutral' pathway does not require a maternal contribution and were it possible to measure urinary oestriol formed by this route it would provide a better means of assessing fetal viability.

Oestriol is the predominant oestrogen excreted in the urine and the output rises during pregnancy and falls rapidly after delivery (Fig. 10.2). Levels of oestriol in maternal blood rise slowly to about 4 μg per 100 ml by 32 weeks after which there is a rapid but variable rise to levels between 8 and 22 μg per 100 ml at term. The relative proportions of the oestrogen fractions in blood differ from that in the urine. In urine oestriol makes up 75–97 per cent of all oestrogens, whereas in blood the proportion is lower, from 25–80 per cent. Again most of the oestrone and oestradiol in urine are present in the conjugated form as glucosidouronates, but in the blood conjugates are present in only trace amounts. In late pregnancy there appears to be a circadian rhythm of blood oestrogen levels, lowest values being seen at 4.30 p.m. In amniotic fluid oestriol levels rise steeply in the last few weeks of pregnancy to values as high as 150–200 μg per 100 ml. The main source of amniotic fluid oestriol is probably from fetal urine.

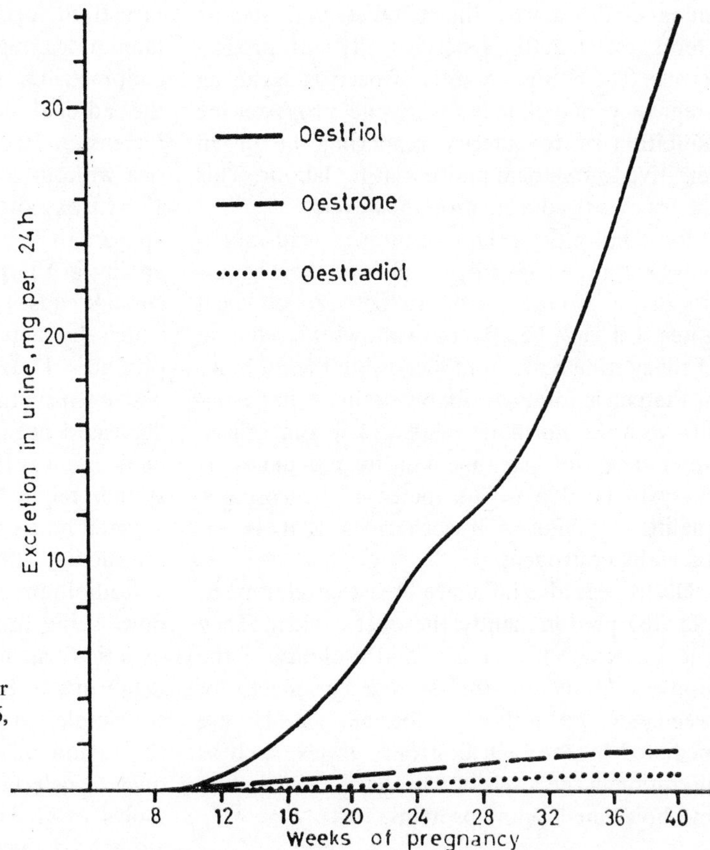

FIGURE 10.2 Excretion of the three major oestrogens in pregnancy (Brown, 1956, from Hytten and Leitch, 1964)

The factors that control oestrogen production during pregnancy are poorly understood but HCG may have some internal regulating role (*see* later). Oestrogen determinations during normal and abnormal pregnancies reflect the function of both the fetus and its placenta, in contrast to determinations such as that of progesterone or placental lactogen, which reflect placental activity alone. Isolated observations are of little value, and serial estimations in a given individual are needed before any conclusions can be drawn. There is a tendency for oestrogen excretion to be low in moderately severe pre-eclamptic toxaemia, in diabetic pregnancies, and in the presence of hydatidiform moles and chorionepithelioma. Fetal death is associated with a fall in urinary oestrogens.

Oestrogens cause a marked increase in RNA, phospholipid, and protein synthesis in the uterus. Puromycin and actinomycin D both interfere with oestrogen action, which suggests that protein synthesis possibly of various types of RNA polymerase may be an early requisite for hormone action. Whatever their primary action, oestrogens control the growth of the decidual lining of the uterus, the myometrium, and its blood vessels, acting synergistically with progesterone. The rising amounts of oestrogen during pregnancy may finally overcome progesterone inhibition of the uterus, rendering the organ sensitive to oxytocin and initiating labour. This theory awaits confirmation, however.

By altering the polymerisation of acid mucopolysaccharides, oestrogens change the properties of the ground substance between collagen fibres. This may be a factor in allowing stretching of the uterine cervix and increasing the mobility of the pelvic joints, probably acting synergistically with the hormone relaxin. The generalised water retention in the skin in pregnancy is likely to be due to the increased hygroscopic qualities of mucopolysaccharides that is induced by oestrogens.

Oestrogens also influence breast development, affecting predominantly the duct system. They also increase both the size and mobility of the nipples. Many of the secondary effects of pregnancy on other endocrine glands are mediated by the high oestrogen levels, such as alteration in the levels of various clotting factors and hormone-binding proteins.

(*c*) HUMAN CHORIONIC GONADOTROPHIN (HCG)

HCG cannot yet be estimated chemically and is assayed by biological or immunological methods. By definition, 1 IU is the activity contained in 0·1 mg of the standard preparation. It is produced exclusively in the trophoblast and can be detected in the serum as early as 10 days after fertilisation. The level rises rapidly at about the 40th day of pregnancy, peaking at the 60th day, and showing a rapid fall by the 80th day to a fairly steady level maintained throughout pregnancy apart from a slight secondary peak between 30 and 36 weeks (Fig. 10.3). Levels in late pregnancy are slightly higher in the presence of a female fetus. Peak values usually range from 20,000–100,000 IU/litre of serum and between 20,000–500,000 IU/24 hr in the urine. The hormone is luteotrophic and can prolong the menstrual cycle by maintaining the corpus luteum leading to a decidual reaction in the endometrium. It also appears to have actions on the adrenal cortex of the fetus, causing an increase in production of dehydroepiandrosterone without an increase in excretion of either 17-hydroxycorticosteroids or oestrogens. There appears to be a feedback system in which a need arising in the placenta for more oestrogen precursors causes an increase in HCG production which by acting on the fetal adrenal cortex produces DHEA which is then available for oestrogen synthesis in the placenta. Conversely a decreased need for oestrogen precursors results in a fall in HCG production. The feedback system might provide an explanation for the lowered oestrogen excretion and increased HCG production in pre-eclampsia.

Radioimmunoassay of HCG in the urine is now being used to follow up women with hydatidiform moles as well as an aid in initial diagnosis. In Britain about 800 women are seen with moles each year and of these, probably in the region of 10 per cent, develop serious sequelae such as more serious forms of invasive moles or choriocarcinoma. In the majority of women delivered of moles, HCG excretion continues for weeks or months indicating that viable trophoblastic tissue may persist for some time. The problem is to identify those who require treatment within six months of evacuation of the mole since treatment of such patients by modern methods is almost always successful. Serial assays of HCG in urine for a two year period is now provided as a service in Britain (Crawford, 1972). Assays are done frequently until normal levels of LH are attained (antisera to HCG cross-react with LH) and then monthly up to 12 months after evacuation of the mole and three-monthly during a second year of follow-up. In patients being treated for choriocarcinoma (or for trophoblastic tumours of the testis), HCG assays provide a sensitive method of monitoring the effectiveness of therapy. HCG output is of little value in the diagnosis of placental failure in various disorders.

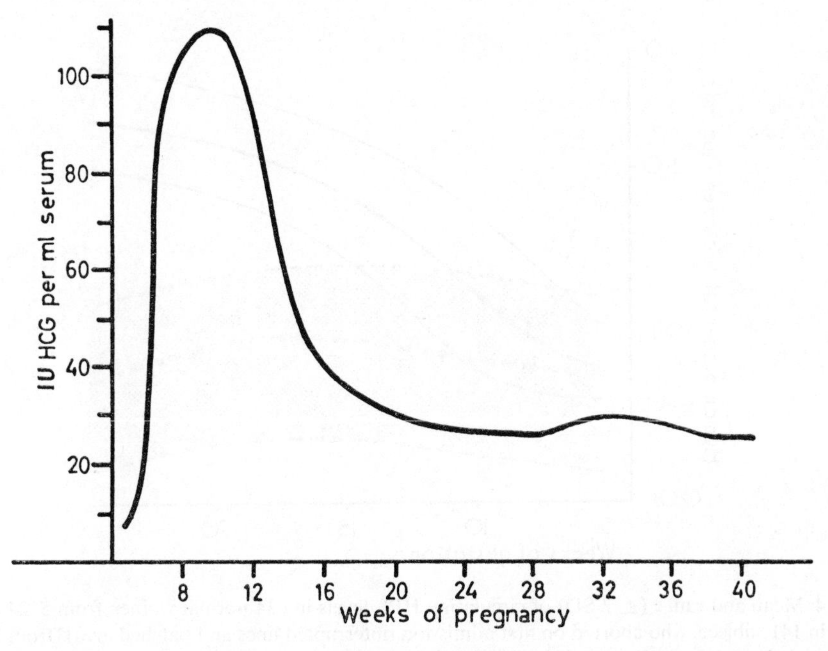

FIGURE 10.3 Concentration of HCG in serum during pregnancy (from Hytten and Leitch, 1971)

The hormone is a glycoprotein with a molecular weight of about 30,000 which shows similarities in structure to LH, FSH and TSH. It comprises α-subunits identical with those in the other glycoprotein hormones and hormone-specific β-subunits. During pregnancy free α-subunits can be detected in the urine and these have been shown to be of placental origin

(*d*) HUMAN PLACENTAL LACTOGEN (HPL), [HUMAN CHORIONIC SOMATOMAMMOTROPHIN, HCS]

HPL is a protein hormone with considerable similarities to growth hormone in molecular weight and amino acid content, and also in immunological and biological properties. It is produced in the placental trophoblast and the amounts produced show a positive correlation with placental weight. Since there is also a direct relationship between the weight of the placenta and that of the fetus, there is also a correlation between HPL levels and fetal weight. It is present largely in the maternal circulation, very little crosses the placenta and no significant amounts can be detected in the maternal urine. Maternal levels fall rapidly after delivery. Amniotic fluid contains levels of about one eighth that found in maternal serum. Factors controlling secretion of HPL are poorly understood but some workers have reported depression of serum HPL in response to glucose and a rise after hypoglycaemia. Although HPL levels reflect only the function of the placenta they are nevertheless a valuable guide to fetal well-being, since the fetus is very dependent on placental function.

The clinical applications of HPL measurements are still being investigated, but so far two major roles have been proposed; first as a guide to the outcome of threatened abortion (Niven *et al.*, 1972); secondly as a screening test for fetal distress and neonatal asphyxia (Letchworth and Chard, 1972). After establishing the normal range of values for the first and second trimesters it was shown that in patients admitted with vaginal bleeding after the eighth week of gestation, low levels of HPL were found in those in whom abortion was completed during the first admission (Fig. 10.4). Women whose pregnancies continued normally or who aborted after their first discharge from hospital had normal levels. In the absence of contra-indicating factors such as maternal age or infertility, low levels might be a factor in deciding whether or not to evacuate the uterus in a women with vaginal bleeding early in pregnancy.

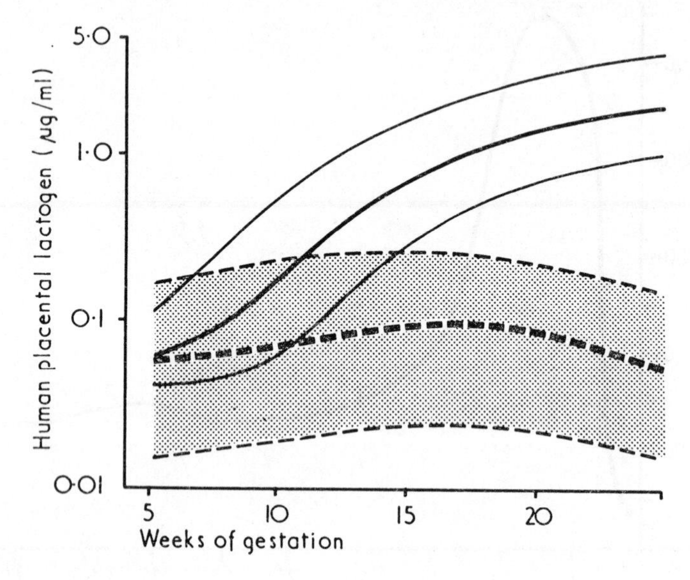

FIGURE 10.4 Mean and range (± 2 SD) of circulating HPL levels in 634 normal women from 5–24 weeks (solid lines), and in 141 subjects who aborted on first admission (interrupted lines and hatched area) (from Niven *et al.*, 1972, by permission of the authors and the Editor of the *BMJ*)

Measurements of HPL levels after the thirtieth week of pregnancy can help to predict subsequent fetal distress and/or neonatal asphyxia. Three or more levels of HPL less than 4 µg per ml between the thirty-fifth and fortieth weeks of pregnancy indicate a 71 per cent risk of fetal distress in labour or neonatal asphyxia, whereas levels above 5 µg per ml were associated with a very low frequency of these complications. If further studies confirm these findings there may be a place for routine HPL screening in late pregnancy and particularly in those where placental function may be at risk, for example, in hypertensive women.

The role of HPL is not yet understood—it may have humoral effects on mother and fetus and a local action on the trophoblast. It may be responsible for:

1. A rise in plasma free fatty acid due to maternal fat mobilisation to meet fetal growth requirements.
2. Increased insulin resistance causing a higher level of circulating insulin.
3. Increased nitrogen storage.
4. Increased amino-acid transport across the placenta.

5. Increased breast growth.
6. An overall metabolic effect on mother and placenta greater than that on the fetus in view of its differential distribution.

(*e*) HUMAN CHORIONIC THYROTROPHIN (HCT) AND HUMAN MOLAR THYROTROPHIN (HMT)

The normal placenta produces two thyroid-stimulating agents termed HCT and HMT, the latter so designated because it is produced in large amounts in some patients with hydatidiform moles or choriocarcinoma when it may be responsible for abnormalities of thyroid function tests and occasionally for overt hyperthyroidism. It is possible that HMT may act as a precursor for HCT but firm evidence for this is lacking. A comparison of the two trophoblastic thyrotrophins is shown in Table 10.1.

TABLE 10.1 *Comparison of HCT and HMT*

Source	HCT Normal placenta	HMT Mole and normal placenta
Reaction with anti-human TSH	Partial	None
Reaction with anti-bovine TSH	Yes	None
Duration of action	Short	Intermediate ($>$TSH, $<$LATS)
Molecular size	~30,000	~70,000

The role of HCT and HMT in normal pregnancy is virtually unknown.

(*f*) RELAXIN

Relaxin is probably a polypeptide which appears in the circulation during pregnancy. Levels rise irregularly as pregnancy proceeds and fall rapidly after delivery. Its source and actions in human pregnancy are unknown. It has been claimed to prevent or halt premature labour and to assist labour by increasing cervical softening and relaxing pelvic joints but the evidence for these actions is as yet unconvincing.

(*g*) PROSTAGLANDINS (PG)

The prostaglandins are a group of chemically-related 20-carbon hydroxy fatty acid derivatives of prostanoic acid which are widely distributed in the body. Their role in human reproduction is uncertain at present. Amniotic fluid collected during labour contains high concentrations of PG, $F_2\alpha$, which causes myometrial contractions whereas fluid collected earlier contains no PG $F_2\alpha$ and only a little PGE_1. $PGF_2\alpha$ has been detected in maternal venous blood immediately before uterine contractions in normal spontaneous labour, but not before the onset of labour. Both PGE_2 and $PGF_2\alpha$ have been used by oral, intravenous, intravaginal and intra-amniotic routes to induce labour. It is likely that the placenta is the major source of PGs found in the amniotic fluid and maternal circulation. Synthesis and release may be controlled by fetal corticosteroids. It is possible that PGs in the maternal circulation are involved in release of oxytocin from the posterior pituitary.

II. *SECONDARY HORMONAL CHANGES*

(*a*) THE ADRENAL GLAND AND PREGNANCY

Cortisol:

In normal pregnancy, plasma 17-OHCS levels average 10 μg per cent at the third month (normal non-pregnant women 9·5 μg per cent) rising to a mean of 24 μg per cent at the ninth month (range 11–42 μg). The normal range is reached 6 days after delivery (Fig. 10.5). Most of the rise of plasma 17-OHCS is due to cortisol. Since the cortisol-binding protein, transcortin, increases in concentration and probably also in binding avidity during pregnancy, it was previously believed that most of the increase in cortisol was in the bound form. However, direct measurements of circulating free cortisol have demonstrated a two to three fold increase in late pregnancy. This has been confirmed by urinary free cortisol measurements which reflect plasma

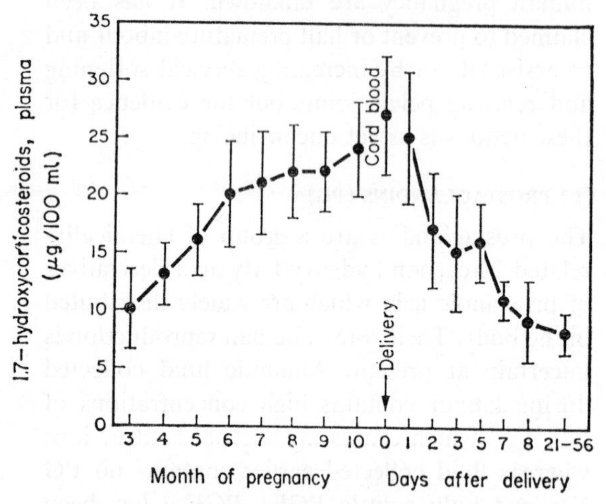

FIGURE 10.5 Mean levels and standard deviations of plasma 17-hydroxycorticosteroids during pregnancy and the puerperium in normal women (from Bayliss *et al.*, 1955)

free cortisol, and from direct estimates of cortisol production rate, which show values two to three times greater than normal in late pregnancy.

The rate of removal of cortisol from plasma is also slowed, possibly due to delayed reduction of ring A or to defective conjugation. Urinary excretion of 17-hydroxycorticosteroids shows little change during the first half of pregnancy, then a steep continuous rise to levels about 50 per cent higher by the end of pregnancy. The consequences of the exposure of tissues to increased free cortisol levels during pregnancy is uncertain, but it may account for the symptomatic improvement in rheumatoid arthritis which is sometimes observed. However, it should be noted that in women with Addison's disease or who have undergone previous bilateral adrenalectomy, no increase in corticosteroid dosage is required during pregnancy, although it is likely that in many replacement regimes cortisol therapy may be 'over-generous'.

Pregnancy can occur normally in patients with Addison's disease who are maintained on routine replacement therapy, using hydrocortisone 20–30 mg/day and fludrocortisome 0·05 to 0·10 mg/day. Replacement therapy should be increased promptly if vomiting, infections, or trauma occur. The stress of delivery should be covered for 48 hours with increased corticosteroid dosage, always in hospital. Caesarian section should be dealt with as any other surgical emergency. Steroid therapy should not be stopped but increased if pre-eclamptic toxaemia develops; there is no evidence that adrenocortical overactivity is involved in this condition. The patient should be given a steroid card, the features of hypoadrenalism discussed, and she should be informed that at no time should steroid therapy be discontinued (*see* Chapter 6).

Aldosterone

There is a marked increase in aldosterone secretion, plasma levels and urinary excretion in normal pregnancy which is apparent from the sixteenth week of gestation. Secretion responds normally to variations in dietary sodium intake. The mechanisms responsible for the increase in aldosterone secretion are unknown. It may be required to compensate for the sodium-losing tendency which would otherwise result from the increase in glomerular filtration rate in late pregnancy from the raised progesterone and oestrogen levels. In addition sodium must be conserved in order to provide for the growing fetus.

The role of the renin-angiotensin system in the stimulation of aldosterone secretion during pregnancy is not entirely clear. There is no correlation between plasma aldosterone levels and plasma renin concentrations in individual pregnant women. There is an increase in renin substrate as well as in renin concentration during pregnancy and a significant positive correlation between the concurrent plasma aldosterone concentration and the product of renin and renin-substrate in late pregnancy. Part of the circulating renin in pregnancy has been shown to exist in an inactive form.

(*b*) THE THYROID GLAND AND PREGNANCY

The thyroid gland enlarges during pregnancy. In Aberdeen, Crooks *et al.* (1964) found 70 per cent of 184 pregnant women to have both visible and palpable thyroid enlargement compared with a figure of 37 per cent of 116 non-pregnant age-matched controls. Many of the clinical features of pregnancy simulate hyperthyroidism but the increased oxygen consumption, tachycardia, heat intolerance, and raised PBI have other explanations. Epithelial hypertrophy in the thyroid is found in pregnancy along with some increase in colloid.

The PBI and T4 iodine is raised by some 3 to 5 μg or more per 100 ml during pregnancy, the elevation being detectable within the first two months. As with transcortin, thyroxine-binding globulin production rate is increased by the hyperoestrinism of pregnancy, and most if not all of the increase in circulating thyroid hormone is bound to protein. The peripheral turnover of thyroxine is also slowed during pregnancy.

Studies of thyroid function during pregnancy by Crooks and his colleagues have confirmed an increased thyroidal radioiodine uptake. Using ^{132}I they carried out serial determinations of several parameters of thyroid function (Fig. 10.6.). Renal clearance of iodide is increased, lowering the plasma concentration of inorganic iodide to less than half normal. The thyroid clearance of iodide is raised, presumably as a result of TSH stimulation in an effort to compensate for the transient decrease in free thyroxine from increased protein binding and the decreased iodine available to the gland. Current TSH assays are not sufficiently sensitive to detect any change in level during pregnancy. Absolute iodide uptake is maintained within the normal range by these compensatory mechanisms. Goitre in pregnancy, therefore, probably results from a conditioned iodine deficiency and from increased thyroxine needs due, at least in part, to the increase of the binding protein. Thyroxine can only cross the placenta from mother to fetus at a slow rate insufficient to allow normal fetal development when the fetal thyroid gland is abnormal. Small amounts of T3 are able to cross the placenta in late pregnancy. Normally, the fetal thyroid produces thyroid hormone by about the fourth month; at an earlier stage only iodotyrosines can be detected in the gland. The role of HCT and HMT in normal pregnancy is unknown (*see* p. 237).

The hypermetabolic state of pregnancy can easily be confused with hyperthyroidism, a misdiagnosis particularly likely in the presence of an anxiety state. During pregnancy, routine thyroidal radioiodine studies are hardly justifiable even when the short-lived isotope ^{132}I is used—serum thyroxine levels are elevated but a free thyroxine index (*see* Appendix) can be obtained from T4 and residual binding capacity measurements (Clarke and Horn, 1965). Elevated values are obtained in hyperthyroidism, lowered values in hypothyroidism, and a normal result is obtained in the euthyroid pregnant patient. The BMR is elevated during pregnancy as is the serum cholesterol.

Opinions vary as to the most suitable form of therapy for hyperthyroidism during pregnancy. In the young non-pregnant woman with a significant goitre the treatment of choice is usually partial thyroidectomy, and recurrence after operation is rare. The authors prefer to treat hyperthyroidism during pregnancy with antithyroid drugs, usually carbimazole, the dose being kept as low as possible, especially during the last few weeks. Goitre is uncommon in the child, but breast feeding should be avoided since antithyroid drugs enter the milk. The alternative form of therapy, namely, partial thyroidectomy during the second trimester, is a satisfactory treatment particularly when an experienced thyroid surgeon is available.

Goitre in the newborn child is usually due to a genetically determined enzyme defect in the gland, often familial, or to an acquired defect resulting from maternal ingestion of goitrogens, e.g. iodides, during pregnancy. Very rarely, goitre in the newborn is due to neonatal Graves' disease, a condition resulting from the transplacental passage of the long-acting thyroid stimulator (LATS) from the maternal circulation. The mother is rarely thyrotoxic but usually

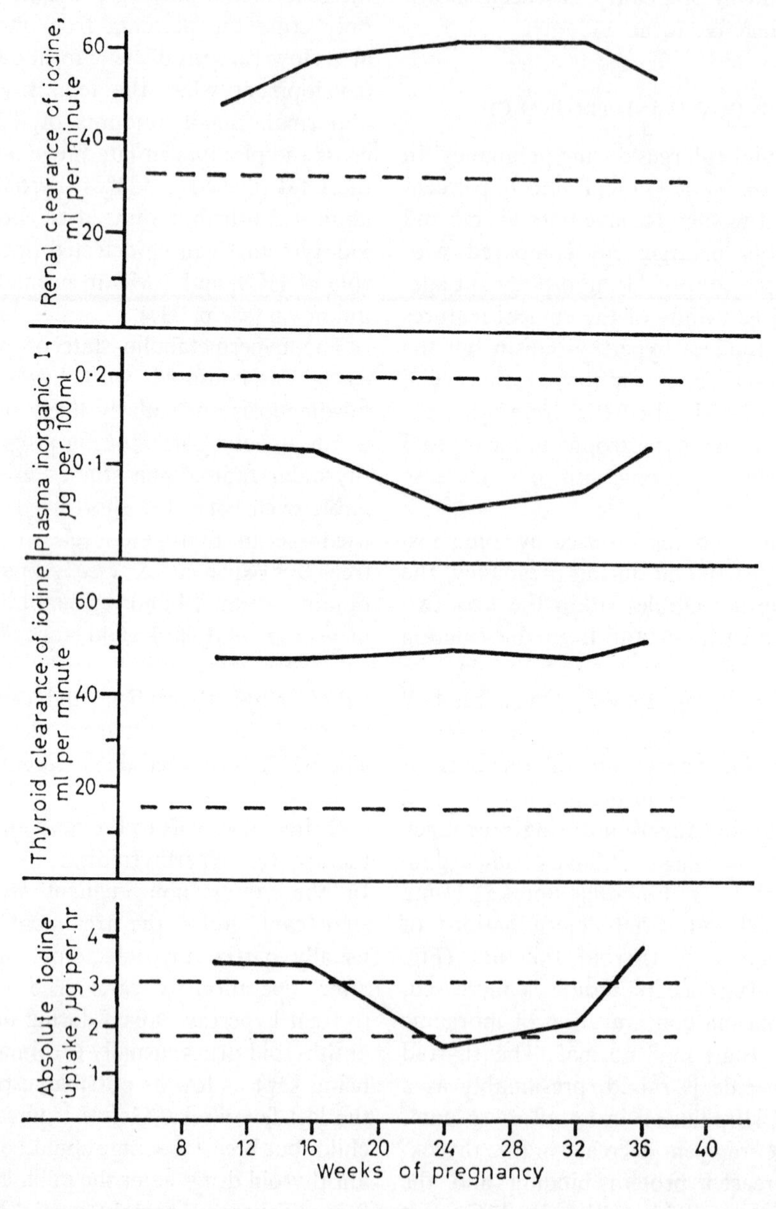

FIGURE 10.6 Iodine metabolism during pregnancy. Dotted lines show usual non-pregnant levels (from Crooks and Aboul-Khair, 1964)

shows the stigmata of Graves' disease—exophthalmos and often pretibial myxoedema. The children of all mothers with Graves' disease should be examined carefully at birth and for the first few weeks of life for this condition. Goitre, swelling of the eyelids, tachycardia, peripheral vasodilatation and other features of hyperthyroidism are indications for urgent therapy with iodides and carbimazole. The condition is self-limiting, improvement paralleling the removal of the maternal LATS gamma-globulin from the circulation, and full recovery occurs in three to four months.

Non-toxic goitres may increase in size during pregnancy and l-thyroxine therapy will prevent this enlargement. Therapy of hypothyroid states varies in no way from that in the non-pregnant woman.

(*c*) THE PITUITARY GLAND IN PREGNANCY

The pituitary gland increases in size and weight during pregnancy, and even in the non-pregnant state multipara have larger glands than childless women. Both acidophilic and basophilic cells increase during pregnancy but detailed histological studies are lacking. There is an increase in prolactin-secreting acidophil cells during pregnancy.

Pituitary gonadotrophins are unnecessary for the maintenance of pregnancy once fertilisation has occurred. In patients with hypopituitarism a short course of pituitary FSH and then HCG can sometimes induce ovulation, and after conception the pregnancy can be carried to term without further gonadotrophin therapy.

Growth hormone levels in pregnancy are difficult to ascertain because of interference by HPL. However using sensitive and specific assays for growth hormone it has been shown that maternal levels are similar to those in the non-pregnant state and respond to stimuli such as insulin-induced hypoglycaemia in the normal way. Levels in the fetus are at least three times those in the maternal circulation. Maternal growth hormone is probably not required for fetal growth and the anencephalic fetus grows in the absence of the fetal pituitary. HPL may prove to be a necessary stimulus for growth.

Increased production of TSH probably occurs during pregnancy though confirmation by critical radioimmunoassays is lacking.

The posterior pituitary peptides, arginine vasopressin and oxytocin, are produced in the hypothalamus. Oxytocin stimulates milk ejection and uterine contractions. Its blood concentration rises during pregnancy and is matched by an oxytocinase of placental origin. It is uncertain whether the hormone is normally required to initiate labour but it can certainly induce labour at the end of pregnancy.

Plasma osmolality falls abruptly in the first eight weeks of pregnancy from a non-pregnant level of about 290 mOsm per kg water to a value of about 280 mOsm per kg which is maintained throughout pregnancy. This change can probably be attributed to a fall in electrolyte concentration. Despite these changes, normal urine volumes and vasopressin activity are found during pregnancy. Women with diabetes insipidus lack vasopressin and usually have poor uterine action without replacement therapy.

III. *ENDOCRINE SEQUELAE OF PREGNANCY*

POST-PARTUM PITUITARY NECROSIS (*see* Chapter 1)

This is usually due to spasm of the infundibular arteries causing stasis and thrombosis in the portal system and necrosis of the anterior pituitary. Spasm results from hypotension due to haemorrhage during or shortly after pregnancy when the hyperplastic pituitary is especially vulnerable.

Very rarely, hypotension following haemorrhage may cause infarction of the pituitary in men or or non-pregnant women. All degrees of hypopituitarism may ensue, the usual clinical features being failure of lactation, amenorrhoea, and variable thyroidal and adrenal insufficiency. Loss or reduction of body hair is usual. Menstruation may occasionally persist with irregular and reduced losses and, very rarely, a further pregnancy can occur, which causes improvement of pituitary function. In countries with a high standard of obstetric practice this is now a rare cause of hypopituitarism.

AMENORRHOEA-GALACTORRHOEA SYNDROME

Persistent lactation without suckling, associated with amenorrhoea following pregnancy, is considered in Chapter 1. It should always raise the possibility of a pituitary tumour, and visual fields and skull X-rays should be carried out at six-monthly intervals if the condition persists.

REFERENCES

Bayliss, R. I. S., Browne, J. C. M., Round, B. P., and Steinbeck, A. W. (1955). *Lancet*, **i**, 62.

Carey, H. M. (Ed.) (1963). *Modern Trends in Human Reproductive Physiology*. London: Butterworth.

Cope, C. L., and Black, E. G. (1955). *Obstet. Gynec. Brit. Empire*, **66**, 404.

Crawford, J. W. (1972). *Brit. med. J.*, **4**, 715.

Crooks, J., Aboul-Khair, S. A., Turnbull, A. C., and Hytten, F. C. (1964). *Lancet*, **ii**, 334.

Diczfalusy, E. (1970). *Symp. Dtsch. Ges. Endokrin.*, **16**, 32.

Fuchs, F., and Klopper, A. (Eds) (1971). *Endocrinology of Pregnancy*. London: Harper and Row.

Hytten, F. E., and Leitch, I. (Eds) (1971). *The Physiology of Human Pregnancy*. Second Edition. Oxford: Blackwell Scientific.

Letchworth, A. T., and Chard, T. (1972). *Lancet*, **i**, 704.

Loraine, J. A., and Bell, E. T. (1966). *Hormone Assays and Their Clinical Application*, 2nd Edition. London: Livingstone.

Niven, P. A. R., Landon, J., and Chard, T. (1972). *Brit. med. J.*, **3**, 799.

Taylor, S. (Ed.) (1965). *Proc. Second Internat. Cong. Endocrinol.*, 17–22 August, 1964, Part I and II. London: Excerpta Medica Foundation.

Wolstenholme, G. E. W., and Porter, Ruth (Eds) (1967). *The Human Adrenal Cortex*, Ciba Foundation Study Group No. 27. London: Churchill.

11

TESTIS

The functions of the testis are:

(*a*) the formation of spermatozoa (spermatogenesis);

(*b*) the synthesis and secretion of testosterone.

The embryology of the testis and the development of the genital ducts and external genitalia are dealt with in Chapter 13. This chapter deals with the physiology of the testis and its secretions and with the diagnosis of hypogonadism in the male resulting from a decrease in testicular function affecting the production of spermatozoa and/or testosterone. This may be due to inherent disease of the testis associated with chromosomal defects or to acquired disease, or to lesions of the pituitary or hypothalamus having secondary effects on the testis.

ANATOMY OF THE MALE REPRODUCTIVE SYSTEM

In the adult, each testis weighs about 25 g (range 10–45 g). The dimensions are easily measured with calipers, the length being 3 to 5 cm and the width 2 to 3 cm. The testes are covered by a layer of connective tissue—the visceral portion of the tunica vaginalis, beneath which is a thick fibrous layer, the tunica albuginea, from which septa enter the gland. Posteriorly, the septa converge at the site of entry of the blood vessels, lymphatics and nerves.The internal spermatic artery supplying the testis arises from the abdominal aorta just below the renal artery. It also supplies the spermatic cord and epididymis. Veins leaving the testis form the pampiniform plexus of the cord which unite to form the testicular veins. The right testicular vein drains into the inferior vena cava and the left into the left renal vein. Nerves from the lumbar sympathetic chain reach the testis via the cord.

The bulk of the testis is made up of fine coiled seminiferous tubules joining at the posterior end of the testis into straight tubules which, in turn, open into a fine network from which efferent ductules lead to the head of the epididymis. The epididymis, attached to the back of the testis, is a coiled tube about 7 metres long that continues from the tail of the epididymis as the vas deferens. The vas forms part of the spermatic cord, entering the abdominal cavity where, at the base of the bladder, it joins the duct of the seminal vesicles to form the ejaculatory duct, which traverses the prostate to open into the prostatic portion of the urethra. Several glands add their secretions to the spermatozoa to form the semen. The seminal vesicles are paired glands that lie between the bladder and the rectum. Their secretion contains a high concentration of fructose and is under the control of testicular androgens. Secretions from the prostate are rich in citrate and enter the prostatic ducts that open into the urethra. The bulbourethral glands secrete mucous, which enters the membranous part of the urethra. Various vestigeal structures on the head of the epididymis and testis represent remnants of the Müllerian and Wolffian duct systems. The scrotum encloses the testes, its main function being to regulate their temperature, which is maintained at a level at least 2°C less than the intra-abdominal temperature. This hypothermia is essential for normal spermatogenesis.

SEMEN

Semen consists of fluid, mainly derived from the seminal vesicles and prostate, and spermatozoa. It varies in composition from day to day even in an individual and the volume of ejaculations may also vary from about 2 to 6 ml. For this reason, it is necessary for diagnostic purposes to do a series of seminal analyses. Secretions of the male accessory glands reflect the action of testicular testosterone, hence chemical analyses, particularly for fructose, are a useful tool in assessing the level of androgenic activity. The fructose concentration and total fructose in the ejaculate is lower in older age groups, but the citric acid content is not age-dependent.

As mentioned before, the prostate secretes citrate and acid phosphatase, and the seminal vesicles and ampulla, fructose. Occlusion of the ejaculatory ducts causes the production of semen without spermatozoa or fructose which contains citrate from the prostate. Inflammatory conditions of the epididymis reduce the content of glycerophosphorylcholine that it normally contributes to semen. Fructose levels in semen also reflect the level of blood glucose, and are increased in diabetes mellitus. Continence for up to four or five days increases the ejaculatory volume and sperm count, whereas frequent emissions cause lowering of the semen content of sperms, fructose, citrate, and acid phosphatase. In ejaculatory disturbances, the normal chemical pattern of the ejaculate may be altered—the earlier portion of the ejaculate normally contains more citrate, and the later, more fructose. Drugs such as amphetamines can also influence the pattern of secretion. Seminal stains on clothing can be identified by their particular chemical composition, which may be of importance in cases of suspected rape. About 95 per cent of men of proved fertility have a sperm population density of over 20 million/ml, though fertility may be present at lower levels. Normally, 60 per cent of the sperms show high-grade motility three hours after ejaculation. With sperm counts greater than 20 million/ml degrees of fertility are more related to motility than to sperm counts. Morphologically, 60–80 per cent of the forms are normal in highly fertile semen.

The fertilising ability of the spermatozoa is enhanced during the time taken to traverse the female genital tract, a phenomenon termed capacitation. Motility of spermatozoa obviously resides in the flagella, and fertilising ability in the head. The head contains a large amount of deoxyribonucleic acid (DNA) which has a constant base composition with the haploid number of chromosomes. Spermatozoa are transported in the epididymis by the action of smooth muscle and the cilia of the epithelium and are moved along the vas by contractions of its muscular coat. Ejaculation is caused by contraction of the seminal vesicles and prostate as a result of sympathetic stimulation. Closure of the bladder neck by sympathetic stimulation prevents reflux of semen into the bladder. Contractions of perineal muscles aid in ejaculation but are not essential.

CONTROL OF TESTICULAR FUNCTION

During fetal life, the interstitial cells of the testis (Leydig cells) develop very early, reaching a maximum at 14 to 16 weeks and largely disappearing by the time of birth. Chorionic gonadotrophin has been shown to be present in significant amounts in fetal tissues and it is likely that the high level of this hormone present from the 6th to 16th week is a major factor in the interstitial cell proliferation. The absence of interstitial cells in anencephalic fetuses that are without a pituitary suggest that the fetal pituitary may also be of some importance, for morphological differentiation in this gland can normally be detected by the

12th week. Histochemical studies show several types of enzymes capable of forming steroids such as testosterone in the fetal testis which are responsible for the differentiation of the male genital tract. A separate humoral agent is responsible for suppression of the Müllerian system (*see* Chapter 13). After about the twentieth week the interstitial cells decrease in number and in activity and do not regain prominence until just before puberty.

The testes gradually descend down the posterior abdominal wall to reach the scrotum shortly before birth. From a few weeks after birth till about four years the histological appearance of the testis is static, the seminiferous tubules being small and measuring about 66 microns in diameter. There is only slight tortuosity of the tubules, which are lined by small, undifferentiated cubical cells. Lumina can be identified in only about half of the tubules, and Leydig cells are absent. From the age of five to nine years the tubules are still small but show increasing tortuosity and have an average diameter of 78 microns, a basement membrane is evident, and spermatogonia and Sertoli cells are present but Leydig cells are still absent.

Prior to puberty, pituitary gonadotrophins can be detected in the circulation and in the urine only in low concentration, although the pituitary can clearly make gonadotrophins much earlier than this, since when synthetic hypothalamic LH/FSH releasing hormone is given to prepubertal children LH and FSH are secreted as in the adult. At the initiation of puberty, presumably under the influence of the hypothalamus, gonadotrophin secretion increases and blood levels rise. Interstitial cell stimulating hormone (ICSH), which is probably the same as luteinising hormone (LH) in the female, causes the Leydig cells to develop and secrete androgens, especially testosterone. The close apposition of the Leydig cells to the tubules may allow high concentrations of androgens to reach the tubules, to stimulate spermatogenesis from the spermatogonia (basal cell) to the spermatid stage as well as causing development of the secondary sexual characteristics of puberty (Table 11.1). Considerable evidence exists (Van Thiel *et al.*, 1972) that tubules secrete a hormone (provisionally called 'inhibin') which is responsible for the negative feedback control of FSH secretion from the pituitary, so that spermatogenetic activity is closely related to FSH levels; in contradistinction LH appears to be controlled by testosterone and dihydrotestosterone levels.

TABLE 11.1 *Pubertal Changes*

Testes:	Increase in size*
Accessory sex organs:	Enlargement and secretion from the prostate and seminal vesicles (secretions contain citrate and fructose).
External genitalia:	Enlargement of the penis and scrotum* which becomes rugose and pigmented.
Hair growth:	Development of hair on the upper lip, chin, axillae, temporal recession of hair, pubic hair* grows towards umbilicus.
Voice:	Enlargement of the larynx with deepening of the voice.
Bone growth:	Increase in rate of linear growth* from about two up to three inches yearly. Maturation of skeletal development leading to fusion of epiphyses.
Psyche:	Increase in libido and potency, male 'drive' appears.

* Earliest signs of puberty.

Follicle-stimulating hormone (FSH) has no effect on prepubertal seminiferous tubules but is essential for the final stages of spermatogenesis after puberty, when the tubular cells have been primed with androgens. The tubules increase in size at puberty until they attain the average adult diameter of 150 to 180 microns. The first evidence

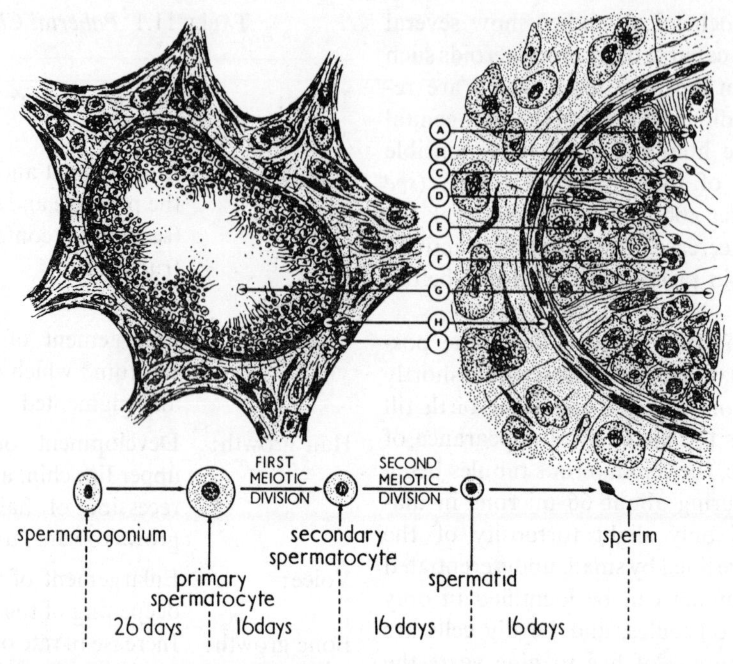

FIGURE 11.1 Histology of the testis (diagrammatic)

A = Spermatozoon
B = Spermatogonium
C = Spermatid
D = Sertoli cell
E = Secondary spermatocyte
F = Spermatid
G = Lumen of seminiferous tubule
H = Basement membrane
I = Interstitial (Leydig) cell

of puberty is the development of the tubular tunica propria and basement membrane which surround the tubules (Fig. 11.1). Attached to the basement membranes are Sertoli cells with their characteristic nucleoli, brush borders, and high glycogen content. They are thought to act as supporting cells which may provide energy substrates for the germinal cells.

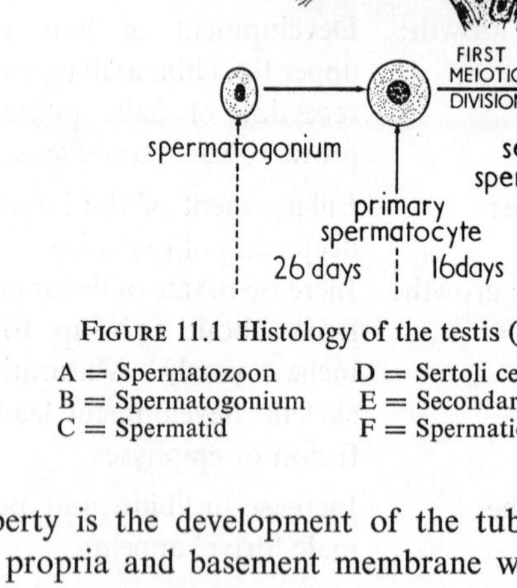

The process of spermatogenesis, which takes between 74 and 90 days, is indicated in Fig. 11.2, which shows the reduction division (meiosis) whereby spermatoza are produced with a haploid number of chromosomes including either one X or one Y chromosome.

FIGURE 11.2 The process of spermatogenesis

CONTROL OF PUBERTY AND THE FEED-BACK MECHANISM

The onset of puberty is triggered by secretion of pituitary gonadotrophins, themselves under the control of releasing factors from the hypothalamus. The factors that initiate the surge of hypothalamic activity at puberty are not known, though from studies in identical twins the timing must be partly under genetic control. There is a good correlation between skeletal maturity and the onset of puberty, both of which may be hastened by androgens. Young children may develop an early puberty after removal of a tumour secreting androgens.

The first sign of puberty in the male is an increase in testicular size, soon followed by wrinkling of the scrotal skin and the growth of a few coarse pubic hairs. These findings often allow the normal onset of puberty to be predicted. The age at which puberty develops varies in different countries and races but in the United Kingdom, in the male, it is usually between 12 and 14 years with a range from 9 to 18 years. Genital development in the male may be assessed in stages by comparison with the standards for genital maturity in boys published by Tanner (*see* Appendix pp. 452–3).

Feedback control between gonadal hormones, hypothalamus, and pituitary gonadotrophins, is complex and not fully elucidated. There is a marked rise in FSH in tubular dysfunctions, being most marked when germinal elements are absent and, therefore, in castration. Reference has already been made to the specific seminiferous tubular factor ('inhibin') which inhibits FSH secretion in man. ICSH levels also rise after castration or in the absence of Leydig cell function but testosterone is relatively ineffective as a suppressor of FSH and suppresses ICSH only in unphysiological doses. Research in this field has been hampered by the lack of specific assays for FSH and ICSH, reliance previously having to be placed on crude bioassays for total gonadotrophins or more laborious and not fully specific bioassays for the separate hormones. However, ICSH (LH) and FSH radioimmunoassays are now available in many centres, and understanding of the hypothalamic—pituitary—gonadal relationships is growing rapidly.

TESTOSTERONE SYNTHESIS, METABOLISM, AND CLINICAL EFFECTS

Testosterone is the major androgen produced by the Leydig cells of the testis. Small amounts of the hormone are also produced by the adrenal cortex in both sexes and by the ovary. Testosterone is a 17β-hydroxylated C-19 steroid, the formula of which is shown in the Fig. 11.3, but it appears to require conversion to an active and much more potent metabolite, dihydrotestosterone, and this can occur both in the circulation and in the peripheral target tissues.

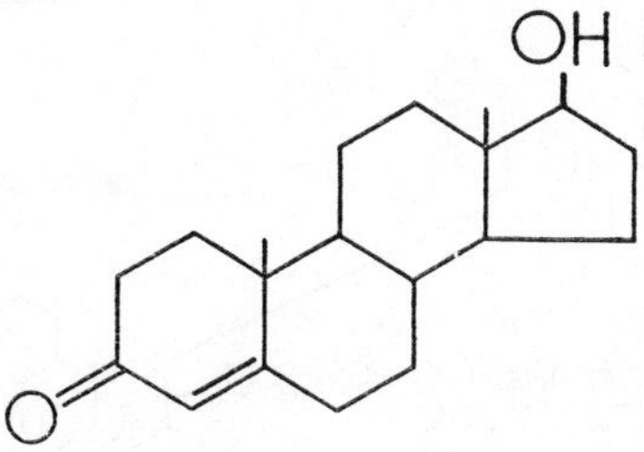

OH

O

FIGURE 11.3 Testosterone

Synthesis (Fig. 11.4). Similar enzymatic processes are involved in the synthesis of steroid hormones in the adrenal cortex, ovary, and testis, In each of these glands the side chain of cholesterol is degraded to form pregnenolone and, hence, dehydroepiandrosterone. Pregnenolone is converted to progesterone which, in turn is converted to androstenedione and then testosterone.

Transport and Fate. Testosterone and dihydrotestosterone are transported in the blood loosely bound to carrier proteins, mainly globulin—'sex hormone binding globulin' (SHBG)—or 'testosterone binding globulin' (TeBG) which also has a high affinity for other 17 β-hydroxyandrogens (17-OHA). Testosterone binding capacity of serum (TeBC) is similar in both sexes before puberty and in the adult female range, but is higher in adult females than in adult males. There is increased TeBC in male hypogonadism, hyperthyroidism, and cirrhosis of the liver. During pregnancy TeBC is raised, but at term a low normal level is found. TeBC is made in the liver and production is increased by oestrogens and also by high levels of thyroid hormones; progestogens have no effect. TeBC levels are low in hirsutism, in obese female patients and in patients with nephrotic syndrome (Vermeulen *et al.*, 1969). Androgenic activity is believed to be a function of the free (unbound) plasma androgen concentration, Disturbances of protein binding of androgens have been incriminated in some cases of hirsutism in the female (Rosenfield, 1971) and a syndrome of gynaecomastia and impotence associated with abnormal testosterone binding has been reported (Anderson *et al.*, 1972). Testosterone is degraded, particularly in the liver, under the influence of 17β-dehydrogenase enzyme systems and then conjugated with sulphates or glucuronic acid to be excreted in the urine as 17-oxosteroids (androsterone, aetiocholanolone and epiandrosterone). The testis contributes about 30 per cent of the 17-oxosteroids in man, the remainder coming from the adrenal cortex (largely dehydroepiandrosterone, but in smaller amount androsterone and aetiocholanolone). Adrenal 17-oxosteroids derived from cortisol are mainly 11-oxy-17-oxosteroids. Testosterone can also be converted to oestrogens, particularly oestrone and oestradiol, but this is only a minor fate of the hormone. Testosterone is converted mainly into dihydrotestosterone in the blood and at the site of its target tissues (Liao and Fang, 1969; Wilson and Gloyna, 1970). The biological action of testosterone can be produced by dihydrotestosterone (Baulieu, Lasnitzki and Robel, 1968). The plasma concentration of dihydrotestosterone is higher in males than in females and in both sexes its concentration is far lower than testosterone. In normal men, the production of dihydrotestosterone is about 0·4 mg per day, 50 per cent being derived from the transformation of plasma testosterone, whereas in normal females the production of dihydrotestosterone is only about 0·05 mg per day, of which only 10 per cent comes from testosterone (Salz *et al.*, 1972). In normal males the production rate of testosterone is 6–7 mg per day, depending on the method used. In normal females testosterone production rate is much lower at 1·5 mg per day.

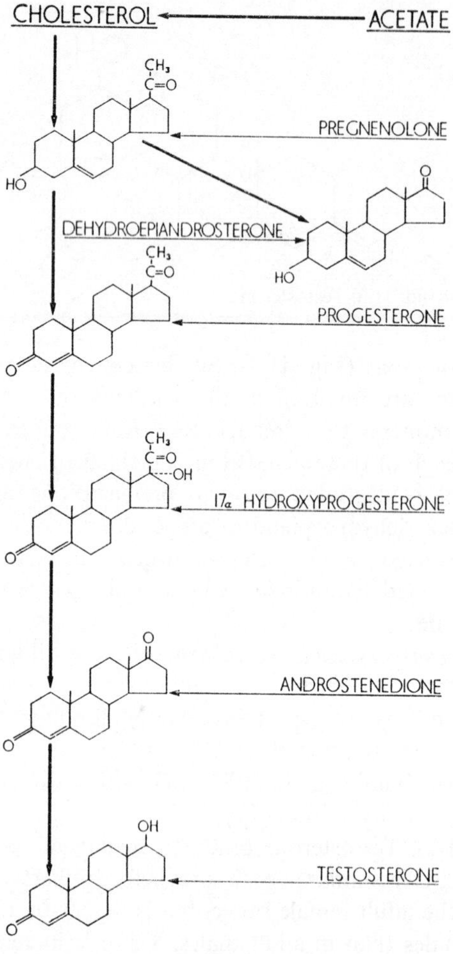

CHOLESTEROL ← ACETATE
PREGNENOLONE
DEHYDROEPIANDROSTERONE
PROGESTERONE
17α HYDROXYPROGESTERONE
ANDROSTENEDIONE
TESTOSTERONE

FIGURE 11.4 Biosynthesis of testosterone

Testosterone Levels in Body Fluids. Testosterone is the most potent naturally occurring androgen but is present in such small amounts in the blood that its estimation is not possible in most routine laboratories. Estimation of the urinary 17-oxosteroids is all that is available to most hospital laboratories. Since the majority of the 17-oxosteroids are metabolic products of precursors other than testosterone they form a poor tool for the investigation of diseases caused by altered androgen metabolism. Recently, new techniques such as double isotope derivative dilution, competitive protein binding and gas-liquid chromatography have allowed testosterone levels to be measured in blood and urine as a research procedure. In the authors' laboratories the mean concentration of testosterone in peripheral plasma using a competitive protein binding technique is 3–11 ng per ml. In women the range is 0·2–0·8 ng per ml, levels being slightly higher in the luteal phase of the cycle suggesting an ovarian source. In boys, testosterone levels tend to rise before there is clinical evidence of puberty. Normal levels are seen in many aged men. Like cortisol, testosterone levels in the blood appear to show circadian rhythmicity with higher levels observed at 8 a.m. and lowest levels between midnight and 4 a.m. (Faiman and Winter, 1971). A decline in testosterone levels is usual with sleep onset but there are subsequently fluctuations leading to an increase in level culminating in the 8 a.m. peak. There appears to be an association of individual fluctuations in testosterone levels with periods of REM sleep (Evans *et al.*, 1971). The circadian rhythm of testosterone is not suppressed by dexamethasone and does not depend on ACTH. However, neither has a close dependence on LH secretion been demonstrated. Levels of testosterone are raised by administration of human chorionic gonadotrophin (HCG), and lowered by oestrogens. Powerful synthetic androgens such as fluoxymesterone and 2α-methyldehydrotestosterone suppress testicular testosterone production, probably by inhibiting ICSH formation since this effect can be overcome by administration of HCG.

Mechanism of Action of Testosterone. Testosterone and other androgens are anabolic and stimulate cell growth and multiplication. They tend to increase body weight and cause nitrogen retention. They also increase sebum secretion and accelerate bone maturation, including fusion of the epiphyses. As with many other hormones, effects on messenger and nuclear RNA have been demonstrated but the primary site of action of the hormones is still uncertain.

MALE HYPOGONADISM

As mentioned previously, hypogonadism in the male may affect the tubules causing infertility, or the Leydig cells causing deficiency of testosterone production. When the tubules alone are damaged after puberty the testes become smaller and softer, though this may give rise to no complaints other than infertility. Normal adult testes measure about 4·5 cm in length (range 3·5 to 5·5) and about 2·5 cm in width (range 2·0 to 3·2).

The sequelae of testosterone deficiency depend on the age of the patient. In the young there is delay in the onset of puberty and eunuchoidal features may develop (Table 11·2). In the adult there is a reduction of libido and potency, and after a variable time, regression of secondary sexual characteristics. Facial hair growth slows down and the patient has to shave less frequently, his skin becomes finer, and his muscle strength may decrease.

Hypogonadism may also occur as a result of mechanical disorders or of gonadotrophin deficiency.

TABLE 11.2 *Eunuchoidal Features*

Skeletal proportions:	Immature bone age and delay in closure of epiphyses. Span more than two inches greater than height; pubis to floor measurement more than two inches greater than pubis to head (some normal persons have very long limbs).
Genitalia:	Infantile penis, small soft testes, scrotum lacks rugosity.
Muscles:	Muscles fine, and muscular strength less than average.
Body hair:	Facial hair fine; shaves infrequently; axillary, pubic, and body hair scanty or absent; no temporal hair recession.
Voice:	High-pitched and effeminate.

CLASSIFICATION AND CLINICAL FEATURES

1. *Testicular Disease*

(*a*) *Tubules and interstitial cells:*

- Testicular agenesis
- Bilateral torsion
- Severe bilateral orchitis (mumps)
- Bilateral cryptorchidism
  - Spontaneous
  - Vascular damage at orchidopexy
- Seminiferous tubule dysgenesis
  - Klinefelter's syndrome and its variants
- Reifenstein's syndrome

(*b*) *Tubules only* (interstitial cells largely intact):

- Sertoli-only syndrome
- Radiation damage to germ cells
- Seminiferous tubule dysgenesis
  - Klinefelter's syndrome and its variants
- Milder degrees of bilateral orchitis, e.g. mumps (interstitial cells are more resistant)
- Environmental and local changes
  - Cryptorchidism, Paraplegia, Varicocoele (bracketed)
  - Autoagglutination
  - Idiopathic
- Tubular sclerosis (dystrophia myotonica)
- Treatment with cyclophosphamide and other cytotoxic drugs

(*c*) *Interstitial cells only:*

- Disorders of testosterone biosynthesis
- Idiopathic failure—'male climacteric'

2. *Mechanical Disorders*

- Duct lesions
  - Congenital absence of vasa
  - Obstruction of epididymes
  - Congenital absence of seminal vesicles
  - Obstruction of ejaculatory ducts
- Ejaculatory dysfunction
  - Neurogenic
  - Semen reflux
  - Impotence

3. *Secondary Testicular Failure*

- Isolated gonadotrophin deficiency (FSH and ICSH)
- Early-onset gonadotrophin deficiency associated with deficiencies of other pituitary hormones due to pituitary or hypothalamic disease
- Fertile eunuch syndrome
- Late-onset gonadotrophin deficiency

1. TESTICULAR DISEASE

(*a*) TUBULES AND INTERSTITIAL CELLS

Testicular Agenesis (anorchia, functional prepubertal castrate syndrome). These patients, with male phenotype, usually attend because they are thought to have undescended testes. The scrotum is underdeveloped and empty apart from small nodules of tissue at the end of the vas or epididymis. Operation may be carried out to exclude cryptorchidism, when the vas is found to end in a small nodule of tissue that may have histological features of Wolffian duct derivatives. It is assumed that the testes have 'atrophied' during intrauterine life after the stage when the male phenotype has been determined, probably after the tenth week of fetal life. The chromosomal sex is invariably male. Urinary gonadotrophins (both FSH and ICSH) are elevated at the time of expected puberty but urinary oestrogens and 17-oxosteroids remain lower than normal. Such patients are inevitably infertile, though, with androgen therapy, secondary sexual characteristics develop normally.

Bilateral Torsion. Torsion of the testis is commoner than is generally believed and is often misdiagnosed as epididymitis. The usual patient is a boy or young man who experiences testicular pain coming on without obvious trauma. There may be lower abdominal pain, nausea, and vomiting. The patient may have had previous attacks which resolved spontaneously or were treated as epididymitis. The testis, and soon the scrotum, are swollen and inflamed and the patient becomes febrile. There are no urinary symptoms or urethritis and the urine is free of albumin and pus cells. When the patient stands, the unaffected testis is seen to lie in a horizontal plane since the responsible congenital anomaly is a bilateral one. The horizontal lie of the testis is due to the two layers of tunica vaginalis, which normally cover only the testis, extending upwards to cover the epididymis and a variable length of the cord. The testis may also be separated from the epididymis by a lengthened mesorchium, longest at the upper pole, which causes the testis to lie horizontally when the patient stands. If the testis is viable at operation, which should follow diagnosis at once, orchidopexy is carried out on both sides to fix the testes in the scrotum. A non-viable testis should be removed and orchidopexy performed on the contralateral side.

Severe Bilateral Orchitis (mumps). Orchitis is best known as a complication of mumps though it also occurs in other infectious fevers, in chickenpox, infections due to Coxsackie virus, and in congenital syphilis. It mainly affects young men (it is very rare before puberty), causing severe pain, fever, and sometimes prostration and delirium. The testis is tender and swollen and the epididymis may be similarly affected. About one case in five of adult mumps is complicated by orchitis, and in 15 per cent the swelling is bilateral. Orchitis usually appears about a week after the parotid swelling but may precede or occur without salivary gland involvement. Sterility or reduced fertility occur only when the lesion is bilateral and followed by testicular atrophy. In many instances there are no apparent sequelae of mumps orchitis. Therapy with corticosteroids may lessen the inflammatory condition but probably does not affect the incidence of sterility.

Cryptorchidism (*undescended testis*). The testes descend into the scrotum at about the seventh month of gestation. Descent is dependent on the gubernaculum testis, a structure consisting of mesenchyme which forms a column in the abdomen, attaching the testis to the inguinal region and, thence, to the floor of the scrotum. As the testis descends, the gubernaculum expands and dilates the scrotum and inguinal canal. For normal testicular descent it is essential for the processus vaginalis and cremaster muscle to precede the testis into the scrotum. If fibrous tissue encroaches on the gubernaculum, anchoring bands of fibrous tissue may prevent normal testicular descent, which results in an ectopic testis. The vas deferens and testicular vessels must also grow in length to allow normal descent. Gonadotrophins from the maternal pituitary and the placenta, acting on the fetal testis to induce the formation of androgens, are necessary for the whole process of testicular descent.

Maldescent may result from alterations in any one of the processes mentioned above. If the testes do not descend before the first year of life, they usually remain undescended till puberty, and even then descent is not achieved in some instances. The incidence of unilateral or bilateral undescended testes is difficult to ascertain because of the problem of the retractile testis which is often mistaken for an undescended testis. The cremasteric reflex is very active in children (though not in the newborn), and causes retraction of the testis out of the scrotum. The overall incidence of undescended testis in full-term children at birth is 3·4 per cent, falling to 1·7 per cent at one month, and 0·7 per cent at one year. After this, the incidence is little changed if retractile testes are excluded from consideration, Unilateral failure of descent is five times commoner than bilateral maldescent.

Retractile testes can usually be coaxed into the top of the scrotum if the patient and the examiner's hands are warm, there is powder on the skin to facilitate movement of the testis, and the patient is relaxed; no therapy is required. Ectopic testes are occasionally difficult to distinguish from retractile testes, and in cases of doubt it is justifiable to give a course of chorionic gonadotrophin 4,000 IU three times weekly for one month. Hormone treatment may increase the blood supply to the testis and cause growth of the spermatic cord even if descent of the testis is not achieved. Subsequent operation—orchidopexy—is made easier. The optimal time for hormone therapy or operation is still a matter of controversy. Up to the age of five years undescended testes usually show normal maturation, but between six and ten years only 8 per cent are normal, and after eleven years none are normal. This evidence suggests that for undescended testes a course of hormone therapy should be given between five and six years and if no response is obtained orchidopexy should be performed. In the case of a single undescended testis it may be justifiable to delay therapy till nine years. Testes that have not descended spontaneously are less likely to function normally even if orchidopexy is carried out early. It should be remembered that many testes fail to descend because they are abnormal, while others become abnormal because of maldescent or vascular insufficiency following surgery. In unilateral cases, biopsy of the descended testis often shows it to be abnormal also. Undescended testes are a significant cause of impaired fertility. The risk of malignancy in an undescended testis is increased, being greater if the testis is intra-abdominal than if the testis is placed in the scrotum but the contralateral descended testis is also at risk for malignant change. Usually, it is advisable to place the cryptorchid testis in the scrotum, where malignant change is easily recognised at an early stage.

Seminiferous Tubule Dysgenesis. Klinefelter's syndrome is characterised by varying degrees of seminiferous tubule failure and decreased Leydig cell function. Many patients with this variety of hypogonadism have chromosomal abnormalities, the buccal smear being chromatin positive and the karyotype showing one or more additional X-chromosomes (*see* Chapter 13). Minor degrees of the syndrome may be shown by patients with mosaicism who have normal as well as abnormal cell lines. The testes are small and firm, after puberty often no larger than the size of a pea, and show hyalinised tubules lined only by Sertoli cells, failure of spermatogenesis, and a variable decrease in the number of Leydig cells. In rare cases, probably mosaics, partial spermatogenesis may be retained. Gynaecomastia is common and may be asymmetrical. Intelligence is often at the lower end of normal or below, and the incidence of behaviour disorders is increased. Development of the secondary sexual characteristics varies considerably, some patients being normal and others showing retarded sexual development and eunuchoid features, the result of lowered testosterone production by the testes; the penis is often adequately developed. Patients with Klinefelter's syndrome have elevated serum FSH levels, related to the lack of spermatogenesis. The LH levels tend to be normal in those patients who are well virilised with normal plasma testosterone levels, or elevated when the patients are poorly virilised with low testosterone levels. Sexual development is easily increased by therapy with male hormone, e.g. testosterone propionate (Testoral) 10 mg sublingually two or three times daily, though almost all patients will remain sterile. A rare variant of Klinefelter's syndrome with XXXXY karyotype is commonly associated with bilateral cryptorchidism.

Reifenstein's syndrome is a hereditary disorder in which there is hypospadias, postpubertal tubular atrophy, azoospermia and variable gynaecomastia, and eunuchoidism. The patients resemble those with Klinefelter's syndrome but their chromosomal constitution is normal. Urinary gonadotrophins are usually raised, oestrogen levels are normal, and testosterone levels low. Histology of the testis shows a variable degree of hyalinisation of the tubules but, unlike the picture in Klinefelter's syndrome, elastic fibres are present around the tubules, suggesting that the tubular damage is largely postpubertal. Leydig cells may be prominent and clumped though their function is less than normal. Replacement therapy with testosterone is indicated along with surgical repair of the hypospadias.

(*b*) TUBULES ONLY

Sertoli-only Syndrome (*germinal cell aplasia*). Patients present with infertility but are found to have normal secondary sexual characteristics. The testes may be normal or reduced in size with normal consistency and there is azoospermia. Testicular biopsy reveals no sperm precursors but only Sertoli cells, though before puberty the appearance is said to be normal. Gonadotrophin levels (particularly of FSH) are raised. No treatment is known to effect fertility.

Radiation Damage of Germ Cells. Accidental or therapeutic radiation to the testes can cause damage to the more sensitive germinal cells.

Seminiferous Tubule Dysgenesis. Some patients with Klinefelter's syndrome have intact or even hyperplastic interstitial cells and produce normal testosterone levels in the blood, with satisfactory virilisation.

Environmental and Local Changes. The increased temperature within the abdomen is one cause for the failure in spermatogenesis in the cryptorchid testis. Degeneration of the tubules following paraplegia may be caused by altered testicular temperature due to denervation of the lumbar spinal nerves passing through the lumbar sympathetic ganglia, increasing the blood supply to the testis.

Varicocoeles are associated with reduced fertility, and some 60 per cent of subfertile men with varicocoeles will have their fertility restored after successful spermatic vein ligation. The mechanism by which varicocoeles reduce fertility was first thought to be due to a rise in testicular temperature, but this has been disproved and it is now uncertain whether cellular anoxia resulting from venous stasis or reflux of steroids from the adrenal to the testis by retrograde venous flow is more important. Varicocoeles are usually left-sided and the larger the varicocoele the more effect it has in reducing fertility.

Autoagglutination of sperms may play a part in some cases of subfertility, for about three per cent of subfertile men have high titres of sperm agglutinins in their semen.

Tubular sclerosis occurs in dystrophia myotonica, a disorder characterised by myotonia, frontal baldness, cataracts, and testicular atrophy. The testes are small and soft, but Leydig cell function is intact and secondary sexual characteristics are within the normal range. Biopsy reveals hyalinisation and fibrosis of the seminiferous tubules though the damage is not always severe. Chromosomal studies reveal no abnormality. The patients are infertile. The pituitary fossa is often small, but pituitary function is intact. Nodular enlargement of the thyroid may occur.

Cyclophosphamide and other cytotoxic drugs are increasingly used in renal and systemic disease. Cyclophosphamide produces testicular atrophy which may be profound on histological examination (Kumar *et al.*, 1972). Regeneration may occur in some patients after cessation of the drug.

(*c*) INTERSTITIAL CELLS ONLY

Leydig cell function can be assessed clinically by the presence of secondary sexual characteristics that result from the action of testosterone. Plasma or urinary testosterone levels will be low if there is deficient function of the Leydig cells and will fail to rise after administration of ICSH (usually HCG is given: Perheentupa *et al.*, 1972; Anderson *et al.*, 1972). Fertility can be restored in some patients in this group by administration of male hormone, which allows the full process of spermatogenesis to be completed. In other patients, fertility is normal in the presence of eunuchoidal features—the 'fertile eunuch' syndrome. Selective failure of ICSH secretion by the pituitary appears to be responsible in the rare patients with this syndrome.

TREATMENT OF HYPOGONADISM DUE TO TESTICULAR DISEASE

Wherever possible, any readily treatable cause such as varicocele or cryptorchidism should be dealt with. Commonly, however, no curative treatment can be given and symptomatic therapy then falls under two headings:

1. *Treatment of Androgen Deficiency*. If Leydig cell function is inadequate, androgen replacement therapy should be given. Some of the different androgen preparations available are listed in Table 11.3.

TABLE 11.3 *Androgen Preparations*

Preparation	Dose (mg)	Route of administration	Dosage schedule
Testosterone propionate* in waxy base (Testoral)	10–40	Sublingual	10 mg one to four times daily
Methyl testosterone	10–40	Sublingual	10 mg one to four times daily
Fluoxymesterone (Ultandren)	5–10	Oral	Daily
Testosterone phenylacetate*	200	IM	Every one–two weeks initially
Testosterone propionate	50	IM	Three times weekly
Testosterone pellets* (unconjugated)	300–500	Subcutaneous implantation (e.g. in abdominal wall or thigh)	Every four–six months
Mesterolone (Pro-viron)	75–100	Oral	25 mg three to four times daily
'Sustanon' (four testosterone conjugates)*	100–250	IM	Every two weeks (100 mg) or every four weeks (250 mg

* The preparations recommended by the authors.

Side Effects. Sublingual testosterone in the form of 'Testoral' is often effective and, unlike methyl testosterone, does not cause cholestatic jaundice. This obstructive type of jaundice is also much less frequent with fluoxymesterone. Histologically, the liver shows biliary stasis with round cell infiltration around the bile ducts but little liver cell damage. Liver function tests show the raised alkaline phosphatase and bilirubin of obstructive jaundice. Improvement soon follows withdrawal of therapy. Methyl testosterone also causes dyspepsia suggestive of peptic ulceration in some patients. All androgen preparations will stimulate the growth of prostatic carcinoma. Occasionally bladder neck obstruction is precipitated in elderly patients, presumably due to pre-existing prostatic hyperplasia. Frequent erections are usually the sign of too vigorous therapy. Stimulation of erythropoiesis with a raised haematocrit is a rare sequel of androgen medication. Testosterone therapy given to males with normal testicular function lowers gonadotrophin production and inhibits spermatogenesis. The testes show decrease in size of the tubules which develop fibrosis and hyaline change, and atrophy of the germ cells and Leydig cells.

2. *Treatment of Defective Spermatogenesis* has become possible following the introduction of preparations of human FSH, with or without ICSH supplements given in the form of HCG. However, some degree of spermatogenesis must be present for treatment to be effective, and to date results are not very reliable, although this form of therapy is still in its early stages.

2. MECHANICAL DISORDERS

DUCT LESIONS

Congenital Absence of Vasa. Absence of the vas deferens is responsible for about 1·5 per cent of male infertility and about 5 per cent of all patients with azoospermia. The condition is easily diagnosed by failure to find the vas in the cord and scrotum. Maldevelopment may effect other genital structures. Treatment is rarely possible, and removal of sperms from the epididymis is of little help because such spermatozoa are not suitable for fertilisation. Surgical anastomosis is more feasible in patients who have previously had normal tubes which have been occluded as a result of gonorrhoea or vasectomy.

Obstruction of the epididymes also leads to azoospermia, which is rarely amenable to therapy. It may result from epididymo-orchitis of tuberculous or other bacterial origin.

Absence of the seminal vesicles or obstruction of the ejaculatory ducts are occasional causes of male infertility. Obstruction of the vas deferens may be diagnosed by vasography.

EJACULATORY DYSFUNCTION

Neurogenic. Parasympathetic nerves from the second, third, and fourth sacral nerve roots pass via the nervi erigentes to produce erection. Sympathetic fibres from the first and second lumbar segments cause contraction of the seminal vesicles and closure of the bladder neck. Contraction of voluntary muscle then causes ejaculation of semen from the urethra. Sympathectomy, sympathetic and ganglion-blocking agents, and, rarely, spinal cord lesions may interfere with these processes.

Semen reflux may be a congenital defect or may follow damage to the internal sphincter of the bladder at transurethral or open prostatic resection. It may also result from posterior urethral strictures or a lumbar sympathectomy. Semen can be retrieved from the bladder and used to achieve fertilisation though sometimes surgical repair is possible.

Impotence. Impotence is defined as inability to obtain or sustain penile erection sufficient to conclude satisfactory sexual intercourse. It is a normal occurrence during some illnesses but most often results from emotional disorders, local causes in the genital tract or its nervous control being rare. Impotence is common in patients with hypopituitarism, but is not often a presenting symptom. Diabetes mellitus may cause impotence as the result of a neuropathic process but most patients who complain of impotence have no local or endocrine disease. Various psychoanalytical views have been expressed as to the cause of this common variety of impotence, most lacking any vestige of scientific proof. Some patients with impotence give a life-long history of neuroticism and the impotence is just another feature of their inadequate personality. If the sexual disorder is present from the first attempts at coitus the prognosis is poor. Conflicts in sexual orientation and homosexual traits may be present. Impotence in males who have previously had satisfactory heterosexual relationships may be of acute or insidious onset. Acute onset impotence usually has a well-defined precipitant, guilt over illicit intercourse, honeymoon impotence, debilitating illness, herniorrhaphy, hysterectomy in the wife or childbirth. If it is not the culmination of more profound sexual disharmony the prognosis is usually good. Insidious onset of impotence in later life is often the result of changing sexual attitudes between the married couple. Loss of attraction or attractions elsewhere, marital conflicts, e.g. precipitated by elderly parents joining the household, may all contribute, and the prognosis is less satisfactory in this group. On the whole, the longer the duration of impotence and the less stable the individual the poorer is the outlook.

Cooper and his colleagues (1970) have differentiated 'psychogenic' from 'constitutional' impotence. In the former the onset is acute, there is usually some temporal relationship to specific stress, the complaint is selective, intermittent and transient, there is evidence of potential to respond erotically and 'sex-drive' is high. In the latter there is an insidious onset without obvious temporal relationships, the condition is persistent and gradually worsens, there is evidence of a premature and progressive waning of sex interest and the 'sex-drive' is low. However, Cooper points out that the psychological and constitutional disorders are seen only comparatively rarely in their pure form and aetiological overlap may occur. Cooper and his colleagues (1970) have shown that urinary testosterone levels are higher in the psychogenic than in the constitutional group and have suggested that testosterone excretion patterns—high, average and low, may be one method of classifying impotence. The prognosis seems better in the high excretion group.

Treatment is usually aimed at defining the personality traits of the partners and attempting to resolve any conflicts. Superficial psycho-therapy, mild sedation, and reassurance may prove sufficient. Abstention from intercourse till desire and self-confidence have been restored is sometimes successful but complicated programmes of sexual stimulation have little to offer. Therapy with testosterone is sometimes worth while even in the absence of any obvious endocrine deficiency. Severe and well-established cases of impotence are usually resistant to therapy and, overall, the results are disappointing.

3. SECONDARY TESTICULAR FAILURE

IDIOPATHIC ISOLATED GONADOTROPHIN DEFICIENCY (FSH and ICSH)

This may be a familial condition and may be associated with other congenital abnormalities, including anosmia or reduction in the sense of smell, cleft palate, hare-lip, and craniofacial asymmetry. Blunted growth hormone responses to arginine and to hypoglycaemia may occur. The association of anosmia and eunuchoidism is very suggestive of this syndrome and in this case is usually called Kallman's syndrome. Since normal puberty may be delayed as late as eighteen years, patients cannot be considered to fall into this category till after this age. Patients remain prepubertal in appearance with lack of secondary sexual characteristics. Growth of the limbs continues because epiphyseal fusion is delayed in the absence of sex hormones, and eunuchoidal proportions are sometimes found. Likewise, the testes are prepubertal in size and consistency, but gynaecomastia is rare. Testicular biopsy reveals immature seminiferous tubules with undifferentiated germinal cells, azoospermia, and no Sertoli cells. Mature Leydig cells are absent, mesenchymal precursors only being present. Gonadotrophin excretion (both FSH and ICSH) is below normal, though in partial forms of the syndrome low-normal hormone levels may be found. Testosterone excretion is reduced but because of the adreno-cortical contribution urinary 17-oxosteroids are usually within the normal range. ICSH production may be tested by administration of clomiphene citrate. This drug is given orally in divided doses using a total daily dose of 3 mg/kg body weight for 10 days. In normal men, serum levels of ICSH (measured as LH) rise by a mean of 107 per cent to above the normal range ($2{\cdot}6 \pm 0{\cdot}56$ mU/ml in adult males) and plasma 17 hydroxyandrogens (as a measure of testosterone) by a mean of 114 per cent to above 11·5 ng/ml in normal men (Anderson *et al.*, 1972). There is no rise in early puberty, panhypopituitarism and isolated gonadotrophin deficiency. In chromatin positive Klinefelter's syndrome and in testicular degeneration the high LH levels remain

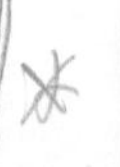

unaltered. This test is of particular value in the diagnosis of gonadotrophin deficiency where basal LH levels may be only borderline low.

Patients with isolated gonadotrophin deficiency usually secrete gonadotrophins promptly if the synthetic gonadotrophin releasing hormone (*see* Chapter 3) is given intravenously (Marshall *et al.*, 1972). This suggests that these patients are deficient in the releasing hormone and have a hypothalamic defect rather than a primary pituitary abnormality. Histological changes within the hypothalamus have been described.

Without therapy, these patients remain eunuchoidal, infertile, and impotent. Ideally, treatment would be given with ICSH combined with FSH, but human pituitary hormones are only just becoming available for routine use, and experience with these preparations is limited. As a compromise, Leydig cell maturity can be achieved by administration of HCG in an intramuscular dose of 4,000 IU three times weekly for six to nine months, after which the dose is halved for a further three to six months. Testosterone is secreted by the Leydig cells, and puberty develops. Spermatogenesis is initiated but usually not completed in the absence of FSH. Therapy is then withdrawn for a further three to six months, and in some patients there is no regression of secondary sexual characteristics and a 'cure' has been produced. Occasionally, several courses of HCG are required before regression is prevented. Full spermatogenesis may not be achieved without later addition of FSH (e.g. "Pergonal' or human pituitary FSH) to the regime. If sexual maturity fails after withdrawal of HCG, permanent therapy with androgens is required.

EARLY-ONSET GONADOTROPHIN DEFICIENCY ASSOCIATED WITH DEFICIENCIES OF OTHER PITUITARY HORMONES

Gonadotrophin secretion may be reduced in association with 'idiopathic' growth hormone deficiency or as a result of organic lesions in the pituitary or hypothalamus. In children, hypopituitarism is commonly due to a craniopharyngioma, chromophobe adenoma, granulomas, or tuberculous meningitis. Gonadotrophin deficiency will not become manifest until the time of puberty.

FERTILE EUNUCH SYNDROME (ICSH DEFICIENCY)

In some patients with eunuchoid features and evidence of testosterone deficiency, spermatogenesis is normal and fertility is achieved. Testicular size is normal or slightly small, and biopsy reveals mainly normal tubules with absent or hypoplastic Leydig cells. It is likely that this is a variant of the previous idiopathic syndrome in which FSH secretion is normal and ICSH secretion reduced but not absent. Sufficient ICSH and androgens may be produced to allow normal spermatogenesis but not for full differentiation of the secondary sexual characteristics. In partial testosterone deficiency it would be reasonable to expect that the adjacent tubules would be exposed to a higher level of hormone than distal body tissues. Treatment is given with testosterone to allow sexual maturation. Alternatively, a course of HCG can be given first.

LATE-ONSET GONADOTROPHIN DEFICIENCY

Rarely, only gonadotrophin secretion by the pituitary fails in a mature fully-developed individual. This is usually the first manifestation of pituitary or hypothalamic disease such as a tumour but occasionally no local lesion can be found. Apart from growth hormone, gonadotrophin secretion tends to be affected earlier than that of other pituitary hormones. In a man, acquired gonadotrophin deficiency leads to impotence (though this is a rare cause of this condition) and reduced fertility. The testes become small and soften, but body hair is only partly reduced so long as ACTH secretion ensures a normal output of adrenal androgens. Gonadotrophin secretion may be reduced as part of the syndrome of panhypopituitarism when other hormonal deficiencies will tend to dominate the clinical picture. Once pubertal development has been attained, gonadotrophin failure is followed by disorganisation and loss of the germinal layers, thickening of the tunica propria which retains its elastic fibres, and degeneration of the Leydig cells. Consequently, response to gonadotrophin therapy is partial or absent unless this is instituted shortly after the pituitary failure. Sterility is difficult to reverse but potency and secondary sexual characteristics are easily restored with male hormone.

SUMMARY OF DIAGNOSIS OF MALE HYPOGONADISM

Reference has already been made to most of the investigations used. Primary gonadal disease may be differentiated from gonadotrophin deficiency by clinical examination and by estimation of plasma and urinary FSH and ICSH (LH) levels which are low in gonadotrophin failure and normal or increased in primary testicular disease. Stimulation tests using clomiphene citrate or HCG may be particularly helpful. If secondary testicular failure is diagnosed, the cause must be ascertained by appropriate investigation of hypothalamic-pituitary function, including clinical examination and skull X-ray.

Investigations useful in the diagnosis of hypogonadism due to testicular failure include:

1 Clinical—history, physical examination (including measurement of height and span and penile and testicular size).
2. Buccal smear and chromosome karyotype.
3. X-rays of left-hand and wrist for bone age (Greulich and Pyle).
4. Semen analysis—sperm count, motility and fructose content (normal 91–520 mg per 100 ml).
5. Plasma or urinary FSH and ICSH (measured as LH), basal and after administration of clomiphene.
6. Plasma 17 OHA after administration of HCG.
7. Plasma and urinary testosterone—basal and after HCG.
8. Testicular biopsy.
9. Vasography.
10. Serum tests for syphilis.

DELAYED PUBERTY

One of the commonest problems presented to an endocrinologist is the teenage boy in whom puberty has not started or is incomplete. When seeing these patients it should be remembered that puberty may be delayed till eighteen years and the individual still develop into a normal fertile man. Such delay of puberty is commonly a familial condition and may be associated with a youthful appearance, some degree of shortness of stature, and delayed bone maturity. By the time the patient attends a hospital out-patient clinic he is usually at least thirteen years of age. A careful history should be obtained from the boy and both parents with reference to any cause of testicular damage or other hormone deficiencies. The boy's height and weight should be recorded. Examination should be directed to the pituitary, the testes, and the secondary sexual characteristics. The fundi should be inspected and visual fields examined. Gynaecomastia may indicate the onset of puberty or the presence of Klinefelter's syndrome. Facial hair tends to develop later than axillary, and that later than pubic hair. Often a few wisps of coarse pubic hair are the first indication of puberty after enlargement of the testes. Usually the testes will be found to be developing, and the early onset of the other manifestations of puberty can be confidently predicted. Obesity will make the penis appear smaller than its true size. Many patients previously labelled as Fröhlich's syndrome were merely obese boys with later than average puberty. Dietary restriction and reassurance is all that is required. Scrotal rugosity is another early sign of puberty. The length and breadth of the testes and penis should be recorded for future comparison. Small, firm testes about the size of a pea suggest a clinical diagnosis of Klinefelter's syndrome. If there are early signs of puberty and the testes are of normal 'prepubertal' or 'pubertal' size the parents and boy can usually be reassured and asked to attend for a final check in six to twelve months, when there will be further development. Other endocrine abnormalities, or a height less than the third percentile, and bone age more than two standard deviations below the mean will indicate that investigations should be directed to other aspects of pituitary function. If puberty is not evident by eighteen years and there is no evidence of other endocrine disease full investigations of gonadal function are indicated, including examination of the chemical composition of the semen, testicular biopsy and pituitary function tests.

MALE INFERTILITY

In all cases of marital infertility both partners should be interviewed and examined. This section deals only with the male aspects of infertility. At least one year of regular intercourse without conception should elapse before considerations of reduced fertility are raised. The patient should be questioned about his libido, the frequency of coitus, and the occurrence of ejaculation. Failure of ejaculation with nocturnal emissions often indicates a psychological disturbance. If there has always been failure of ejaculation, androgen deficiency, congenital absence of the seminal vesicles, or congenital dilatation of the bladder neck should be considered. Acquired failure of ejaculation may also indicate androgen deficiency or may follow sympathectomy, resection of the bladder neck as at prostatectomy, or tuberculous or other causes of obstruction of the ejaculatory duct. Testicular maldescent, injury, operation or disease should be enquired for. Examination should be directed to the secondary sexual characteristics, and for evidence of eunuchoidism or gynaecomastia. The presence of the vas deferens on either side should be confirmed by palpation. Past or present prostatitis or epididymitis should be excluded. The testes should be located in the scrotum and their size measured. Very small firm testes suggest Klinefelter's syndrome, very small fibrous testes without sensation are found after testicular torsion, and small soft testes may be seen in primary or secondary testicular disease. Cryptorchidism is easily recognised but unilateral maldescent may be associated with maldevelopment of the descended testis. Varicocoeles should always be looked for with the patient standing up.

Investigations as outlined for the diagnosis of hypogonadism should be performed. *Semen*, obtained by masturbation into a glass container after four days of abstinence from sexual intercourse, should be examined within one hour of production. At least three separate specimens should be examined for sperm count, motility and abnormal forms. The volume of semen on each occasion should exceed 1·5 ml. *Testicular biopsy* is indicated in all cases of azoospermia or oligospermia where the cause is not obvious. It should be emphasised that the appearance of the Leydig cells is not always a very good indication of their ability to synthesise testosterone. *Specific assays for FSH* and *ICSH* (*LH*) are often of value, both basal and after clomiphene stimulation. Finally, *serum and urine testosterone levels*, reduced in Leydig cell malfunction, should be estimated before and after HCG stimulation.

In all cases, the patient's wife should also be examined, and, if necessary, investigated.

TREATMENT OF MALE INFERTILITY

1. *Prophylaxis*. Early treatment of cryptorchidism with achievement of the scrotal position by

ten years may sometimes prevent irreversible tubular damage. Torsion of the testis should be treated early and the unaffected side should be fixed in the scrotum.

2. *Therapy*. Aspermia of mechanical origin is rarely amenable to therapy. Azoospermia from mechanical obstruction is rarely suitable for surgery unless obstruction is in the tail of the epididymis, usually from old gonococcal epididymitis. Varicocoeles can be treated by high ligation; hot baths and close fitting pants should be avoided. In some patients with tubular dysfunction of unknown cause testosterone therapy may increase sperm motility by an action on the accessory organs, and may prime the tubules for endogenous FSH and increase semen volume. Testosterone rebound therapy has been employed, giving large doses which temporarily suppress gonadotrophins, in theory to 'rest the tubules'. Withdrawal of therapy after three months may 'cause' an increase in sperm count. Therapy with HCG and FSH has already been mentioned in the case of early onset gonadotrophin deficiency. On the whole, gonadotrophin therapy has so far proved disappointing in the treatment of male infertility, and clomiphene has not been as successful as in female infertility.

Androgen Replacement Therapy. When Leydig cell function is inadequate due to primary testicular disease or secondary to gonadotrophin deficiency, androgen replacement therapy may be required (Table 11.3).

ENDOCRINE ASPECTS OF TESTICULAR TUMOURS

Nomenclature. For the nomenclature of testicular tumours in Britain and North America the reader is referred to Dayan (1966). Testicular tumours can be divided simply into five groups:

1. Seminoma
2. Teratoma
3. Combined seminoma and teratoma

(1–3: Germinal cell origin)

4. Sertoli cell tumours
5. Leydig cell tumours

Incidence. The incidence of testicular tumours is between two and three per 100,000 men/year, making up one or two per cent of all malignant tumours in men. The highest incidence occurs between the ages of 20 and 35 years.

CLINICAL FEATURES

1. *Local*. The commonest complaint is of a lump in the testis, which is usually painless. Often, patients ascribe the lump to recent trauma, thereby misleading the unwary. Sometimes the history suggests an acute inflammatory lesion that resembles torsion or epididymitis. Infertility is another common complaint.

2. *Metastases* to the liver, abdominal glands or bone are a later sign.

3. *Endocrine*. Gynaecomastia may be associated with any variety of testicular tumour. Gonadotrophins are found in the urine in about one-third of patients with testicular tumours. When HCG-like activity can be detected in plasma or urine it is likely that functioning chorionic elements will be found in the tumour, the prognosis then being poor. Response to therapy can sometimes be monitored by following the levels of HCG. In some patients with seminomas, pituitary gonadotrophin-like activity is found in the urine and persists after removal of the tumour (in the absence of metastases). It is, thus, likely that these gonadotrophins are produced by the pituitary although the reason for this phenomenon is uncertain. It could represent response of the pituitary to testicular damage of germinal or Leydig cells, or augmentation of the pituitary gonadotrophin assay by very small amounts of HCG. Sertoli cell tumours and Leydig cell tumours

secrete oestrogens, though the latter sometimes secrete androgens.

PROGNOSIS AND TREATMENT

Treatment consists of orchidectomy followed by radiation to the areas of lymphatic drainage and abdominal glands. In patients with certain varieties of teratomas, chemotherapy with actinomycin D, methotrexate, and chlorambucil may be useful. Sertoli cell tumours are exceptionally rare and are benign. Leydig cell tumours are also uncommon and a proportion of them are benign. Some 80 per cent of patients with seminomas survive for five years after therapy. Teratomas are more malignant and the survival rate is lower.

REFERENCES

Anderson, D. C., Marshall, J. C., Galvão-Teles, A., and Corker, C. S. (1972). *Proc. roy. Soc. Med.*, **65**, 787.

Anderson, D. C., Marshall, J. C., Young, J. L., and Russell Fraser, T. (1972). *Clin. Endocr.*, **1**, 127.

Baulieu, E. E., Lasnitzki, I., and Robel, P. (1970). *Nature* (London), **219**, 1155.

Cooper, A. J., Ismail, A. A. A., Smith, C. G., and Loraine, J. A. (1970). *Brit. Med. J.*, **3**, 17.

Coppage, W. S., Jr., and Cooner, A. E. (1965). *New Eng. J. Med.*, **273**, 902.

Ellis, J. D. (1968). *Brit. J. Hosp. Med.*, **2**, 654.

Evans, J. I., Maclean, A. M., Ismail, A. A. A., and Love, D. (1971). *Proc. roy. Soc. Med.*, **64**, 841.

Faiman, C., and Winter, J. S. D. (1971). *J. Clin. Endocr.*, **33**, 186.

Johnson, J. (1968). *Brit. J. Hosp. Med.*, **2**, 661.

Kumar, R., Biggart, J. D., McEvoy, J., and McGeown, M. (1972). *Lancet*, **i**, 1212.

Liao, S., and Fang, S. (1969). *Vitamins Hormones*, **27**, 16.

Mann, T. (Ed.) (1964). *The Biochemistry of Semen and of the Ma e Reproductive Tract*. London: Methuen.

Marshall, J. C., Harsoulis, P., Anderson, D. C., McNeilly, A. S., Besser, G. M., and Hall, R. (1972). *Brit. med. J.*, **4**, 643.

Perheentupa, J., Dessypris, A., and Adlercreutz, H. (1972). *Clin. Endocr.*, **1**, 141.

Prunty, F. T. G. (1966). *Brit. med. J.*, **ii**, 605.

Rosenfield, R. L. (1971). *J. Clin. Endocr.*, **32**, 717.

Saez, J. M., Forest, M. G., Morera, A. M., and Bertrand, J. (1972)l *J. Clin. Invest.*, **51**, 1226.

Stuart Scott, L. (1968). *Brit. J. Hosp. Med.*, **2**, 644.

Van Thiel, D. H., Sherins, R. J., Myers, G. H., Jr., and De Vita, V. T., Jr. (1972). *J. Clin. Invest.*, **51**, 1009.

Vermeulen, A., Verdonck, L., Van der Straeten, M., and Orie, N. (1969). *J. Clin. Endocr.*, **29**, 1470.

Wilson, J. D., and Gloyna, R. E. (1970). *Recent Progr. Hormone Res.*, **26**, 309.

Wolstenholme, G. E. W., and O'Connor, M. (Eds) (1967). *Endocrinology of the Testis*, Ciba Foundation Colloquia on Endocrinology, Vol. 16. London: Churchill.

12

PRECOCIOUS PUBERTY

When sexual development begins before the age of ten in boys and eight in girls, the term precocious puberty may be used. This term includes true precocious puberty, in which normal hypothalamic-pituitary maturation occurs early, and pseudo-precocious puberty where secondary sexual characteristics develop in the absence of gonadal maturation. The latter condition is caused by overproduction of androgenic or oestrogenic hormones due to disease of the adrenals or gonads, or to tumours containing gonadal components, e.g. teratomas. In pseudo-precocious puberty, normal testicular or ovarian development does not occur, whereas in true precocious puberty the patient may be fertile at an early age. Pseudo-precocious puberty has largely been dealt with in Chapters 6 and 13 (adrenal tumours, congenital adrenal hyperplasia), in Chapter 11 (testicular tumours, and in Chapter 7 (ovarian tumours). Virilisation in the female and feminisation in the male are also considered elsewhere. In males, precocious sexual development is, on the whole, more serious than in females, where the cause is often unknown and the progress benign. More than 60 per cent of affected boys have significant organic disease (of the brain, adrenals or gonads) whereas only 20 per cent of girls are so affected.

Incomplete varieties of precocious puberty are termed 'precocious thelarche' (breast development) and 'precocious pubarche' (pubic and axillary hair development). They may represent a early manifestation of true precocious puberty but on other occasions occur as solitary phenomena. Their cause is unknown but they are usually benign.

VARIETIES OF TRUE PRECOCITY

1. *Constitutional*

2. *Symptomatic*

   (*a*) 'Pineal tumours', hypothalamic hamartomas, neurofibromas, astrocytomas, ganglioneuromas, ependymomas, infundibulomas, and chorionepitheliomas.

   (*b*) After encephalitis, after meningitis, arrested hydrocephalus, toxoplasmosis, tuberose sclerosis and degenerative encephalopathy.

   (*c*) Polyostotic fibrous dysplasia (Albright's syndrome).

   (*d*) Hypothyroidism.

   (*e*) Hepatomas and hepatoblastomas.

1. CONSTITUTIONAL

This is much more common in girls and is presumably due to early maturation of the hypothalamus.

Since the pituitary is capable of producing gonadotrophins and the gonads of producing sex hormones from an early age, it is assumed that the normal delay in the onset of puberty occurs because early in life the hypothalamus is very sensitive to gonadal hormones. Maturation of the hypothalamus may then be associated with reduced sensitivity to this feedback process. Some 10 per cent of cases of precocious puberty are familial, and this has been reported to occur in several generations where males were affected. Transmission appeared to be as a Mendelian dominant. In some patients with true precocious puberty, minor abnormalities can be detected by electroencephalography, increased slow waves, and/or paroxysmal activity being found.

2. SYMPTOMATIC

'*Pineal tumours*'. Tumours in the region of the pineal gland most often cause precocious puberty by causing pressure on the hypothalamus. They include pineal tumours such as pineocytomas or pineoblastomas, and teratomas which are found more often in this region than true pineal tumours.

Hypothalamic hamartomas are collections of nerve cells in the posterior hypothalamus. They may cause precocious puberty and, later, evidence of hypothalamic compression with all its sequelae. Whether they have any hormonal capacity, e.g. to secrete gonadotrophin-releasing factors, is as yet unknown.

Polyostotic fibrous dysplasia associated with precocious puberty is commoner in girls. Bony abnormalities at the base of the skull are unlikely to be responsible. The condition is recognised by the typical X-ray appearances of the bones (which may be localised), by areas of skin pigmentation and occasionally by hyperthyroidism.

Hypothyroidism in children is very rarely associated with precocious puberty, and occasionally enlargement of the pituitary fossa, increased skin pigmentation, and galactorrhoea may also be present. The underlying pathogenesis of these features is unknown, but a likely possibility is that hypothyroidism interferes with hypothalamic function and impairs the normal tonic inhibition exerted by this area on the pituitary. Reduced secretion of prolactin-inhibiting factor (PIF) may lead to galactorrhoea, and a reduction of melanocyte-stimulating hormone inhibitory factor (MSH-IF) may cause increased skin pigmentation.

CLINICAL FEATURES AND DIAGNOSIS

The manifestation of precocious sexual development may appear shortly after birth. In boys, penile growth or the development of pubic hair are the earliest findings. Muscular and skeletal development progress rapidly and there may be precocious sexual activity, though this is not invariably the case. Premature epiphyseal fusion leads to a reduction in the ultimate height. In girls, premature breast development, growth of pubic hair, and even menstruation may be seen at an early age.

The first step is to distinguish between true and pseudo-precocious puberty. In the latter, testicular development in the male is not advanced, and spermatogenesis cannot be demonstrated by prostatic smears or testicular biopsy. Evidence of lesions in the hypothalamic region should be sought. A history of headache, somnolence, polyuria, mental retardation or epilepsy may be observed. Very rarely, obesity may be seen. The visual fields and fundi should be examined and the cranial nerves should be tested with particular care. Reduction of upward gaze or ocular palsies may indicate pressure on the upper brain stem. Hormonal studies may be helpful. Elevation of the urinary 17-oxosteroids is found in most variants of congenital adrenal hyperplasia though levels approaching those found in pubertal males are seen in some children with true precocious puberty. In children with true precocious puberty levels of serum LH and FSH are significantly higher than in normal prepubertal children.

The bone age should be determined and a skull X-ray performed looking for evidence of raised intracranial pressure, suprasellar calcification or of Albright's syndrome. An electroencephalogram may help to localise a cerebral lesion. Air encephalography is sometimes indicated, particularly in boys, if there is any hint of an organic brain lesion.

Tumours of the testis are usually obvious on clinical examination, and tumours of the adrenal causing pseudo-precocious puberty will also increase 17-oxosteroid output. Tumours of the adrenal may sometimes produce oestrogens causing pseudo-precocity in the female and feminisation in the male, but these are very rare. The investigations to be carried out in a patient suspected of having an adrenal tumour are discussed in Chapter 6, and include flat X-ray of the abdomen, intravenous pyelogram with tomography, and peri-renal oxygen insufflation. In both sexes, precocious puberty may rarely be caused by the highly malignant chorion-epithelioma, a type of teratoma affecting the testis or ovary. In both cases a tumour mass will usually be evident. The urinary gonadotrophin levels are grossly elevated and pregnancy tests based on the effects of chorionic gonadotrophin are positive. Such tumours are highly malignant and radical surgical removal should be carried out. Metastases may be treated palliatively by radiotherapy or cytotoxic drugs.

In the female, the tumours that may produce pseudo-precocity by their secretion of oestrogens are the granulosa and, more rarely, the theca cell tumours, and the luteoma. An abdominal mass may be palpable, but apart from this, the signs present are simply those of sexual precocity. Rectal examination, under sedation or under general anaesthesia if necessary, should be done to exclude ovarian lesions and to assess uterine size. The diagnosis depends on the demonstration of persistently elevated urinary oestrogen levels with low or absent urinary gonadotrophins. In the absence of an abdominal mass, these findings should be confirmed on several occasions before laparotomy is recommended. Rarely, signs of precocity or of feminisation may be produced by exogenous oestrogens. These will seldom, if ever, be given therapeutically to pre-pubertal children, but pharmaceutical preparations may occasionally be contaminated by oestrogens, particularly if oestrogen-containing compounds have been made in the same tablet press. A little 'detective work' on the part of the physician may be necessary to elucidate this cause of pseudo-precocity.

TREATMENT

Whereas pseudo-precocious puberty is commonly amenable to therapy, albeit palliative, true precocious puberty is rarely treatable. The constitutional variety requires no specific therapy once organic disease has been excluded, beyond reassurance of the parents and child. Psychological management is important but need not necessarily involve more than sympathetic handling of the problem by the physician. It should be remembered that some children are fertile, and care should be taken to avoid the consequence of this. A trial of long-acting progestational agents may sometimes arrest precocious sexual development by suppressing gonadotrophin output. Agents such as 17-hydroxyprogesterone caproate have been used, particularly to suppress menstruation. Organic brain lesions are usually so inaccessible as to be unamenable to surgery, though, rarely, pineal tumours respond to external radiation or local implantation with radioactive seeds. Hypothyroidism is the one treatable variety of precocious puberty, development halting with the institution of thyroid hormone medication.

REFERENCE

Raiti, S. (1970). *Brit. J. Hosp. Med.*, June, p. 873:

13

DISORDERS OF SEX DIFFERENTIATION

It is difficult to formulate a satisfactory definition of male or female, and in most countries there does not appear to be any clear legal definition. Maleness or femaleness may be assessed from at least five viewpoints, namely, chromosomal constitution or karyotype, gonadal type, bodily configuration or phenotype, chemical or hormonal make-up, and psychological attitude. Humans are, in fact, bimodally distributed so that the majority form clusters in approximately equal proportions about the areas known as 'male' and 'female', but between these areas there is a continuum in which particular individuals exhibit mixed characteristics, some of which would be called 'male' and some 'female'. In order to understand this situation, and in particular in order to unravel the various clinical problems that may present, it is necessary to understand various general principles as they affect the human. Although of great importance, the psychological aspects will not be specifically dealt with, for as knowledge stands at present, they lie to a large extent outside the subject matter of this book. It should be noted that hormonal influences undoubtedly play a part in the increase in sexual drive and activity that occurs at puberty. There is no evidence that the *direction* of sexual orientation is influenced in the human by the sex hormones at puberty, or in adult life. However, there is evidence that the direction of sexual orientation after puberty may be determined by the hormonal situation during fetal life in monkeys (Young *et al.*, 1964), or about the time of birth in rats (Harris and Levine, 1965).

The development of the organs of sex in embryonic life, and at puberty, is dependent on a series of events that occur in an orderly sequence. It is usual to distinguish between *sex determination* and *sex differentiation*, the former being decided by the sex chromosome content of the fertilising sperm.

SEX DETERMINATION

Normal spermatoza have 23 chromosomes, including either one X or one Y chromosome. Normal ova have 23 chromosomes, including a single X chromosome. The fertilised ovum or zygote is, therefore, normally either 46XY = 'male' or 46XX = 'female'. Abnormalities due to the presence of abnormal numbers of chromosomes are seen from time to time. Anomalies of structure of the chromosomes also occur.

The 46 chromosomes of the somatic cells form

the diploid set, and can be regarded as 23 homologous pairs, the ovum having contributed one haploid set of 23 chromosomes, and the spermatozoon a genetically equivalent haploid set. During *mitosis*, the members of each pair act independently, but in *meiosis* they behave as a pair, first meeting and then moving to opposite daughter cells as the cell divides. The cycle of chromosome activity in *mitosis* is as follows. After cell division, i.e. in interphase, each chromosome is a single, very long strand or thread. The process of DNA replication divides their length. It is this stage that is usually chosen to make illustrations of the human chromosomes (Fig. 13.1). As the cell begins division, the centromere of each chromosome divides and the chromatids of each are pulled to opposite poles of the cell (the centromere leading) and so to opposite daughter cells arising from the division. The process of DNA replication is then repeated and the chromosome becomes double-stranded again. Nondisjunctional anomalies arise when both chromatids of a chromosome move into the same daughter cell at cell division, or when one chromatid moves too slowly, 'lags', and fails to become included in the nucleus of its daughter cell and so, failing to be replicated, is lost. Thus, a cell that had an X and a Y chromosome could give rise to two daughter cells, one being XYY and the other XO, 'O' indicating absence of a chromosome. Or, in the case of chromatid lagging, a dividing XY cell could produce an XY cell and an XO cell. Nondisjunctional anomalies of mitosis will produce 'mosaics' in which some cells have one chromosome constitution and some cells another, e.g. 45*XO*/46*XY*, unless the abnormal division occurs very early in development, when one cell line may be included entirely in extra-embryonic tissues—amnion, chorion, etc. (Fig. 13.4). One form of structural anomaly occurs at mitosis, isochromosome formation. The defect arises because the centromere divides horizontally instead of longitudinally. The effect is to give both chromatids from one side of the centromere to one daughter cell, and both chromatids from the other side to the other (Figs. 13.5 and 13.6). It frequently happens that one product is lost. An isochromosome has one arm of the normal chromosome represented twice (duplicated) while the other arm is absent (deleted)'

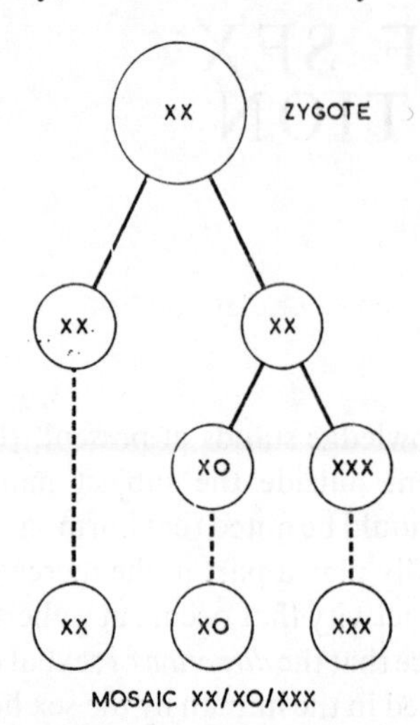

FIGURE 13.4 Diagrammatic representation of possible results of nondisjunction involving an X chromosome in an XX cell

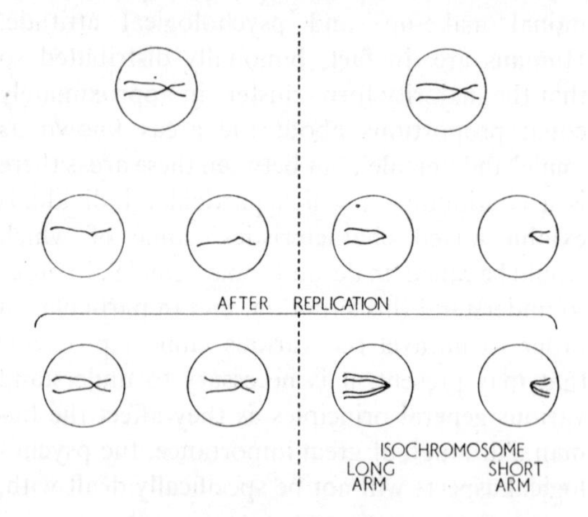

FIGURE 13.5 Normal chromosome division on the left and isochromosome formation from horizontal division of the centromere on the right

Other structural anomalies arise during interphase. The simplest case is when part of a chromosome is broken off and, failing to reunite before the cell divides, the part is lost. 'Deletions' are

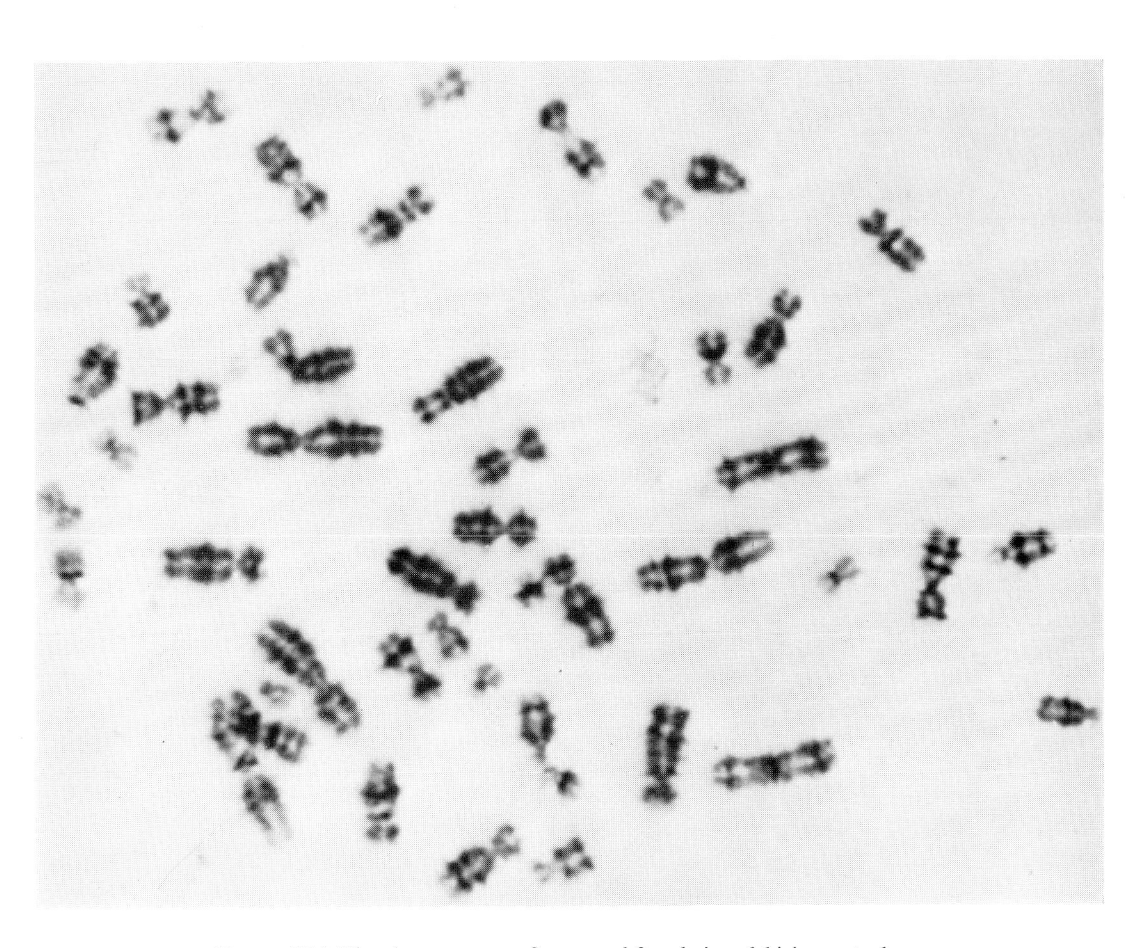

FIGURE 13.1 The chromosomes of a normal female in colchicine metaphase, stained by a 'banding' technique

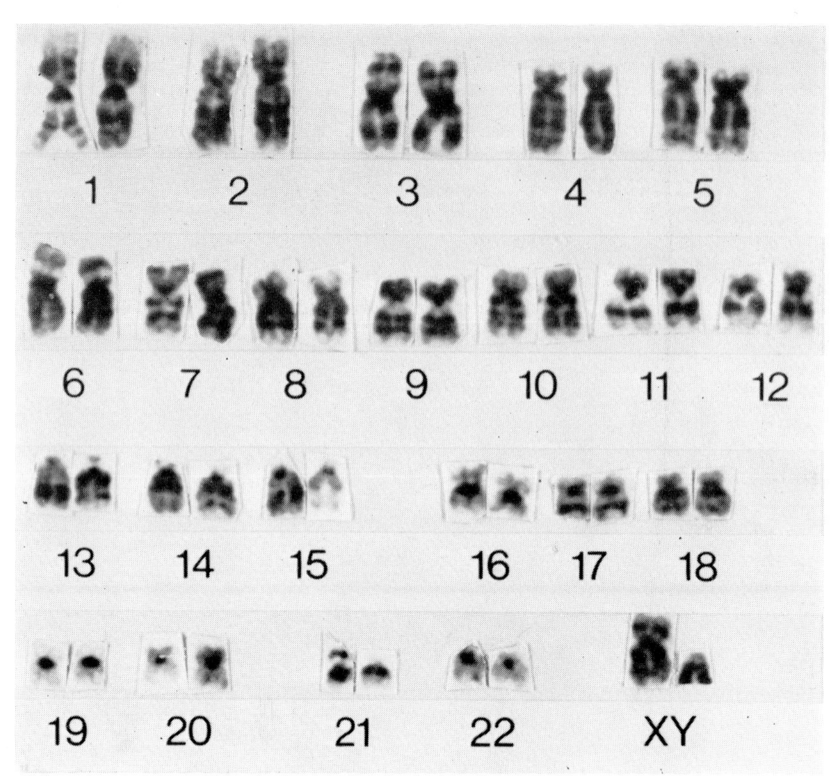

FIGURE 13.2 The chromosomes of a normal male

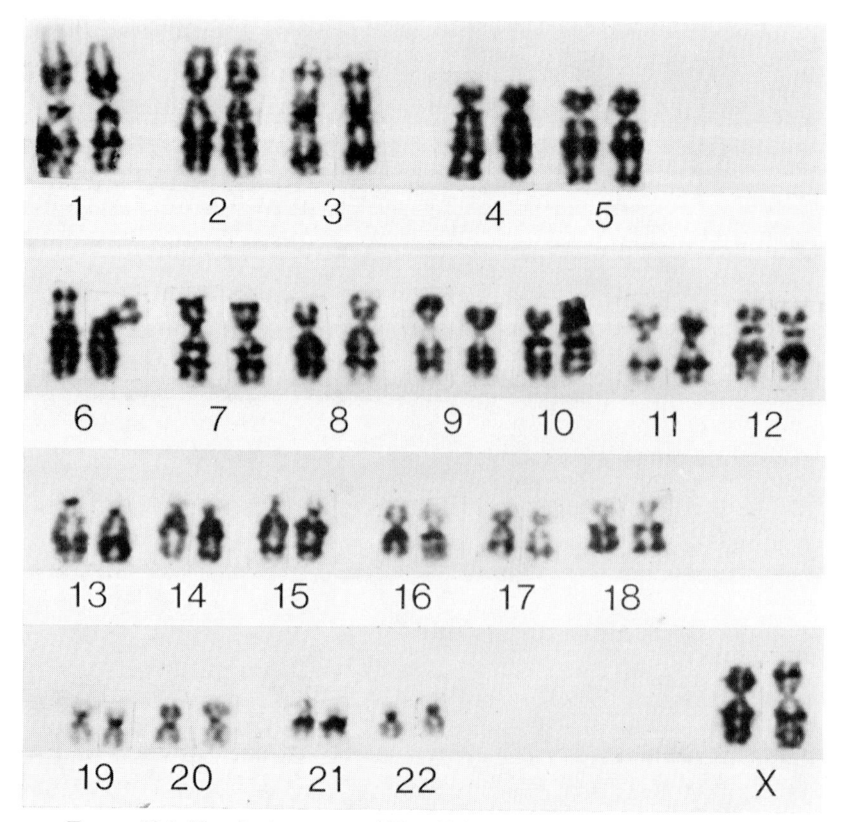

FIGURE 13.3 The chromosomes of Fig. 13.1 arranged to show the karyotype of a normal female

formed in this way. Two-break events produce more complex anomalies. When one chromosome suffers two breaks, one on each side of the contromere, the 'raw ends' of the piece containing the centromere may unite, so forming a ring chromosome; the fragments without the centromere are lost at the next cell division. If one break

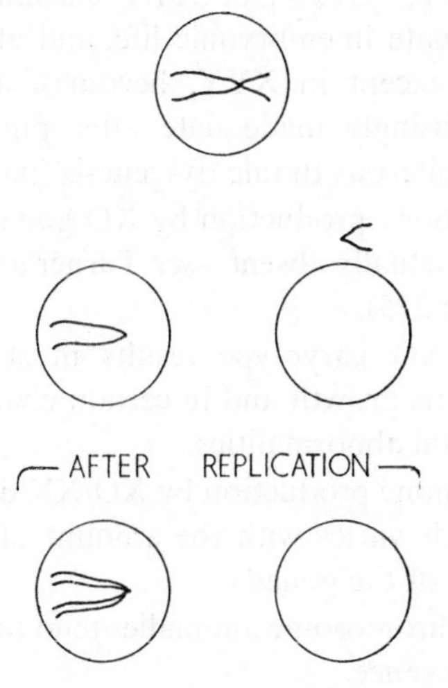

FIGURE 13.6 Isochromosome formation with loss of one of the products of division resulting in a mosaic

occurs in one chromosome and another break in a different chromosome the fragments may reunite to the 'wrong' chromosome, so producing a translocation or interchange.

The two successive divisions preceding the formation of the ovum or spermatozoon form the *meiotic* divisions—meiosis I and meiosis II. The essentials of meiosis I are: (i) pairing of homologous chromosomes, (ii) interchange of material between chromatids of homologues at 'chiasmata', (iii) movement of whole chromosomes to opposite poles of the cell, thus separating members of homologous pairs when the cell divides. This reduces the number of chromosomes from 46 to 23 and, in the male, separates X and Y. The next division, or meiosis II, resembles mitosis in that each chromosome divides into its two chromatids which move into opposite daughter cells, but, because of the interchange or crossing over that occurred in the chiasmata in meiosis I, the chromatids are not genetically identical.

In the female, all cells of the sex line (the primary oocytes) have entered the pairing stage of meiosis I by the 5th month of fetal life. The chromosomes remain paired until the 'ovum' is about to be shed at ovulation. The remaining stages of the first meiotic division are completed just before ovulation. Meiosis II occurs after penetration by the fertilising spermatozoon. In the male, meiosis I is closely followed by meiosis II. The spermatids arising from meiosis II mature over some weeks without further division into spermatozoa. The pairing of X and Y is precarious, in fact they touch only at their ends instead of throughout their length, as in the case of the X pair in the female, or the autosomes in either sex. For this reason, the X and Y may separate prematurely and, not moving reciprocally, may move to the same daughter cell at meiosis I.

Nondisjunctional abnormalities of meiosis I or II in spermatogenesis or öogenesis may lead to formation of zygotes with abnormal sex chromosomes, as shown in the table

TABLE 13.1

Karyotype or sex chromosomes of abnormal zygote	Gonad	Estimated frequency at birth
XO	Fibrous 'streak'	1:2,500 female phenotypes
XXX	Ovary	1:1,500 female phenotypes
XXXX	Sterile ovary	Very rare—female phenotype
XXXXX	Sterile ovary	Very rare—female phenotype
XXY	Sterile testis	1:700 male phenotypes
XXXY	Sterile testis	Rare—male phenotypes
XXXXY	Sterile testis	Very rare—male phenotype or intersex
XXYY	Sterile testis	1:5,000 male phenotypes
XYY	Fertile testis	1:500 male phenotypes

Abnormalities of cell division during very early development of the embryo can also lead to loss or gain of a chromosome. In this case, the embryo may be formed of two or three cell lines of different chromosome content and is called a mosaic, the commonest type in relation to the sex chromosomes being XO/XY; XO/XX is also relatively common.

Loss of *part* of a sex chromosome may also occur with effects broadly the same as loss of a whole sex chromosome.

Analysis of cases of sex chromosome anomaly has led to the following conclusions:

1. At least one X chromosome is necessary for life.
2. The action of the sex chromosomes in sexual development is exerted solely on the gonad.
3. Two X chromosomes are necessary for a functioning ovary.
4. A Y chromosome will form a testis if one, two, three, or even four X chromosomes are present, but if more than one X is present the testis will be structurally abnormal and sterile.
5. In mosaics, the development of the gonad depends on the sex chromosome content of the gonad, e.g. an XO/XY mosaic may have fibrous streak gonads (both being XO) or have one testis (XY) and one streak gonad (XO).
6. Hormone production by testes with XXY, XXXY, XXYY, or XYY chromosomes is adequate in embryonic life, and at puberty, but, except in XYY, becomes, as a rule, increasingly inadequate after puberty—*see* seminiferous tubule dysgenesis (page 252).
7. Hormone production by XO gonads is usually virtually absent—*see* Turner's syndrome (page 275).
8. The XO karyotype results in stunting of somatic growth and in certain characteristic skeletal abnormalities.
9. Hormone production by XO/XX or XO/XY gonads varies with the amount of development of the gonads.
10. Sex chromosome anomalies tend to diminish intelligence.

SEX DIFFERENTIATION AND EMBRYONIC SEX DEVELOPMENT

Development of the organs of sex apart from the gonads is not directly dependent on the sex chromosome content of the cells. Three stages of development are described each with its own type of control (Fig. 13.7).

STAGE I: THE UNDIFFERENTIATED STAGE (Figures 13.8, 13.9, 13.10)

The gonad shows no differentiation into testis or ovary until the 8th week of development. The other primordial organs of sex are undifferentiated until the 9th week. At this conception age (11th week menstrual age) the state of development is as follows:

1. There is a comparatively large phallus (penis/clitoris and labia minora).
2. There are swellings at each side of the phallus called the labioscrotal folds.
3. The urinary bladder and proximal part of the urethra are recognisable but the latter opens to the exterior at the base of the phallus—as in the adult female. A deep groove extends forwards on the ventral aspect of the phallus, foreshadowing the later inclusion of the distal part of the urethra in the penis in the male.
4. Running down the posterior wall of the abdomen on each side there is a duct—the mesonephric duct (Wolffian duct—WD)—which opens into the posterior part of the urethra. The lower part of this duct occupies a position like the end of the adult vas deferens; its upper part is anterior to the ureter. The WD has already given off a bud which has grown

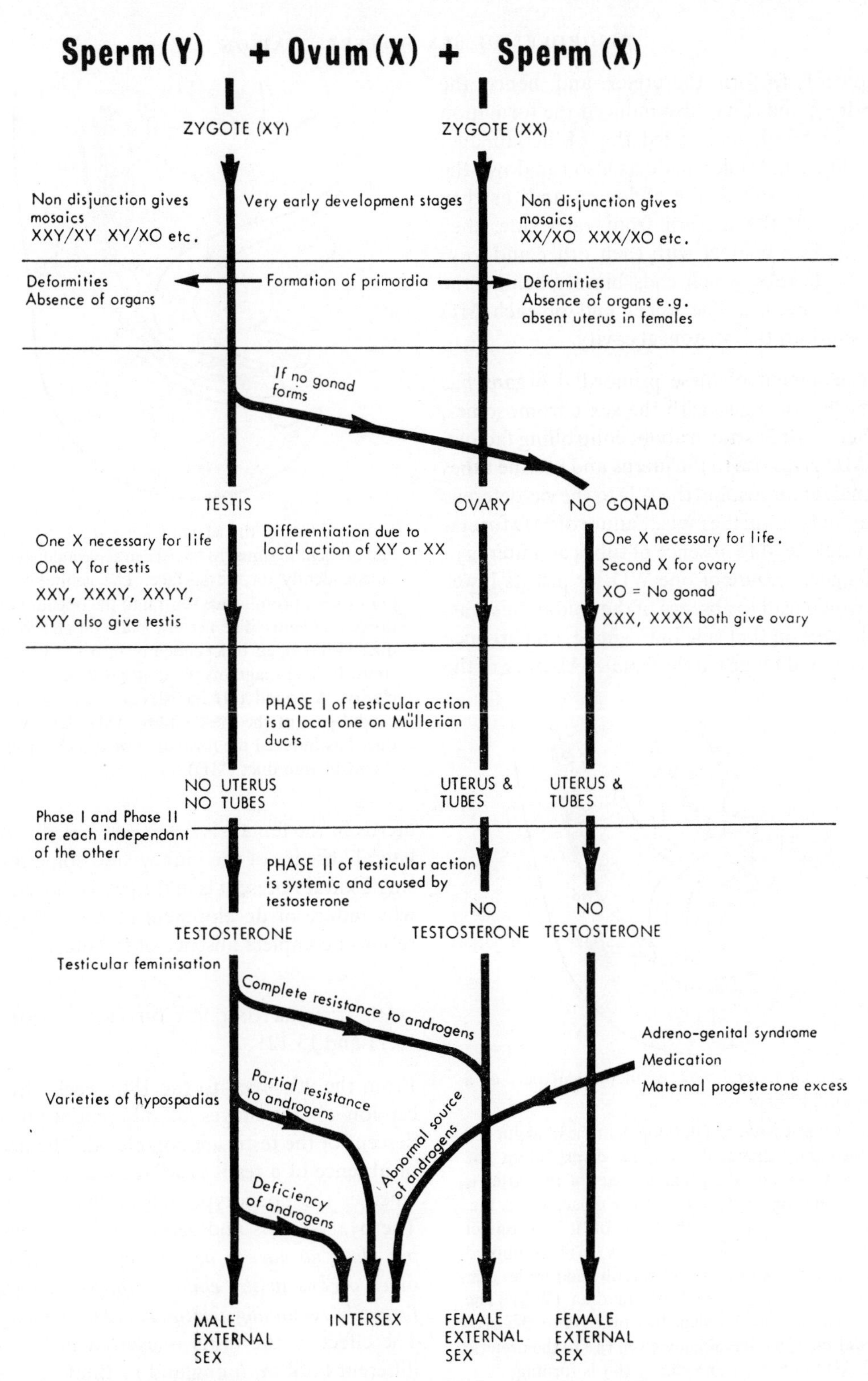

FIGURE 13.7 Summary of the stages of sexual development, the controlling factors involved and abnormalities that may arise

upwards to form the ureter, and, hence, the kidney, and it has also induced the formation of a second duct called the Müllerian duct (MD). The Müllerian ducts also run down the posterior wall of the abdomen and, as they approach the urethra from each side, they come into contact with each other and form a single tube which ends blindly behind the lower urethra. The upper end of each MD opens into the peritoneal cavity.

Development of these primordial organs has not been associated with the sex chromosomes, and very little is known about controlling factors. The MD gives rise to the uterus and uterine tubes in female embryos, and the WD to the vas deferens and epididymis in the male. Failure of MD formation would lead to absence of tubes and uterus in the female. Failure of one WD, or just its lower end, would lead to absence of the epididymis, vas, and kidney on that side in the male, and absence of uterus and kidney in the female. Absence of the uterus in the female is often associated with unilateral absence of the kidney, and sometimes the single kidney present is in the pelvis. It is not clear why failure of development of one MD should result in complete absence of the uterus.

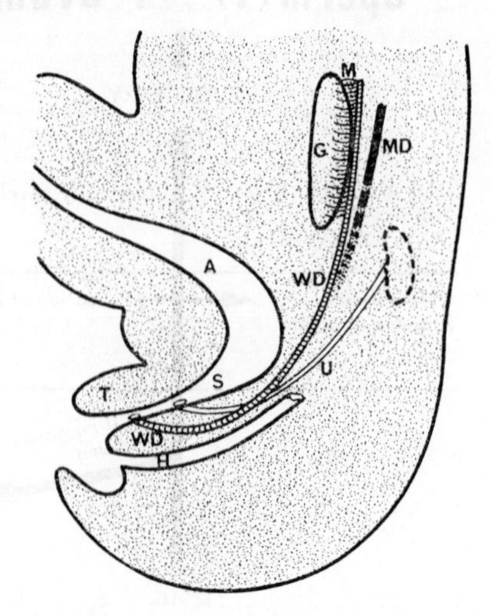

FIGURE 13.9 By the seventh week the hind gut (H) and urogenital sinus (S) have been separated and open independently on the surface. The genital tubercle (T) forms a prominence ventral to the opening of the urogenital sinus. The ureteric bud (U) and Wolffian duct (WD) open independently into the urogenital sinus. In later diagrams the ureter will be omitted for clarity. A gonad (G) has developed alongside the caudal part of the mesonephros (M). The Wolffian duct has induced the formation of the upper part of the Müllerian duct (MD)

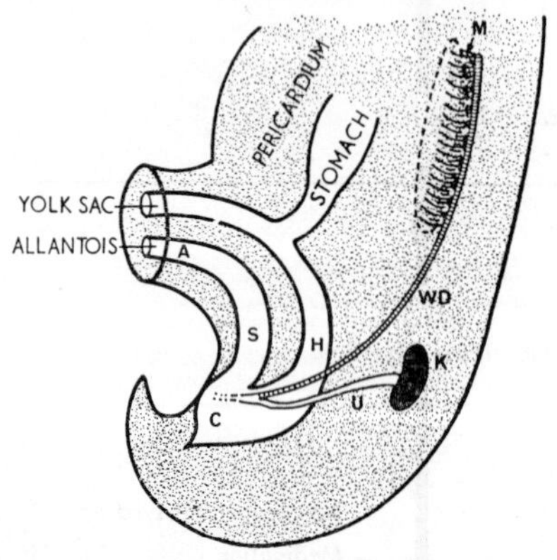

FIGURE 13.8 Lateral view of the caudal part of a fifth week embryo

During the fifth week of development the hind gut (H) is becoming separated from its diverticulum the allantois (A), and the proximal part of the latter is called the urogenital sinus (S). The cloaca (C) is the, as yet, undivided part of the hind gut; it is in contact with the exterior. The mesonephros (M) is composed of a number of kidney-like glomeruli and tubules that open into its duct, the Wolffian duct (WD). The lower end of the Wolffian duct opens into the urogenital sinus and has already given rise to the ureteric bud (U) from which the kidney (K) is forming

STAGE II: EMBRYONIC SEX DIFFERENTIATION (Figs 13.11 and 13.12)

From the 9th week to the 18th week after conception all the stages of differentiation except descent of the testis are completed. The presence or absence of a testis is what usually determines whether the phenotype will be male or female. The ovary forms and grows in female embryos *but plays no part in organising differentiation of other organs in the embryo, for when no gonad forms the remaining genitalia take the female form.* The effect of the testis is exerted in two ways, different both in timing and method.

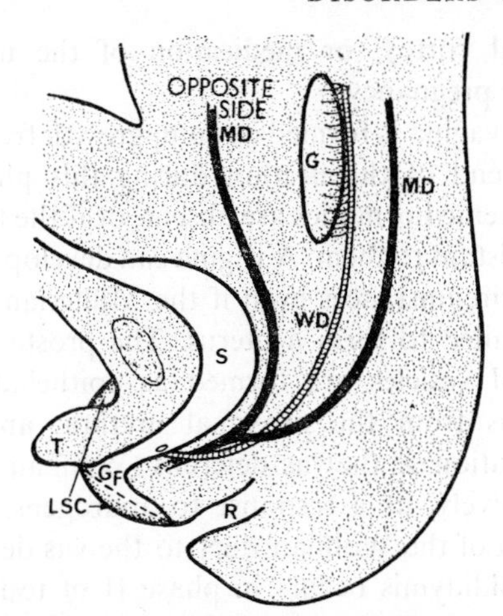

FIGURE 13.10 At the end of the indifferent stage (eighth week) the WD has completed the induction of the Müllerian duct (MD). The upper end of each MD opens into the primitive peritoneal cavity while the lower ends meet, fuse and lie behind the lower part of the urogenital sinus (S). The genital tubercle (T) has continued to grow, has split antero-posteriorly on its caudal aspect forming the genital folds (GF). A fold of skin, the labio-scrotal fold (LSC) surrounds the genital tubercle and the opening of the urogenital sinus. The lower end of the hind gut now forms the rectum (R)

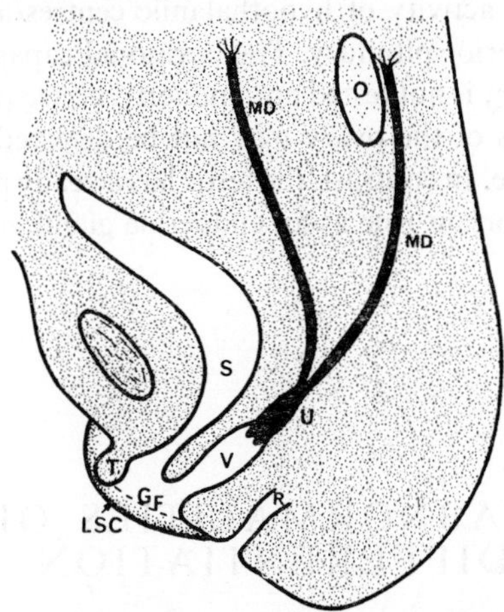

FIGURE 13.11 When a testis has not formed, female development is well advanced by the end of the fourth month. An upgrowth from the urogenital sinus has formed a vagina (V) and the fused Müllerian ducts have formed a uterus which opens into the vagina. The openings of the urethra and vagina to the exterior are flanked by the genital folds (labia minora) and labio-scrotal folds (labia majora). The genital tubercle has formed the clitoris

Phase 1 of testicular action is exerted on the Müllerian ducts and leads to their suppression. This action is local, i.e. each testis acts on its own side only. The suppressive action is not mediated by testosterone or other androgenic hormones, and Jost (1950) demonstrated in the rabbit that

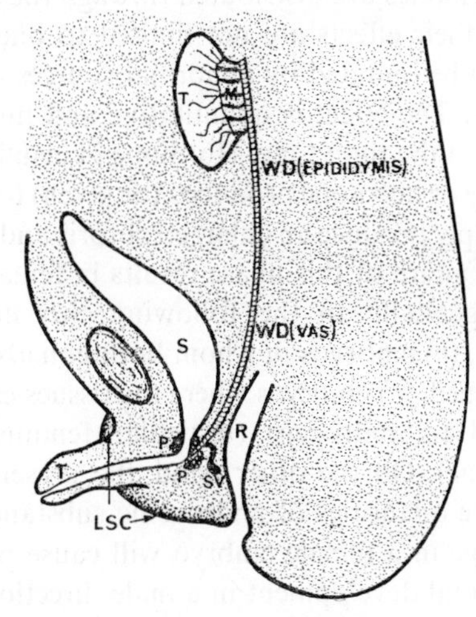

FIGURE 13.12 When testes have formed the normal male fetal development is almost complete by the fifth month. The split part of the genital tubercle (T) has 'healed' so forming the proximal penile urethra. The latter has joined an ingrowth from the tip of the genital tubercle so that the urethra traverses the glans penis. The urogenital sinus has given off buds to form the prostate (P) and the WD has differentiated to form the vas deferens and epididymis. The seminal vesicle (SV) is a bud from the lower end of WD. The seminiferous tubules of the testis (T) have anastomosed with the tubules of the mesonephros (M). The testis will descend into the scrotum (LSC) after the seventh month

implantation of testicular tissue into distant sites was ineffective in suppressing the Müllerian duct. This phase occurs between the 9th and 10th week of development. Isolated failure of this phase in a male embyo (with subsequent testicular development) leads to an apparently normal male child with a uterus; the testes would be attached to the uterus by the gubernaculum (cf. ligament of ovary), and usually only one descends to the scrotum, although it can sometimes pull the other testis and the uterus after it into a hernia.

Phase 2 of testicular action runs from the end of the 10th week and is complete at the 18th week, except for descent of the testis in the 8th month. This phase is dependent on androgenic hormones produced by the fetal testes, which have by now developed conspicuous clumps of interstitial cells. The hormones are distributed through the circulation; their effects are not limited to one side, and can be imitated by abnormal sources of androgens. The effect is quantitative and must be exerted at the right time. Hormone in insufficient quantity or hormone produced (or given) too late will simply produce an enlarged clitoris and not a penis. Failure of this phase results in female external genitalia in the following: (*a*) normal females, (*b*) embryos in whom both gonads have not formed, (*c*) embryos where the tissues cannot respond to androgens (testicular feminisation syndrome). On the other hand, the presence of excessive quantities of androgenic substances at this stage in a female embryo will cause phallic and scrotal development in a male direction.

Thus, examination of the external genitalia in cases of indeterminate sex, cannot give enough information to decide between the three possibilities: (*a*) the child is 'male' but production of fetal testicular androgens was insufficient for normal development; (*b*) the child is 'male' but the tissues are incapable of making an adequate response to androgens; (*c*) the child is 'female' but there has been an abnormal source of androgens, e.g. adrenal cortex, or medication of the mother during pregnancy.

The vagina is formed as an upgrowth from the lower end of the urethra during this phase if androgenic hormones are absent, or if the tissues are resistant to them. A vagina can develop under these circumstances even if the Müllerian ducts have failed to form a uterus. The prostate and seminal vesicles are formed as epithelial outgrowths from the proximal urethra, and the termination of the vas deferens (Wolffian duct), respectively, as a response to androgens. Conversion of the Wolffian duct to the vas deferens and epididymis occurs in phase II of testicular action.

STAGE III: PUBERTY

The immediate causes of the changes of puberty are androgens from the testis in the male, and oestrogens and progestogens in the female, though androgens from the adrenal cortex also play a part. These glands are stimulated by increased activity of hypothalamic centres and of the anterior pituitary. The hormonal capacity of the ovary is not tested until puberty, consequently agenesis of the ovary may not be detected until this time. In contrast, the testis has already played an important role as an endocrine gland, in fetal life.

CLINICAL FEATURES OF THE ABNORMALITIES OF SEX DETERMINATION AND DIFFERENTIATION

DETECTION OF CHROMOSOMAL ABNORMALITIES

The first step in the detection of a sex chromosome abnormality in man is to examine a smear from the oral mucosa, suitably fixed and stained. According to the strictness of the criteria and methods used, some 30 per cent or more of the nuclei of the cells from normal females show a separate mass of chromatin near the nuclear membrane (Fig. 13.13). This appearance was first described by Barr and Bertram (1949) in nerve cells of female cats, and the body is known as a 'Barr body'; individuals in whom many cells contain a Barr body are said to be chromatin positive (not female). Normal males are chromatin negative, for hardly any of their cells contain a separate chromatin mass resembling a Barr body; but chromatin-negative persons are not necessarily male. Occasionally, patients are found whose cells contain more than one Barr body and, in general, chromosomal analysis reveals that the maximum number of Barr bodies is always one less than the number of X chromosomes (Fig. 13.14). It is almost certain that the Barr body represents a large activated part of an X chromosome. Barr bodies of abnormal size may occur in individuals with morphologically abnormal X chromosomes. It has been suggested by Lyon (1961) that one of the X chromosomes is inactivated in female cells and that two different lines of cells may occur, one of which has the paternal and the other the maternal X chromosome inactivated. All females may thus be regarded as mosaics in respect of the X chromosome. The Y chromosome may be displayed in buccal smears that have been stained, by, e.g. quinacrine, and examined under ultra-violet light. It appears as a brightly fluorescent body.

The second step in the detection process is to determine the karyotype. Cultures of peripheral blood lymphocytes, or fibroblasts, or

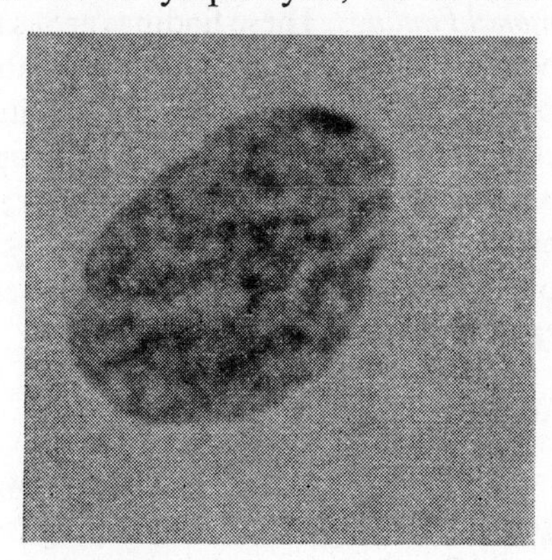

FIGURE 13.13 The nucleus of a female cell showing the Barr body

other cells in appropriate media are made to provide large numbers of dividing cells—or blood-forming bone marrow may be examined without culture. When the culture contains many dividing cells they can be processed to display their chromosomes. The steps usually taken are: (1) colchicine is added in order to prevent cells completing cell division; (2) a few hours later the cells are transferred to hypotonic KCl solution in order to make the cells swell by imbibing water; (3) after a few minutes, when the chromosomes will have dispersed in the swollen cell, the material

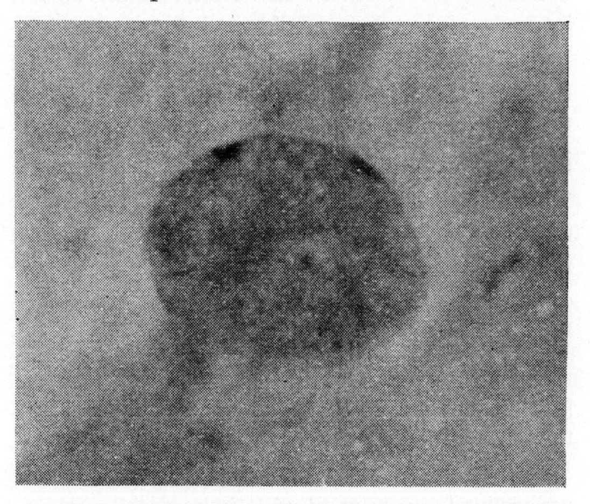

FIGURE 13.14 The nucleus of a cell from an XXXY male showing two Barr bodies

is fixed by transferring it to a mixture of methanol and acetic acid; (4) a drop of cells suspended in fixative is placed on a clean dry slide. As the fixative evaporates, the cell is stretched and flattened so that in many cells the chromosomes may be seen clearly under the microscope.

The chromosomes (Fig. 13.2) are classified according to their length '1' being the longest and '22' the smallest. The position of the centromere provides an additional method of identification, although these criteria do not allow identification of all chromosomes. In routine preparations, only the 1st, 2nd, 3rd, 16th pairs and the Y are individually recognisable, the remainder fall into groups, i.e. B = 4th and 5th, C = 6th–12th, D = 13th–15th, E = 17th–18th, F = 19th–20th, and G = 21st–22nd. The X chromosome is indistinguishable from other members of the C group (Fig. 13.3). There are specialised techniques which allow identification of all the chromosomes individually.

ABNORMALITIES ASSOCIATED WITH A MALE PHENOTYPE

SEX CHROMOSOME ANOMALIES

KARYOTYPE 47XXY

These are cases of chromatin positive Klinefelter's syndrome (*see* p. 252) (Klinefelter *et al.*, 1948). Surveys of new-born children indicate that the karyotype 47XXY is present in 1:700 of all male births. Testicular function is adequate during fetal life so the cases will usually be unsuspected during infancy and childhood. Non-descent of the testes, with or without hypospadias, may lead to their discovery before puberty although the association is probably fortuitous. The extra sex chromosome commonly causes some diminution of intelligence but frank mental deficiency is rare. Testosterone secretion is less than normal during and after puberty, and virtually all cases are sterile, but they are not impotent. These patients often marry. Homosexuality is not a feature but some subtle difference from normal male behaviour, perhaps lack of aggression and drive, seems to be the most likely reason for the frequency with which their mothers or wives initiate investigation. The only constant sign is the extremely small testes.

MOSAIC KARYOTYPE 47XXY/46XY

The presence of some cells of normal male karyotype tends to reduce the severity of the syndrome. Mosaics may be fertile.

KARYOTYPES 48XXXY AND 49XXXXY

The extra X chromosomes usually cause mental deficiency. Patients with four X chromosomes are very rare.

KARYOTYPE 46XX IN MALES

A few per cent of cases of chromatin-positive Klinefelter's syndrome are found to have a normal female karyotype. They differ from the 47XXY cases in two respects: intelligence is likely to be normal, and they are shorter rather than taller than average. But in general they resemble other cases of Klinefelter's syndrome.

It may be that these patients have a crucial part of a Y chromosome translocated into one of their X chromosomes. It is interesting to note, however, that in goats and mice, XX males also occur as an abnormality, and in these animals genetic analysis has shown that an abnormal autosomal gene of a classical Mendelian type is responsible, having as it were usurped the action of Y. In goats the gene is recessive, in mice it is a dominant.

MALE TURNER'S SYNDROME

A few patients have been described who are phenotypically male, but who possess some of the somatic abnormalities characteristic of Turner's syndrome (*see* p. 275). The testes are usually small and show changes somewhat similar to those found in tubular dysgenesis. Chromosomal analysis shows them to have a sex chromosome content of XY. Presumably, there are abnormalities in a sex chromosome that cannot be detected by present methods.

Hormonal Findings. These findings are as might be expected when the gonads are unable to develop fully. There is a tendency for the pituitary to secrete increased quantities of gonadotrophins, and measurements of the production rate of testosterone in a number of cases have shown them to be below normal or at the lower end of the normal range.

TREATMENT

Most individuals with these syndromes will require treatment with a testosterone preparation. This should be done, not only to bring about further sexual maturation, but because of the generally beneficial metabolic effects of the hormone, particularly on muscle, bone, and other tissues. The preparations can be given orally, by injection, or by subcutaneous implantation in the form of pellets (*see* Chapter 11).

ABNORMALITIES ASSOCIATED WITH A FEMALE PHENOTYPE

OVARIAN DYSGENESIS (TURNER'S SYNDROME)

Turner (1938) described a series of patients with diminished sexual development, webbing of the neck, and bilateral cubitus vulgus, and Wilkins and Fleischmann (1944) found that such individuals had no ovaries, the gonad being represented merely by a whitish streak of tissue on the posterior surface of the broad ligaments. The majority (80 per cent) of individuals with this syndrome are chromatin negative, and chromosomal analysis shows that most have a sex chromosome constitution consisting of only one X chromosome (45, XO).

Although this condition may sometimes be recognised at an early age because of the associated somatic defects, the commonest presenting complaint is primary amenorrhoea. Very occasionally menstruation occurs, and there have been two well-documented patients who became pregnant. As pointed out elsewhere, perfectly normal girls may not start to menstruate until about the age of 17 or 18 years, but patients with Turner's syndrome who present earlier than this will often have features that lead one to suspect the real underlying aetiology. In the first-place they are nearly always of short stature (about 4 ft 1 in. to 4 ft 10 in. at age of 14 years) and a number of characteristic skeletal abnormalities are often present. Cubitus valgus, as described by Turner, may be evident, the carrying angle being increased (Fig. 13.15); X-ray of the wrist (Fig. 13.16) may also reveal an abnormal carpal angle (mean 118° ± 6.6, normal 131.5° ± 7·2) as described by Kosowicz (1962), and there may be enlargement and deformity of the medial tibial and femoral condyles. There may be shortening of one or more of the metacarpals. The chest is often abnormal in shape, commonly being described as shield-like. The epiphyses are less developed and fuse later than in normal girls, i.e. the bone age is retarded. Apart from these skeletal abnormalities there is generally less secondary sexual development than might be expected for the age, and the breasts are usually strikingly undeveloped, the

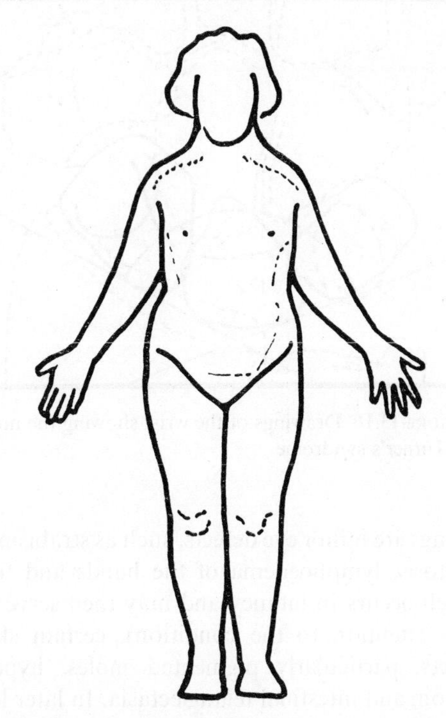

FIGURE 13.15 Diagram of patient with Turner's syndrome showing the increased carrying angle and webbing of the neck

nipples being placed wider apart on the chest than in the normal immature female. Webbing of the neck may be found (Fig. 13.15) but is by no means constantly present. Cardiovascular abnormalities are present in about 20 per cent of cases. Coarctation of the aorta has been particularly associated, but atrial, or ventricular septal defects, and aortic valvular stenosis are not unusual. There may be other congenital anomalies. Red-green colour blindness, which is an X-linked recessive character, occurs as frequently in cases of Turner's syndrome as it does in males, and therefore, is at least ten times commoner than in chromosomally normal females. Although the finding is of little diagnostic value it has been used to discover whether the single X chromosome of a case of Turner's syndrome has been inherited from her father or from her mother. Other less frequent

or XX/XO or when a ring chromosome or isochromosome is present, some gonadal development is more likely to occur. In cases of XY/XO or X ring Y karyotype there is some danger of development of seminoma in the rudimentary gonad, which could form some testicular tissue (Polani, 1968).

The internal genital organs, apart from the gonads, are usually normal, though they may be small.

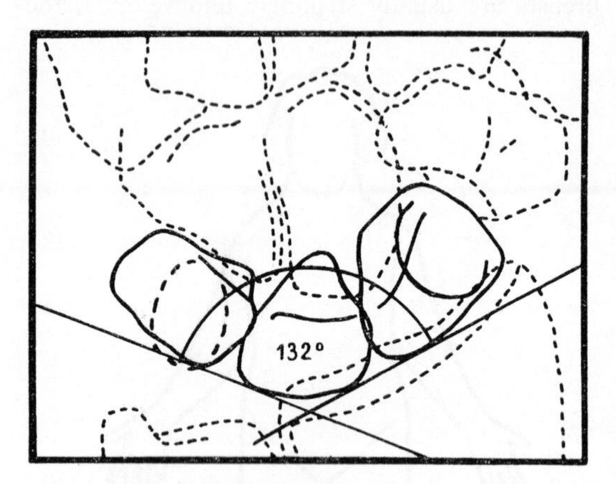

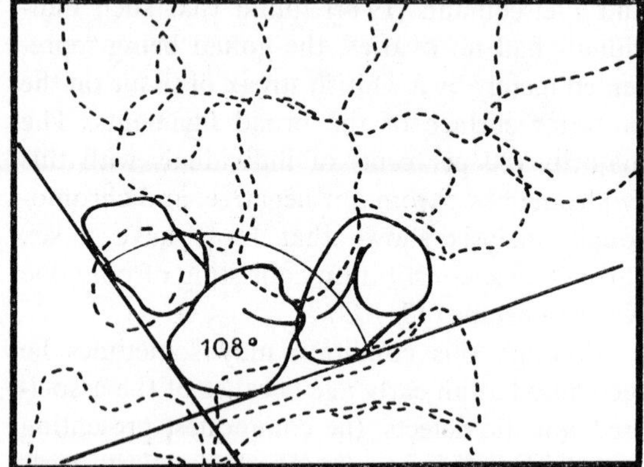

FIGURE 13.16 Drawings of the wrist showing the normal carpal angle and the reduced carpal angle characteristic of Turner's syndrome

findings are minor eye defects, such as strabismus or ptosis, lymphoedema of the hands and feet (which occurs in infancy and may then serve to draw attention to the condition), certain skin defects, particularly pigmented moles, hypertension, and intestinal telangiectasia. In later life there is a tendency for these patients to develop osteoporosis, and they assume a senile appearance at a relatively early age.

Histologically the gonads consist of longish stromal cells arranged in a wavy pattern, an appearance closely resembling the ovarian stroma. In the vast majority of patients no follicles can be found but a few are occasionally present, a finding which explains the occasional patient who menstruates, and obviously the pregnancies referred to above must have resulted from an ovulation. When the karyotype is a mosaic XY/XO

Hormonal Findings. As might be expected with diminished ovarian function, the output of gonadotrophins may be greater than normal, but this is not a universal finding. Urinary output of oestrogens is low, and sometimes a low output of 17-ketosteroids has been found, which may lead the unwary to suspect hypopituitarism. In general, studies of hormonal secretion are not of great diagnostic help.

CLINICAL DIAGNOSIS

Ovarian dysgenesis should be suspected if any of the associated somatic defects are present and in any girl of short stature with primary amenorrhoea. Only very occasionally is it found in girls of normal height with primary amenorrhoea. The crucial investigations are examination of the buccal smear and examination of the karyotype. In Turner's syndrome it will be found either that all cells examined have less than two complete sex chromosomes, or that some cells have less than two sex chromosomes. The commonest karyotype is 45XO, but mosaics 46XX/45XO or 46XY/45XO occur. In some cases a structural anomaly of an X chromosome, e.g. loss of most of the short arm may be present. Loss of the short arm of the Y chromosome in cases who would otherwise be 46XY normal male results in a female with Turner's syndrome. In general, the somatic signs are more severe in 45XO cases. The mosaic karyotype 46XX/45XO may allow some ovarian development and puberty may occur and these mosaics may be fertile. The 46XY/45XO mosaic is a special case because any gonadal development that does occur will form testicular tissue and consequently masculinisation of the genitalia may occur in these mosaics, and there is a possibility of seminoma developing. 46XY/45XO mosaics may have only 'streak' gonads with no masculinisation, the critical factors being the proportions of the two cell lines and whether any 46XY cells have formed the primordial gonad.

TREATMENT

There are usually three main problems in the management of patients with ovarian dysgenesis: (1) sexual immaturity, (2) short stature, and (3) amenorrhoea. Later, they may suffer from generalised osteoporosis, the spine in particular being affected.

The amenorrhoea is easily treated with cyclical oestrogen and progestogen therapy, and this also will produce quite a striking increase in sexual maturity, with development of the breasts and increased growth of pubic hair. However, if these hormones are given in full doses there is rapid fusion of the epiphyses and it is probably desirable, by using minimal amounts, to stimulate development more slowly and to allow growth to continue for as long as possible. Obviously, one has to achieve as satisfactory a compromise as possible in this situation. The authors usually use ethinyl oestradiol in a daily dose of 0·02 mg or 0·05 mg for cycles of twenty-four days, a progestogen such as norethisterone being given in addition for the last ten days of each cycle—a daily dose of 5 mg of norethisterone is satisfactory. Just enough ethinyl oestradiol is given to provoke withdrawal bleeding. Stilboestrol is avoided because it tends to cause deep pigmentation of the nipples (Dodd's nipples) which is cosmetically undesirable. When it seems that no further growth will occur, of if the patient does not mind her shortness and wishes mainly to achieve a greater degree ot sexual development, then somewhat higher doses of oestrogen may be used.

KARYOTYPE 47XXX

This karyotype is compatible with normal ovarian development. The patients tend to be tall and their intelligence is likely to be diminished. Occasionally cases come to light because they develop a premature menopause. Mosaics 47XXX/45XO occur. The clinical status of the patient will depend on which of the two cell types predominate in the somatic cells and in the gonads respectively. Patients with four and even five X chromosomes have been described. They are mentally defective.

PURE GONADAL DYSGENESIS

When there is very early failure of gonadal development, the other organs of sex are female whatever the chromosome constitution. When the karyotype is normal female, 46XX, the patients present with complete or partial failure of puberty depending on the degree of development of the gonad. These eunuchoid young women have raised gonadotrophin and low oestrogen levels. The failure of ovarian development can be confirmed by laparoscopy. Treatment by oestrogens and progesterone as in Turner's syndrome p. 277 is indicated.

The karyotype 46XY in association with pure gonadal dysgenesis is more dangerous for the patient because any gonadal development that does occur produces tissue potentially capable of transforming into a metastasising seminoma. The degree of development of the gonad varies. Both gonads may be absent, they may be fibrous streaks, perhaps with a few tubules resembling the seminiferous tubules of a cryptorchid testis. In some cases, testicular development has advanced far enough to produce some masculinisation. Cases are seen in whom the gonads produce enough hormones to induce the changes of female puberty at the usual age of puberty, usually, but not always without any masculinisation. In these cases the gonads appear to be gonadotrophin-sensitive. They may be a few cms in diameter and display a mixture of clumps of interstitial cells, and solid rods of cells that are supposed to include Sertoli cells and spermatogonia. The proportions of these cell types vary from case to case. These gonads often display large masses of fibrous tissue and some calcified areas are usually present. There may be cysts. The term gonadoblastoma has been used to describe these gonads. One case in whom a metastasising dysgerminoma developed is known to the authors. The 46XY cases of pure gonadal agenesis are easily distinguished from the testicular feminisation (TF) syndrome because the former have a uterus, and sexual hair growth keeps pace with other pubertal development whereas TF syndrome cases have neither uterus nor sexual hair. 46XY pure gonadal agenesis has been observed in two members of the same sibship. Usually both have had the same type of gonads but cases with differing gonadal types have also been observed.

The treatment of 46XY cases of pure gonadal agenesis who have been raised as girls is to remove both gonads and to institute oestrogen/progesterone therapy.

TESTICULAR FEMINISATION

These individuals are superficially normal females except that pubic and axillary hair does not grow at all or is scanty in amount. Psychologically they are completely female. Breast development is usually quite normal, though the nipples may be hypoplastic, and there is primary amenorrhoea. The external genitalia are completely female. A vagina is present, usually ending as a blind pouch, but there is no uterus. Occasionally, the clitoris may be somewhat larger than normal.

A buccal smear examination shows these patients to be chromatin-negative, and karyotyping reveals an XY sex chromosome complement. The gonads are testes, and they may be either intra-abdominal, associated with inguinal herniae, or palpable in the labia. A gonad may be extra-abdominal on one side only. Histologically the appearances are similar to those found in undescended intra-abdominal testes in phenotypical males. There is no spermatogenesis, there may be peritubular fibrosis, and there may be Leydig cell hyperplasia. Sometimes the testes are larger than normal. The Müllerian duct structures may be absent or rudimentary.

The TF syndrome is probably an X-linked characteristic (Sanger *et al.*, 1969). It is likely that the tissues either do not respond, or have a diminished response to androgens. Many recent studies have shown that testosterone is produced at the same rate as in normal males (Southern *et al.*, 1965a; Southern *et al.*, 1965b; French *et al.*, 1965; French *et al.*, 1966). Wilkins (1957) mentions a patient who failed to masculinise when treated with methyl testosterone.

Treatment. These patients complain of primary amenorrhoea, coupled, if they are married, with infertility. Occasionally, the condition may be noted in early life because of the presence of gonads in the inguinal region or in the labia. Obviously nothing can be done to right the amenorrhoea or infertility, but once the diagnosis is made or suspected it is generally advocated that the testes should be removed because of the high incidence of neoplastic change in these organs. Menopausal symptoms will follow the castration, and these should be anticipated and treated with oestrogens.

PHENOTYPICALLY INDETERMINATE INTERSEX

A group of cases of different aetiologies possess the same disability, namely that their 'true sex' cannot be decided by simple inspection at birth. It is important that correct decisions should be made soon after birth, so that the child may be fitted as well as possible to a role either as a man or woman, but it sometimes happens that the cases present as older children, at puberty, or even as adults. As time passes, the freedom of choice becomes constrained by previous decisions and treatment, and the patient's own idea of his or her sex becomes increasingly the dominant feature of the case.

When the external genitalia are neither normal male nor normal female at birth, investigations should be initiated urgently to decide on the sex of rearing and to lay down the programme of treatment. The plan will include the following:

1. Careful clinical examination. This will disclose whether the genitalia are intermediate in development between male and female or whether the anomaly is a deformity of the sex organs. Examination may disclose the presence of testes in the groin. When the infant is a few days old a blood-stained mucoid discharge from the genital orifices may indicate that a uterus is present.
2. Buccal smear will give indirect information about the nature of the gonad. Chromatin positive cases may be tentatively presumed to have ovaries.
3. The chromosomes should be examined—a few millilitres of cord blood received into a sterile bottle provide a suitable source of lymphocytes.
4. Hormone investigations are less useful, except in congenital adrenal hyperplasia where they are of vital importance.

The information obtained from these measures has then to be considered in the light of the stages of development outlined at the beginning of this chapter. The case can then nearly always be fitted into one of the following types:

1. DEFORMITIES OF SEXUAL ORGANS

These may be bizarre, tragic, or trivial. The buccal smear and karyotype will indicate the nature of the gonad. It is nearly always correct to bring the child up according to the chromosome sex and presumed gonadal sex, performing such reconstructive surgery as is likely to be helpful.

2. INTERMEDIATE DEVELOPMENT OF THE EXTERNAL GENITALIA

(*a*) *The buccal smear is chromatin negative, the karyotype is 46XY.* Testes are assumed to exist. Unless the phallus is very small and a vagina is present the case is classified as a male with hypospadias, and corrective surgery is performed as required to fit the child for the male role. Difficulty arises when the phallus is very small for a penis and there is a vagina. In these cases, the tissues may be capable of only a minimal response to androgens and attempts to 'correct' the hypospadias may produce a man whose penis is too small either for copulation, or for micturition in the manner customary for men. These cases should probably be treated as testicular feminisation (*see* above) and reared as girls. There is a great need for some *in vitro* test whereby tissue response to androgens could be accurately assessed.

(*b*) *The buccal smear is chromatin negative, the karyotype is a mosaic* 46*XY*/45*XO*. Because some development in the male direction has occurred, testicular tissue is assumed to exist. The degree of masculinisation will indicate the amount of testis present. Minimal masculinisation, e.g. a slightly enlarged clitoris only, with a vagina and uterus, will best be treated as a case of Turner's syndrome and the patient reared as a female. More extensive masculinisation would indicate rearing as a 'male', correcting the hypospadias, removing a uterus if present, and correcting the position of the testes.

(*c*) *The buccal smear is chromatin positive, and the karyotype is* 46*XX*. Ovaries should be presumed to exist. Masculinisation has occurred from an abnormal source of androgens. The most likely cause is congenital adrenal hyperplasia (page 282), and investigations must be pursued urgently to confirm or refute that diagnosis. Less commonly, an extrinsic source of androgens, or perhaps true hermaphroditism (*see* below), is the cause. In virtually all these cases the female sex is selected.

(*d*) *The buccal smear is chromatin-positive and the karyotope is* 47*XXY*. The patient is treated as a male with hypospadias and seminiferous tubule dysgenesis (Klinefelter's syndrome). These conditions sometimes occur in the same individual.

(*e*) *There are some cells* 46*XY and some* 46*XX*. The patient is a chimera. True hermaphroditism is likely. The sex of rearing should be that best suited to the development of the external genitalia.

Cases presenting for the first time later in life, or being reassessed later, are capable of being analysed in the same way but, as already stated, the sex of rearing and the psychological orientation of the patient increasingly dominate the choice of treatment. Thus, a patient of karyotype 46XX with congenital adrenal hyperplasia, and considerable masculinisation who has been reared as a male and who seeks advice because of menstrual bleeding from the urethra, or 'gynaecomastia', may best be treated by mastectomy, hysterectomy, and correction of hypospadias so that he may remain as the male he believes himself to be.

TRUE HERMAPHRODITISM

This is an extremely rare condition characterised by the presence in the same patient of both testicular and ovarian tissues. The cases present with phenotypically indeterminate intersex at birth, but they are described separately because of the variety of sub-types that exist. Published cases where there has been adequate anatomical investigation can be placed into one of three categories: (1) *lateral*, where there is an ovary on one side and a testis on the other; (2) *unilateral*, where there is an unequivocal testis or ovary on one side and an ovotestis (a gonad containing both ovarian and testicular components) on the other; (3) *bilateral*, where an ovotestis is found on both sides.

When a testis is present it is usually in the scrotum or scrotolabial fold, but it may be in the inguinal canal, or be intra-abdominal. Usually, on the side of the testis the Müllerian structures have been suppressed and the Wolffian duct structures developed, so that there is no Fallopian tube, and a vas deferens and epididymis are present; if the other gonad is an ovary—the patient having lateral hermaphroditism—the Wolffian structures are not apparent and there is a Fallopian tube and a uterine horn. Given the different gonads, this is the appearance that might be expected from the principles of embryonic development previously discussed. Histologically, the testis usually resembles the cryptorchid testis. The seminiferous tubules usually show absent or incomplete spermatogenesis, though occasionally complete spermatogenesis has been observed. Sometimes there has been hyalinisation of the tubules. Leydig cells are present and may be prominent.

An ovary is usually intra-abdominal and placed in the expected situation; it may sometimes be found, however, in the inguinal canal. Histologically, the appearances are usually those of a normal ovary; ova surrounded by a corona of granulosa cells are present, but occasionally they have been absent and the gonad more closely resembles that seen in Turner's syndrome. The picture with an ovotestis is more variable. The position of the gonad is usually intra-abdominal, but it is sometimes found in the inguinal canal or even in the scrotum. There is also a wide variation in the development of the various internal sexual organs. Usually, the Müllerian system has developed, but sometimes not fully, so that, for example, in bilateral hermaphroditism (an ovotestis on both sides) there may be Fallopian tubes and a uterus, though the latter may be small or bicornuate. In about one-third there are also Wolffian duct structures present—a vas deferens and an epididymis. From patient to patient great differences have been found in the relative development of these structures. The proof of an ovotestis by histology may be somewhat difficult, for a biopsy may not be sufficiently extensive to contain both types of tissue.

The development of the external genitalia in a true hermaphrodite is usually ambiguous, there being a phallus intermediate in size between a clitoris and penis, usually a perineal urethra with either a separate vaginal orifice, or a rudimentary vagina joining the urethra. Sometimes, however, it has been impossible to tell that an individual was not a normal male, though most will not have a normal penile urethra; on the other hand, a number have closely resembled normal females except for clitoral enlargement, very occasionally so great that it would have been possible for the individual to take either a male or a female role in intercourse. Usually, after puberty there is breast development though sometimes this is entirely lacking (Armstrong *et al.*, 1957).

The question arises how both types of gonad can develop in one individual. When chromosomal analysis first became available a few cases were reported to have a normal female karyotype, 46XX, but there were also reports of 46XY cases, mosaicism XO/XY, and XX/XXY/XXYYY. As technical methods have improved it has become evident that most true hermaphrodites are whole body chimeras, i.e. they are composed of a mixture of 46XX and 46XY cells (Gartler *et al.*, 1962; Benirschhke *et al.*, 1972). The two cell lines differ in other genetic markers, e.g. in blood groups and it is often possible to demonstrate that both parents have each made two contributions to a single child. The exact mechanism is unknown but fertilisation by separate sperms of an ovum and its second polar body has been suggested. It is convenient to regard a whole body chimera as having arisen by fusion of dizygotic twin embryos at an early stage, and this may be the method of formation. The term 'chimera' is used in preference to 'mosaic' p. 268 to emphasise the widespread genetic disparity in the two cell lines.

It can be seen from the above descriptions, that it is quite impossible to categorise accurately any individual with ambiguous external genitalia without careful and detailed study. It is necessary both to have chromosomal analysis carried out, often on more than one tissue, and to delineate accurately the precise anatomical configuration of the internal sexual organs. Hormonal studies are usually unhelpful diagnostically except in the case of congenital adrenal hyperplasia (page 282). Diagnosis of this syndrome is of some urgency because a fatal electrolyte crisis may occur a few days after birth if appropriate treatment is not started in time. For a more detailed description of the chromosomal abnormalities reference should be made to the Medical Research Council Report (1964), *Abnormalities of the Sex Chromosome Complement in Man* by Court Brown *et al.*, and a great deal of fundamental information on the subject of intersexuality will be found in *Intersexuality in Vertebrates and Man* by Armstrong and Marshall (1964).

CONGENITAL ADRENAL HYPERPLASIA

Hyperplasia of the adrenal cortex can result from inherited defects in the enzymes responsible for corticosteroid biosynthesis, when the lowered cortisol production causes an increased output of ACTH. The severity of the enzyme deficiencies vary; in some cases the deficiency is so severe that virtually no cortisol is produced, while in others basal corticosteroid production by the enlarged gland may be normal. There are various forms of congenital adrenal hyperplasia, depending on the particular enzyme that is deficient. The syndrome is one of the commonest inborn errors of metabolism, the gene frequency for the common 21-hydroxylase defect being as high as 1/50 in some regions. Consanguinity in the families is not uncommon, siblings are often affected, and the pattern of inheritance is generally accepted to be as an autosomal recessive. The commonest defects interfere with cortisol production and ACTH and β-MSH levels are consequently high, occasionally high enough to cause pigmentation of the skin. Since ACTH stimulates early in the chain of adrenal steroid synthesis, there is an increased output of cortisol precursors synthesised prior to the enzyme block. Many of these precursors are androgenic and cause virilisation, hence the effects are most marked in the female, and the clinical effects depend on the stage of intrauterine development that the fetus is exposed to the androgens. The androgens produced by the adrenal in the female fetus modify the external genitalia to the male pattern to a greater or lesser extent though such patients have a normal uterus, tubes, and ovaries because there is no testis to produce the suppressor of the Müllerian structures.

ENZYMATIC DEFECTS

The number of defects described is increasing and deficiencies of almost all of the enzymes of the corticosteroid biosynthetic pathway have been described (Fig. 13.17). Depending on the site of the block, the synthesis of cortisol, aldosterone and of androgens may be impaired.

1. LIPOID HYPERPLASIA (C-70 BLOCK)

This is the most severe defect in steroid biosynthesis interfering with the formation of aldosterone, cortisol, and androgens. Cortisol biosynthesis is effected at a very early stage possibly in the desmolase reaction in which the cholesterol side chain is removed from the basic steroid nucleus. It has been suggested that the defect affecting the fetal adrenal cortex may result from some intrauterine disorder such as erythroblastosis. The adrenal cortex is filled with lipid, largely cholesterol. Patients with this syndrome rarely survive, dying of hypoadrenalism soon after birth. The enzyme in the ovaries and testes is also affected and because of the absence of androgens, external genitalia of male fetuses

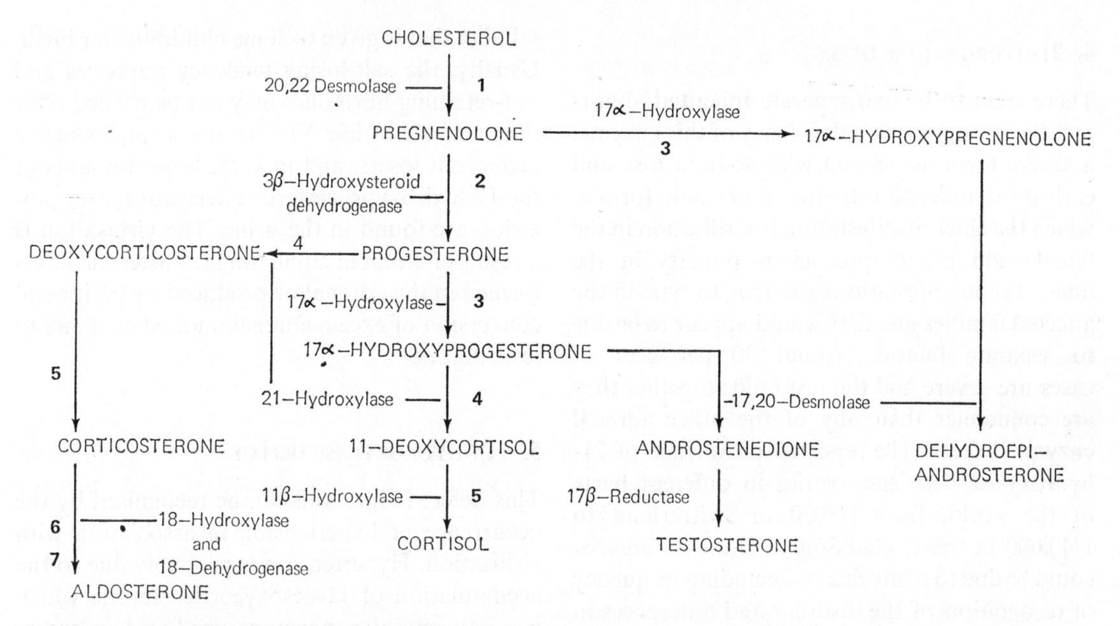

FIGURE 13.17 Enzyme defects in congenital adrenal hyperplasia
1 lipoid hyperplasia (C-20 block). 2 3β-hydroxysteroid-dehydrogenase deficiency. 3 17α-hydroxylase deficiency. 4 21-hydroxylase deficiency. 5 11β-hydroxylase deficiency. 6,7 18-hydroxylase and 18-dehydrogenase deficiencies

develop along female lines. At birth, all affected children appear as phenotypic females but differentiation can easily be made by buccal smear. The early administration of cortisol, mineralocorticoids and saline is essential for survival.

2. 3β-HYDROXYSTEROID-DEHYDROGENASE DEFECT

This rare defect interferes with the production of cortisol and aldosterone. There is also a reduced conversion of dehydroepiandrosterone (DHEA) to androstenedione and hence to testosterone, a defect shared by the ovaries and testes. The children present with a severe salt-losing syndrome. In male patients the external genitalia are ambiguous whereas in females there is mild virilisation probably due to the weak androgenic action of DHEA. Early treatment with cortisol, a salt-retaining steroid and salt supplements is required. Surgical correction of genital abnormalities and androgen supplements will be required in boys at the time of puberty.

3. 17α-HYDROXYLASE DEFECT

This rare defect impairs the production of cortisol and other 17-hydroxycorticosteroids but not the synthesis of corticosterone and desoxycorticosterone. Because of the increased ACTH drive, levels of corticosterone and desoxycorticosterone rise and salt retention and hypertension result. The hypervolaemia causes suppression of renin and angiotensin production and aldosterone levels are low. Adrenal androgen production is impaired and the defect may also effect androgen synthesis in the testes and oestrogen synthesis in the ovaries. Affected females present with primary amenorrhoea, lack of secondary sexual characteristics, hypertension and hypokalaemia. Affected males, when the testicular biosynthetic pathways are also affected, present with pseudohermaphroditism and gynaecomastia. The testes do not respond to HCG but the patients become masculinised with testosterone administration. It is likely that this rare defect is also transmitted as an autosomal recessive trait.

4. 21-HYDROXYLASE DEFECT

There seem to be two separate inherited abnormalities giving rise to a deficiency of this enzyme, a severe form associated with sodium loss and early death unless it is treated, and a mild form in which the chief manifestation is virilisation in the female and pseudo-precocious puberty in the male. The manifestations run true to type in the affected families and they would appear to be due to separate factors. About 30 per cent of cases are severe and the rest mild; together they are commoner than any of the other adrenal enzyme defects. The reported prevalence of 21-hydroxylase deficiency varies in different parts of the world, from 1/5000 in Switzerland to 1/40,000 in the United States. These differences could be due to many factors including frequency of recognition of the disorder and differences in consanguinity. Heterozygotes for 21-hydroxylase deficiency do not usually show any abnormalities, but some can be recognised by their increased excretion of urinary pregnanetriol after the combined administration of ACTH and metyrapone. Amniotic fluid pregnanetriol levels in women bearing an affected fetus are elevated near term; earlier elevation may sometimes be due to non-specific fetal distress.

In the *sodium losers* there is low basal production of both cortisol and aldosterone and little rise after stimulation with ACTH. The juxtaglomerular apparatus is hypertrophied and plasma levels of renin and angiotensin are increased. Angiotensin may play a part in increasing salt loss. Patients present usually between 7 and 14 days after birth with severe hypoadrenalism, pigmentation, and virilisation. In the *non-salt losers* basal production of both aldosterone and cortisol may be within the normal range and there is a further rise after administration of ACTH. Patients may present shortly after birth with hyponatraemia but adrenal crises rarely occur. The hyponatraemia may be due to the high levels of 17α-hydroxyprogesterone and its metabolites which act as an aldosterone antagonist on the renal tubules. The effect is aggravated by the low salt diet that is given to some children after birth. Usually, the salt-losing tendency improves and salt-retaining hormones may not be needed after the first year of life. Virilisation occurs as in the severe salt losers, and in both, large amounts of the 17-hydroxyprogesterone derivative, pregnanetriol, are found in the urine. The virilisation is a result of elevated circulating testosterone levels formed in the adrenal or produced by peripheral conversion of excess adrenal androstenedione to testosterone.

5. 11β-HYDROXYLASE DEFECT

This defect is rare and can be recognised by the occurrence of hypertension in association with virilisation. Hypertension is probably due to the accumulation of 11-desoxycorticosterone which is a salt-retaining hormone produced in excess because the block in cortisol synthesis results in considerable ACTH stimulation of the adrenal cortex. There is no hyperplasia of the juxtaglomerular cells and plasma renin levels are low despite the low production rate of aldosterone. Cortisol production is impaired and 11-desoxycortisol accumulates. The defect can be characterised by the excretion in the urine of large amounts of the tetra-hydro derivative of 11-desoxycortisol, tetrahydro-S. Pregnanetriol excretion is not usually so high as in the 21-hydroxylase defect. Virilisation and occasionally skin pigmentation occur as in the other examples of the syndrome. Virilisation is due to increased circulating testosterone levels as in the 21-hydroxylase variety. Hypertension is not invariable, suggesting some heterogeneity of the syndrome. The urinary findings can be mimicked by the administration of metyrapone which inhibits 11β-hydroxylation.

6. 18-HYDROXYLASE DEFECT

This syndrome results from a deficiency of hydroxylation of the methyl group at C-18, the penultimate stage of aldosterone biosynthesis. Aldosterone production is low and the patients present with a salt-losing syndrome. The patient may show some improvement with age as a consequence of the salt-retaining properties of DOC and corticosterone, both of which are produced in increased amounts. Salt supplements or a sodium-retaining steroid such as fludrocortisone may be required at first, but later no treatment may be needed if the sodium intake is adequate. Production of cortisol is normal, as are plasma ACTH levels and hence virilisation and pigmentation do not occur in patients presenting with this defect.

7. 18-DEHYDROGENASE DEFECT

This syndrome results from a deficiency of the dehydrogenation of 18-hydroxycorticosterone to aldosterone, the final stage in the aldosterone biosynthetic pathway. The biochemical abnormalities, clinical features and management are similar to those in patients with the 18-hydroxylase defect. It is possible that some of the patients who present with the rare condition of hypoaldosteronism in adult life may represent late-onset variants of defective C-18 hydroxylation or dehydrogenation.

CLINICAL DIAGNOSIS

Variants of the common clinical picture have been mentioned under the enzymatic defects. In the male there may be no abnormalities at birth, but premature sexual development results in the syndrome of pseudo-precocious puberty. There is growth of the penis, frequent erections, early development of pubic hair, increased musculature, and rapid growth in height. Unlike true precocious puberty there is no enlargement of testicular tissue though, occasionally, ectopic adrenal tissue may cause apparent testicular enlargement. If the level of androgens is not reduced by therapy the epiphyses fuse early and the ultimate height is less than would have been expected.

The salt-losing defect may affect either sex shortly after birth, causing all the features of an adrenal crisis—hyponatraemia, hyperkalaemia, hypotension, vomiting, collapse, coma, and death. Pigmentation is more frequent in severely affected patients.

In the typical affected female, virilisation begins before the twelfth week of intrauterine life and the external genitalia usually show labial fusion and clitoral hypertrophy. Severe cases may show persistence of the urogenital sinus, with the vagina opening into the urethra, which may itself open at any point along the course of the phallus, but usually at the base. The external genitalia may therefore resemble those of a male with hypospadias and undescended testes. In more mildly affected females there may merely be clitoral hypertrophy. Occasional cases have been described where virilisation occurs after birth or even after puberty, the patient presenting with hirsuties. Since androgens do not inhibit the development of the Müllerian ducts, female infants have normal internal genitalia, the virilisation effecting only the urogenital sinus and external genitalia. Similar virilisation of the external genitalia in the female may result from exposure to androgens from extra-adrenal sources during intrauterine life. Maternal androgen-secreting tumours, e.g. an ovarian arrhenoblastoma, may be responsible, as may various androgens given to the mother. Many of the synthetic progestogens administered for habitual abortion are androgenic.

INVESTIGATIONS

Any child with ambiguity of the external genitalia ranging from slight clitoral hypertrophy, on the one hand, to a 'boy' with bilateral undescended testes, on the other, should have a buccal smear and, if indicated, a chromosomal analysis. If a masculinised girl or apparent boy is chromatin positive and has an XX sex chromatin complement, then congenital adrenal hyperplasia is a distinct likelihood. The next step is to estimate the twenty-four hour excretion of urinary steroids. An elevated output of 17-oxosteroids will usually be found when this is the cause of virilisation, and partition of the various steroids will help to delineate which enzyme defect is present.

Elevated 17-oxosteroid excretion is found in cases with impaired cortisol synthesis but no interruption of androgen formation, because of overproduction of ACTH. In lipoid hyperplasia and in defects specific to the aldosterone biosynthetic pathway the oxosteroid excretion will not be raised, and it is in these groups that virilisation is absent. In the more common varieties increased oxosteroid output occurs, except during the first week of life in some cases where the excretion may normally range from 2 to 5 mg a day. After this period, the daily excretion is normally less than 2 mg up to the age of six years. There is then a gradual rise in excretion, reaching about 9 mg every 24 hours by puberty in both sexes, and adult levels are reached by 17 to 20 years. When the 17-oxosteroids are fractionated in the disease an increase in androsterone, aetiocholanolone, 11-oxoaetiocholanolone, 11-hydroxyandrosterone, and DHA are found, with virtual absence of 11-hydroxyaetiocholanolone, an oxosteroid arising from cortisol degradation. A further marked rise in 17-oxosteroid output can be produced in most cases by injections of ACTH.

Pregnanetriol and 11-oxopregnanetriol are normally present in very small amounts in the urine up to the age of two years; in older children, levels of pregnanetriol up to 1·5 mg/day may be found, and in adults never more than 3·5 mg daily. Marked increases in pregnanetriol output are found in the commoner 21-hydroxylase defect. This test is of value in determining those very rare cases of hirsuties that are due to congenital adrenal hyperplasia of late onset. Pregnanetriol is estimated in some assays for urinary 17-hydroxycorticosteroids, so in these circumstances excretion of both 17-oxosteroids and 17-hydroxycorticosteroids will be increased. In the 11-hydroxylase defect large amounts of tetrahydro-S are excreted in the urine.

In defects specific to the aldosterone synthetic pathway, precursors prior to the enzymatic block, e.g. desoxycorticosterone, along with their particular degradation products are excreted in the urine. Complex biochemical techniques are required to determine the precise site of the enzyme defect.

TREATMENT

In the salt-losing varieties, treatment is urgent, giving cortisol in a dose of 0·3 mg/lb of body weight per day in divided doses, along with a salt-retaining hormone, e.g. fludrocortisone, 0·1 to 0·2 mg/day and intravenous saline to correct the water and electrolyte imbalance.

In the male with pseudo-precocious puberty the aims of therapy are to correct cortisol deficiency if present, provide extra cortisol under conditions of stress and to reduce the level of androgens, which in time will:

1. slow the rate of bone maturation and allow normal height to be attained.
2. allow normal gonadotrophin secretion at puberty with normal spermatogenesis
3. decrease libido and premature interest in the opposite sex, and
4. reduce the aggressive behaviour seen in some cases.

To achieve these aims therapy with cortisol must be started as soon as possible in a dose up to 50 per cent more than the normal physiological requirements, but is reduced to the normal replacement dose as soon as control is obtained. The dose is titrated against the fall in 17-oxosteroid excretion to lower the 17-oxosteroid excretion to the normal range for age. The height and weight must be charted frequently. If the dose of cortisol is too high, growth hormone action will be suppressed and linear growth will cease; if the dose is too low the accelerated growth in height and rapid bone maturation will persist. Since the main requirement of cortisol therapy is to suppress ACTH production, the daily dose should be divided and spread throughout the day. The last dose should be given as close to midnight as possible and should consist of 50 per cent of the total daily dose, since administration of corticosteroids at this time of the twenty-four hour ACTH cycle is the most effective method of suppressing ACTH secretion. Intramuscular cortisone acetate can be injected daily or on alternate days in a dose related to body weight to give a smoother suppression of ACTH output. The synthetic steroid prednisolone may be used and has the advantage that it does not interfere with urinary steroid assays. A dose of 2·5 mg on waking and 5 mg on retiring is usually satisfactory. After growth has ceased in males, it is probably wise to continue a maintenance dose of cortisol since most patients with congenital adrenal hyperplasia will have impaired adrenal reserve and infertility may well arise if the condition persists uncontrolled.

In the female, the aims of therapy will be to treat salt deficiency, to correct any lack of cortisol, and to suppress androgen output which, in turn, will:

1. slow the rate of bone maturation;
2. restore gonadotrophin output and allow normal puberty to occur;
3. reduce virilisation, especially excessive body hair, male configuration, and masculinisation of the external genitalia;
4. allow normal menstruation, intercourse, and pregnancy.

Cortisol therapy should be continued permanently, otherwise signs of virilisation will recur. Plastic surgery may be required to correct the abnormalities of the external genitalia but this should be conservative till the effects of cortisol are assessed. Removal of the enlarged clitoris should be avoided, as with labial maturation at puberty the clitoris will not appear so large and in any case can be partially buried to render the appearance more aesthetic. Plastic repair of the vagina may be required to allow normal menstruation and intercourse. The female with congenital adrenal hyperplasia who has been reared as a boy for several years presents a difficult problem. Some workers believe that reassignment of sex even at an early age constitutes a profound psychological hazard, and should be avoided. They advocate administration of additional androgens, castration, and plastic surgery to make the external genitalia more perfectly male. Other workers, ourselves included, advise a more flexible approach, believing that sex can be reassigned, even after many years of rearing in some cases, and that it is usually better to produce a fertile woman than a male castrate. Older patients with 'wrongly' assigned sex require careful assessment of their psycho-sexual orientation before a decision on their final sexual assignment is made.

REFERENCES

Armstrong, C. N., Gray, J. E., Race, R. R., and Thompson, R. B. (1957). *Brit. med. J.*, **2**, 605.

Armstrong, C. N., and Marshall, A. J. (Eds) (1964). *Intersexuality in Vertebrates including Man.* London and New York: Academic Press.

Barr, M. L., and Bertram, E. G. (1949). *Nature* (Lond.), **163**, 676.

Benirschke, K., Naftolin, F., Gittes, R., Khudr, G., Yen, S. S. C., Allen, F. H. Jr. (1972). *Am. J. Obstet. Gynecol.* **113**, 449.

Court Brown, W. M., Harnden, D. G., Jacobs, A., MacLean, N., and Mantle, D. J. (1964). *Abnormalities of the Sex Chromosome Complement in Man.* Medical Research Council, Special Report Series No. 305. London: HMSO.

French, F. S., Baggett, B., Van Wyk, J. J., Talbert, L. M., Hubbard, W., Johnston, F. R., and Weaver, R. P. (1965). *J. clin. Endocrinol.*, **25**, 661.

French, F. S., Van Wyk, J. J., Bagget, B., Easterling, W. E., Talbert, L. M., Johnston, F. R., Forchielli, E., and Dey, A. C. (1966). *J. clin. Endocrinol.*, **26**, 493.

Gartler, S. M., Waxman, S. H., and Giblett, E. (1962). *Proc. nat. Acad. Sci.* (Wash.), **48**, 332.

Harris, G. W., and Levine, S. (1965). *J. Physiol.*, **181**, 379.

Jost, A. (1950). *Gynec. Obstet.* (Paris), **49**, 44.

Keats, T. E., and Burns, T. W. (1964). 'The Radiographic Manifestations of Gondal Dysgenesis'. *The Radiologic Clinics of North America*, Vol. II, No. 2 (Ed. G. S. Lodivick). London: Saunders Co.

Klinefelter, H. F., Reifenstein, E. C., and Albright, F. (1942). *J. clin. Endocrinol.*, **2**, 615.

Kosowicz, J. (1962). *J. clin. Endocrinol.*, **22**, 949.

Lyon, M. F. (1961). *Nature* (Lond.), **190**, 372.

Rice, B. F., Cleveland, W. W., Sandberg, D. H., Ahmad, N., Politano, V. T., and Savard, K. (1967). *J. clin. Endocrinol.*, **27**. 29.

Russell, A., Moschos, A., Butler, L. J., and Abraham, J. M. (1966). *J. clin. Endocrinol.*, **26**, 1282.

Sanger, R., Tippett, P., Gavin, J., Gooch, A., and Race, R. R. (1969). *J. med. Genet.*, **6**, 26.

Southern, A. L., Tochimoto, S., Carmody, N. C., and Isurgi, K. (1965a). *J. clin. Endocrinol.*, **25**, 1441.

Southern, A. L., Ros, H. Sharma, D. C., Gordon, G., Weingold, A. B., and Dorfman, R. I. (1965b). *J. clin. Endocrinol.*, **25**, 518.

Swyer, G. I. M. (1955). *Brit. med. J.*, **2**, 709.

Turner, H. H. (1938). *Endocrinology*, **23**, 566.

Wilkins, L., and Fleischmann, W. (1944). *J. clin. Endocrinol.*, **4**, 357.

Wilkins, L. (1957). In *The Diagnosis and Treatment of Endocrine Disorders in Childhood and Adolescence.* Oxford: Blackwell, p. 276.

Young, W. C., Goy, R. W., and Phoenix, C. H. (1964). *Science*, **143**, 212.

Hamilton, W. (1972) 'Congenital adrenal hyperplasia', in *Clinics in Endocrinology and Metabolism, Diseases of the Adrenal Cortex* (Ed. A. Stuart Mason), Vol. 1, Number 2, Saunders Co. Ltd., London, p. 503.

Rimoin, D. L. and Schimke, R. N. (1971). *Genetic Disorders of the Endocrine Glands*, C. V. Masby Co., Saint Louis, p. 225.

14

HORMONAL CONTROL OF CARBOHYDRATE, PROTEIN, AND FAT METABOLISM

This chapter opens with a brief review of the metabolism of carbohydrate, fat, and protein. The metabolic pathways whereby the body derives energy from food sources are not separate and distinct but interrelated, and any study of carbohydrate metabolism, and any fault involved therein, necessarily involves the metabolism of protein and fat as well.

GENERAL PRINCIPLES

The purposes of tissue metabolism are to maintain function, to promote cell growth and to synthesise new substances such as proteins and enzymes. Energy must also be provided to enable these tasks to be carried out. The metabolic pathways involved in these processes are so ordered and integrated that the functions of cell growth, synthesis of new material and energy production are carried out in the most efficient way, providing safeguard and 'first-aid' mechanisms in order that abnormal and emergency situations can be adequately dealt with, and cellular metabolism maintained under all circumstances.

The requirements necessary to ensure the performance of these functions are:

1. basic 'raw materials' that can be converted to or used as 'cell fuels' or substrates for synthetic purposes;
2. functional units to utilise the fuels and substrates;
3. provision for storage of substances necessary to cellular economy—either for day-to-day working or for emergency situations;
4. factors that will control and integrate the supply and utilisation of energy sources, enabling the metabolic processes to keep pace with the needs of the body and with the amount of raw material supplied;
5. provision of an adequate supply of the vitamins and minerals concerned in intermediary metabolism.

The '*raw materials*' are supplied in the form of food—carbohydrate, fat, or protein. The main dietary *carbohydrates* are starch and disaccharides. Digestion of starch begins almost immediately after mastication of food, since saliva contains ptyalin, a starch-splitting enzyme. The digestion of carbohydrates in the lumen of the small bowel is due chiefly to the enzyme amylase which is secreted in the pancreatic juice, and starch and glycogen are broken down to their component disaccharides and to oligosaccharides. These, together with dietary disaccharides, are absorbed into the mucosa of the small bowel where they come into contact with disaccharidases and are split into monosaccharides which are absorbed into the portal blood. Hexose sugars that are ingested as such are absorbed unaltered through the wall of the small intestine by a process of active transport, which requires energy. *Fat* is supplied in the diet in the form of neutral fat (triglyceride), free fatty acids (FFA), sterols, and other complex lipids. The most abundant dietary fat is triglyceride. The molecule is hydrolysed to free fatty acids, lower glycerides and glycerol by pancreatic lipase, and to a lesser extent by intestinal lipase. This reaction is facilitated by the emulsifying action of bile salts. The breakdown products of fat digestion are absorbed into the cells of the intestinal villi in a highly emulsified form either by passing through the cell membrane or by the process of pinocytosis ('drinking in'). Lower glycerides and FFA are converted within the mucosal cell to triglyceride, which along with preformed triglyceride is then incorporated into a chylomicron by the addition of lipoprotein, phospholipid and cholesterol ester. The chylomicrons are discharged into the intestinal lymphatics and from there pass to the systemic circulation. Short-chain fatty acids which are water soluble, and some glycerol pass unchanged through the mucosal cell into the portal circulation. After absorption, lipids are available for metabolism in the liver and adipose tissue to forms in which they can be conveniently stored or utilised by other tissues such as muscle. During digestion, *protein* foods are broken down by hydrolysis into their component amino-acids and peptides. Some of the amino-acids are actively transported across the intestinal cell membrane while others diffuse across the mucosa. It is now generally accepted that peptides are absorbed into the cell as such and are then hydrolysed by peptidase enzymes in the mucosal cells into their constituent amino-acids before passing into the portal circulation. The amino-acids are utilised for protein synthesis in the liver and other tissues. Amino-acids may also contribute their carbon atom chains for fatty acid synthesis or for use as energy. Most of the amino-acids are, in addition, glycogenic, i.e. they can contribute to the formation of glucose or glycogen. Some amino-acids are also ketogenic, i.e. they may give rise to acetoacetate and other ketone bodies.

The basic *'fuels'* that may be utilised in the body by the *individual functional units* (the cells) are glucose and free fatty acids. Glucose is vital for the functioning of the brain, which has no significant stores of glycogen, and which does not normally metabolise other substrates. The blood glucose concentration must therefore be maintained at an adequate level for this purpose, but the exclusive use of glucose as fuel for assimilation by other cells in the body under all conditions is rather inefficient and uneconomical, and free fatty acids act as an important energy source. Free fatty acids provide as much as 1,200–1,800 kcal daily for energy purposes. If balance is maintained, as much free fatty acid will enter fat, or be synthesised, to be stored as triglyceride. In the fasting state and under basal conditions free fatty acids supply about 50 per cent of the energy requirements, while during exercise, when energy demands are high, glucose becomes an important energy source. During prolonged starvation, free fatty acids assume the major role since glucose utilisation will then be largely confined to the brain. Glucose serves as a substrate that can be used promptly in an emergency situation, and that is immediately available for energy metabolism after absorption. The amount of carbohydrate that can be stored in the body is strictly limited, and glucose metabolism provides the basic two carbon atom fragments used in fatty acid synthesis, α-glycerol phosphate for the esterification of the fatty acids, and the factors and co-factors necessary for the synthesis of lipid.

Free fatty acids both *in vitro* and *in vivo* cause inhibition of glucose uptake by muscle, and Randle *et al.* (1963) have suggested that plasma FFA, under the influence of insulin and growth hormone, may play a major part in the homeostasis of blood glucose. When blood glucose levels fall, FFA are mobilised from fat, and plasma levels rise. Free fatty acids are preferentially oxidised by muscle and, thus, glucose uptake by muscle is inhibited. This 'glucose sparing effect' will prevent hypoglycaemia, and when blood glucose levels rise after a meal, or as a result of release of glucose from the liver, mobilisation of FFA from adipose tissue is diminished. This sequence of events, which has been termed the *glucose-fatty acid cycle*, is initiated once more as blood glucose levels fall. Thus, the level of blood glucose may be maintained largely by these reciprocal fluctuations in glucose and FFA levels. There is evidence that the concentration of ketones in the blood may also be concerned in the normal homeostasis of blood glucose (Jenkins, 1967).

It will be apparent that since the tissues require a continuous supply of 'fuel', and since the 'raw materials' are consumed intermittently, the body must have mechanisms for *storage*. These body stores must be able to take up material when there is excess metabolic substrate available, and must be able to release fuel when there is an increased demand. Carbohydrate is stored in the form of glycogen, in muscle and in liver, and lipid is stored in the form of triglyceride in the fat depots. The liver is the principal source of glucose replacement to the blood, and this is made available either by glycogen breakdown or by synthesis from amino-acids (gluconeogenesis) and other substrates such as pyruvate and lactate (glucogenesis). The amount of glycogen that can be stored is, of course, strictly limited, and only about six per cent (100 g) of the liver's weight can be used in this way. Since muscle lacks the enzymes necessary for the conversion of glycogen to free glucose, glucose is not available to the bloodstream from that source. Lactate, however, may be released into the circulation from muscle, and this, in turn, can be converted to glucose in the liver. While pyruvate and lactate may be converted by the liver to glucose, it must be remembered that the protein reserve of the body (i.e. the maximum amount that may be lost on starvation beyond which survival is unlikely) is only 2 to 3 kg. The body can, therefore, supply little glucose directly on demand. It has been estimated that the body of a 70 kg man contains only about 370 g of available carbohydrate—enough to supply basal caloric needs for only about twelve hours. On the other hand, there is little limit to the amount of triglyceride that can be stored in the fat deposits of the body. The calorific value of adipose tissue, allowing for the small amounts of extracellular and intracellular fluid and protein present, is in the region of 7 to 7·5 kcal/g. Adipose tissue is, therefore, a source of relatively water-free fuel that is metabolically in a constant dynamic state. Even when the total amount of depot fat remains constant, triglyceride is constantly being broken down and replaced. A 150 kg obese man may contain in his storage depots as much as 100 kg of adipose tissue—equivalent to about 700,000 kcal and, theoretically eight months calorie supply. Protein in excess of the body's requirements may also contribute to the synthesis of fat, but the principal precursors come from carbohydrate and pre-formed lipid.

Intermediary metabolism is regulated by the cellular enzymes, many of them under hormonal control. The supply of the energy sources, and the integration of metabolic function in the intact animal, is also under the influence of circulating hormones—particularly insulin, growth hormone, glucagon and adrenaline, though the autonomic nervous system plays a part. The intake of food is regulated at hypothalamic and cortical levels.

PATHWAYS OF INTERMEDIARY METABOLISM

The Metabolism of Glucose. The rate of entry of glucose into the muscle or fat cell is the rate-limiting step in their metabolism, and is increased by insulin. The liver cell is less dependent on insulin for the uptake of glucose (*see* below). When glucose enters the cell, it is first phosphorylated to glucose-6-phosphate. It may then be converted to glycogen, be metabolised via the hexose monophosphate (HMP) shunt (this occurs mainly in fat), or be metabolised via the Embden Meyerhof (EM) pathway.

Glycogen Synthesis and Glycogenolysis. There is very little glycogen synthesis and storage in adipose tissue, these functions occurring principally in liver and muscle. Glycogen is a polysaccharide of high molecular weight made up of α-D-glucose units linked to one another in a branching structure (Fig. 14.1). After phosphorylation of glucose to glucose-6-phosphate and the conversion of this compound to glucose-1-phosphate, uridine diphosphoglucose is formed (Fig. 14.2). The enzyme glycogen synthetase then catalyses the formation of long non-branched

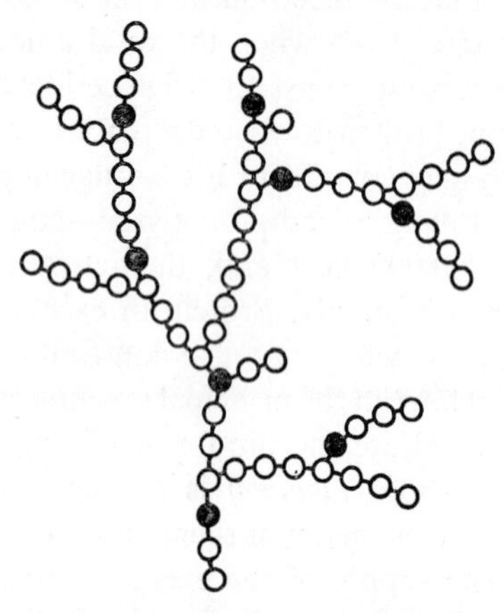

FIGURE 14.1 Structure of glycogen
1,6 linked glucose unit = ●
1,4 linked glucose unit = ○

chains of glucose which form glycogen under the influence of 'brancher' enzyme. In glycogenolysis, the molecule is first attacked by phosphorylase, which is converted from its inactive to its active form by cyclic 3′5′ AMP. Phosphorylase removes the glucose units of the outer branches in 1,4 linkages to yield glucose-1-phosphate, but stops short at the 1,6 linkages occurring at the branch points, which are attacked by 'debrancher' enzyme, yielding free glucose. Phosphorylase then continues the splitting off of the 1,4 linkages until the next branch point. Breakdown of glycogen therefore yields mainly glucose-1-phosphate, and some free glucose. The glucose-1-phosphate may be converted to glucose-6-phosphate and, thence, to free glucose if the enzyme glucose-6-phosphatase is present. This enzyme is normally absent from muscle; it is also absent from the liver in one type of glycogen storage disease.

HMP Shunt (Fig. 14.3). Here the oxidation of glucose-6-phosphate to the corresponding acid phosphogluconate is followed by oxidative decarboxylation to a series of pentose compounds, with the elimination of the original C-1 atom of glucose as carbon dioxide. By the action of dehydrogenase enzymes, the coenzyme reduced nicotinamide adenine dinucleotide phosphate (NADPH) is generated—this is an essential co-factor for fatty acid synthesis (Fig. 14.4). The pentose phosphate compounds are transformed by a complicated series of reactions back to hexosephosphates or, alternatively, they may be used for the synthesis of nucleotides. The degree of lipogenesis in adipose tissue is directly related to metabolism via the HMP shunt, and oxidation of glucose in the shunt is preferentially stimulated by insulin (Winegrad and Renold, 1958).

Embden Meyerhof Pathway (Fig. 14.5). The metabolism of glucose to pyruvate by this pathway (glycolysis) may occur under anaerobic or aerobic conditions. If oxygen is absent, the pyruvate is converted to lactate, and no further metabolism occurs. Nicotinamide adenine dinucleotide (NAD^+) is the coenzyme necessary for the oxidative stage in this glycolytic pathway. If oxygen is present, further transformation of pyruvate

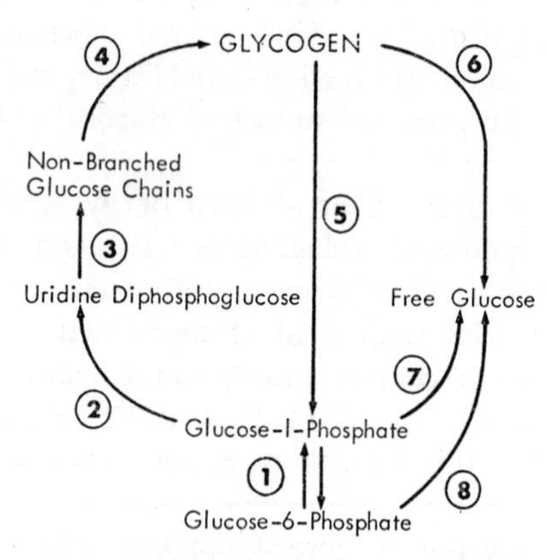

FIGURE 14.2 Glycogen synthesis and glycogenolysis
Enzymes involved: 1 phosphoglucomutase, 2 UDP pyrophosphorylase, 3 'glycogen synthetase', 4 'brancher enzyme', 5 phosphorylase, 6 'debrancher enzyme', 7 glucose-1-phosphatase, 8 glucose-6-phosphatase (only in liver)

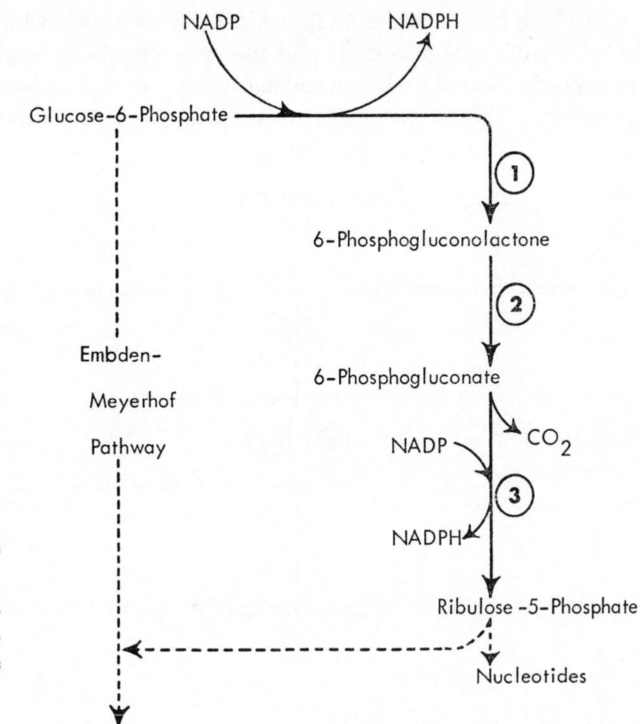

FIGURE 14.3 The hexosemonophosphate shunt

Enzymes involved: 1 glucose-6-phosphate dehydrogenase, 2 phosphogluconolactonase, 3 6-phosphogluconate dehydrogenase

occurs on the mitochondrion where pyruvate is first oxidatively decarboxylated to acetyl coenzyme A (acetyl CoA) with the release of carbon dioxide. The further oxidation of acetyl CoA to CO_2 and water by way of the citric acid cycle of Krebs involves many complex enzyme systems, including those involved in hydrogen transport and in oxidative phosphorylation. During these processes energy is released for storage in compounds such as ATP, where it can be made available for other biochemical reactions in the cells. The complete aerobic metabolism of two molecules of pyruvate (one glucose unit) results in the generation of 38 ATP molecules of which 24 are produced in the Krebs cycle. The yield of useful energy is considerably smaller under anaerobic

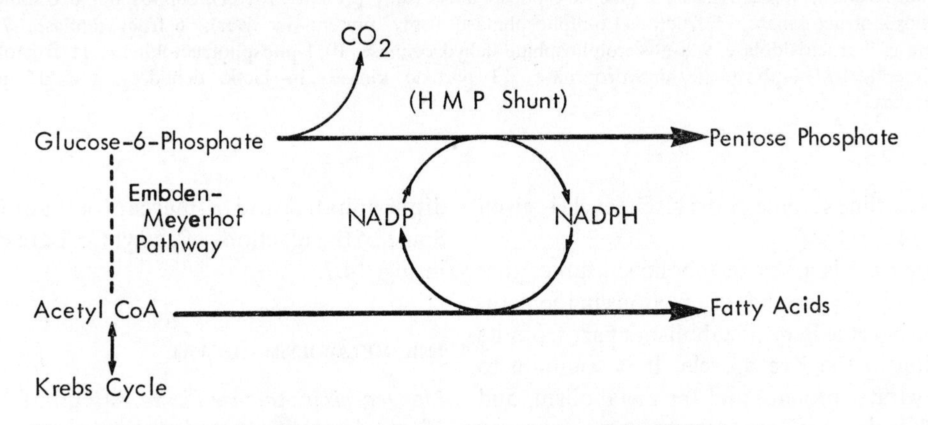

FIGURE 14.4 The relationship between fatty acid synthesis and the HMP shunt

conditions where lactate is the final product. A detailed review of the Krebs cycle and the processes of oxidative phosphorylation and hydrogen transport is beyond the scope of this book. However, an outline scheme of the Krebs cycle is given in Fig. 14.6.

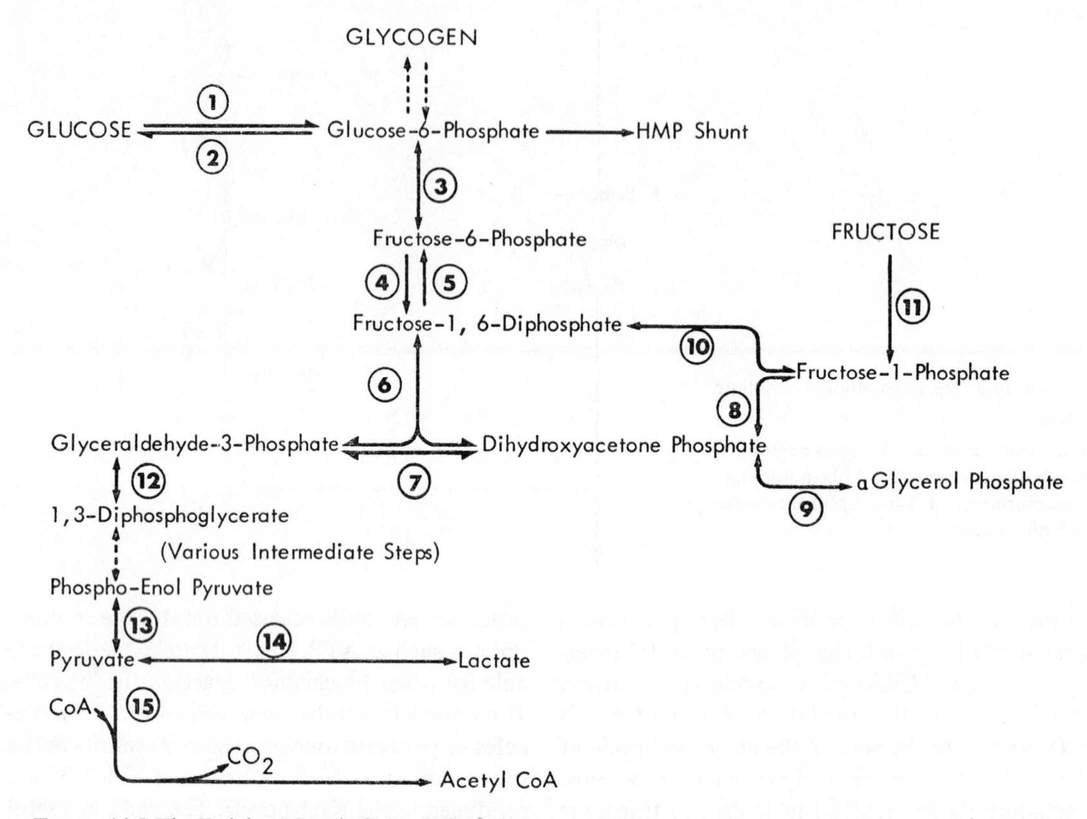

FIGURE 14.5 The Embden-Meyerhof glycolytic pathway

Enzymes involved; 1 glucokinase, 2 glucose-6-phosphatase (only present in liver), 3 phosphoglucoisomerase, 4 6-phosphofructokinase, 5 fructose-1,6-diphosphatase (only present in liver), 6 fructoaldolase, 7 triose isomerase, 8 fructoaldolase, 9 α-glycerolphosphate dehydrogenase, 10 1-phosphofructokinase, 11 fructokinase, 12 glyceraldehyde-3-phosphate dehydrogenase, 13 pyruvic kinase, 14 lactic dehydrogenase, 15 pyruvic hydrogenase

Acetyl CoA is a key metabolic substance that may enter into a number of reactions in the pathways of intermediary metabolism apart from its oxidation in the Krebs cycle. It is common to carbohydrate, protein, and fat metabolism, and through it the acetyl group can enter a common pathway which may lead to oxidation (supplying the body with energy) or to reduction (to supply or replace body materials). The coenzyme A molecule is composed of pantothenic acid, adenosine diphosphate, and β-mercaptoethanolamine. Some of the reactions of acetyl CoA are depicted in Fig. 14.7.

THE METABOLISM OF FAT

Lipogenesis in Adipose Tissue. After the formation of acetyl CoA, fatty acid synthesis can proceed in one of two directions: (*a*) by a mitochondrial pathway (minor importance), (*b*) by an extramitochondrial pathway (major importance). The extramitochondrial pathway starts with the carboxylation of acetyl CoA to form malonyl CoA under the influence of the enzyme acetyl CoA carboxylase. Palmityl CoA is built up from one molecule of acetyl CoA and seven of malonyl CoA, each molecule of the latter losing one molecule of CO_2 and of coenzyme A in the process (Fig. 14.8). After release of coenzyme A, the 16-carbon-atom palmitate may be further elongated

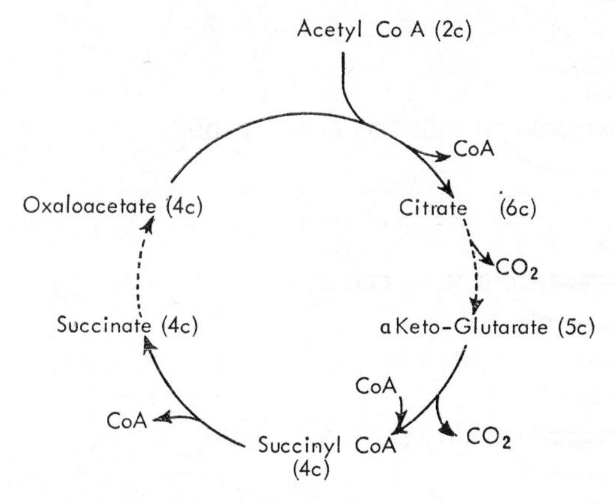

FIGURE 14.6 The Krebs cycle

by the mitochondrial pathway. The provision of free hydrogen is an essential factor during the process of fatty acid synthesis by both pathways—this is supplied mainly by the oxidation of NADPH which has been generated in the HMP shunt, $NADP^+$ being released for further reduction in the shunt. The generation of NADPH in the HMP shunt is dependent on glucose uptake by the cell. In liver, the enzyme acetic thiokinase, which is necessary for the synthesis of acetyl CoA, appears to be a regulatory step in lipogenesis in addition to acetyl CoA carboxylase (Murthy and Steiner, 1972; 1973).

Esterification of Fatty Acids. Fatty acids are esterified with glycerol to produce predominantly triglyceride. Free glycerol cannot be utilised for esterification; it must first be converted to α-glycerol phosphate which is the molecule to which fatty acids are added to yield eventually mono-, di-, and triglycerides. The enzyme necessary for the conversion of glycerol to α-glycerol phosphate

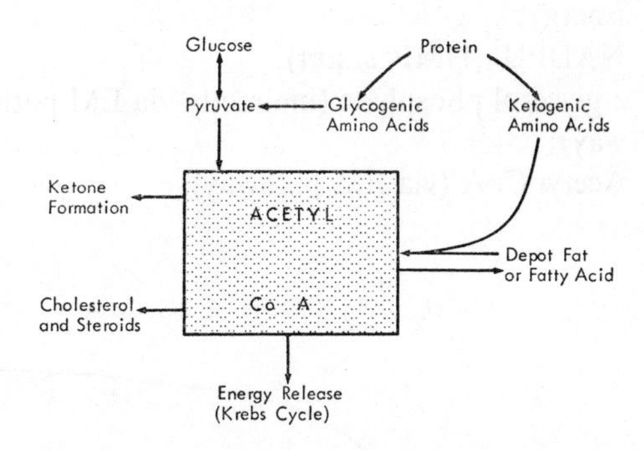

FIGURE 14.7 The reactions of acetyl coenzyme A

is glycerol-phosphokinase, which is absent from adipose tissue, although it is present in the liver. It is essential therefore, that for the esterification of fatty acids in adipose tissue there should be an

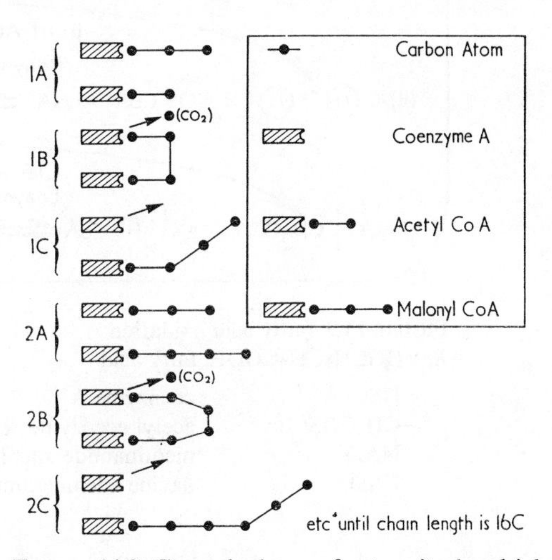

FIGURE 14.8 General scheme of extramitochondrial fatty acid synthesis

adequate supply of α-glycerol phosphate, and this is provided during glycolysis—dihydroxyacetone phosphate being converted to α-glycerol phosphate under the influence of α-glycerolphosphate dehydrogenase.

It can be seen that the metabolism of glucose by the fat cell yields all the factors necessary for the formation of triglyceride fat:

1. Energy;
2. NADPH (HMP shunt);
3. α-glycerol phosphate (indirectly via EM pathway);
4. Acetyl CoA (via EM pathway).

hormone sensitive and attacks the 2-carbon position of glycerol. Free glycerol is released, which then leaves the fat cell to be metabolised in the liver. The fatty acids released may be re-esterified, may be released into the circulation to be metabolised elsewhere, or may be broken down by the process of β-oxidation, each 2-carbon atom unit contributing to one molecule of acetyl CoA (Fig. 14.9). Growth hormone also increases mobilis-

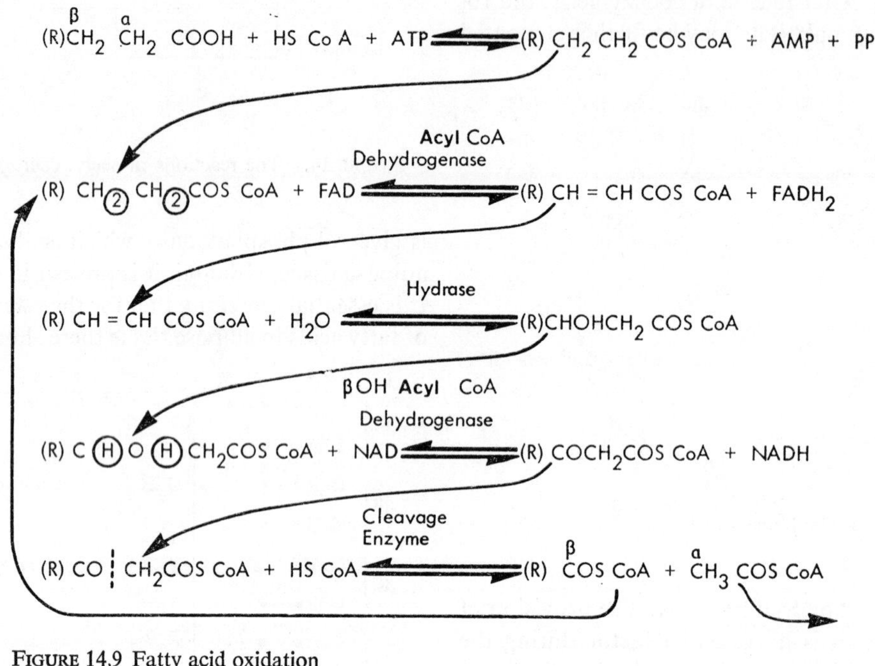

FIGURE 14.9 Fatty acid oxidation
Key (R)CH_2CH_2COOH fatty acid

HSCoA	coenzyme A
$CH_3COSCoA$	acetyl coenzyme A
NAD	nicotinamide adenine dinucleotide
FAD	flavine adenine dinucleotide

Lipolysis. The triglyceride is first attacked by the enzymes, triglyceride and monoglyceride lipase. The former enzyme, which is released on fasting, is hormone sensitive (adrenaline and glucagon, etc.) and is activated by cyclic 3′5′ AMP. It attacks the 1- and 3- carbon positions of the glycerol molecule. Monoglyceride lipase is also released on starvation but does not appear to be

ation of FFA but does not act through triglyceride lipase. Its effect may be to prevent re-esterification of FFA. In the intact organism, the lipolytic response to fasting is probably initiated and maintained by the interactions of a number of different hormones—adrenaline, growth hormone, corticotrophin and glucagon.

The Fatty Acid-Triglyceride Cycle in Fat. The

amount and composition of triglyceride in adipose tissue results from a balance of:

1. The input of preformed lipids from the gut, which have been processed in the liver.
2. The input of preformed lipids synthesised in the liver.
3. *De novo* synthesis of lipid in the fat cell from glucose.
4. Mobilisation of free fatty acids.

Preformed lipid is carried in the circulation as lipoprotein and is hydrolysed before entry into the cell by lipoprotein lipase. The synthesis of lipid in the cell is indirectly controlled by insulin which regulates glucose entry into the cell. The lipolysis of triglyceride is constantly taking place. This reaction involves the lipase enzymes mentioned above and is accelerated by the catecholamines and by corticotrophin. The fatty acids liberated on lipolysis are either re-esterified, oxidised, or liberated into the circulation (by a process of simple diffusion) where they are bound to albumin and carried to the tissues. There is a constant cycle between FFA and triglyceride in the fat cell (Fig. 14.10), the speed and direction of the cycle depending on the circumstances and the needs of the body. When

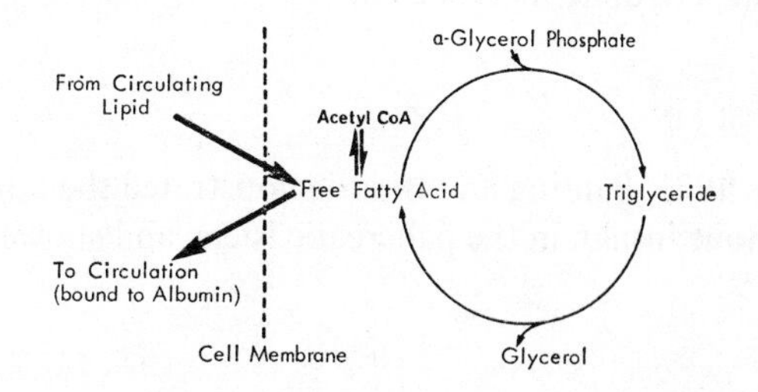

FIGURE 14.10 The free fatty acid—triglyceride cycle

there is a free supply of glucose, fatty acids are synthesised and esterified to triglyceride. On starvation, the cycle favours lipolysis, followed by oxidation or release of fatty acids, due to activation of triglyceride lipase and to deficiency of glucose and, hence, of the essential factors necessary for lipogenesis.

THE PANCREAS AND ITS HORMONES

Anatomy

The pancreas is a compound racemose gland, which is flattened and elongated, and measures 12 to 15 cm in length. The head is lodged within the curve of the duodenum, and sometimes a small portion of the head is actually embedded in the duodenal wall. The boundary between the head and the neck is marked anteriorly by a groove for the gastro-duodenal artery, and the anterior surface of the neck and body is covered with peritoneum. The posterior surface is in contact with the aorta and the origin of the superior mesenteric artery, the left adrenal gland and the left kidney and its vessels. The tail is narrow and is contained within the two layers of the lienorenal ligament, together with the splenic vessels. The arteries of the pancreas are derived from the splenic and the pancreaticoduodenal arteries. Venous drainage is into the portal, splenic and superior mesenteric veins.

Structure and Functions

The normal human pancreas weighs between 50 and 75 g, of which only about one gramme is islet tissue. It possesses between a quarter and one and three-quarter million islets of Langerhans which are scattered throughout the organ, increasing in number towards the tail. Individual islets vary from about 75 to 175 microns in diameter, and the different cells composing the islet may be identified by their staining and morphological characteristics. In the human pancreas the two cell types of importance are the α and β cells—the latter predominate, accounting for 70 to 80 per cent of the total. The α cells are subdivided into α_1 and α_2 cells. It is thought that the α_1 cells may be the source of gastrin which is present in small quantities in the islets; the α_2 cells are the source of glucagon. The β cells secrete insulin, and both glucagon and insulin participate in the control of carbohydrate metabolism.

INSULIN

In 1921, Banting and Best demonstrated the hormone insulin in the pancreatic islets, and showed that it lowered blood sugar. Within a year, extracts suitable for clinical use were prepared. Insulin is a small polypeptide with a molecular weight of about 6,000 in the monomer form, composed of two chains, A (glycyl) and B (phenylalanyl), held together by disulphide linkages. The structure of the molecule was established by Sanger in 1956 (Fig. 14.11), and its synthesis in low yield has been achieved by Katsoyannis (1964). Human, bovine, and porcine insulins differ from one another, and antibodies are invariably present in patients treated with insulins of animal origin.

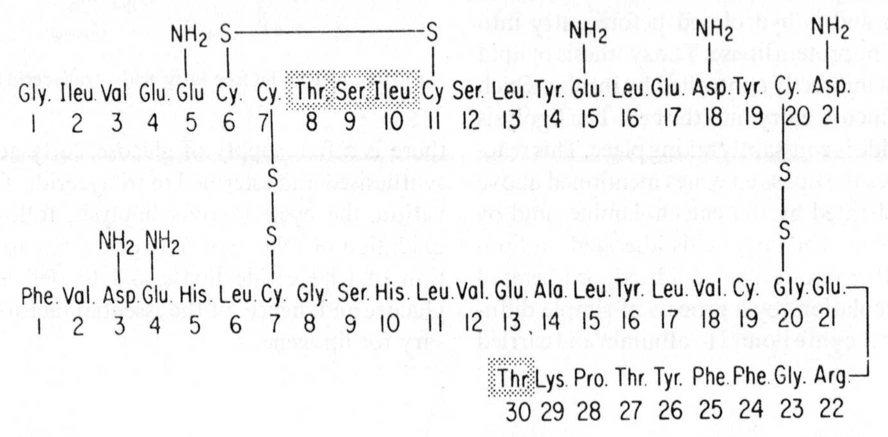

Structure of human insulin. The structures of certain animal species differ only as follows:

	Chain A			Chain B
	8	9	10	30
Man	Thr	Ser	Ileu	Thr
Pig	Thr	Ser	Ileu	Ala
Rabbit	Thr	Ser	Ileu	Ser
Beef	Ala	Ser	Val	Ala

FIGURE 14.11 The structure of insulin (from *Textbook of Endocrinology* (1968), Ed. Williams)

Proinsulin

Proinsulin, which is a precursor in the biosynthesis of insulin, has been demonstrated in pancreatic islet cells. It has been suggested that proinsulin is a normal constituent of all insulin-secreting cells, and the hormone has been demonstrated in blood and urine in normal individuals (Rubenstein *et al.*, 1968). Human proinsulin is a single-chain polypeptide with a molecular weight of about 9,000 and its structure is shown in Fig. 14.12. The composition of the connecting peptide, which connects the N-terminal of the A chain to the C-terminal of the B chain varies greatly from species to species and may contain 30–40 amino-acid residues. The terms connecting peptide and C peptide are not synonymous. The C peptide is proteolytically derived from the connecting peptide during the formation of insulin and has four basic residues less in its structure than the connecting peptide. Two of these residues are lost at its N-terminal and two at its C-terminal. Human C peptide contains 31 amino-acids and has a molecular weight of 3,021. Since proinsulin contains the intact amino-acid sequence of the insulin molecule, it is not surprising that it cross-reacts with antibodies produced against various species of insulin. It may therefore interfere with the insulin radioimmunoassay, although it has different electrophoretic properties to insulin. Proinsulin exerts an insulin-like effect *in vitro* and *in vivo* (Lazarus *et al.*, 1972; Toomey *et al.*, 1970; Lazarus *et al.*, 1970), although its activity is considerably less than that of insulin. There is no evidence that proinsulin must be converted to insulin to exert its biological effect. The C peptide appears to be biologically inactive.

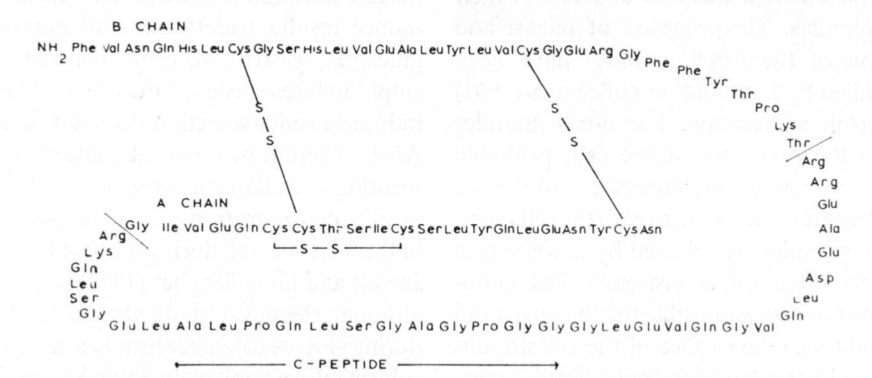

FIGURE 14.12 The structure of human proinsulin (from Taylor, 1972). Reproduced by permission of the author and publishers

The fasting concentration of proinsulin-like material in normal subjects ranges from 0–0·4 ng/ml and represents 0 to 40 per cent of the insulin concentration; the percentage of proinsulin present in the pancreas is much less—1 to 2 per cent (Lazarus, 1972). The plasma concentration of proinsulin, like that of insulin, rises after oral glucose or intravenous tolbutamide stimulation. Obese subjects show a greater rise of proinsulin after glucose stimulation than do normal subjects, although since insulin levels are also raised the proportion of proinsulin to insulin remains the same. High levels of proinsulin (30 to 85 per cent of total immunoreactive insulin) are found in the plasma of patients with islet cell tumour, and this is the only condition in which an absolute increase in the level of proinsulin has been found. Serum proinsulin-like material comprises less than 20 per cent of the total immunoreactive insulin in diabetic patients (Goldsmith, Yalow and Berson, 1969) and there is no evidence that a defect in the insulin hydrolysis mechanism plays any role in the aetiology of diabetes mellitus. The high level of proinsulin observed in patients with islet cell tumours is a secondary phenomenon, and the increased concentration (but normal proportion) in obesity appears simply to reflect an increased rate of insulin turnover.

Synthesis, Storage and Secretion of Insulin

Insulin is synthesised in the endoplasmic reticulum of the β cell as a single chain precursor, proinsulin, from which the two-chain structure is split-off by a trypsin-like enzyme (Steiner *et al.*, 1969). The rate of insulin synthesis is highly dependent on glucose concentrations and the synthesis of proinsulin is also glucose-dependent. Islets respond to an increased concentration of glucose in their environment with increased rates of metabolism of glucose and of insulin secretion.

The effect of glucose in stimulating insulin synthesis does not seem to be related to an increase in newly formed RNA. The newly synthesised material is transported to the Golgi complex and insulin is stored in the β-cell granules in a crystalline form, possibly combined with zinc to form a stable insoluble complex. The morphology of the granules as observed on electron microscopy differs from species to species, and this may be related to the different chemical structure of their insulin molecules. The processes of release and reformation of the β-cell granules have been closely studied by Lacy and his colleagues (1961) using electron microscopy. The β-cell granules migrate to the periphery of the cell, probably guided by a system of microtubules, and the sac in which they are enclosed fuses with the cell membrane. The granules are released by margination and granule extrusion, a process called emiocytosis. The factors responsible for the migration of the granules to the surface of the cell are unknown. β-cell granulation indicates insulin storage, and degranulation indicates increased insulin output. Degranulation may also be observed when the insulinogenic capacity of the β-cell is lost, as in alloxan-treated animals and in animals with diabetes secondary to the chronic administration of adrenocortical or growth hormones. Once the cell is degranulated, an interval is necessary before regranulation can occur, and before further release of insulin is possible. Both transport and secretion of insulin involve glucose utilisation and control of secretion may be exercised at the level of glucose phosphorylation or possibly through a reaction involving the early stages of the hexosemonophosphate pathways.

Recently it has been shown that there are two phases of insulin secretion. After glucose stimulation, an acute release of insulin within the first one to three minutes after the stimulus, amounting to about two per cent of the total insulin stored, is followed by a sustained and more prolonged increase in secretion over the next 30 to 60 minutes (Grodsky *et al.*, 1969). This phenomenon has been explained by assuming that there is a small labile pool of insulin which can easily be released on stimulation. It is thought that after synthesis insulin is transferred to a second compartment within the β-cell from which release may take place over an extended period of time. Tolbutamide produces release only from the more labile compartment. Many of the agents which stimulate insulin secretion do so through the mediation of cyclic AMP, which is elaborated in the cell membrane and which in some way causes insulin secretion to take place. Substances which induce insulin secretion in this manner include glucagon, gastrin, secretin, corticotrophin and sulphonylurea drugs. Glucose and amino-acid induced insulin secretion does not involve cyclic AMP. There is now considerable evidence documenting circadian variation in blood glucose and insulin concentrations, both in the fasting and in the fed state and during glucose tolerance tests. Jarrett and his colleagues (1972) have shown that although the mean blood glucose levels obtained during glucose tolerance tests in a group of normal subjects were similar during tests carried out in the afternoon and in the evening, these levels were significantly higher than those seen in tests carried out in the morning. Plasma immunoreactive insulin levels, however, were highest in the morning tests. These results support the hypothesis that diurnal variation in glucose tolerance is secondary to a circadian rhythm in the islet cells.

Factors Stimulating Pancreatic Insulin Release

1. *Hyperglycaemia*. The rate of insulin release is largely controlled by the blood glucose level. When this rises the rate of insulin secretion rises, and the rate of secretion falls with a fall in blood glucose. Glucose stimulates the reformation of the β-cells granules, i.e. the synthesis of insulin, as well as their release. The reappearance of normal granulation is seen some six hours after degranulation has been induced by glucose.

2. *Amino-acids*. Leucine, arginine, lysine and phenylalanine stimulate pancreatic insulin release, and in some cases there is a synergistic effect between two amino-acids (e.g. arginine and leucine).

Little is known about the intracellular mechanism for insulin release by amino-acids.

3. *Hormonal factors.* (*a*) *Glucagon.* Samols *et al.* (1965) have demonstrated a rise in plasma insulin after glucagon injection and have shown that this is due to a direct effect on the pancreas, and is not secondary to the hyperglycaemia produced by glucagon. This action of glucagon in stimulating insulin secretion is now well documented, and is used as the basis of a test for the diagnosis of islet cell tumour.

(*b*) *Enterohumoral Factors.* Oral glucose produces a more striking rise in plasma insulin than the same dose given intravenously, despite the lower blood glucose levels resulting from oral administration. This effect is not dependent on the liver, as it occurs in patients with end-to-side porto-caval anastomoses. The most likely explanation for these observations is that oral glucose causes the release of a humoral substance which stimulates the pancreatic islets to release insulin. A number of small molecular weight peptides, including secretin, pancreozymin and gastrin, stimulate insulin secretion and each has been proposed as the enterohumoral stimulus to insulin secretion which supplements the effect of oral carbohydrate. Glucagon-like material, secreted by cells in the upper gastrointestinal tract and cross-reacting with glucagon in an immunoassay, ('enteroglucagon'), is another candidate for this role. However, other polypeptide factors derived from the gut wall may also be elaborated in response to food and may then travel by the blood to the β-cell to increase the effectiveness of insulin-release under these circumstances. One such substance, which is distinct from 'enteroglucagon', has been described by Turner and Marks (1972).

(*c*) *Growth Hormone.* Administration of growth hormone leads to a continuously maintained increase in insulin secretion, and an exaggerated insulin response to hyperglycaemia. However, there is no convincing evidence that growth hormone directly or immediately affects insulin secretin and it seems likely that the effect of growth hormone on the islets is either indirect or is delayed. The results of growth hormone treatment appear to be a sensitisation of the islets to the effects of secretory agents such as glucose.

It has been shown that continued injections of growth hormone produce morphological changes in the β-cells consistent with increased insulin secretion, leading finally to β-cell degeneration and atrophy. It appears, therefore, that diabetes due to prolonged administration of growth hormone may be due to β-cell overstimulation and eventual exhaustion atrophy. There is evidence that continuous infusion of glucose into suitable animals will produce similar changes in the β-cells.

(*d*) *Corticotrophin.* It has been shown in adrenalectomised rabbits that administration of purified corticotrophin results in a five to tenfold rise in immunoassayable insulin secreted from the pancreas. A direct stimulatory effect has also been shown using *in vitro* preparations.

4. *Sulphonylurea Compounds.* These also induce insulin release, but do not stimulate granule reformation. Thus, the reappearance of normal granulation after sulphonylurea discharge takes much longer than after glucose discharge.

5. *Other Substances.* In man, medium chain triglycerides and in some animals ketone bodies and fatty acids have been shown to stimulate insulin secretion. A growing number of other substances have been reported to have similar effects, but in most cases these are not physiologically important.

6. *Neurogenic Control of Insulin Release.* The pancreas is innervated by the sympathetic nervous system and by branches of the right vagus. Insulin-induced hypoglycaemia has been shown to result from right vagal stimulation. Insulin is also released under vagal stimulation in conditions of severe stress, although the hypoglycaemia may be seen only when adrenalectomy is performed to prevent compensatory hyperglycaemic mechanisms from operating.

Inhibition of Insulin Release

Adrenaline inhibits insulin release and this effect is abolished *in vitro* by ergotamine. The beta effects of adrenaline are stimulatory, involving an accumulation of cyclic AMP, and the alpha effects are inhibitory, resulting in lowered cyclic AMP levels. The beta blocking-agent propranolol produces a fall in β-cell cyclic AMP and reduces insulin secretion, whereas the alpha blocking-agent phentolamine increases cyclic AMP and causes insulin release. In pancreatic islets the alpha receptor mechanism predominates, so that adrenaline acts as an inhibitor of insulin secretion. This action is of importance in any state where adrenaline concentrations in the blood are raised and may result in hyperglycaemia in the non-diabetic and increased rise of blood glucose in the diabetic.

The benzothiadiazine compound diazoxide is diabetogenic and reduces islet cell concentrations of cyclic AMP. Diazoxide may also promote adrenaline release, and this could in turn inhibit insulin release from the islets. Other related thiazide compounds, frequently used as diuretics, have a definite but milder diabetogenic action.

Insulin-like Activity in the Blood

After secretion, insulin enters the portal circulation and then passes to the liver. As much as 40 per cent of the insulin entering the liver may be split into its constituent A and B chains by the enzyme Glutathione-insulin transhydrogenase (G.I.T.).

The total insulin-like activity (ILA) in plasma is a variable quantity that depends on the biological technique used to measure it (*see* below). The hormone that reacts with anti-insulin serum in the immunoassay technique for insulin accounts for only a small part of the total ILA in plasma. This immunologically active insulin (a proportion of which is proinsulin) can be neutralised by adequate amounts of anti-insulin serum *in vitro*, and has been termed by Froesch (1963) suppressible ILA. Immunologically active insulin migrates as a homogenous band on electrophoresis just ahead of albumin and appears to circulate in a virtually free state. Its concentrations rise and fall in response to alterations in blood glucose level, and it is no longer detectable in plasma after total pancreatectomy. That fraction of ILA in plasma that is not suppressed by antibody, non-suppressible ILA, is probably not (by contrast with suppressible ILA) a distinct entity, and various forms have been described. Vallance-Owen (1958 and 1961a) has identified an insulin antagonist that circulates associated with plasma albumin—the synalbumin antagonist. This substance, which is present in excess in the plasma of diabetics and prediabetics, antagonises the effect of insulin on muscle but not on fat; it appears to have an insulin-like effect on fat. It has been used as a genetic marker to detect those of the population who are constituted as diabetics, and Ensinck *et al.* (1965) have suggested that the synalbumin antagonist may be the B chain of insulin, produced in the liver by cleavage of the insulin molecule by G.I.T. Another form of non-suppressible ILA, 'bound' insulin, has been described by Antoniades and his colleagues (1961, 1965) who postulate that it is derived by conjugation of insulin to a basic protein in the liver. 'Free' insulin, according to Antoniades, corresponds in all biochemical respects to immunologically active insulin, whereas 'bound' insulin has a higher molecular weight and does not react with insulin antisera. Antoniades claims that the fasting level of 'bound' insulin in plasma is eight times greater than that of 'free' insulin, and that full insulin activity can be demonstrated only when insulin is dissociated from its complexes. 'Free' insulin is active on muscle and fat, whereas 'bound' insulin produces a metabolic effect only on fat. However, when 'bound' insulin is pre-incubated with fat, an action can subsequently be demonstrated on muscle—it is claimed that fat 'unbinds' the complex, releasing 'free' insulin. Not all workers have been able to demonstrate 'bound insulin' in human serum (Meade *et al.*, 1968). A similar concept to that of Antoniades has been put forward by Samaan and his colleagues (1963), who have described 'typical' and 'atypical' forms of insulin in the blood. 'Typical' insulin is 'free' or immunologically active insulin, for it can be removed by addition of an appropriate insulin antibody, while 'atypical' insulin bears considerable resemblance to 'bound' insulin.

It seems reasonable to conclude that circulating insulin-like activity consists of two components—insulin (including proinsulin) directly comparable to the hormones of pancreatic origin, and a second component which is distinct from insulin by physicochemical and physiological criteria. The precise role of non-suppressible ILA in normal physiology and disease states is not yet fully understood but possible relationships are discussed further in Chapter 15.

Insulin Antagonists, Resistance, and Antibodies

Vallance-Owen (1960) has defined an insulin antagonist as any substance or fraction that can modify or combine with insulin to render it inactive or counteract its effect *in vivo* or *in vitro*. A number of hormones, particularly the adrenocortical steroids and growth hormone, are regarded as physiological insulin antagonists. In addition, a number of other substances such as the synalbumin antagonist have been identified in plasma. They are probably not hormones, but they may be hormone-dependent and have an anti-insulin effect. A polypeptide which is antagonistic to insulin and which is of a similar nature to the growth hormone derived polypeptide In-G (*see* below) has been detected in the plasma of normal subjects and, in higher concentrations, in the plasma of diabetics (Zimmet *et al.*, 1971). The polypeptide is absent from the plasma of hypophysectomised diabetic patients and appears to be of pituitary origin, but its significance in the pathogenesis of diabetes is unknown.

Insulin Resistance in Diabetic Ketosis. Very large amounts of insulin may sometimes be needed to reverse diabetic ketosis. This resistance is short-lived, and an antagonist that migrates electrophoretically with the α_1-globulin fraction has been described, although the factor responsible has not yet been identified. In diabetic ketosis there is some inhibition of cellular glucose uptake secondary to the ketosis, but this does not necessarily indicate insulin antagonism as defined above.

Insulin Antibodies. Insulin binding antibodies can almost invariably be identified in the plasma of diabetic or normal subjects who have received insulin for more than three months. Such antibodies may occasionally cause insulin resistance in diabetics, when treatment with adrenocortical steroids may be beneficial. They do not play a major part in determining insulin requirements in most patients, and cannot be implicated in the aetiology of diabetes. Apart from these antibodies there is no evidence that other plasma proteins bind insulin, although Arquilla (1966) has reported the isolation of a heat-labile insulin-binding factor which is present in normal plasma, which may be an α_2-globulin and which is not a component of complement. These findings remain to be confirmed. Insulin in insulin-treated diabetics is bound to IgG.

The Metabolic Effects of Insulin

The major effect of insulin is to increase the utilisation of glucose by most body tissues, and it does so by increasing the transportation of glucose across the cell membrane. Insulin acts mainly upon those tissues that offer a high resistance to glucose penetration—muscle, fat, the lens, and the leucocyte. In these tissues, the rate of entry of glucose is the limiting step in their metabolism of carbohydrate. The liver is much less dependent on insulin for the transport of glucose, while brain, kidney, intestinal mucosa and red cells are almost completely independent of insulin.

Insulin has the following metabolic actions:

1. *Blood Glucose.* The hypoglycaemia following insulin injection could be due either to a reduction of glucose output from the liver, or to an increase in the uptake by peripheral cells. It is now generally accepted that the latter effect is mainly responsible for insulin hypoglycaemia, although diminished hepatic output of glucose may play a part.

2. *Glucose Transfer.* Insulin increases the rate of glucose transfer across certain cell membranes. The mechanism of action is still uncertain but a number of theories have been propounded. It has been suggested that glucose might enter the cell by a process resembling pinocytosis (or 'drinking in'), although presumably much fluid would need

to accompany the sugar into the cell interior. Any theory must take into account the specificity of insulin action, since the hormone acts only on sugars with the same configuration as glucose in the C-1, -2 and -3 positions. In order to explain the phenomena of chemical specificity and competition for entry observed between glucose and other sugars, the presence of a specific insulin-dependent carrier has been postulated, which forms a sugar-carrier complex involved in transport of glucose across the cell membrane. It has been postulated that insulin may maintain this carrier in its active state.

3. *Muscle and Liver.* The most important quantitative effects of insulin in the intact animal are to increase the rate of glycogen formation in muscle and in liver and to increase the rate of oxidation of carbohydrate in muscle. Insulin increases the activity of the enzyme glycogen synthetase in muscle and liver, and of liver glucokinase, while inhibiting both gluconeogenesis and hepatic glycogenolysis. Insulin reduces the hepatic output of glucose.

4. *Adipose Tissue.* Glucose uptake and oxidation by fat is increased by insulin. Lipogenesis and the esterification of fatty acids are stimulated and the rate of release of free fatty acids is much reduced. The classical studies of Winegrad and Renold (1958) demonstrated that in the presence of insulin, the rate of oxidation of glucose via the HMP shunt is increased to a much greater degree than is its oxidation via other pathways, thus making available NADPH necessary for the synthesis of the long chain fatty acids (*see* Fig. 14.4). It has in the past been difficult to demonstrate a consistent effect of insulin on human adipose tissue *in vitro*. More recently, it has been shown that human fat is quite sensitive to physiological doses of insulin, although sensitivity diminishes with age (Gries and Steinke, 1967).

5. *Anti-ketotic Effect.* Insulin reverses ketosis largely by increasing glucose uptake and cellular metabolism, by stimulating lipid biosynthesis from glucose, by reducing the rate of fatty acid oxidation, and by reducing gluconeogenesis in the liver.

6. *Serum Potassium and Phosphate.* The reduction in serum potassium observed with insulin and glucose therapy is presumably related to the increased rate of entry of glucose into the cell, potassium entering the tissues in proportion to the amount of carbohydrate taken up. In the insulin-deficient diabetic organism, the serum phosphate level is abnormally high, and returns to normal on treatment with insulin.

7. *Protein Synthesis.* Insulin has important effects on protein synthesis, both by increasing the transport of amino-acids into the cells and by stimulating nucleic acid synthesis. These effects are not entirely dependent on an increased rate of carbohydrate utilisation, and may be observed in the absence of glucose. The mechanism by which insulin increases amino-acid transport across the cell membrane is unknown. However, this effect persists in the presence of inhibitors of protein and RNA synthesis, and the stimulation may therefore result from an activation of formerly inactive effector molecules or from an increased rate of operation of the pre-existing effector complex (Guidotti, 1971).

Thus, the overall effect of insulin is to increase the synthesis of cellular materials, the storage units *glycogen*, *fatty acids*, and *triglyceride*, and the structural and functional units *protein* and *RNA* which are also involved in growth.

The Assay of Insulin in Body Fluids

Early assays relied on the effects of serum or serum extracts on the blood sugar level of small animals rendered more insulin-sensitive by removal of various endocrine glands. Later assays depended upon the metabolic effects produced by insulin on suitable isolated tissues. The biological systems most commonly used at present are:

1. Glucose uptake by the rat epididymal fat pad.
2. Rate of oxidation of ^{14}C-labelled glucose by the fat pad.
3. Glucose uptake by the isolated rat diaphragm.

When these bioassay techniques are used, it is assumed that serum will behave in the experimental system in the same way as crystalline insulin standards, and that only insulin will significantly influence glucose metabolism. These assumptions are not completely valid, and it has therefore become usual to speak of insulin-like activity (ILA) when insulin is assayed by these methods. Reference has already been made to suppressible and non-suppressible ILA. There are marked differences in the results using different bioassay methods, and those obtained using the fat pad assay are considerably higher than those obtained using rat diaphragm.

Yalow and Berson (1959) introduced a radioimmunoassay for insulin, which measures only insulin that can be bound to specific antibody (suppressible ILA). This assay has been modified by several later workers. However, it remains uncertain whether the immunoassay technique measures all the physiologically active insulin present in biological fluids, and it does, of course, measure proinsulin. The results obtained by the immunoassay technique in normal subjects by various workers are indicated in Table 14.1. It will be seen that there is considerable variation in the results from different laboratories. The results obtained in the authors' laboratory are very similar to those of Welborn *et al.* (1966). It is usual to measure insulin in a fasting state and serially after a glucose load.

The radioimmunoassay has setbacks and the two chief disadvantages are that when labelled antigen is used a large proportion of the unknown remains unreacted, and that a change in the amount of free or bound labelled hormone is measured against a large 'background', giving a small relative change in count rate for what may be a very large relative change in the amount of unlabelled hormone bound to antibody. In addition, the procedure of labelling a hormone causes damage to it. To overcome such difficulties, Miles and Hales (1968) have utilised an immunoradiometric assay in which they labelled the insulin antibodies that had been purified on an immunoabsorbent, rather than the antigen. This assay appears to be more sensitive than the radioimmunoassay. Nevertheless, immunoassays measure immunological rather than biological properties, whereas the clinician is concerned with the latter. Recent developments using biological membranes suggest that a specific method for measuring the biological potency of circulating insulin can be developed (Freychet, Roth and Neville, 1971). The subject of biological membrane assays has been reviewed by Lazarus (1972).

TABLE 14.1 *Ranges of Plasma Insulin in Normal Subjects Estimated by Immunoassay*

Author	Date	Dose of glucose	Range of insulin values (μu/ml) at			
			Fasting	30 min	60 min	120 min
Yalow and Berson	1960	100 G	0–66	39–294	18–342	21–233
Hales and Randle	1963	100 G	10–27	45–320	20–100	—
Welborn *et al.*	1966	50 G	3–26	15–125	13–131	6–60

GLUCAGON

Glucagon is secreted by the granular α_2 cells of the pancreatic islets. It is a small protein composed of twenty-nine amino-acid residues with a molecular weight of 3,485 (Fig. 14.13), the structure being quite different from that of insulin. Glucagon is broken down chiefly in the liver by proteolysis, and its half-life in tissues appears to be less than ten minutes. A substance which shares some of the immunological and possibly physiological properties of glucagon is produced and secreted by endocrine cells in the gut (glucagon-like material or 'enteroglucagon').

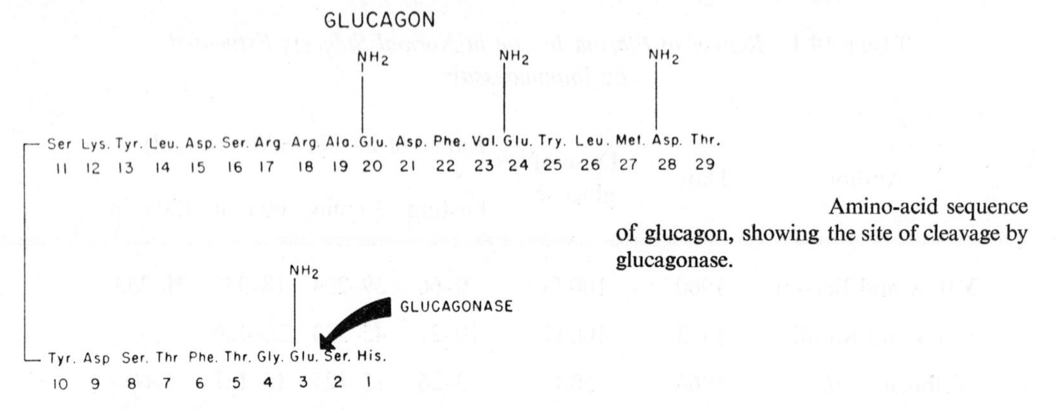

Amino-acid sequence of glucagon, showing the site of cleavage by glucagonase.

FIGURE 14.13 The structure of glucagon (from *Textbook of Endocrinology* (1968), Ed. Williams)

Metabolic Effects

1. *Insulin Secretion.* Glucagon stimulates insulin secretion by the pancreas.

2. *Blood Glucose.* The major metabolic effect of glucagon is to cause a rise in blood glucose levels by breaking down liver glycogen. Glucagon is secreted in response to lowered blood sugar levels, when it enhances the conversion of inactive liver phosphorylase B into active phosphorylase A, which increases liver glycogen breakdown. This conversion of inactive to active phosphorylase is brought about by a phosphokinase enzyme, and glucagon increases the production or release of 3′, 5′ cyclic AMP which is a vital coenzyme for the phosphokinase. The glycogenolytic effect serves to increase blood glucose, which is then utilised in extra-hepatic tissues under the influence of insulin. Glucagon itself has no readily demonstrable effect on the extra-hepatic utilisation of glucose, although repeated treatment with large doses impairs carbohydrate tolerance, probably due to β-cell exhaustion. Glucagon does not cause breakdown of muscle glycogen since it is unable to activate muscle phosphorylase. Glucagon also stimulates hepatic gluconeogenesis, its effects in this direction being counteracted by insulin.

3. *Lipolysis.* The hormone has a pronounced lipolytic effect on rat adipose tissue *in vitro*, and a similar effect may be observed in intact dogs. An unequivocal lipolytic action in man has been demonstrated, although up to three days of fasting may be necessary before this effect becomes apparent, presumably due to inhibition of the insulinotropic effect of glucagon.

4. *Lipid Lowering Effects.* Intravenous administration of glucagon produces a significant depression of total plasma lipids, triglyceride and cholesterol, and this may be due to transfer of plasma lipids to blood platelets, which release the lipid back to plasma when the action of glucagon ceases (Caren and Corbo, 1970). Plasma immunoreactive glucagon levels are abnormally high in Type III and Type IV hyperlipoproteinaemia, and in these conditions there may be endogenous glucagon resistance.

5. *Other Effects.* Glucagon lowers the serum calcium in animals, and it is possible that the raised glucagon levels observed in clinical and experimental pancreatitis are responsible for the

hypocalcaemia commonly observed in these conditions. Glucagon given intravenously is a potent stimulus to adrenaline release and has been used as a diagnostic test in phaeochromocytoma. The hormone reduces gastrointestinal motility and may produce a feeling of satiety, although this effect has proved of little value in the treatment of obesity. Glucagon also causes the release of growth hormone which occurs as the blood sugar level falls about two hours after subcutaneous administration. This effect has been used to assess growth hormone reserve.

Glucagon increases the rate and force of the cardiac contraction and has been used, in large doses given intravenously, in the treatment of refractory heart failure.

The Assay of Glucagon

Glucagon in plasma has been estimated by a radioimmunoassay technique. The assay is difficult, since glucagon is of low antigenicity and labelled glucagon is rapidly degraded in plasma. Many assays lack specificity and the presence of glucagon cross-reacting material produced in the gut further interferes with the assay. Because of this, conclusions drawn from studies utilising this technique require confirmation, and should be viewed with circumspection.

The Physiological Role of Glucagon

An excellent monograph has recently summarised current knowledge on glucagon (Lefebvre and Unger, 1972). The physiological role of glucagon appears to be to ensure, in association with insulin, a steady supply of metabolic substrates such as glucose, free fatty acids and ketones, under a wide range of circumstances (Unger and Lefebvre 1972). It appears that the molar ratio of insulin to glucagon in the blood is more important in ensuring homeostasis than the absolute concentrations of either. Glucagon is released in increased amounts from the pancreas during short periods of fasting, exercise and acute hypoglycaemia (conditions associated with a reduced secretion of insulin), ensuring an acceleration of hepatic glucose release and of free fatty acid release from adipose tissue, and an increase in gluconeogenesis. A fall in plasma free fatty acids stimulates pancreatic glucagon secretion, which is also stimulated by those amino-acids which stimulate insulin secretion and by diazoxide, pancreozymin and catecholamine. Neural factors are also important in the control of glucagon secretion and most physiological conditions under which glucagon secretion increases are associated with increased sympathetic nervous activity. Following oral glucose there is a significant fall in glucagon concentrations in normal individuals, although this fall is not observed in diabetics, and in severe insulin-dependent diabetics there is a significant rise in glucagon concentrations after oral glucose (Buchanan and McCarroll, 1972). Glucagon secretion is also inhibited by high plasma levels of free fatty acids and of insulin.

In discussing the relationships between insulin and glucagon, the effect of glucagon in stimulating insulin secretion must be considered. Conditions favourable to the stimulation of insulin secretion by glucagon occur normally only during and shortly after the ingestion of a mixed meal, which produces an increase in blood amino-acids, stimulates pancreozymin secretion and causes a fall in plasma free fatty acids, all of which stimulate pancreatic glucagon secretion at a time when its insulinotropic effect is favourable and desirable. Under all other circumstances which cause increased glucagon secretion such as starvation, muscular exercise and hypoglycaemia, the insulinotropic effect is inhibited by adrenergic activity or by intracellular substrate deficiency, while glucagon increases the availability of metabolisable substrate to active tissue. Insulin itself inhibits glucagon secretion, although it is uncertain whether this is a direct effect on the α_2 cells of the islets. When insulin secretion is reduced there is an increased secretion of glucagon. This is most marked in diabetic ketosis, and contributes to biochemical deterioration by accelerating lipolysis and increasing hyperglycaemia.

It has recently been suggested (Marks, 1972), that glucagon is casually related to the increased protein breakdown which follows surgical or other trauma and this would be consistent with what is known about the secretion and actions of glucagon.

THE ACTIONS OF OTHER HORMONES ON THE METABOLISM OF CARBOHYDRATE AND FAT

Vallance-Owen and Lilley (1961b) have stated that synalbumin insulin antagonism is dependent on an intact pituitary-adrenal axis. Thus, acromegaly and Cushing's syndrome may lead to impaired carbohydrate tolerance or to frank diabetes by increasing the level of synalbumin or other antagonism in those genetically constituted as diabetics (prediabetics). Apart from this possible relationship, however, most naturally occurring hormones have significant direct effects on carbohydrate and fat metabolism.

GROWTH HORMONE

The actions of growth hormone on carbohydrate and fat metabolism are complex, and will be dealt with in three parts:

(*a*) Metabolic effects.

(*b*) Physiological effects in the intact animals.

(*c*) Diabetogenic effects.

(*a*) *Metabolic Effects of Growth Hormone.* Early and late effects of growth hormone on the metabolism of glucose by fat have been described (Goodman, 1965). The early effects represent an insulin-like action, with stimulation of glucose uptake by fat, increased oxidation of the glucose and increased incorporation of the substrate into lipid. A further early action is an anti-lipolytic effect (Goodman, 1970). The late actions, which are observed three hours after injection of growth hormone in hypophysectomised rats, produce a diabetogenic or hyperglycaemic effect with reduced glucose uptake and fatty acid synthesis, and markedly increased lipolysis. Bornstein and his colleagues have described two polypeptides prepared from growth hormone by hydrolysis which by their actions on certain enzymes of the glycolytic pathways appear capable of accounting for both the early insulin-like and the later hyperglycaemic actions of the hormone (Bornstein *et al.*, 1968). The first of these fractions has been named acceleratory polypeptide growth hormone (Ac-G) and the second, inhibitory polypeptide growth hormone (In-G). All the known actions of growth hormone on carbohydrate and fat metabolism may be accounted for by the actions of these polypeptides. In-G inhibits glycolysis and fat synthesis and accelerates breakdown of fat, Ac-G causes hypoglycaemia and increased glucose metabolism by fat, and also reverses the inhibition produced by In-G. It is thought that In-G acts by inhibiting the enzyme triosephosphate dehydrogenase. The respective effects of these polypeptide fractions have been demonstrated in man (Armstrong *et al.*, 1969).

Growth hormone stimulates protein synthesis in muscle and fat, and a considerably greater effect is obtained when insulin is present in addition to growth hormone. The effect of growth hormone on protein synthesis *in vivo* is thought to be largely mediated through the action of insulin. Hepatic gluconeogenesis and ketone production is increased in the presence of growth hormone. These effects presumably reflect the actions of the In-G fraction.

(*b*) *Physiological Effects of Growth Hormone in the Intact Animal.* The interaction of growth hormone and insulin which has been suggested to follow a mixed meal is as follows:

Blood glucose rises and insulin is secreted, the secretion of growth hormone being depressed. Under the influence of insulin, glucose enters the cell and is metabolised, lipogenesis is stimulated and release of free fatty acid from adipose tissue is much reduced. Insulin secretion in response to the carbohydrate fraction of the meal is magnified by the effects of pancreatic glucagon and the enterohumoral factors. As the blood glucose level falls, the secretion of growth hormone and glucagon increases and rapid synthesis of protein results from the combined actions of growth hormone and insulin. As the blood glucose returns to fasting levels, the secretion of insulin ceases and the output of growth hormone and glucagon rises further. As a result of this, lipolysis is stimulated and plasma FFA levels rise. The preferential uptake and oxidation of FFA by muscle has a glucose-sparing effect, thus avoiding too great a fall in blood glucose levels until the next meal is taken. Growth hormone therefore has the effect, in the intact animal, of reducing glucose utilisation by muscle. If this scheme is the correct interpretation of the physiological situation, it is apparent that under normal conditions physiological levels of growth hormone do not stimulate insulin release in the presence of a normal or low blood glucose. In other words, the depressant effect of a low blood glucose level on insulin secretion predominates over any stimulatory effect of growth hormone.

(*c*) *Diabetogenic Effects of Growth Hormone.* Growth hormone is a physiological insulin antagonist, and 25 per cent of acromegalic patients show carbohydrate intolerance after a glucose load. Since the studies of Houssay, is has been apparent that growth hormone aggravates the severity of diabetes mellitus and that hypophysectomy alleviates the condition. Injection of human growth hormone in normal individuals results in a rise in plasma free fatty acid levels and impairment of carbohydrate tolerance. In these and other acute experiments, it seems likely that the effect of the In-G polypeptide fraction, particularly the lipolytic effect, is largely responsible for the diabetogenic action of the hormone. Young showed, in animal studies, that prolonged growth hormone administration can induce permanent diabetes in some species, particularly the dog, and this effect is largely due to β-cell exhaustion and atrophy. Animals on a low carbohydrate diet treated with growth hormone for long periods do not develop diabetes and, presumably carbohydrate restriction protects the β-cells. There is also evidence that somatomedin (otherwise known as the sulphation factor), a growth-promoting protein produced by the action of growth hormone on the liver, competes with insulin for binding to receptors on the fat cell membrane. It seems possible that the anti-insulin action of growth hormone may, at least in part, be due to this action of somatomedin.

CORTICOTROPHIN

This hormone mobilises free fatty acid, reduces blood sugar levels and has a ketogenic effect. It is also potentially diabetogenic by stimulating secretion of corticosteroids.

CORTICOSTEROIDS

Cortisol, like growth hormone, is a physiological insulin antagonist. About 25 per cent of patients with Cushing's syndrome show impaired carbohydrate tolerance or overt diabetes, whereas hypoadrenalism produces an amelioration of the diabetic state. When Addison's disease and diabetes occur together, there is extreme sensitivity to exogenous insulin, but insulin requirements are increased as steroid replacement therapy is given. The glucocorticoids increase hepatic output of glucose, increase protein catabolism and gluconeogenesis, and may decrease peripheral glucose utilisation in both muscle and fat. These may be the reasons for the diabetogenic action of these hormones and would explain the insulin sensitivity seen in hypoadrenal states.

ADRENALINE

Adrenaline inhibits insulin secretion (*see* above). Adrenaline increases the breakdown of liver glycogen by an action similar to that of glucagon (p. 306), but it is of interest that while glucagon only activates liver phosphorylase, adrenaline stimulates the activity of the enzyme in both liver and muscle. Adrenaline also mobilises free fatty acid by activating the hormone-sensitive triglyceride lipase in fat, again through the mediation of cyclic 3′5′ AMP—an action that takes place through the β-adrenergic receptors (Pilkington *et al.*, 1962). This lipolytic effect will help to maintain blood glucose levels as FFA will be preferentially metabolised by muscle. It seems likely that under physiological conditions, the lipolytic effect of adrenaline reinforces that of growth hormone.

NORADRENALINE

Noradrenaline has no effect on liver phosphorylase, but has a similar lipolytic effect to adrenaline. Like adrenaline, noradrenaline inhibits insulin secretion.

ALDOSTERONE

A high percentage of patients with aldosteronism have abnormal glucose tolerance curves, and there may be a very small number of diabetic patients who have an undiagnosed aldosterone secreting tumour of the adrenal. The impaired carbohydrate tolerance in aldosteronism is reversible by potassium loading, and Conn (1965) has suggested that it is due to the effects of chronic potassium depletion rather than to the glucocorticoid action of aldosterone.

THYROID HORMONES

Carbohydrate tolerance is often impaired in thyrotoxic patients, and overt diabetes is aggravated. Blood glucose levels in abnormal thyroid states are influenced principally by the effects of excess or deficient hormone on the gastro-intestinal tract, absorption of hexose sugars being decreased in thyroid deficiency and increased when thyroid hormone is present in excess. Thyroid hormone increases gluconeogenesis and also increases the rate of carbohydrate utilisation by peripheral tissues.

OESTROGEN

Oral contraceptives induce a complex series of changes in carbohydrate metabolism, and the magnitude of the alterations depends on the integrity of the β cells in providing adequate compensatory hyperinsulinism (Yen and Vela, 1969).

Impaired glucose tolerance may be observed to develop in potential and latent diabetics during therapy with oestrogen containing ovulatory suppressant drugs, and the renal threshold for glucose may be decreased. In patients with established diabetes there is little change in insulin requirements during the administration of oral contraceptives. Javier *et al.* (1968) have shown that 85 per cent of women taking oral contraceptives develop abnormal cortisone stressed glucose tolerance tests and that administration of the oestrogen alone produces these changes. In the early stages of treatment, insulin secretion tends to increase, but with prolonged therapy insulin secretion may decrease in some women. The reason for these changes is unknown, but they may be related to alterations in hepatic function or to humoral and enzymic factors in the entero-hepatic system.

REFERENCES

Antoniades, H. N. (1961). *Endocrinology*, **68,** 7.

Antoniades, H. N., Huber, A. M., Boshell, B. R., Saravis, C. W., and Gershoff, S. N. (1965). *Endocrinology*, **76,** 709.

Armstrong J. McD., Bornstein, J. Ng, F. M. and Taft, H. P. (1969) *Brit. Med. J.*, **2,** 157.

Arquilla, E. R (1966) *Diabetes*, **15,** 281.

Banting, F. G., and Best, C. H. (1922). *J. lab. clin. Med.*, **7,** 251.

Bornstein, J., Krahl, M. E., Marshall, L. B., Gould, M. K. and Armstrong, J. McD. (1968). *Biochim. Biophys. Acta*, **156,** 31.

Buchanan, K, D. and McCarroll, A. M. (1972). *Lancet*, **ii,** 1394.

Caren, R. and Corbo, L. (1970). *Metabolism*, **19,**, 598.

Conn, J. W. (1965). *New Eng. J. Med.*, **273,** 1135.

Ensinck, J. W., Mahler, R. J., and Vallance-Owen, J. (1965). *Biochem. J.*, **94,** 150.

Freychet, D., Roth, J. and Neville, D. M. Jr. (1971). *Proc. Nat. Acad. Sci.*, **68,** 1823.

Froesch, E. R., Bürgi, H., Ramseier, E. B., Bally, P., and Labhart, A. (1963). *J. clin. Invest.*, **42,** 1816.

Goldsmith, J. J., Yalow, R. S., and Berson, S. A. (1969). *Diabetes*, **18**, 834.
Goodman, H. M. (1965). *Endocrinology*, **76**, 1134.
Goodman, H. M. (1970). *Metabolism*, **19**, 849.
Gries, F. A., and Steinke, J. (1967). *Metabolism*, **16**, 693.
Grodsky, G. M. *et al.* (1969). *Acta diabet. lat.* **6** (Suppl. 1), 554.
Guidotti, G. G. (1971). *Acta diabet. lat.* **8**, 1201.
Hales, C. M., and Randle, P. J. (1963). *Lancet*, **i**, 790.
Jarrett, R. J., Baker, I. A., Keen, H., and Oakley, N. W. (1972). *Brit. med. J.*, **1**, 199.
Javier, Z., Gershberg, H., and Hulse, M. (1968). *Metabolism*, **17**, 443.
Jenkins, D. J. A. (1967). *Lancet*, **ii**, 338.
Katsoyannis, P. G. (1964). *Diabetes*, **13**, 339.
Lacy, P. E., Williamson, J. R., and Grisham, J. W. (1961). *Diabetes*, **10**, 463.
Lazarus, N. R. (1972). In *Clinics in Endocrinology and Metabolism*, **1:3**, (Ed. D. A. Pyke). London: Saunders, p. 623.
Lazarus, N. R., Gutman, R. A., Penhos, J. C. and Recant, L. (1972). *Diabetologia*, **8**, 131.
Lazarus, N. R., Penhos, J. C., Tanese, T., Michaels, L., Gutman, R., and Recant, L. (1970). *J. Clin. Invest.*, **49**, 487.
Lefebvre, P. J., and Unger, R. H. (Eds) (1972). *Glucagon—Molecular Physiology, Clinical and Therapeutic Implications.* Oxford: Pergamon.
Marks, V. (1972). In *Clinics in Endocrinology and Metabolism*, **1:3** (Ed. D. A. Pyke). London: Saunders, p. 829.
Meade, R. C., Brush, J. S., and Klitgaard, H. M. (1968). *Diabetes*, **17**, 369.
Miles, L. E. M., and Hales, C. N. (1968). *Biochem. J.*, **108**, 611.
Murthy, V. K., and Steiner, G. (1972). *Metabolism*, **21**, 213.
Murthy, V. K., and Steiner, G. (1973). *Metabolism*, **22**, 81.
Pilkington, T. R. E., Lowe, R. D., Robinson, B. F., and Titterington E. (1962). *Lancet*, **ii**, 316.
Randle, P. J., Garland, P. B., Hales, C. N., and Newsholme, E. A. (1963). *Lancet*, **i**, 785.
Rubenstein, A. H., Cho, S., and Steiner, D. F. (1968). *Lancet*, **i**, 1353.
Saaman, N. A., Fraser, R., and Dampster, J. (1963). *Diabetes*, **12**, 339.
Samols, E., Tyler, J., Marri, G., and Marks, V. (1965). *Lancet*, **ii**, 1257.
Sanger, F. (1956). *Ciba Found. Coll. Endocrinol.*, **9**, 110.,
Steiner, D. F., Clark, J. L., Nolan, C., Rubenstein, A. H.. Margolish, E., Aten, B. and Oyer, P. E. 1969). *Rec prog. Hormone Res.*, **25**, 207.
Taylor, K. W. (1972). In *Clinics in Endocrinology and Metabolism*, **1:3** (Ed. D. A. Pyke). London: Saunders p. 601.
Toomey, R. E., Shaw, W. N., Reid, L. R. Jr., and Young, W. K. (1970). *Diabetes*, **19**, 209.
Turner, D. S., and Marks, V. (1972). *Lancet*, **i**, 1095.
Unger, R. H., and Lefebvre, P. J. (1972). In *Glucagon* (Ed. P. J. Lefebvre and R. H. Unger). Oxford: Pergamon.
Vallance-Owen, J. (1960). *Brit. med. Bull.*, **16**, 214.
Vallance-Owen, J., Dennes, E., and Campbell, P. N. (1958). *Lancet*, **ii**, 336.
Vallance-Owen, J., and Lilley, M. D. (1961a). *Lancet*, **i**, 214.
Vallance-Owen, J., and Lilley, M. D. (1961b). *Lancet*, **i**, 804.
Welborn, T. A., Rubenstein, A. H., Haslam, R., and Fraser, R. (1966). *Lancet*, **i**, 280.
Winegrad, A. I., and Renold, A. E. (1958). *J. Biol. Chem.*, **233**, 269, 273.
Yalow, R. S., and Berson, A. S. (1959). *Nature* (Lond.), **184**, 1648.
Yalow, R. S., and Berson, S. A. (1950). *J. clin. Invest.*, **39**, 1157.
Yen, S. S. C., and Vela, P. (1969). *J. Reproduct. Med.*, **3**, 6.
Zimmet, P., Ng, F. M., Bornstein, J., Armstrong, J. McD., and Taft, H. P. (1971). *Brit. Med. J.*, **1**, 203.

15

DIABETES MELLITUS

Diabetes mellitus is the name given to a syndrome that has as its most prominent feature an elevation in the concentration of glucose in the blood, with consequent glycosuria. This abnormal elevation of blood glucose level may occur only after the intake of carbohydrate and may not be associated with any symptoms. When a high concentration is sustained, however, considerable quantities of glucose are lost in the urine, and this is associated with polyuria, the result of an osmotic diuresis, with consequent thirst and lack of energy, and with weight loss resulting, in part, from the loss of calories in the urine.

Although the disturbance in carbohydrate metabolism is obvious and easily measured and can be reasonably controlled, other biochemical abnormalities undoubtedly exist since there is a great tendency even for well-controlled patients to develop complications, the most serious and characteristic being related to the vascular system.

Von Mering and Minkowski in 1889 reproduced the syndrome of diabetes mellitus in animals by total pancreatectomy and, since it was subsequently shown that loss of acinar tissue was not responsible, it was suggested that deficiency of an internal secretion from the Islets of Langerhans might be the cause of the human disease. The name insulin was later suggested for this secretion by Knowlton and Starling in 1912, and in 1921 Banting and Best obtained a pancreatic extract which lowered the concentration of glucose in the plasma, a finding that was to revolutionise the treatment of patients with diabetes mellitus. Evidence has since accumulated, however, which suggests that a simple deficiency in insulin secretion is only one cause of the syndrome of diabetes mellitus.

CLASSIFICATION

The overt syndrome is conventionally classified as idiopathic (or essential), where the condition is inherited, and secondary when it is related to some other disease or is precipitated by certain drugs. This division is somewhat unsatisfactory, as a number of patients with 'secondary' diabetes already have a hereditary disposition to develop the syndrome (prediabetics or potential diabetics) and should more properly be classified as having 'idiopathic diabetes precipitated by superadded factors'. Bearing in mind that diabetes mellitus is the same clinical syndrome whatever the causation or associations, the following classification is suggested:

A. Hereditary idiopathic diabetes mellitus

1. Prediabetes
2. Latent diabetes
3. Asymptomatic (chemical) diabetes

} sub-clinical

4. Overt diabetes—'juvenile onset' (insulin-dependent) type
'maturity onset' type with or without obesity

B. *Diabetes mellitus due to demonstrable pancreatic disease*

1. Chronic pancreatitis
2. Haemochromatosis
3. After pancreatectomy
4. Tumours
5. After acute pancreatitis
6. After removal of an islet cell tumour

C. *Diabetes mellitus related to other endocrine syndromes*

1. Cushing's syndrome
2. Acromegaly
3. Phaeochromocytoma
4. Aldosteronism
5. Thyrotoxicosis

D. *Diabetes mellitus precipitated by drugs*

1. Thiazide diuretics
2. Steroids
3. Ovulatory suppressant compounds
4. Diazoxide
5. Alloxan, streptozotocin and other substances toxic to the β cells.

E. *Diabetes mellitus related to non-endocrine disease*

1. Chronic renal failure
2. Liver disease

A. TYPES OF IDIOPATHIC DIABETES MELLITUS

1. *Prediabetes or Potential Diabetes* is the state of those individuals who may eventually develop the overt syndrome, but in whom no abnormality of carbohydrate metabolism is demonstrable on glucose tolerance test, even after steroid administration (Camerini-Davalos, 1964). There is, therefore, an inherent abnormality that the body is able to resist for a variable number of years—perhaps even until death.

Situations in which the prediabetic state may be suspected are:

(*a*) The identical non-diabetic twin of a diabetic.
(*b*) An individual with both parents diabetic.
(*c*) An individual with one diabetic parent whose other (non-diabetic) parent has, or had, either a diabetic parent, sibling or offspring or a sibling having a diabetic child.
(*d*) Patients with an abnormal obstetric history characterised by:
  (i) A tendency to large live or stillborn babies (60 per cent of mothers with diabetes have in the prediabetic years produced at least one baby over 10 lb at birth).
  (ii) Frequent miscarriages.

In each of these groups there is a higher incidence of diabetes than in a population without these features. There is also an increased incidence of diabetes in the obese, in women with endometrial carcinoma and in patients with atherosclerosis. It has recently been suggested that perhaps not all identical non-diabetic twins of diabetics are in fact themselves potentially diabetic (Tattersall and Pyke, 1972).

There is no certain way of diagnosing the prediabetic state, which is usually diagnosed retrospectively although Vallance-Owen has claimed that the presence of excessive synalbumin antagonism indicates prediabetes.

There is still controversy regarding plasma insulin levels in prediabetics and both low concentrations with a deficient response to glucose (Cerasi and Luft, 1967; Hales *et al.*, 1968; Cerasi *et al.*, 1973) and high insulin levels (Chlouverakis *et al.*, 1967; Khurana *et al.*, 1971) have been reported. Jackson and his colleagues (1972) have published studies which indicate that the earliest biochemical lesion in diabetes is associated with insulin excess rather than insulin deficiency, and it is generally agreed that the pancreatic islets are hypertrophied in the potential diabetic (Bloodworth, 1970). It is quite possible that patients classified as prediabetics present a heterogeneous group of insulin responses.

2. *Latent Diabetes* refers to those normal individuals who may develop glycosuria and impairment of carbohydrate tolerance after any form of stress or after the administration of steroids. The development of the frank diabetic state may be delayed for many years. This abnormality is frequently found in obese individuals and, if successful weight reduction is achieved the overt syndrome may never occur. Elevated plasma immunoreactive insulin levels are often observed during a glucose tolerance test.

3. *Asymptomatic* (*Chemical*) *Diabetes*. About 25 per cent of patients referred to diabetic clinics are asymptomatic at the time of referral, although they have glycosuria, hyperglycaemia, and impaired carbohydrate tolerance during a glucose tolerance test. Many of these patients will admit upon reflection that they have had some symptoms such as slight weight loss, nocturia or thirst which they overlooked or to which they had attached no significance. It is well recognised that patients may present with diabetic complications before the true diagnosis of diabetes is made.

4. *Overt Diabetes Mellitus*. The typical features of the two main clinical syndromes are listed below.

Juvenile onset (*Insulin dependent*)	*Maturity onset*
Underweight	Overweight or of normal weight
Young	Older age groups (after middle age)
Ketotic if treatment is withheld	Ketotic only if acute or severe infections are present
Low or absent endogenous insulin secretion. In the earliest stages and in prediabetes, insulin secretion may be temporarily increased	Normal or increased endogenous insulin secretion in earliest stages; in the more advanced cases insulin secretion low
Treatment with insulin necessary	Respond to diet alone, oral drugs needed in some cases; insulin may be required temporarily during infections or surgery
Insulin sensitive	Tendency to insulin resistance.

Although many patients with diabetes mellitus fall into one or other of these categories, many intermediate cases occur and it should be realised that these are merely the two extremes of the clinical syndrome of diabetes mellitus, and are not necessarily two distinct diseases of different aetiology. Thus, young people may be seen who are overweight and who respond to diet, elderly people may be diagnosed who are ketotic and require insulin, and other patients of all ages are seen who do not respond to weight reduction alone and who, while not ketotic, require either oral compounds or insulin to control blood sugar levels and symptoms. In the early stages of juvenile onset diabetes, insulin requirements may fluctuate markedly, and it is not unusual for insulin requirements to fall to very low levels for some weeks or months after the initial acute ketotic episode has been corrected. The insulin injections should be continued in such patients, even in very low dosage, and frequent observation continued, since sooner or later insulin demands will rise and may do so suddenly, causing a further episode of ketosis if the requirements are not promptly met.

B. DIABETES DUE TO DEMONSTRABLE PANCREATIC DISEASE

The most common causes of this rare type of diabetes are haemochromatosis and chronic pancreatitis, and other features of these diseases are usually present. Insulin production is limited by a reduction in the β-cell population due to pancreatic fibrosis. In haemochromatosis, diabetes may rarely be improved by venesection. In pancreatic diabetes the diabetes may not be severe, but it cannot usually be controlled by diet alone. Oral drugs may be effective if some normal pancreatic tissue remains, but insulin is commonly needed. The daily dose of insulin does not usually exceed 40 to 50 units, and may be much smaller. If higher doses are necessary, it should be suspected that the disease has occurred in a patient who is already a potential or a latent idiopathic diabetic. Diabetes may also follow acute pancreatitis (Johansen and Ørnsholt, 1972) or removal of an islet cell adenoma (*see* Chapter 16). Pancreatic carcinoma is much commoner in diabetics than would be expected (Bell, 1957) but it is not certain whether this is merely due to the high incidence of diabetes in patients with this tumour.

C and D. DIABETES RELATED TO OTHER ENDOCRINE SYNDROMES OR PRECIPITATED BY DRUGS

The pathogenesis of carbohydrate intolerance in thyrotoxicosis, Cushing's syndrome, acromegaly, and in patients treated with steroids or contraceptive preparations, is discussed in Chapter 14. Growth hormone and cortisol are diabetogenic, and although overt diabetes does not occur in all cases of acromegaly or Cushing's syndrome, asymptomatic abnormalities of glucose tolerance are present in the majority. In some cases, the glandular hyperfunction appears to precipitate diabetes in pre- or latent diabetic individuals. Carbohydrate intolerance in association with an excess of catecholamines is discussed elsewhere. The carbohydrate intolerance that may occur in patients with aldosteronism may be related to chronic potassium depletion, and a similar mechanism could contribute to the diabetogenic action of the thiazide diuretics, which may also have pancreatic and peripheral effects.

E. DIABETES RELATED TO OTHER DISEASES

Carbohydrate tolerance is impaired, often to a considerable degree, in the majority of patients with chronic renal failure. There is considerable evidence that improvement in carbohydrate metabolism occurs after haemodialysis, and is associated with a rise in plasma immunoreactive insulin concentrations, suggesting that the carbohydrate intolerance of uraemia is due to a dialysable substance either inhibiting insulin release or increasing insulin degradation.

Carbohydrate intolerance is occasionally seen in association with liver disease such as cirrhosis

—in a series of unselected patients with chronic liver disease, 32 per cent had unequivocal 'diabetes mellitus' and 25 per cent had impaired glucose tolerance (Megyesi *et al.*, 1967). The authors postulated that chronic liver disease in some way produces endogenous insulin resistance, causing hyperinsulinaemia before glucose tolerance is impaired, and that diabetes follows when β-cell decompensation occurs.

AETIOLOGY OF IDIOPATHIC DIABETES MELLITUS

The precise aetiology of diabetes mellitus is unknown, but the disease can only occur when insulin activity (although not necessarily pancreatic insulin secretion) is deficient. Possible factors in the aetiology of diabetes which merit serious consideration may be mentioned.

HEREDITY

The tendency for diabetes to run in families is an undisputed fact. The observations of geneticists suggest that the inheritance of diabetes is of polygenic or multifactorial type, rather than as a simple Mendelian dominant or recessive involving predominantly a single gene.

PARITY

There is a definite association between parity and the incidence of diabetes: the incidence in single or nulliparous females is similar to that in males and each of these groups has a lower incidence of the disease than have married or widowed women with children.

AGE

Diabetes becomes more common as age increases. The peak blood glucose response to an oral glucose load rises steadily with increasing age, but it appears that there is a true increase in the prevalence of diabetes as age rises, rather than a generalised deterioration in glucose tolerance in the whole population.

OBESITY

There is a strong association between obesity and diabetes (*Lancet*, 1971a). Plasma insulin levels are higher in obese than in lean individuals and this is related in most cases to adipose tissue insensitivity to the action of insulin (*see* p. 373). It seems, therefore, that the obese have to produce more insulin than those of ideal weight to preserve normal glucose tolerance. Those with a defect in pancreatic β-cell function (perhaps the hereditary component) are unable to maintain this extra production and become diabetic. Weight reduction causes a fall in plasma insulin concentrations and an improvement in impaired carbohydrate tolerance, although this is not invariable. In the majority of patients, improvement in the diabetic state may be achieved as a result simply of carbohydrate restriction without weight loss (Wall *et al.*, 1973), although weight loss will inevitably follow if carbohydrate restriction is associated with a reduction in overall caloric intake, which will almost invariably be the case.

INFECTION

Pancreatitis is a well-recognised complication of mumps: diabetes may follow. A possible causative relationship between congenital rubella infection and diabetes mellitus has been suggested (Forrest *et al.*, 1971). There is also circumstantial evidence that links Coxsackie B4 infection with diabetes in man (*Lancet*, 1971b). Gamble *et al.* (1969) found a significantly raised titre of antibodies to this virus in the serum of acute-onset diabetics who were tested within three months of developing the disease, and Gamble and Taylor (1969) reported a significant correlation between the seasonal incidence of Coxsackie B4 infections and the incidence of diabetes in patients under 30. There is as yet no *direct* evidence that infection with this virus may cause diabetes in man.

AUTOIMMUNITY

It has long been recognised that there is a clinical association between vitiligo, thyroid disease, pernicious anaemia and diabetes, and antibodies to thyroid and to gastric parietal cells are found more commonly in diabetes than in age and sex-matched controls. Although lymphocytic infiltration in the islets has been observed in patients with juvenile onset diabetes, the significance of this finding is unknown. Autoimmune diseases are generally accepted to be inherited, and it seems possible that this genetic factor may be linked with that of diabetes mellitus.

INSULIN SECRETION IN DIABETES MELLITUS AND INSULIN ANTAGONISM

The normal human pancreas produces the equivalent of 30 to 40 units of crystalline insulin daily, though many insulin-dependent diabetics require much more than this for adequate control, a finding that is not due simply to the presence of circulating antibodies to the injected insulin. The question of insulin secretion and plasma insulin levels in diabetes is still unresolved. All agree that in insulin-dependent diabetes and in established overt maturity onset diabetes insulin secretion is deficient; but there is considerable evidence (Yalow and Berson, 1961; Yalow *et al.*, 1965) that some maturity onset diabetics in the earliest stages of their disease have normal or even increased amounts of circulating insulin and are capable of increasing the circulating insulin concentration in stimulation tests. Jackson *et al.* (1972) have also shown evidence that the initial biochemical lesion in diabetes is associated with insulin excess rather than insulin deficiency, and reactive hypoglycaemia preceding the onset of diabetes, both in the child and in the adult, is well recognised. Seltzer *et al.* (1967), Cerasi and Luft (1967), Kipnis (1968) and Cerasi *et al.* (1973) have suggested that an initial delay in the insulin response to hyperglycaemia is a feature of prediabetes, of the earlier and milder degrees of diabetes and also of overt clinical diabetes, but this suggestion has been refuted by Johansen (1972). The observations of normal or increased circulating insulin concentrations in some patients in the presence of carbohydrate intolerance and the large doses of insulin required to achieve control in some diabetics have led to the concept of 'resistance' to the action of endogenous insulin as playing a key role in the aetiology of diabetes mellitus, and if these observations have any validity it is difficult to escape this conclusion. This 'resistance' may be due to a specific circulating antagonist to insulin, to abnormal binding of insulin in plasma, to peripheral tissue resistance, or to some other mechanism as yet undefined. The theory of insulin antagonism or resistance is that the abnormality initially results in a compensatory increased production of insulin from the pancreas, later to be followed by β-cell exhaustion and deficient pancreatic insulin production. There is thus the concept of a spectrum of hereditary idiopathic diabetes mellitus, ranging from the patient without symptoms, signs, or detectable abnormalities of carbohydrate metabolism who may be shown only by special testing to have insulin antagonism, increased tissue insulin-insensitivity or abnormal binding of insulin in the plasma, to the patient with mild diabetes of late onset who is usually obese, and thence to the young patient with severe diabetes who requires large doses of insulin. On the basis of this concept the juvenile diabetic is one whose pancreas has been rapidly exhausted by increasing demands leading to an almost complete failure of insulin production. The maturity onset diabetic has a pancreas that is *almost* able to supply the increased demands for insulin—sufficient to prevent ketosis and to deal with a smaller carbohydrate load when the patient's dietary carbohydrate intake is restricted, but insufficient to prevent carbohydrate intolerance under all circumstances when a free diet is allowed. The nature of the defect of the β cell and the mechanisms leading to rapid β-cell failure in some diabetics are unknown. It is presumed that, if a patient is genetically constituted as a diabetic, the further progress of the abnormality and its manifestations depend mainly on the ability of his pancreas to respond to increased demand for insulin and on environmental factors; for example, if a predia-

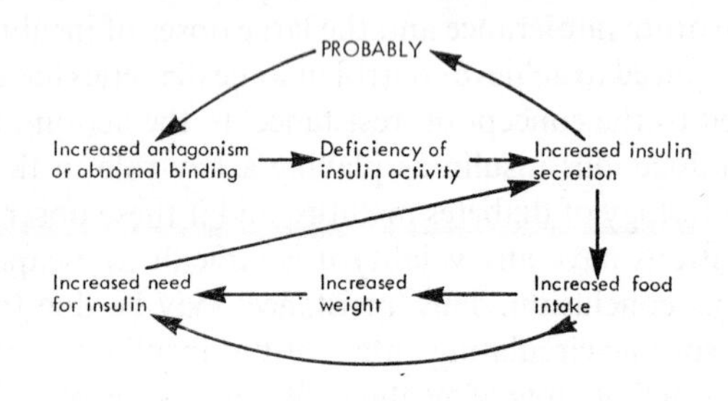

FIGURE 15.1 Obesity and insulin antagonism

betic is exposed to excess growth-hormone or cortisol, or allows himself to gain weight excessively, he may manifest the overt syndrome that would otherwise have lain dormant. On this basis, it has been suggested that the obese diabetic could be obese because he is 'diabetic'—the possible sequence of events in maturity onset obese diabetes would then appear to be related as shown in Fig. 15.1. The sequence postulated appears to be dependent on a free supply of carbohydrate and thus will be alleviated if carbohydrate intake is reduced, unless pancreatic β-cell exhaustion has supervened.

However, although a reduction in the biological effectiveness of insulin in obese people is generally accepted there is considerable controversy at present regarding the various theories of insulin antagonism. Nevertheless, interest continues and it is important to consider the theories which have been proposed, if only because they have led to a new way of thinking about the aetiology of diabetes as being very much more complex than a simple deficiency disease analogous to hypothyroidism or Addison's disease. These factors have already been mentioned in Chapter 14.

Synalbumin Antagonism (Vallance-Owen, 1966). Vallance-Owen considers the synalbumin antagonist to be the B-chain of insulin, circulating in association with serum albumin. Bajaj and Vallance-Owen (1971) have postulated that diabetic and normal albumin differ in their ability to bind insulin B-chain, which is one possible explanation why excessive circulating B-chain bound to albumin is seen in diabetes. Synalbumin antagonism is dependent on pituitary-adrenal function and appears to be inherited as an autosomal dominant. Vallance-Owen's suggestion that increased synalbumin antagonism is inherited as an autosomal dominant is at variance with the generally accepted idea that the inheritance of diabetes mellitus is polygenic. It must be remembered that while Vallance-Owen postulates that 25 per cent of the population are genetically constituted as diabetics (i.e. have inherited a gene determining increased synalbumin antagonism) the incidence of the overt syndrome is much lower. Providing all the facts are confirmed, it is suggested that either the gene determining the Vallance-Owen antagonist is only one of the genes involved in the polygenic mode of diabetic inheritance, and others, not yet identified are just as important, or that the gene determining the synalbumin antagonist does in fact determine the *prediabetic* state, which is inherited as an autosomal dominant. The development of overt disease in an individual constituted genetically as a prediabetic may then depend on the action of other genes as well as on environmental factors.

The synalbumin antagonist is said to inhibit the action of insulin on muscle, but not on fat, and there is evidence that the antagonist itself has an insulin-like effect on fat. Vallance-Owen has found excessive insulin antagonism in albumin prepared from the plasma of pre- and latent diabetics, maturity onset diabetics and insulin-dependent diabetics. Excessive synalbumin antagonism may also be found in some of the normal relatives of diabetics. Work carried out by Davidson and Poffenbarger (1970) has revealed serious obstacles to the acceptance of a role for the synalbumin antagonist in diabetes mellitus, although does not absolutely deny a physiological role for the antagonist. The further results of Vallance-Owen's continuing studies are awaited with interest.

'Free' and 'Bound' Insulin (Antoniades 1961, 1965). 'Bound' insulin is inactive on muscle, but fat is considered to release 'free' insulin from the 'bound' form. In diabetes, it is postulated that there is increased binding, or some physiological difficulty in the unbinding of insulin. Not all workers have succeeded in demonstrating 'bound' insulin in human serum (Meade *et al.*, 1968).

Free Fatty Acid (Randle *et al.*, 1963). Free fatty acids are preferentially oxidised by muscle and when plasma free fatty acid levels are high, glucose uptake by muscle may be diminished. This interrelationship has been termed the glucose-fatty acid cycle (Randle *et al.*, 1963). Randle and his colleagues have suggested that in diabetes an early development may be an abnormality of lipid metabolism, perhaps mediated through an abnormality of growth hormone secretion, which leads to excessive mobilisation of free fatty acid with consequent inhibition of glucose uptake by muscle, rise in blood sugar levels and pancreatic stimulation with increased secretion of insulin, free fatty acid thus acting as an insulin antagonist. Jenkins (1967) has extended this theory and has suggested that raised plasma levels of ketone bodies may also contribute to the production of increased plasma insulin levels and of insulin resistance in such patients. However, restriction of carbohydrate intake in obese diabetics improves glucose tolerance even though plasma free fatty acid levels remain elevated, and in insulin-sensitive juvenile diabetics insulin lowers both glucose and free fatty acid levels. It has been suggested, therefore, that the observed changes in the glucose-fatty acid cycle in diabetics might be secondary rather than primary abnormalities and recent work indicates that it is unlikely that excessive secretion of growth hormone is involved primarily in the aetiology of idiopathic diabetes mellitus (Baird *et al.*, 1973).

HISTOLOGY OF THE PANCREAS IN DIABETES

The pancreatic islets appear histologically 'normal' in 40 to 50 per cent of diabetics when sections are stained by routine techniques such as haematoxylin and eosin (Warren, LeCompte, and Legg, 1966), although if examined from the quantitative point of view, using granule stains, hardly any diabetic pancreas is in fact normal. Such quantitative studies usually demonstrate a diminution in the number of β cells, those present showing partial or complete degranulation—such changes are particularly frequent in established juvenile onset diabetes. There is little correlation between the quantitative and qualitative changes observed in the pancreas at autopsy and the severity of diabetes during life.

Hyalinisation of the islets of Langerhans is the most common qualitative lesion observed in diabetics and is seen in about 30 per cent of patients. The hyaline material is an acid mucopolysaccharide which may be derived from the endothelium of the islet capillaries, and hyalinisation is a non-specific finding of unknown significance. It is chiefly seen in patients with the maturity onset syndrome and is more closely related to age than to the duration of diabetes. It may be an unassociated phenomenon and does not appear to be a cause of diabetes.

Fibrosis of the islets is seen in a smaller proportion of patients (about 20 per cent) and, like hyalinisation, tends to occur in older individuals although it is not infrequently seen in young patients. Fibrosis and hyalinisation may both occur in the same pancreas and, sometimes, the same islet.

Hydropic degeneration of β cells characterised by degranulation, swelling, and vacuole formation, which is associated with glycogen deposition and which is commonly observed in experimental diabetes, is rarely seen in the human pancreas. The change is observed most frequently in fulminating diabetes of short duration and seems to be reversible. Hydropic degeneration appears to be the result of extreme functional strain and has been interpreted as an insulin exhaustion phenomenon although it has also been suggested that it may be an example of the abnormal distribution and deposition of glycogen, which is found in various tissues in diabetes.

Hypertrophy of the pancreatic islets is sometimes observed in prediabetics, obese diabetics and in the earliest stages of juvenile onset diabetes. In the latter, islet hypertrophy rapidly declines as the disease progresses and, eventually, there is a marked reduction in islet cell mass. This may also occur, although more slowly and to a lesser degree, in maturity onset obese diabetics. Islet hypertrophy is frequently seen in infants born to diabetic mothers.

Lymphocytic and fatty infiltration in and around the islets are rare findings which have raised the possibility of an autoimmune basis for the disease in these patients.

INCIDENCE

Idiopathic diabetes mellitus is a common disease although the incidence varies considerably in different countries. The incidence appears similar in the United Kingdom and in the USA, but studies on mixed populations in the West Indies and South Africa have shown an increased incidence in East Indians as compared with Negroes and Europeans, who have a similar incidence. Surveys in the UK and in the USA have given an incidence of 1–1·5 per cent, of whom half were previously undiagnosed. In a study in Birmingham (Diabetes Survey Working Party, 1962) nearly 20,000 patients were screened. The incidence of known diabetes was 0·64 per cent, and of previously unknown diabetes 0·69 per cent, although it has been suggested that this estimate may be too low (Butterfield, 1964). Most new diabetics discovered in such surveys show the maturity onset type of syndrome. The incidence of idiopathic diabetes increases with age. The number of males diagnosed before the age of forty exceeds the number of females; after the age of forty the sex incidence is reversed. The number of prediabetics cannot be estimated but it has been suggested that some 25 per cent of the population are so constituted.

SYMPTOMS AND SIGNS OF DIABETES

The presenting features of diabetes may be:

(*a*) Thirst, polyuria and tiredness
(*b*) Weight loss—particularly with a good appetite
(*c*) Pruritus vulvae or balanitis, moniliasis, furunculosis and boils
(*d*) Cataracts, visual disturbances, retinopathy
(*e*) Peripheral vascular disease
(*f*) Nephropathy, neuropathy (including autonomic features such as impotence and nocturnal diarrhoea)
(*g*) Glycosuria.

Sometimes the symptoms will develop dramatically within a few hours; in other cases the onset may be insidious. The presentation in juvenile diabetes is much more sudden than in maturity onset cases and the diagnosis is commonly made when the patient presents with ketosis. In about 90 per cent of the juvenile patients a spurt of linear growth immediately precedes the onset of the syndrome, and during this stage hypoglycaemia may occur. There are no specific *signs* of diabetes, except those associated with its complications or those consequent upon metabolic disturbances such as dehydration and ketosis. Some patients will, however, observe that drops of urine on the clothing or shoes dry leaving a white stain.

DIAGNOSIS

Once the suspicion of diabetes has arisen the diagnosis may be confirmed by some of the following investigations:

Urine testing
Random blood sugar
Fasting blood sugar
Two-hour post-prandial blood sugar
Oral glucose tolerance test
Intravenous glucose tolerance test.

Urine Testing. The 'Clinitest' has replaced Benedict's and Fehling's solutions for the detection of glycosuria. As with all tests involving the reduction of copper salts, the 'Clinitest' reacts to reducing substances other than glucose. Clinistix and Tes-tape are now in general use as specific screening tests for glycosuria. These reagents consist of filter paper impregnated with glucose oxidase, a peroxidase, and an indicator. Any glucose absorbed by the paper after dipping into urine is rapidly oxidised under the catalytic action of glucose oxidase. The hydrogen peroxide then formed produces a blue colour by acting on the indicator in the presence of peroxidase. Neither method is suitable as a quantitative test. Ketonuria may be detected by the use of ferric chloride but this test is non-specific. Acetest tablets, containing a mixture of sodium nitroprusside, glycine and disodium phosphate, are specific for the detection of β-hydroxy-butyrate and acetoacetate, but quantitation is difficult. The simultaneous detection of glycosuria and ketonuria is highly suggestive of diabetes mellitus, but it must be remembered that the detection of ketonuria alone, particularly in childhood, does not necessarily indicate diabetes.

Random blood sugar estimations may in themselves be diagnostic. A result greater than 200 mg per cent is association with the symptoms described above is diagnostic of diabetes.

Fasting blood sugar estimation is often not possible at the first visit; but if the patient does happen to be in the fasting state a value in excess of 120 mg per cent is diagnostic of diabetes mellitus, and figures between 100 and 120 mg per cent are suggestive. In early diabetes the fasting blood sugar may be normal.

Two-hour post-prandial blood sugar. If this is in excess of 140 mg per cent, the diagnosis is confirmed, and if the result is between 120 and 140 mg per cent there is strong suspicion of the disease, and a glucose tolerance test is indicated. The two-hour blood sugar value after a standard carbohydrate load has been frequently used in population surveys and detection drives. A coca-cola flavoured glucose drink is very popular in the USA as the carbohydrate load used to challenge the patient.

A glucose tolerance test is not always necessary to make the diagnosis of diabetes mellitus. The test is of value:

(*a*) to establish the diagnosis in patients in whom the fasting or post-prandial blood sugar level is equivocal;
(*b*) in disorders suggestive of diabetes but without unequivocal hyperglycaemia, i.e. retinopathy, neuropathy, nephropathy;
(*c*) in the evaluation of 'patients at risk', i.e. the obese, mothers with large babies or other suggestive obstetric features, or those with diabetic relatives;
(*d*) in patients with unexplained and asymptomatic glycosuria;
(*e*) in some patients, to define the renal threshold for glucose.

The test must be performed under standard conditions (Fitzgerald and Keen, 1964). The most important of these is the provision of an adequate carbohydrate intake (at least 300 g/day) for three days preceding the test. Many patients referred as possible diabetics will have been on a low calorie diet prior to being seen and minor abnormalities in glucose tolerance tests under these conditions are meaningless. The patient fasts overnight and before the test sits quietly for 30 minutes. After capillary blood has been taken for glucose estimation, he is given 50 g of glucose in 200 ml of water favoured with lemon juice to drink in five minutes. Capillary blood specimens are then taken for glucose estimation at $\frac{1}{2}$ hr, 1 hr, $1\frac{1}{2}$ hr, and 2 hr. The subject remains seated during the test and does not smoke.

The standards of normality usually accepted are a fasting level and a 2-hour value of less than 120 mg per cent, and a 1-hour value of less than 180 mg per cent. If venous blood specimens are used, the corresponding glucose values are 110 mg and 160 mg per cent. It is conventional to set the standards a little lower when venous blood is used, although Lind and his colleagues (1972) have failed to show a constant relationship between capillary and venous blood glucose concentrations. All of these blood glucose values refer to estimation by either the glucose oxidase method or by the ferricyanide method after dialysis, using the autoanalyser. Capillary blood glucose levels between 110 and 120 mg per cent either fasting or at two hours are suspicious. There is a progressive rise in the blood glucose response after carbohydrate with increasing age, which affects mainly the height of the peak. It is possible to analyse the blood glucose curve statistically and to calculate an 'index of homeostasis' (H) which quantifies the shape and time course of the curve and which correlates well with the degree of carbohydrate tolerance or intolerance (Billewicz, Anderson and Lind, 1973).

The *intravenous glucose tolerance test* has little place in the routine diagnosis of diabetes mellitus although one major advantage is the elimination of differences in the alimentary absorption of glucose, which makes the test more reproducible. While it is mainly used to study the rate of disappearance of glucose from the plasma under various experimental conditions, relying on mathematical analysis of the blood glucose curve obtained after the rapid intravenous administration of glucose, it may also be valuable in the diagnosis of mild diabetes.

Diagnosis of Latent Diabetes Mellitus. Several tests have been used to detect the latent diabetic; all depend on the observation that steroids impair carbohydrate tolerance in these individuals.

1. The cortisone-augmented oral glucose tolerance test (Fajans and Conn, 1961).
2. The prednisone glycosuria test (Joplin *et al.*, 1961).

1. *Cortisone Test*

Cortisone acetate is given orally 8½ and 2 hours before a glucose tolerance test. A dose of 50 mg is given on each occasion if body weight is below 160 lb, and 62·5 mg if body weight is greater. A fasting venous blood specimen is taken for glucose estimation by a specific glucose oxidase method, and an oral load of 1·75 g glucose/kg of ideal body weight is given as a 25 per cent solution in water. Ideal weight is defined as the average weight of normal persons of the same height, age, and sex. As in the standard test, the patient is given a 300 g carbohydrate diet prior to the test. A positive test is shown by a one-hour blood glucose level of 160 mg/100 ml or more, a 1½-hour level greater than 150 mg/100 ml, and a 2-hour level above 140 mg/100 ml. Fajans (1963) has stressed that these criteria apply *only* to otherwise healthy, ambulant, non-pregnant individuals under the age of forty-five, and Conn 1958) considers that, within these limitations, the test 'seems to separate nondiabetic relatives of diabetics into groups (26 per cent abnormal) which are distinctly different from the groups which are found when the same test is applied to people with no known family history of diabetes (4 per cent abnormal)'. Other workers have not obtained such consistent and clear-cut results as Fajans and Conn.

2. *Prednisone Glycosuria Test*

(*a*) The patient has three days on a 300 g carbohydrate diet.
(*b*) A standard glucose tolerance test is performed.
(*c*) On the following day 20 mg of prednisone is given orally at 12 noon, 4 p.m., and 8 p.m. The patient fasts from 7 p.m. to 6 a.m. the next day.
(*d*) Urine is collected from 10 p.m. to 6 a.m., and glucose content is estimated by a glucose oxidase method. Hibitane 1/2,000 is used as preservative.
(*e*) Blood is taken for glucose estimation at 12 midnight and 1 a.m.

Latent diabetes is indicated by:

1. Overnight urinary glucose greater than 60 mg/hour (in the presence of a normal renal threshold as shown by standard oral GTT).
2. Blood glucose levels at midnight or 1 a.m. greater than 133 mg per cent (the mean blood glucose level at this time in normal individuals without glycosuria is 111 mg per cent with a standard deviation of 11).

Prednisone increases the hepatic output of glucose and lowers the renal threshold for glucose, probably by increasing glomerular filtration. These actions are enhanced in the latent diabetic. This test is simple to perform but has not been satisfactorily compared with the cortisone glucose tolerance test.

TREATMENT

In diabetes, perhaps more than in any other metabolic disease, there are many different opinions as to therapy, mainly concerned with the type of insulin routinely used, the type of diet, and the type of patient who is given oral drugs. We have, therefore, attempted to discuss the aims and principles of therapy in broad terms, making specific recommendations only when the great balance of opinion and evidence support them.

Aims of Treatment

To enable the patient to live his normal life-span as a useful and productive member of society without radically altering his habits, his way of life or those of his family.
To alleviate symptoms.
To restore body weight to the ideal level and, in children, to maintain normal growth.
To achieve biochemical normality.
To prevent complications.

There can be little disagreement that these reflect the ideal, but the first three aims should certainly be achieved if control is to be considered at all adequate. The patient is most concerned with the alleviation of symptoms; the doctor is, in addition, concerned with the prevention of complications. It is as important to restore body weight towards normal in the thin diabetic as it is to reduce weight in the obese. Most clinicians would agree that the weight of the juvenile onset diabetic should be kept slightly below the mean for age and height, although the temptation to place *all* diabetics regardless of type on a sub-caloric diet so that the dosage of insulin or oral hypoglycaemic agents may be kept to a minimum should be resisted.

Opinions vary as to what is meant by 'biochemical normality'. There is, however, general agreement that in the maturity onset diabetic whether he be treated by diet alone or by diet with oral drugs, control is inadequate unless the blood sugar levels are kept within the normal range throughout the 24 hours. There are two schools of thought as regards the control of the diabetic on insulin: one (now happily in the minority) is satisfied if symptoms are relieved and ketonuria corrected and is not too concerned with glycosuria or hyperglycaemia; the other insists on as complete biochemical normality as possible. In practice, the most one can hope to achieve is to reduce the blood sugar to within normal limits during the period of maximal insulin action. The duration of the normal blood sugar level will vary from individual to individual, depending on the frequency of injection, the type of insulin given, the dose used, and the patient's occupation, dietary requirements, and eating pattern. Obviously, the more frequently insulin is given, the more nearly does the blood glucose approach physiological levels throughout the day, but there are few diabetics who would agree to taking more than two injections a day. Constant ideal control is difficult to achieve because insulin and caloric requirements vary from day to day, particularly in the young diabetic. It is usually impossible to avoid postprandial hyperglycaemia in all except the mildest cases, and recognition of this fact is of prime importance in the avoidance of hypoglycaemia, which may be almost inevitable if too heroic attempts are made to produce glucose-free urine and normoglycaemia after meals.

For the patient on insulin, acceptable control consists of:

1. Glycosuria in 24 hours not exceeding 5 per cent of the total carbohydrate intake.
2. Urine free from ketones.
3. Majority of blood glucose levels less than 150 mg per cent three or more hours after the preceding meal.

The 'brittle' (labile) diabetic is one who is prone to ketosis and who experiences hypoglycaemia with only slight overdosage of insulin. With rare exceptions, all persons with diabetes diagnosed before the age of twenty are 'brittle', but such instability can be seen in older patients. It is impossible to achieve continuous normoglycaemia during normal daily activity without causing frequent hypoglycaemia. 'Brittle' diabetics are characterised by a complete absence of insulinogenic reserve (Cremer *et al.*, 1971) and there are also differences in the pattern of insulin antibodies in the labile diabetic—such patients have very small amounts of antibody compared with stable diabetics, although these are avid binders of insulin compared with the insulin-binding antibodies of low affinity in the stable patient (Dixon *et al.*, 1972). The antibodies in the labile diabetic are less effective in buffering changes in free insulin concentration which occur when exogenous insulin enters the vascular space. It is unlikely that abnormalities of growth hormone secretion or of an exaggerated responsiveness to endogenous growth hormone play a primary role in the aetiology of brittle diabetes. Although in some patients at least, improved control significantly lowers the plasma growth-hormone concentration, in these patients the increase in growth hormone secretion observed during periods of poor control appears to be a secondary phenomenon. In 'brittle' diabetes it is reasonable to compromise, accepting moderate hyperglycaemia and glycosuria, and even transient ketonuria, in an effort to avoid hypoglycaemia. It is important that in diabetic children normal growth should be maintained.

A number of workers have stressed that poor control is associated with an increased incidence of complications, particularly retinal changes (Colwell, 1966). Others, however, have not found any clear correlation between the degree of control and freedom from or progression of complications (Downie and Martin, 1966; Adnitt and Taylor, 1970). There seems no doubt that some complications such as retinopathy and neuropathy may be improved, if they have not progressed too far, by long periods of rigid control (Dollery and Oakley, 1965), but in general the evidence that strict control can postpone or prevent the common vascular complications is no more than circumstantial, and the onset of these complications seems more closely related to the duration of the diabetes than to the degree of control achieved, although it must be admitted that perfect biochemical control in the insulin-dependent diabetic is only rarely achieved on a long-term basis unless the patient is admitted to hospital for a lengthy period. Nevertheless, the circumstantial evidence is sufficiently strong that any scheme of treatment must include this as one of its aims. There is some evidence that strict control during the first five years after the diagnosis is made might delay the onset of chronic complications, but the degree of control achieved and the ease with which it is achieved may simply reflect differences in the severity of the diabetes—more 'severe' diabetics may be at greater risk of developing vascular complications. Prospective studies are badly needed. At the present time, however, it must be re-emphasised that strict control is the only hope of avoiding or delaying serious complications; unfortunately, this is less frequently achieved than might be hoped.

An Outline of Therapy

Before undertaking treatment of a diabetic, the following considerations should be borne in mind:

1. Obesity is, in general, a contra-indication to the use of insulin for long-term control (although obesity may occur as a complication in insulin-dependent diabetics).

2. Ketosis is a contra-indication to oral drugs and necessitates the use of insulin.
3. Juvenile-onset patients require insulin therapy and a diet appropriate to their needs.
4. Maturity-onset patients with obesity are best treated by a low-calorie, low-carbohydrate diet and, if this fails, with a biguanide given in addition to the diet.
5. Maturity-onset patients of average weight and those who have lost weight to an ideal level on diet but who have persistent symptoms and/or glycosuria are best treated with a weight-maintaining (measured carbohydrate) diet with, if necessary, a sulphonylurea.
6. Maturity-onset patients of average weight whose diabetes is not controlled by oral hypoglycaemic drugs, singly or in combination, must be considered for insulin therapy.

DIETARY THERAPY

The basic nutritional requirements are the same in a diabetic as in a non-diabetic person and dietary carbohydrate restriction is the most important aspect of treatment in mild diabetes.

In maturity-onset diabetics with obesity a low-calorie, low-carbohydrate diet is indicated. Wall *et al.* (1973) have shown that 80 per cent of obese diabetics can be controlled by diet alone, and control is dependent on carbohydrate restriction and independent of the degree of weight loss achieved. Many diets are available, but usually the stricter the diet, the less likely is the patient to stick to it. Marriott's weight-reducing diet is probably the easiest to follow and the most attractive, although careful supervision is necessary. Strict adherence will result in weight loss of at least 1½ to 2 lb a week (*see* Chapter 17). This diet has the advantage that the carbohydrate allowance is very low, but in some patients even stricter carbohydrate restriction may be necessary. Diabetic foods, which commonly use sorbitol as a sweetener, should not be used by diabetics on weight-reducing diets since they contain calories.

In maturity onset diabetics of average weight the purpose of dieting is to keep the weight at or slightly below the ideal level for the patients' age, height, and sex. Such a diet is prescribed in accordance with the needs of the patient. Once the correct diet has been established, additional therapy in the form of oral hypoglycaemic agents may be needed.

In insulin-requiring diabetics, weight loss prior to treatment is almost invariable. For these patients, a diet based on the energy requirements for normal day-to-day activity and desired weight should be given, so that optimal nutrition will be obtained when control is achieved by the use of insulin. Since injected insulin provides only a relatively crude control of blood sugar levels it, it is best to avoid wide fluctuations in caloric intake.

It is conventional in the United Kingdom to measure, and, if necessary, to restrict only carbohydrate in the diet, allowing freedom of choice as regards protein and fat. This seems reasonable, since carbohydrate is the main caloric variable in the diet. In the UK the calorie intake derived from carbohydrate in patients of normal weight with 'normal' eating habits accounts for some 40 to 45 per cent of the total caloric intake. Most young insulin-dependent diabetics require between 120 and 300 g of carbohydrate daily, depending on age, sex, initial weight and desired weight, activity and occupation. Once the total daily carbohydrate allowance is decided, it is apportioned to each meal, depending on the patient's normal eating habits. It is usually considered advisable to allow more carbohydrate in the meals that immediately follow the insulin injections, and in those on soluble insulin small "buffer" snacks about 3 to 4 hours after the injection are a wise precaution. The diet should contain an adequate amount of protein—not less than 1 g/kg body weight/day for patients of average weight. Proteins are very satisfying and, therefore, a high-protein diet may be used to advantage when calorie restriction is desired. The amount of fat in the diet will, under normal circumstances, depend on the carbohydrate and

TABLE 15.1 *Dosages of Sulphonylurea Compounds*

Drug	Biological half-life	Frequency of dose	Initial dose	Effective daily dosage range
Tolbutamide	4 hours	3–4 times daily	1·5 g daily	1–3 g
Chlorpropamide	35–40 hours	Once daily	100–250 mg daily	100–500 mg
Tolazamide	7 hours	Once or twice daily	100–250 mg daily	100–1,000 mg
Glibenclamide	12 hours	Once or twice daily	2·5–5 mg daily	2·5–20 mg

protein components. The amount of carbohydrate can be explained to the patient in terms of 10 g quantities, which will allow latitude and variety as regards 'exchange' portions.

Alcohol does not require insulin for its metabolism but has a high calorie content (7 Cals per g). Diabetics should be advised against taking alcohol, which is almost certain to be an addition to the rest of the diet, encouraging weight-gain. Also, alcoholic intoxication may mimic hypoglycaemia, causing difficulty in diagnosis, and may indeed precipitate hypoglycaemia. Patients who find alcohol indispensable may be advised that an *occasional* measure of spirits, dry wine or dry sherry can usually be taken with impunity; on the other hand, half a pint of beer contains 10 g of carbohydrate and half a pint of cider 15 g. *Fructose* and *sorbitol* also do not require insulin for their metabolism and may be used by the diabetic as sweetening agents. However, about 30 per cent of fructose is converted into glucose, and it is recommended that diabetics do not use more than 60 g of this sugar per day, taken in small quantities throughout the day.

It is sobering to remember that only 30 per cent of diabetics follow their diets accurately to within 10 per cent of the allocated daily quantity of carbohydrate, and in as many as 32 per cent there is little or no adherence to the prescribed diet (Tunbridge and Wetherill, 1970). Dietary accuracy is more reliable in younger diabetics, in those on insulin and in those on higher calorie diets.

THE ORAL HYPOGLYCAEMIC COMPOUNDS

Sulphonylurea Compounds

These act by stimulating the production of insulin by the β cells of the pancreas. They also have a secondary effect in reducing hepatic glucose output. Preparations include tolbutamide, chlorpropamide, tolazamide and glibenclamide. The dosage regimes are indicated in Table 15.1, and the structures of the compounds are shown in Fig. 15.2.

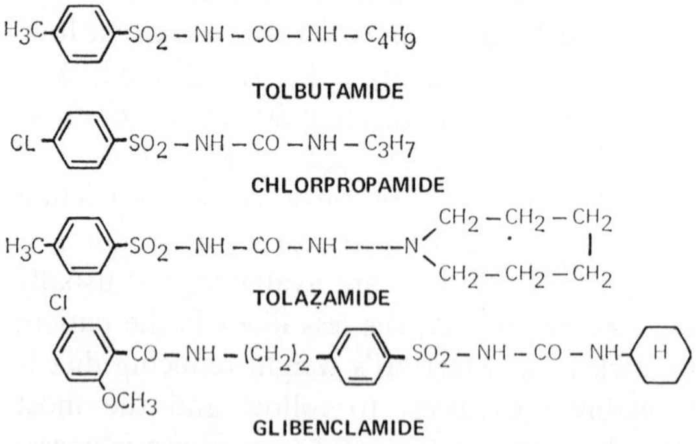

TOLBUTAMIDE

CHLORPROPAMIDE

TOLAZAMIDE

GLIBENCLAMIDE

FIGURE 15.2 Structure of sulphonylurea compounds

An initial loading dose is not required; indeed, in the case of chlorpropamide, tolazamide and glibenclamide this may induce hypoglycaemia. An advantage that used to be claimed for tolbutamide was its short duration of action; thus, the physiological fluctuations in insulin secretion might be reproduced. It is now apparent that after discharge of β-cell granules, there is a considerable delay during which granular reformation takes place, and before further discharge may occur; some would, therefore, regard the short action of this drug as a disadvantage. The convenience of the once daily dosage of chlorpropamide may be outweighed by the possibility of nocturnal hypoglycaemia due to its prolonged action. The maximum effect of these drugs may not be reached for two to three weeks, so they should not be dismissed as ineffective without fair trial. However, the most potent sulphonylurea, glibenclamide, has a more rapid blood glucose-lowering effect than the others, and shows maximal hypoglycaemic action within a few days. Glibenclamide appears to stimulate the synthesis of insulin as well as its release, although all sulphonylureas have been shown to have a β-cytotrophic action in that prolonged treatment causes islet hypertrophy and increased insulinogenic potential in many patients. All four drugs are relatively free from unwanted effects and the choice between them is largely a matter of individual preference. Some patients may, nevertheless, fail to respond to one drug, but respond to another preparation. Sulphonylureas have been used in patients with subclinical diabetes and in these they appear to delay the onset of the overt syndrome (Stowers, 1970). There is no evidence that sulphonylureas might accelerate β-cell failure.

Secondary failures are not uncommon, and while some of these may be due to pancreatic β-cell atrophy the majority probably result from poor initial selection or relaxation of the diet.

Indications for Sulphonylureas. Patients for whom sulphonylurea therapy may be considered are:

1. Maturity-onset diabetics of average weight.
2. Diabetics of normal weight stabilised on doses of insulin usually not in excess of 20–30 units a day, who have never been ketotic and who do not become ketotic on discontinuation of their insulin during observation in hospital.

Sulphonylureas are contraindicated in patients with ketosis, and are of no value in juvenile diabetics. Given in association with insulin any beneficial effect is marginal, and they are no longer used in this way.

Patients who developed their diabetes under the age of forty, whose diabetes is of long duration or who are underweight, often show a poor response to sulphonylurea therapy. In obese patients, every effort must be made to bring about weight reduction before oral therapy begins, and sulphonylurea drugs should *not* be given alone. In such cases a biguanide is the drug of first choice, although a sulphonylurea may usefully be added if the diet and biguanide alone fail to control hyperglycaemia and related symptoms.

Unwanted Effects of Sulphonylureas

1. Hypoglycaemia
2. Dyspepsia
3. Skin rashes
4. Alcohol sensitivity
5. Impairment of liver function
6. Cholestatic jaundice (chlorpropamide)
7. Blood dyscrasias.

Side effects with all of the sulphonylurea compounds are rare and are usually reversible. Hypoglycaemia may occur with all compounds, particularly if meals are missed, but is most troublesome and dangerous with chlorpropamide, when, due to the long biochemical half-life of the drug, hypoglycaemia is prolonged and recurrent despite treatment. Fatalities have been recorded. A number of drugs in common use, including phenylbutazone, sulphaphenazole, probenecid, salicylates and monoamine oxidase inhibitors may potentiate the hypoglycaemic effect of the sulphonylureas. Metabolites of chlorpropamide, tolazamide and glibenclamide have some hypoglycaemic effect and are normally excreted by the kidneys, so that the drugs should be used with great caution in the presence of renal failure. The most troublesome side effect is alcohol sensitivity, which presents as facial flushing after the ingestion of alcohol and which occurs in 10 to 20 per cent of patients taking chlorpropamide. It seems to be much less frequent with tolbutamide and appears to be very rare with tolazamide. The mechanism of the reaction, which resembles that of antabuse, is unknown. Toxic effects on the liver and on the bone marrow are exceedingly rare.

An extensive prospective study of diabetics on various treatment regimens, the University Group Diabetes Program (UGDP) (1970), has been carried out in the USA. This study appeared to indicate that patients treated with tolbutamide had a higher mortality from cardiovascular deaths than those on diet alone or on diet and insulin. This study has provoked considerable controversy and criticism, and both randomisation and the selection of the control group appeared faulty (Bloom, 1972). Other important criticisms have been made, particularly since similar prospective studies carried out in Europe have yielded conflicting results (Keen and Jarrett, 1970; Paasikivi, 1970). In both of these studies it appeared that tolbutamide had a protective effect on the vascular system. Both European studies were concerned with somewhat smaller figures than the UGDP, but had the advantage that all patients were followed by the same observers throughout. Nevertheless, more recent papers from Belfast describing both retrospective and prospective studies of adult-onset diabetics (Boyle *et al.*, 1972; Hadden *et al.*, 1972) appeared to support the UGDP findings, by indicating that patients treated with oral hypoglycaemic agents had a frequency of myocardial infarction twice as great as those treated by diet alone, although these workers make the important point that patients who cannot be controlled by diet alone may select themselves as a group with an inherently greater risk of myocardial infarction. Discussion and controversy still rages but one conclusion which did emerge from the UGDP study was that there was no obvious benefit in the long term from treating mild overt diabetics routinely with oral hypoglycaemic agents. The study has also drawn attention to the fact that these are potent drugs which should only be prescribed in suitable patients who are likely to benefit from them.

As many as one-third of patients established on long-term sulphonylureas are able to discontinue their drugs and maintain satisfactory control on diet alone (Tomkins and Bloom, 1972).

Biguanide Compounds

In 1957, Ungar and his colleagues published a study of phenethylbiguanide (phenformin) and, shortly afterwards, dimethylbiguanide (metformin) was isolated (Fig. 15.3). Both these compounds lower blood glucose levels in diabetics but there are some points of difference between them. Metformin is not metabolised in the body, whereas phenformin is metabolised into several substances. Neither causes hypoglycaemia in the normal adult nor stimulates the islets of Langerhans, though both are inactive in the absence of insulin. Both compounds increase cellular glucose uptake in the presence of insulin, reduce hepatic glucose synthesis, reduce the absorption of glucose from the gut and reduce elevated plasma insulin levels in the obese non-diabetic or early mild-diabetic. Phenformin in high concentrations may stimulate anaerobic glycolysis and increase production of lactate; these changes have not been observed with metformin even in high doses. Weight loss occurs with both compounds, and this is not entirely due to loss of appetite. Both metformin and phenformin have been shown to have a fibrinolytic effect.

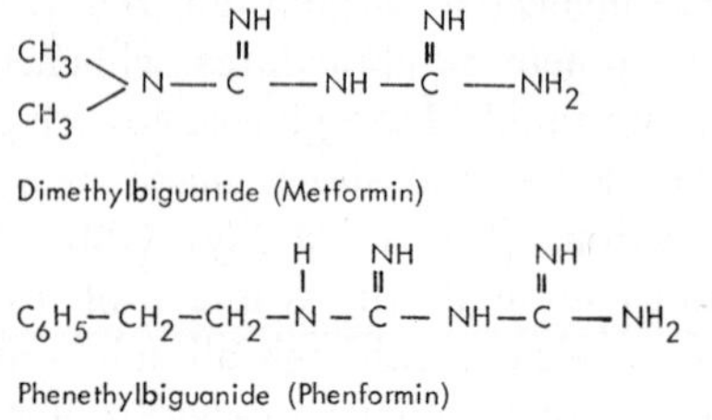

$$(CH_3)_2N-C(=NH)-NH-C(=NH)-NH_2$$

Dimethylbiguanide (Metformin)

$$C_6H_5-CH_2-CH_2-NH-C(=NH)-NH-C(=NH)-NH_2$$

Phenethylbiguanide (Phenformin)

FIGURE 15.3 Structure of biguanide compounds

Indications for Biguanide Therapy

1. Treatment of the maturity-onset obese diabetic who has failed to lose weight on diet.
2. In combination with sulphonylureas.
3. As an adjunct to insulin therapy.

Contra-indications to Biguanide Therapy

1. Diabetic ketosis.
2. Infantile and juvenile diabetes without concomitant use of insulin.
3. Pregnancy.
4. Phenformin but not metformin is contra-indicated in the presence of hepatic or renal disease.
5. Impaired diabetic control due to increase in insulin demands resulting from infection or trauma.
6. Both drugs are best avoided in any potentially hypoxic state such as heart failure or acute or chronic lung disease.

Most clinicians reserve the biguanides for the treatment of the maturity-onset diabetic who remains obese despite all attempts at dieting. A sulphonylurea is preferred for the initial treatment of maturity-onset cases of average weight, a biguanide being used in addition only if the patient fails to respond. The hypoglycaemic effects of a sulphonylurea and a biguanide are additive, and biguanides appear sometimes to potentiate the effect of a sulphonylurea drug. Their use may allow oral therapy to be maintained in patients who would otherwise have required insulin. The biguanides may also be used to supplement the action of insulin in 'brittle' diabetics, in older patients who require a moderately large dose of an intermediate acting insulin, or in patients on insulin who are overweight. Given alone, they will not reduce blood glucose, but they may replace as much as 30 per cent of the insulin requirement. These smaller doses of insulin are less likely to produce hypoglycaemia and excessive weight-gain but are sufficient to prevent ketosis. Variability of blood sugar levels may remain, but lower blood glucose levels can be tolerated without symptoms in patients receiving biguanides, possibly because the drugs increase the permeability of the brain cells to glucose.

Dosage. Phenformin begins to lower blood sugar within 2 to 3 hours, reaches a maximum effect at 4 to 6 hours, and ceases to act after 8 hours. A sustained-release preparation is available which lowers blood glucose for 12 to 14 hours. Metformin also has a relatively short duration of action, and must usually be given three times daily. The initial dose of phenformin is 25 mg four times a day, or 50 mg twice daily of the sustained-release capsule. Metformin is prescribed initially in a dose of 500 mg three times a day, rising to a maximum of 2,000 mg daily. It is usual to advise that the tablets are taken *with* a meal to reduce gastric irritation. Much smaller doses of phenformin or metformin may be required when given in combination with insulin or sulphonylureas.

Unwanted Effects of Biguanides

1. General malaise.
2. Dyspepsia, anorexia, nausea.
3. Diarrhoea.
4. Lactic acidosis (phenformin).
5. Toxic effects on liver and kidney (phenformin).

Lactic acidosis is a definite hazard of phenformin treatment, although it is usually precipitated by some intercurrent illness. There is no convincing report of lactic acidosis occurring as a result of metformin therapy. The commonest unwanted effects are nausea and dyspepsia. There is evidence that prolonged treatment with a biguanide may lead to vitamin B_{12} malabsorption. Metformin and the sustained-release preparation of phenformin are better tolerated than phenformin alone. Biguanides do not protect a diabetic from ketosis—indeed, ketosis may be precipitated if the unwanted effects of anorexia and vomiting are prominent. The UGDP study showed that patients treated with phenformin appeared to have a higher mortality from cardiovascular disease than those treated with diet or with diet and insulin.

INSULIN THERAPY

Insulin is essential in the treatment of children and adolescents and in all adults who are ketotic when first seen. It may sometimes be needed in the maturity-onset diabetic as a temporary measure in those patients whose diabetic control has been severely upset by acute stress as during an infection or an occlusive vascular episode, or to cover a surgical operation. It is also indicated in those maturity-onset patients of or below average weight who are not adequately controlled by diet and oral hypoglycaemic compounds. The aim using insulin is to achieve normoglycaemia, but this cannot usually be maintained at all times and under all conditions in severe diabetics. In the United Kingdom a number of different regimens are used for the control of insulin-requiring diabetics. Some of the properties of the various types of insulin in common use are shown in Table 15.2.

Single-dose Regimens. One of the intermediate-acting insulins such as lente, isophane, or globin may be used to provide control of blood sugar levels throughout the day following a single morning injection, and this regimen is satisfactory for some mild diabetics. Further modification can be made by mixing ultralente and semilente in different proportions, or by supplementing isophane with soluble insulin, both preparations given as a morning injection. Insulin zinc suspension preparations should not be mixed with soluble insulin B.P. It is generally agreed that preparations with a long or intermediate duration of action should not be used in the following situations:

1. Diabetic ketosis.
2. The 'brittle' diabetic.
3. The adolescent diabetic.
4. The pregnant diabetic.
5. The diabetic with a severe infection.
6. The diabetic whose daily insulin requirements much exceed 40 units.
7. The diabetic who requires an operation.

TABLE 15·2 *Properties of Insulin Preparations*

	Type	Protein modification	Time of maximum action (hours)	Duration of action (hours)
Fast acting	Soluble	None	4–6	6–12
	Semilente	None	4–6	12–18
Intermediate acting	Globin	Globin	6–10	18–32
	Isophane (NPH)*	Protamine	8–12	18–32 or more
	Lente†	None	8–12	18–36
Long acting	PZI‡	Protamine	14–20	36 or more
	Ultralente	None	16–18	36 or more

* NPH is neutral protamine Hagedorn.
† 3 parts of semi-lente; 7 parts ultra-lente.
‡ PZI is protamine zinc insulin.

Another single-dose regimen is to give soluble insulin and PZI by separate injections at the same time in the morning. Due to the prolonged action of PZI, hypoglycaemia is not uncommon and large doses of this preparation are not recommended—it is preferable to use isophane rather than PZI in this situation.

Soluble Insulin Regimens. In the severe diabetic, and when long-acting insulins are contra-indicated (*see* above), morning and evening injections of soluble insulin form the basis of most satisfactory treatment regimens. However, the hypoglycaemic action of this preparation is short, and even when given twice daily there may be fairly prolonged periods when little or no insulin effect is present. This situation will be aggravated in the highly insulin-sensitive 'brittle' diabetic, who can tolerate only relatively small doses of soluble insulin without hypoglycaemia and who thus has hyperglycaemia before the next dose of insulin. A number of workers have suggested modifications to the basic twice daily soluble insulin regimen in an attempt to avoid hypoglycaemia at mid-morning or in the late evening, in association with hyperglycaemia in the fasting state. The first modification, suggested by Lawrence and Oakley in 1944, involves the addition of a small amount of PZI (4 to 12 units) to the evening dose of soluble, the injection being given before tea instead of before the main evening meal. The two insulins are sometimes measured and mixed in the same syringe, but are best given by separate injections. Since PZI contains an excess of protamine and buffering agents, the addition of soluble insulin is followed by further precipitation of protamine zinc insulin. The addition of PZI to the evening dose of soluble insulin therefore smooths out and prolongs its action, avoiding nocturnal hypoglycaemia and fasting hyperglycaemia. With this regime, hypoglycaemia still tends to occur in the mid-morning due to the prolonged effect of the PZI, and many patients who are unable to take their second injection until they return home from work find the arrangement unsuitable. A further disadvantage of this regimen is the unpredictable and variable. effect of a mixture of soluble and PZI, and some have stated that it is unwise to mix PZI and soluble insulin. If the insulins are not mixed, then it means that the diabetic must take three injections a day, and many find this unacceptable. Oakley (1966) has suggested the use of combined injections of soluble and isophane insulin. The latter type has a shorter duration of action than PZI and its use in this situation has now superseded that of PZI. Since isophane insulin contains no excess of protamine or buffering agents, the effect of the combination is virtually the same as that following separate injections of the two insulins if it is given within three minutes of mixing. The soluble insulin controls the blood sugar for the first six to eight hours, and for the remainder of the time the isophane is effective. No adjustment of the times of meals or injections is necessary, and the isophane insulin may be given with both the morning and evening doses of soluble, if these are evenly spaced, with the evening dose if this is taken early and the morning dose late, or with the morning dose if this is taken early and the evening dose late. It is suggested that this regimen provides the most satisfactory control for most diabetics.

The Newer Insulins

1. *'Nuso' Neutral Insulin*. Soluble insulin BP has an acid pH whereas 'Nuso' insulin is neutral (pH of 7·2). The latter is said to be more stable than soluble insulin, and seems less likely to give rise to local irritation and fibrosis at the injection site. The potency and duration of action appear to be identical with soluble insulin, and neutral insulin can be used as a substitute for soluble insulin BP.

2. *Pork Insulin*. The great majority of insulin preparations commonly in use in the U.K. until recently have been of bovine origin. Preparations of pork insulin have now become available, some of them being combined with beef insulin. Two such preparations are available—neutral porcine insulin ('Actrapid') and biphasic insulin ('Rapitard'), which is a mixture of 25 per cent pork and 75 per cent bovine insulins, with no added protein. One advantage of pork insulin is that it may be used in the rare diabetics who are allergic to or who have developed high titres of antibodies to beef insulin, which may result in very high insulin requirements. Initially, in such patients much lower doses of pork insulin are required. Even in patients without high titres of antibodies to beef insulin, hypoglycaemia may occur if pork insulin is inadvertently used in the same dose as the previously used bovine preparation. This is a very real danger, and pharmacist, patient, and doctor should constantly be on the alert to avoid it.

Insulin Strengths

In the United Kingdom insulin is available in strengths of 40 and 80 units per ml; soluble is also available as 20 units per ml. Each type and each strength of insulin used in the UK has a standard colour code. The strength most commonly used in this country is 40 units per ml; it is therefore unfortunate that the British Standard insulin syringe (B.S. 1619) is calibrated for 20 units per ml. and this has caused confusion to patients, nurses and doctors alike. In an attempt to ensure standardisation, it is proposed in the USA to introduce a single insulin strength of 100 units per ml, to be used with syringes calibrated to contain 30 units or 100 units.

THE INITIAL STABILISATION OF DIABETICS WITH INSULIN

In all except the mildest cases this is best carried out in hospital, for there is much for the patient to learn. In the patient who has never previously had insulin the diet is first agreed between patient, physician and dietitian, and apportioned throughout the day according to the patient's requirements and habits along the lines previously discussed. Soluble insulin is used for initial stabilisation of all but the mildest, who may be given an intermediate-acting insulin once daily. The initial dose of soluble insulin will usually be in the region of 12 to 20 units twice daily—it is convenient for the patient to measure his dose when it is given in multiples of 4 units if 40 units/ml strength insulin is used. The insulin dosage may then be cautiously increased according to the patient's response, and any modifications such as the addition of isophane insulin may be made as necessary. Urine samples are tested for sugar and ketones before each meal, and blood glucose estimations are performed with the patient fasting, at 11 a.m. (maximal insulin effect) and 3 p.m. (insulin effect subsiding). Samples taken at 9 p.m. or later may also be of value in stabilisation, particularly if isophane or PZI are used with the evening dose. The precise timing of the blood sugars must be modified depending on the times of injection and meals and the type of insulin used.

It is most important during the process of diabetic stabilisation in hospital to reproduce, as far as possible, the timing of meals as taken at home and the patient should be encouraged to be as active as possible even to the extent of regarding the hospital as a hotel where he simply eats, sleeps and has blood glucose samples taken. The transition from hospital to home is thus made easier and there is less likelihood of any marked change in insulin requirements. Because it may be difficult to ensure as much exercise in hospital as the patient will take at home, and because with exercise less insulin may be needed, it is usual to make a slight reduction in the insulin dosage when the patient leaves hospital, final adjustment being carried out on an out-patient basis.

The giving of insulin and discussion of diet are only part of the management of a diabetic, and it is important that instruction and advice on the following subjects should also be given:

1. Technique of urine testing, so that the patient may be able to test his urine correctly for glucose and acetone. He should be encouraged to carry out and record pre-prandial and fasting urine tests several times each day on his return home and to adjust his insulin dosage according to the tests—reducing the dose if no glucose is detected or increasing it if all tests show one per cent glucose or more. Ketonuria which persists for more than a single urine specimen should be reported. Best control is achieved if about half the urine specimens are negative and half show a trace or ½ per cent glycosuria. Later, this frequent testing may be relaxed if control is good.
2. Technique of insulin injection:
   (*a*) care of syringe and needles
   (*b*) measurement of insulin and types used
   (*c*) the injection technique including preparation of skin and the rotation of injection sites to include the arms, legs and possibly abdomen, ensuring that the injections are *not* always given in the same site.
3. Instructions as to what can be done and where advice may be sought in an emergency such as acute infection or a gastro-intestinal upset. In such cases the insulin dosage must never

be reduced and will usually need to be increased. If the patient is unable to maintain an adequate carbohydrate intake, even in fluid form, treatment in hospital is needed.

4. The patient should be provided with a card which prominently indicates his diabetic state and gives his name and address, that of his general practitioner, and that of the hospital. Most cards have a statement such as: 'I am a diabetic. If found drowsy or confused please attempt to give me glucose or milk drinks by mouth and contact immediately Dr. . . .' The patient should always carry with him some glucose to use in an emergency.

In addition to regular review of diabetic control, routine physical examination should be carried out at yearly intervals to detect the onset of complications, and should include detailed retinoscopy. Care of the feet should be stressed.

Having considered insulin therapy in some detail, it is sobering to realise what patients actually do in practice. Stowers, in an excellent appraisal of insulin therapy (1972), has drawn attention to the work of Watkins and his colleagues (1967). These workers in North Carolina found that no less than 58 per cent of 115 patients of different social levels taking insulin made errors of dosage, and in over one-third of these the error was of more than 15 per cent, sometimes because the wrong strength of insulin was used. The frequency of errors increased with the duration of treatment. As Stowers points out, it is incumbent on doctors treating patients with insulin to give very clear instructions and to make sure that the patient understands them.

THE COMPLICATIONS OF DIABETES MELLITUS

ACUTE COMPLICATIONS

COMPLICATIONS OF THERAPY

Insulin

(*a*) *Insulin Allergy*. Erythema at the injection site is usually due to either contaminants or infection. True insulin allergy is very rarely seen with soluble crystalline insulin and usually represents an allergy specifically dependent on the beast of origin of the insulin. If this occurs with the most commonly used bovine preparation, the porcine form should be substituted. Allergy is not uncommon in patients who use an insulin preparation modified by the addition of a protein, e.g. PZI, isophane, globin. The usual manifestation is urticaria, although severe anaphylactic shock may occur. If such reactions are seen with these modified insulins, the most sensible course of action is to discontinue their use and to rely on soluble or lente insulin. The allergic reactions may be treated symptomatically with antihistamines, or if severe, with hydrocortisone. In the very rare cases of true allergy to insulin, desensitisation will be necessary.

(*b*) *Hypoglycaemia* and its clinical manifestations are discussed elsewhere (*see* Chapter 16). The treatment consists of the administration of glucose or sucrose orally, or glucose intravenously if this is not possible. Diabetics should be warned to carry with them glucose, sugar lumps, or some other simple and accessible source of utilisable carbohydrate. Glucose may be given intravenously in any concentration from 10 to 25 per cent. The higher concentrations have a tendency to cause venous thromboses, though they may be convenient if the patient is struggling or violent. If intravenous glucose is not available, then glucagon given subcutaneously in a dose of 0·5 to 1·0 mg or adrenaline subcutaneously in a dose of 0·5 to 1 ml of a 1 in 1,000 solution may be helpful. These, however, are an indirect way of treating hypoglycaemia and the patient may in any case have mobilised much of his liver glycogen under the influence of his endogenous adrenaline. Recurrent and severe hypoglycaemia may produce permanent cerebral damage or a psychopathic state. Hypoglycaemia with PZI may be particularly dangerous; it is often slow of onset, and commonly relapses after the patient is thought to have recovered. It must be remembered that propranolol make provoke hypoglycaemia in diabetic patients who take insulin. There should be no difficulty whatsoever in differentiating hypoglycaemic coma from the coma of diabetic ketosis. The two conditions are entirely different, though it is vitally important to remember that they may co-exist, as in the over-enthusiastic treatment of diabetic ketoacidaemia. Features of coma as a result of diabetic ketoacidaemia and as a result of hypoglycaemia are shown in Table 15.3.

TABLE 15.3 *Features of Ketoacidaemic and Hypoglycaemic Coma*

	Ketoacidaemic	Hypoglycaemic
May be preceded by:	Infection, trauma, errors in dosage of insulin	Undue exercise, missed meal, errors in dosage of insulin
Rate of onset:	Hours or days	Minutes
Breathing:	Deep and rapid: 'air hunger'	Stertorous
Hydration:	Marked dehydration	Normal
Sweating:	Absent	Usually marked
CNS signs:	No change apart from perhaps diminution of reflexes	Almost anything. Characteristically bilateral extensor plantar responses
Urine:	Marked ketonuria. Usually marked glycosuria	Not helpful

DIABETIC KETOACIDAEMIA (KETOSIS)

This is essentially due to insufficient insulin activity and results in 'starvation' at a cellular or tissue level. Consequences of the basic metabolic defect are dehydration and electrolyte abnormalities.

The causes of inadequate insulin action are:

Insufficient insulin available	*Increased insulin requirements*
Patients stopped or reduced insulin	Illness, infection, trauma and 'stress'
Doctor stopped or reduced insulin	
Errors in insulin dosage	
Incorrect injection technique (including leaky syringe)	
Previously untreated diabetes.	

Metabolic Changes. In the condition of diabetic ketoacidaemia one of the cardinal features is hyperglycaemia. This is mainly due to decreased peripheral glucose utilisation, but increased hepatic output of glucose and increased gluconeogenesis also contribute. The sequence of events leading to ketone body production is briefly as follows:

(*a*) Impaired carbohydrate utilisation.
(*b*) Increased lipolysis and oxidation of fatty acids, with reduced fatty acid biosynthesis and esterification.

(*c*) Increased accumulation of acetyl coenzyme A and acetoacetyl coenzyme A. The main site of ketone body production via these substrates is the liver, but there is a contribution also from fat. The main source of the fatty acids which are ultimately converted to ketone bodies is adipose tissue. In fat, because of suppression of the glycolytic pathways resulting from decreased cellular uptake of glucose, with consequent lack of pyruvate and oxaloacetate, acetyl CoA and acetoacetyl CoA cannot be effectively metabolised by the normal routes, i.e. Krebs cycle and fatty acid biosynthetic pathways. Liver can to some extent metabolise fatty acids by normal pathways in the absence of insulin, but the substrate load thrown on the liver in uncontrolled diabetic ketoacidaemia is far greater than this organ can handle. The supply of acetyl CoA exceeds the available oxaloacetate, since there is a relative deficiency of oxaloacetate in diabetic ketoacidaemia (Wieland, 1965).

(*d*) This leads to accumulation of:
- (i) acetoacetyl CoA→ketone bodies (acetone, acetoacetate and β-hydroxybutyrate)
- (ii) acetyl CoA→β-hydroxy β-methyl glutaryl CoA→ketone bodies and cholesterol (Fig. 15.4).

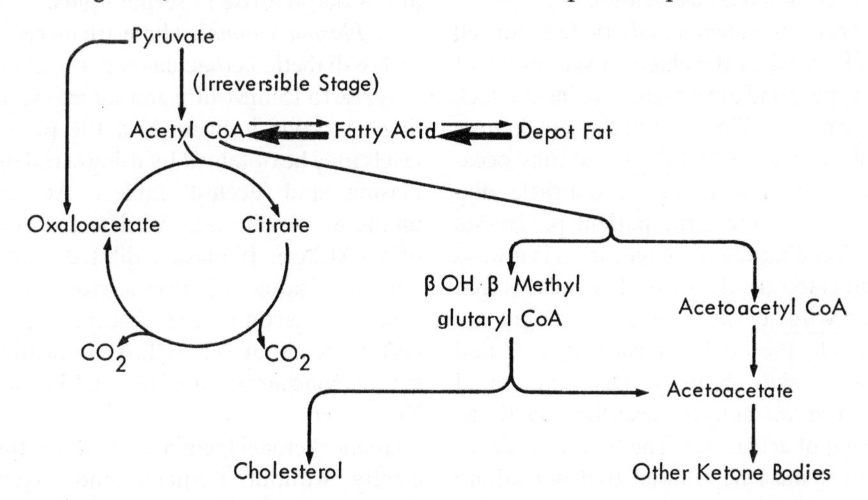

FIGURE 15.4 The pathogenesis of ketosis

(*e*) The ketone bodies themselves induce a degree of insulin resistance, probably by further inhibiting glucose uptake. There is also evidence that the ketone bodies inhibit the activity of the enzyme phosphofructokinase—an essential step in glycolysis. The principal site of metabolism of ketone bodies is in muscle, where they are normally oxidised to provide energy.

The Role of Glucagon

Plasma glucagon concentrations rise markedly, in part as a result of insulin deficiency (Buchanan and McCarroll, 1972; *Lancet*, 1972a) and under the influence of this hormone a vicious circle is established whereby accelerated lipolysis leads to exaggerated ketogenesis, accelerated gluconeogenesis and further hyperglycaemia. The changes in water and hydrogen ion metabolism consequent upon diabetic ketoacidaemia activate the sympathetic nervous system (Marks, 1971), thereby enhancing glucagon secretion and inhibiting still further any residual insulin secreting capacity of the pancreas.

In consequence of the impaired carbohydrate utilisation and ketonaemia there occur, therefore:

1. Non-respiratory acidaemia.
2. Rise in plasma lipids.

3. Excretion of partly neutralised keto acids via the kidney with loss of cations such as sodium and potassium.
4. Hyperglycaemia and glycosuria leading to osmotic diuresis and further loss of water. There is also loss of carbohydrate and, hence, glucose depletion, despite the high blood glucose concentration.

As a result of the acidaemia there is loss of intracellular fluid and electrolytes, and acidotic breathing, which will produce further loss of water. In addition, vomiting is almost invariable, and will further accentuate the dehydration and electrolyte abnormalities.

Lowering of red cell 2,3-diphosphoglycerate (2,3-DPG) levels occurs in diabetic ketoacidaemia. There is a strong positive correlation of 2,3-DPG, with arterial blood pH, and a negative correlation with total ketone bodies (Alberti *et al.*, 1972). A fall in 2,3-DPG by itself causes impaired oxyhaemoglobin dissociation, which may result in tissue anoxia. However, in diabetic ketoacidaemia a balance is reached between the effect of the lowered 2,3-DPG levels and that of the lowered pH on the oxyhaemoglobin dissociation curve, so that there is little net effect on tissue oxygen supply. This has important implications when the use of bicarbonate solutions to correct acidaemia is considered (*see* below).

Clinical Features. When a diabetic feels unwell and particularly when the classical symptoms of diabetes reappear and are progressive insulin lack should be suspected. The onset of diabetic ketosis is usually slow, over several days, but may occasionally occur in a few hours in the 'brittle' diabetic. Without treatment the patient progresses into coma. Some degree of dehydration is always present, and is frequently gross. The pulse is thin and of poor volume, the mouth and tongue are dry and rough, the ocular tension is low, and there is loss of skin elasticity. Deep and rapid respiration, the 'air-hunger' described by Kussmaul, is a sign of acidaemia. The breath smells of acetone, but it must be realised that not all are able to smell this compound and every physician should know whether or not he is able to do so. Abdominal pain may be severe, and nausea and vomiting are almost invariable when the ketonaemia and acidaemia are well advanced.

Biochemical Features. 1. *Hyperglycaemia.* This is always present, although the level of blood glucose is not always correlated with the degree of ketonaemia.

2. *Glycosuria and Ketonuria.* Invariable unless renal function is grossly impaired.

3. *Low Plasma Bicarbonate.* If less than 10 mEq/litre, it is usual to regard the acidaemia as 'severe', although this is purely arbitrary.

4. *Low Blood pH.*

5. *Plasma Electrolytes.* There is loss of sodium, chloride (largely in vomit), and potassium from the body, the latter usually of severe degree. Since the rate of transfer of potassium from cells to extracellular fluid is more rapid than its urinary loss the concentrations of potassium in the plasma may be higher than normal; in the most severe cases with copious vomiting the plasma potassium may, however, be low. There is always a total body deficit of sodium, sometimes of severe degree, but this may go unrecognised because of a normal plasma sodium level in the presence of a diminished volume of extracellular fluid.

6. *Plasma Free Fatty Acids.* These are markedly elevated because of increased lipolysis. There is also a marked rise in serum lipids.

7. *Plasma Ketones.* These are increased and, in severe diabetic ketoacidaemia, the concentration may rise to 15 mM/litre and sometimes to 30 mM/litre. A crude indication of the plasma ketone levels may be obtained by using serial dilutions of plasma, and 'acetest' tablets. Acetoacetate in undiluted plasma may be detected at a dilution of 1 mM/litre. If plasma diluted with an equal volume of saline produces a strong 'acetest' reaction at 30 seconds, the concentration of acetoacetate is about 5 mM/litre, indicating a total ketone concentration of about 15 mM/litre.

Treatment

Diabetic ketoacidaemia cannot be treated efficiently without frequent and accurate biochemical control. Each patient presents an individual problem, and only principles and guidelines can be given. The principles of therapy are:

1. Normal carbohydrate metabolism must be re-established by the administration of insulin.
2. Deficiencies of water and intracellular as well as extracellular electrolytes must be corrected.
3. Glucose depletion must be replenished in order that normal carbohydrate metabolism may be maintained.

Two excellent reviews of the treatment of diabetic ketoacidaemia have recently been published (Malins, 1971; Hockaday and Alberti, 1972). Complete bed rest is essential, and the patient must be attended by a nurse, if possible until recovery is assured. Unless the patient is fully conscious and is not vomiting a nasogastric tube should be passed and it may be necessary to catheterise the unconscious patient. In the older patient it is wise constantly to monitor the central venous pressure to avoid fluid overload.

Blood is first taken for glucose and electrolyte estimations and cross matching and an arterial sample is taken for measurements of pH and pCO_2. An ECG should be recorded and the patient attached to a cardiac monitor. An initial dose of soluble insulin is then given and the size of this first dose depends on:

1. the route of administration;
2. whether or not the patient is a known diabetic;
3. if a known diabetic, his normal daily dose of insulin;
4. the presence of coma, severe dehydration, serious infection or other complications.

Some guide as to the initial dose of insulin is given in Table 15.4.

TABLE 15.4

New diabetics or children		Known diabetics	
No evidence of severe dehydration or infection. Not in coma.	Severe dehydration, infection or coma present.	No evidence of severe dehydration or infection. Not in coma.	Severe dehydration, infection or coma present
40–50 units	80–100 units	60–80 units	100–120 units

Insulin. The first step is to give soluble insulin, for the patient is severely insulin-deficient and, in addition to a degree of insulin resistance brought about by the ketosis and dehydration, an insulin antagonist that migrates with the α_1-globulin fraction of plasma protein is present in the plasma in severe cases. Massive doses of insulin may be needed to overcome this antagonism, which disappears rapidly when effective treatment is given. Adrenocortical overactivity may also be a factor in causing increased insulin resistance.

If the initial blood glucose exceeds 800 mg per cent an additional 100 units should be given as soon as the blood glucose result is obtained. It is usual to give one-third or one-half of the insulin by the intravenous route and the remainder intramuscularly. The half-life of insulin following a single intravenous injection is four minutes. Some suggest that a constant intravenous infusion of insulin using low doses may be useful in treatment (Sönksen *et al.*, 1972) and an alternative regimen is to give smaller doses of insulin hourly by intramuscular injection (Alberti *et al.*, 1973), but experience with these regimens is at present limited.

A second blood sample is obtained for glucose estimation about one hour after the initial dose has been given. If this level is higher than the first, the further dose of insulin given should be double the initial amount. If the level is the same, the initial dose is repeated, and if a significant fall in blood glucose has occurred the dose may be reduced or even omitted. Blood glucose estimations and the administration of insulin are continued at approximately hourly intervals until blood glucose is less than 300 mg per cent. At this time urine tests may begin to give adequate information. Some physicians assess insulin dosage and response to treatment by estimating serial plasma ketone concentrations.

It is important to note that the patient's clinical response does not always parallel the improvement in his blood glucose levels.

Intravenous Fluids. An intravenous drip must be erected when the patient is first seen. If the systolic blood pressure falls below 80 mm/Hg and signs of peripheral vasoconstriction due to oligaemic shock appear, infusion of whole blood (or of plasma if blood is not available) should be commenced. In the absence of hypotension and shock, normal saline is favoured for infusion, and large volumes must be used. One litre should be given in the first 30 minutes, and then one litre every 60 minutes. One gram of potassium chloride should be given in the first hour after insulin is given, unless the patient is old, has renal failure or is extremely ill. The quantity of fluid given and the rate of administration are judged according to the clinical state and response of the patient. Rapid correction of the acidaemia will aggravate potassium depletion and may correct plasma pH without completely restoring that of the CSF—thus the patient continues to show acidotic respiration with a normal plasma bicarbonate. Great caution should be exercised in the use of bicarbonate infusions, and these are best avoided unless the pH is below 7·1. Even then, care should be taken since rapid correction of pH will shift the oxygen dissociation curve further to the left which, in the presence of low red cell 2,3-DPG levels, could result in poorer oxygen supply to the tissues. Ideal treatment (i.e. adequate amounts of insulin to prevent excessive ketone body formation) must cut off the supply of hydrogen ions, but alkali can afford symptomatic relief to the severely acidaemic patient. It is therefore suggested that if the pH is below 7·0, 125 mMol of sodium bicarbonate (375 ml of 2·74 per cent solution) should be infused over about 30 minutes. Since correction of pH will cause rapid movement of potassium into the cells, 1·5 g of KCl is given in the infusion. If the pH is 7·0–7·1, 50 mMol of sodium bicarbonate (150 ml of 2·74 per cent solution) is given over 15 minutes with one gram of KCl, repeating the infusion after 30 minutes. The pH is measured after one to two hours and further alkali given as required until the pH is returned to about 7·2 (Hockaday and Alberti, 1972). Lactate has no place in the modern treatment of ketoacidaemia.

Potassium and phosphate are lost in the urine, but if renal function is depressed (as it is in diabetic ketosis secondary to dehydration) the rate of release from the cells during the acidotic phase exceeds the rate of excretion in the urine. Thus, initially the plasma potassium may be high despite an overall body deficit of about 500 mEq. The correction of the acidaemia and the resynthesis of glycogen and cellular uptake of glucose which occurs when carbohydrate metabolism is re-established, and the correction of cellular dehyduration leads to the transfer of potassium into the cells and, hence, to a rapid fall in the plasma level. Large amounts of potassium must therefore be given during treatment. It used to be suggested that the administration of potassium should be delayed until four hours after the initial dose of insulin was given or until a significant fall in blood glucose had been observed, but it is now agreed that potassium should be given much earlier than this. As soon as the blood glucose has started to fall potassium will be needed, but awaiting biochemical confirmation of blood glucose fall may be too late, and most now agree that intravenous potassium should be given from the outset unless renal failure is present (Hockaday and Alberti (1972). An infusion rate as rapid as three grams KCl per hour ($\equiv$ 40 mEq of K^+) may be necessary although usually one to two grams per hour will suffice. Frequent estimations of the plasma potassium must be carried out, and in severe cases continuous cardiographic monitoring may be used, for death may occur from hypo- or hyperkalaemia. However, many ECG changes are non-specific, and the recording must never be thought equivalent to determining the plasma potassium biochemically, although it provides a rapid assessment of cardiac excitability and is a useful precaution against hyperkalaemia occurring during potassium infusion. The most dangerously ill patients may present a low plasma potassium. Here potassium must be given in large quantities from the outset, and monitoring of the electrocardiogram is mandatory.

Phosphate. During the development of diabetic ketosis there is a significant loss of inorganic phosphate, which will also enter the cells when effective treatment is underway. The lowered red cell, 2,3-DPG levels observed in diabetic ketoacidaemia take up to five days to return to normal after treatment of the ketoacidaemia (Alberti *et al.*, 1972), and this seems to be secondary to phosphate deficiency—plasma levels may remain very low for some days. It is theoretically possible, therefore, that the introduction of phosphate into intravenous infusion regimens might be beneficial. One such infusion solution is given below.

Glucose must be given at a later stage of treatment, since the body is depleted of glucose and carbohydrate metabolism must be maintained, furthermore the risk of hypoglycaemia is also minimised. Glucose should be given when the blood glucose level has fallen below 300 mg per cent. A convenient intravenous infusion is 4·0 per cent glucose in 0·18 per cent saline given at the rate of 500 ml every 4 to 6 hours, usually with potassium added, and usually with additional intravenous or oral glucose supplements. There is no place for the use of fructose in the treatment of diabetic ketoacidaemia—lactic acidaemia may be precipitated.

An alternative intravenous infusion for use at this stage has been based on Butler's solution by Nabarro, and has the following ionic constitution:

NaCl	1·17 g	Na	20 mEq/litre
K_2HPO_4	0·87 g	K	30 mEq/litre
KCl	1·49 g	Cl	45 mEq/litre
$MgCl_2$	0·24 g	PO_4	10 mEq/litre
Glucose	50 g	Mg	5 mEq/litre
Water to one litre		Glucose = 5 per cent	

It is usually given at the rate of 500 ml every 4 to 6 hours and is based on the observed amounts of these substances that must be given to repair the deficits that have occurred as a result of the ketosis.

Dangerous Situations which may arise during the correction of diabetic ketoacidaemia include hypokalaemia, hyperosmolality, hypoglycaemia, extreme insulin resistance and cerebral oedema, due to osmotic disequilibrium (*Lancet*, 1971c; Clements *et al.*, 1971). Cerebral oedema appears to be due to accumulation of sorbitol and fructose in the brain cells during the period of hyperglycaemia, although dehydration, haemoconcentration, acidaemia (or its rapid correction), all promote cerebral anoxia, which may also lead to cerebral oedema. The physician must be aware of these hazards of therapy, and must anticipate and, by carefully controlled and rational treatment, prevent their possible development. As regards cerebral oedema, one therapeutic implication is that the correction of plasma hyperosmolality should not be made too rapidly. If it occurs, massive doses of dexamethasone may be life-saving, although plainly this will further impair the metabolic state.

Treatment of Cause. In all cases the precipitating cause of the episode should be sought, and appropriate therapeutic measures undertaken. If due to an error in insulin dosage, the patient must be carefully instructed about his maintenance treatment regimen in the convalescent phase.

The Treatment of Milder Degrees of Ketosis. Patients with mild ketosis who are alert, without severe dehydration or infection, and who have blood glucose levels less than 400 mg per cent and bicarbonate levels above 15 mEq/litre do not always need the intensive treatment described above and may often be treated with a 'graduated scale' insulin and glucose regimen, perhaps after an initial higher dose of insulin than is allowed by the scale is given. This may also be used in patients recovering from more severe ketosis in the interim period after initial therapy has controlled the situation but before twice daily insulin is recommended. Carbohydrate is given regularly, and insulin according to the apparent needs of the patient as assessed by urinary examination.

Two alternative regimens, differing in the amount of carbohydrate and insulin given are used, and the outline of these is shown in Table 15.5. The younger, heavier, more active, and more ketotic patient would be given the second regimen; the older, thinner, sedentary, and milder case will usually be adequately controlled by the first. The carbohydrate may be given intravenously, orally, or by a combination of routes, and additional potassium is given as required. In the mildest cases a six-hourly schedule can be used.

TABLE 15.5 *Graduated Scale Regimens of Insulin and Carbohydrate Therapy in Mild Diabetic Ketosis*

Regimen 1:	*Carbohydrate:*	20 g every 4 hours
	Insulin:	Every 4 hours as indicated below:
		Urine Sugar (tested every 4 *hours using 'Clinitest' tablets and colour chart*)
	0 insulin given	0
	5 units soluble	trace to + ($\frac{1}{4}$ to $\frac{1}{2}$ per cent)
	10 units soluble	++ ($\frac{3}{4}$ per cent)
	15 units soluble	+++ (1 per cent)
	20 units soluble	++++ (2 per cent or more)

An additional 5 units soluble is given every 4 hours if urinary ketones are present.

Regimen 2:	*Carbohydrate:*	30 g every 4 hours
	Insulin:	Follow general scheme above but use 8 units soluble insulin per 'plus' of sugar with an additional 8 units for ketones

This procedure depends on a normal or near-normal renal threshold, and there is a danger of hypoglycaemia if it is followed when there is a low renal threshold. Accurate timing is mandatory, and a 'fresh' urine sample should be obtained whenever the urine is to be tested—this means that the patient should empty his bladder half an hour before the test is due and again at the time of the test.

Lactic Acidaemia

Lactic acid accumulates during treatment with phenformin, but rarely to an excessive degree. The syndrome of severe non-ketoacidotic lactic acidaemia usually occurs in diabetic patients who have serious cardiac or renal disease and who are commonly in a terminal state. In these circumstances lactic acidaemia may occur both in patients treated with phenformin and those taking insulin, although it is more commonly seen in the former. There is severe acidaemia, as indicated by low plasma bicarbonate and blood pH, without ketosis. The blood glucose is moderately elevated, and the patient is usually dehydrated. The condition is treated with intravenous isotonic bicarbonate and with insulin, supported as necessary with intravenous glucose. If shock is present, an adequate circulation must be restored using saline and isoproterenol, which has no lactatogenic effect, unlike adrenaline and noradrenaline. Severely ill or dehydrated patients or those with renal failure or severe congestive heart failure should not be treated with phenformin, or indeed with any other oral drug.

Hyperosmolal Non-ketotic Diabetic Coma

Attention was first drawn to this syndrome in 1957, and it was well described by Gerich *et al.* (1971). Hyperosmolal non-ketotic coma (HNC) occurs in the older maturity onset diabetic who is often obese and whose diabetes is usually mild, or even previously undiagnosed. The clinical features are severe dehydration and viscous blood with hypernatraemia, but the blood pressure is usually maintained and ketosis is absent. Potassium depletion may occur rapidly and is commonly severe. Blood sugar levels are very greatly raised (typically exceeding 1,000 mg/100 ml) and there is a very large blood/CSF glucose difference. The coma is usually precipitated by superadded infection or gastro-intestinal upset in a patient who is too weak, ill, or elderly to replace fluids adequately by the oral route. Another frequent precipitating factor is the use of diabetogenic drugs, particularly thiazide diuretics. Dehydration and hyperosmolality therefore play significant roles in the pathogenesis of HNC, although the precise aetiology of the syndrome is unknown. Water loss induced by glycosuria is an important trigger mechanism but this does not tell the whole story—in all cases it should be assumed that there is also some impairment or inefficiency of central osmoregulation, which in some cases may be the main cause of the syndrome (*Lancet*, 1972b). Convulsions may occur and a peculiar reversible syndrome of dysphagia, dysphonia, and mental confusion has been observed. Arterial and venous thromboses frequently occur. The condition has a mortality of at least 20 per cent. Normal saline must not be used in treatment. In general, patients with HNC require less insulin than in the keto-acidaemic form of coma, although insulin requirements tend to vary. Potassium replacement is necessary and large amounts may be needed—the plasma potassium level should be measured frequently. Hypotonic saline (0·45 per cent; 77 mEq/1) is the replacement fluid of choice, and although patients with HNC require more fluid than those with ketoacidaemia, the infusion should be given less rapidly to reduce the risk of cerebral oedema and to allow osmolality to return to normal slowly.

Acute Infections

The diabetic, particularly if poorly controlled, is prone to develop acute infections. Those most frequently seen are pyogenic infections of the skin and urinary infections, and occasionally, the grave syndrome of acute papillary necrosis which may rapidly lead to renal failure and uraemic coma. In the presence of such infections the control of the diabetic deteriorates. Candidal infections are, of course, common in both male and female.

Acute Neuropathy

Several acute neurological syndromes may occur in diabetes. Acute neuropathy is usually seen when the diabetes is badly stabilised, but may precede or follow an episode of poor control. The commonest type of neuropathy involves the motor and sensory nerves of the lower limbs, and severe pain and paraesthesiae, muscular weakness, and loss of reflexes are prominent. Less commonly, there may be generalised acute polyneuropathy affecting both sensory and motor nerves in all four limbs, or the syndrome of mononeuritis multiplex. Segmental demyelination of nerves is found, and there is widespread slowing of nerve conduction velocity. Another acute neural syndrome in diabetes is the diabetic amyotrophy described by Garland (1955). This is predominantly a motor disorder affecting principally the legs, and signs of an upper motor neurone lesion may also be present. Despite this, muscle-wasting is common, and the characteristic lesion on muscle biopsy is single fibre atrophy. This is readily distinguishable from the motor unit type of atrophy sometimes seen in diabetic peripheral neuropathy. Nerve conduction velocities have shown that this syndrome of amyotrophy is due to a proximal radiculopathy. The isolated cranial nerve palsies that sometimes occur in diabetes are probably of vascular origin. Treatment of acute neuropathy is essentially symptomatic, and improvement usually follows better control of the diabetes (*Lancet*, 1972*c*). Diphenylhydantoin and carbamazepine (Tegretol) have been reported to be of value in the treatment of the painful manifestations of diabetic neuropathy.

CHRONIC COMPLICATIONS

COMPLICATIONS OF THERAPY

1. *Insulin Lipodystrophy*

(*a*) *Hypertrophy*. This presents with soft, lipoma-like swellings at the site of injection, and it may become severe enough to affect the fitting of clothes. In the affected areas total lipid is increased and the fat cells are hypertrophied. There may be increased glycogen deposition, but this is mainly seen in experimental situations. The hypertrophy is presumed to be due to the effect of insulin on lipogenesis. Fat hypertrophy is more common under the age of twenty and, in contrast to fat atrophy, is more frequent both below and above this age in the male. There is little effective treatment for fat hypertrophy; therapy is essentially preventive by ensuring that injection sites are changed daily so that a given area is not used more than about once a week. Areas of lesser cosmetic importance and those not in public view (often difficult to find in the female) should be used for the injections. The condition is completely benign, and the prospects for spontaneous recovery are high, although this may take a long time.

(*b*) *Atrophy*. This is usually reported at the site of insulin injection and is due to disappearance of fat tissue. It is more common under the age of twenty, when it seems to affect the sexes equally; but in the adult, although it occurs frequently in females, it is only very rarely seen in males. Only insulin and glucagon have been observed to produce the abnormality and the mechanisms by which they do so are unknown. Fat atrophy is less likely to improve spontaneously than fat hypertrophy, but marked improvement is reported if neutral porcine or biphasic insulin is used, and injected directly into the atrophic areas (Watson and Calder, 1971), although recovery has been reported even when neutral insulin was injected into areas remote from the lesions. Such improvement might well have occurred spontaneously.

2. *Fibrosis at Injection Sites*

This is not infrequent. It may follow localised infection or may be due to the long continued use of the same site for the injection of soluble insulin, which is of acid pH. The condition is of importance, as injection into a fibrosed area, as well as being painful and technically difficult, leads to considerable variation in the rate of insulin absorption, and may thus affect control. Attempts to improve the control may result in hypoglycaemia when the dose of insulin is increased and a different, non-affected site is used for the injection. Poor injection technique of this sort seems to be one of the commonest causes of chronic instability, and is often neglected by the doctor. The condition may be prevented or greatly minimised by rotation of injection sites and careful injection technique. It seems reasonable to suppose that the use of neutral pH insulin will be less likely to result in fibrosis.

THE SYSTEMIC CHRONIC COMPLICATIONS OF DIABETES

In general, these fall into two main groups:

1. Those not specifically related to diabetes but which appear earlier and occur more extensively in diabetics.
2. Those characteristic of the diabetic state.

This distinction is not always clear cut, but is best exemplified when the vascular complications of diabetes are considered. These complications may be due to atherosclerosis, which may affect the peripheral limb vessels, the visceral vessels (producing, for example, glomerulosclerosis or ischaemic heart disease), the retinal vessels, or the vasa nervorum (producing neuropathy). All these manifestations of atherosclerosis tend to occur earlier and with increased frequency in diabetics.

On the other hand, the characteristic vascular lesion in diabetes is microangiopathy, which is responsible for diabetic nephropathy and retinopathy, as well as playing some part in the aetiology of neuropathy and possibly of some skin complications. The characteristic initial lesion in these sites is thickening of the basement membrane (BMT), which appears to affect all arterioles, venules and capillaries in the body to a greater or lesser extent.

In the juvenile diabetic BMT is only rarely seen in the first few years after the diabetes is diagnosed, but is usually found when the diabetes has been present for seven or more years, although even then is not seen in all patients. The presence or absence of BMT is not related to the age at onset, the degree of hyperglycaemia, the residual ability to secrete insulin, a history of frequent episodes of ketosis or hypoglycaemia or the type of treatment given (Danowski *et al.*, 1972). In the adult, BMT is more common and may occur before the diabetes is clinically evident. Basement membrane thickening affecting the small blood vessels may also occur in non-diabetic conditions such as systemic lupus erythematosus. The mechanisms involved in the development of this earliest sign of microangiopathy are not known, and basement membrane thickening might result from: (*a*) overproduction, (*b*) impaired removal, (*c*) leakage and local accumulation of blood constituents, or (*d*) deposition of some substances or complexes on normal membrane. Similarly, the aetiology of BMT is unknown, and impaired phagocytic activity of the basement membrane cells, increased vascular permeability and immunological mechanisms have all been postulated as causing or contributing to the lesion. Beaumont and his colleagues (1971) and other workers have suggested that excessive secretion of growth hormone might be the cause of diabetic capillary disease, and these workers have suggested that growth hormone secretion might lead to an accumulation of sorbitol by inhibiting glucose metabolism, which in turn might be expected to cause osmotic imbalance resulting in damage to tissues (Beaumont *et al.*, 1971). The presence or absence of small vessel disease seems more closely related to the duration of the diabetes than to the degree of control, and may therefore be an almost inevitable and inherent part of the syndrome of diabetes mellitus rather than a true complication. Diabetics who are constantly very well controlled biochemically fare better in general than those who are very badly controlled, but this distinction is not absolute, and may in any case simply reflect the 'severity' of the syndrome.

Atheroma and microangiopathy may occur simultaneously in the same patient and in the same organ. Because of this overlap the complications of diabetes are discussed mainly on the basis of the organ or tissue involved, rather than being divided into specific and non-specific divisions which, although histologically distinct, may not easily be distinguished on clinical grounds. The complications are discussed under the following headings: Atherosclerosis, Renal, Chronic neuropathy, Ophthalmic, Dermatological, Chronic infections, The Feet in diabetes and Diabetic osteopathy.

ATHEROSCLEROSIS

This occurs earlier and more extensively in the diabetic than in the non-diabetic. The effects of atherosclerosis, such as peripheral vascular disease, myocardial infarction, and occlusive cerebrovascular disease are therefore more common. As mentioned above, atherosclerosis may also affect the small vessels of the kidney, the nerves, and the retinae. Cardiovascular disease has become an increasing cause of disability and death in diabetics since ketosis became a readily treatable condition. 'Diabetic' gangrene differs in no way from that in a non-diabetic, although the lesions are more liable to infection. If amputation is necessary, it is now accepted that attempts to save tissue of dubious viability in order to make the amputation as conservative as possible usually lead to poor healing, prolonged morbidity, and the prospect of repeated operations. The surgeon should aim to provide a healthy stump that heals rapidly and to which a suitable prosthesis may be fitted soon after operation.

RENAL

Proteinuria is present in about 4 per cent of patients with diabetes of less than one year's duration, increasing to a frequency of 16 per cent or more in patients who have been known to have the disease for more than 10 years (Miki *et al.*, 1972), and in a significant number is due to lesions such as pyelonephritis, nephrosclerosis or hypertension. There are, however, a number of glomerular lesions characteristic of diabetes, and it has been estimated that such changes are present at least 10 per cent of patients who have had diabetes for more than twenty years. Histological changes of diabetic glomerulosclerosis are observed in 40 per cent of all diabetics at autopsy. The lesions of diabetic glomerulosclerosis are four in number:

1. Dilatation and aneurysm formation in the glomerular capillaries
2. Diffuse glomerulosclerosis
3. The Kimmelstiel-Wilson (KW) nodular lesion
4. Exudative glomerulosclerosis.

1. *Dilatation and aneurysm formation* affecting the glomerular capillaries is an early change which usually precedes the development of the other lesions.

2. *Diffuse glomerulosclerosis* is non-specific. There is more or less uniform thickening of the basement membrane of the glomerular capillaries with deposition of polysaccharides and reticulin. The lesion is an early one.

3. *The Kimmelstiel-Wilson nodular lesion.* The nodules, which contain polysaccharide and sometimes lipid, appear to be specifically related to the diabetic state. They vary in size, are often multiple, and lie in close relationship to the walls of the capillaries in the glomerular tuft. Such lesions are present in half the patients who show diabetic glomerulosclerosis at autopsy. Diffuse glomerulosclerosis is always present in patients who show KW nodules on histology, and these appear to develop simply as an extension of the diffuse lesion.

4. *Exudative glomerulosclerosis*, like the diffuse lesion, is non-specific. Masses of homogeneous fibrinoid material composed of protein and lipid are present between the endothelial cell membrane and the basement membrane of the capillary. Similar changes are also seen in the capsular spaces, in the basement membrane of the capsule, and in the proximal convoluted tubule.

Histological renal changes may be present before any clinical or biochemical evidence of diabetes is apparent. The nodular, diffuse, and exudative lesions all lead ultimately to capillary obstruction and obliteration of the whole glomerulus.

Aetiology of the renal lesions is unknown. It is almost invariably associated with a degree of retinopathy and commonly neuropathy, suggesting a common pathogenesis.

The clinical course of the renal complications may be insidious, proteinuria appearing about ten years after the onset of the diabetes. At first, the protein loss is slight and intermittent, later it becomes massive, consisting mainly of albumin and causing a lowering of the serum albumin and oedema. Hypertension is a late feature. Progress may remain slow even with the onset of renal failure, when there is often some amelioration of the diabetes and a fall in insulin requirements. In established cases there is also an increase in α_2-globulin and cholesterol characteristic of any form of nephrotic syndrome, and birefringent lipid material may be seen in the urinary deposit. Neither renal function nor proteinuria are closely related to the histological changes observed on renal biopsy. Although all patients with heavy proteinuria have advanced renal changes, some patients with serious biopsy lesions have no proteinuria (Watkins *et al.*, 1972). Heavy proteinuria is an ominous finding and the worst prognosis is seen in those patients with marked biopsy changes when these are associated with heavy proteinuria (more than 3 g per 24 hours). When proteinuria is less the prognosis is variable, regardless of the histological changes, and renal function may remain unaltered for many years (Watkins *et al.*, 1972). The factors responsible for the onset of rapid deterioration of renal function are not known.

There is no specific therapy for diabetic glomerulosclerosis of the nodular, diffuse, or exudative type, although in all cases it is important to exclude associated lesions such as pyelonephritis which might respond to specific treatment. Although there is no specific treatment for diabetic glomerulosclerosis an improvement in diabetic control may slow its progression. The use of cyclophosphamide in the treatment of diabetic nephropathy is only just being evaluated. It appears that this therapy may be beneficial in some cases. The presence of advanced diabetic retinopathy, which is found in most cases, and the frequent association of coronary heart disease makes the value of chronic dialysis or renal transplantation in such patients of uncertain value.

CHRONIC NEUROPATHY

Vascular insufficiency, vitamin deficiency, and hyperglycaemia may all contribute to the aetiology of diabetic peripheral neuropathy. The complication is often present in patients with established glomerulosclerosis and retinopathy, and some authors have demonstrated what appears to be an undoubted microangiopathy of the type seen in the retinal and renal vessels affecting the vasa nervorum in such patients, although this finding has not been generally confirmed. Atherosclerotic changes are frequently seen in the vasa nervorum and the larger vessels, but there does not appear to be good correlation between vascular disease and neural change and although atherosclerosis or microangiopathy does seem to be the primary aetiological factor in some patients, vascular insufficiency is unlikely to be the sole factor responsible for diabetic neuropathy.

A conditioned deficiency of vitamins of the B group has been suggested as contributing to the development of the neuropathy, but while a few patients show a striking improvement when given aneurine or pantothenic acid, the overall response to vitamin B preparations is disappointing.

Marked improvement of the symptoms of diabetic neuropathy is often obtained when the diabetes is adequately controlled and blood sugar levels lowered but the reason for this is unknown. It must be remembered that peripheral neuropathy in a diabetic is not always due to diabetes, and other conditions such as neoplasm, vitamin B_{12} deficiency, and spinal cord lesions must always be excluded.

Histology of Nerves. The most consistent finding detected at post mortem in the peripheral nerves of patients with neuropathy is patchy demyelination, with no sign of any significant inflammatory response, involving a few fibres of a nerve. In severe and advanced cases there is also disruption of the axon cylinders.

Clinical Features. Chronic diabetic neuropathy is common, and may occur in patients of any age. As an isolated finding in the older mild diabetic it is often of atherosclerotic origin, and in these patients the symptoms are mainly confined to the lower limbs, consisting of painful paraesthesiae in the feet with loss of ankle jerks.

This syndrome apart, the clinical manifestations of diabetic neuropathy may take the form of symmetrical sensory or autonomic polyneuropathy or of isolated peripheral nerve lesions (mononeuropathy) or multiple isolated lesions (multiple mononeuropathy). There is a close association between the symmetrical sensory polyneuropathy and autonomic neuropathy: over 90 per cent of patients with autonomic neuropathy have been shown to have an associated symmetrical sensory or sensorimotor polyneuropathy (Osuntokun, 1971). It is evident that vascular lesions are important in the pathogenesis of isolated oculomotor nerve palsy, and possibly in many other cases of mononeuropathy. The clinical features of diabetic neuropathy may be summarised:

(*a*) *Sensory Nerve Involvement.* Paraesthesiae are usually the first complaint, to be followed by loss of tendon jerks in the legs and reduction in vibration sense. Loss of pain sensation tends to occur much later, and in association with autonomic involvement may eventually lead to trophic ulceration or neuropathic arthropathy.

(*b*) *Motor nerve involvement* usually occurs later and results in muscle weakness and wasting.

(*c*) *Autonomic nerve involvement* may lead to: Pupillary changes—presenting the picture of the Argyll-Robertson pupil.

Dependent oedema of lower limbs.
Reduced sweating.
Bladder disturbance, commonly incontinence.
Bowel disturbance, particularly nocturnal diarrhoea.
Impotence.
Instability of blood pressure (postural hypotension).
In association with sensory changes, autonomic neuropathy contributes to the development of trophic ulcers and neuropathic arthropathy.

Diabetic neuropathy may occur independently of the control, the severity or duration of diabetes, and may be the presenting clinical manifestation of the syndrome. The only consistent laboratory feature is a modest elevation of the CSF protein to between 60 and 100 mg per cent which is observed in about 80 per cent of patients with neurological involvement. Diabetic neuropathy is usually slowly progressive. Complete recovery is virtually unknown in established cases, but in earlier cases remissions are not uncommon, particularly if hyperglycaemia is corrected, preferably by insulin. Otherwise, treatment is merely supportive and symptomatic. Broad spectrum antibiotics are of value in the treatment of diabetic diarrhoea. Androgens are best avoided in the treatment of impotence, since they may only increase libido (which may not be impaired in any case) without improving potency.

OPHTHALMIC

A number of these complications may occur acutely, but since they are part of a chronic process, all are considered together in this section. They give rise to more distress than any other complication in the diabetic. Diabetes is at all ages the most important known systemic condition causing blindness. Diabetic retinopathy is responsible for 7 per cent of all new blind registrations in England and Wales, and for 20 per cent of new cases of blindness in middle-aged women.

The ophthalmic complications consist of disturbances in visual acuity, cataracts, iridopathy, and retinopathy.

Disturbances in Visual Acuity

These consist mainly of alterations in accommodation and refraction. In young diabetics, particularly those with widely fluctuating blood glucose levels, these changes are due to differences in osmotic pressure between the lens and the extra-cellular fluid, but in some cases there are also metabolic alterations in the ciliary bodies. All these changes tend to be corrected rapidly when the diabetic control is improved.

Cataracts

Cataracts specifically due to diabetes are rare, being found more often in the younger patient. They may occur rapidly and are usually bilateral, and have a snowflake appearance usually first observed in the subcapsular region of the lens. Spontaneous improvement is rare even with adequate control of the diabetes, and cataract extraction may be necessary. Senile cataracts occur more frequently and at an earlier age in diabetes, differing in no way from the senile cataract of the non-diabetic. Cataract extraction is usually required, but the prognosis for visual recovery depends on the degree of underlying retinopathy.

Iridopathy

In poorly treated younger diabetics, glycogen may be deposited in the pigment epithelium of the posterior surface of the iris leading to its depigmentation and causing the iris to have a 'moth-eaten' appearance. At a later stage, a meshwork of new blood vessels appears over the anterior surface of the iris involving the pupillary zone and the root of the iris (rubeosis iridis), giving eventually the appearance of a wreath of blood vessels encircling the pupil. Haemorrhagic glaucoma appears sooner or later. Little treatment is possible, and complete blindness invariably results.

Retinopathy

Hypertensive and atherosclerotic changes may be observed in the retinae of diabetic patients but the lesions associated with diabetes are quite distinctive.

The Lesions of Diabetic Retinopathy. 1. *Venous Changes*. Generalised dilatation and fullness of veins is an early change. Later, beading, tortuosity, varicosities, and sheathing may precede the appearance of microaneurysms. The venous changes are non-specific and have also been reported in Eale's disease and systemic lupus erythematosus.

2. *Arterial Changes*. In the juvenile diabetic the arteries are usually normal, but in the older patient hyalinisation and narrowing may be seen. These changes commonly reflect associated atherosclerosis and/or hypertension, but a characteristic endothelial proliferation has also been described.

3. *Microaneurysms* form the characteristic feature of diabetic retinopathy and they are the earliest specific change seen. They resemble pinpoint or punctate haemorrhages of variable size and are usually scattered throughout the posterior pole or in the macular region. Microaneurysms also occur after retinal vein occlusion, where they are grouped around the occluded vein, and in Eale's disease where they occur only in small numbers, and never in the posterior pole. Microaneurysms develop in the deepest layer of the retinal capillary plexus which resides in the outer molecular layer of the retina, on the venous side of the network. On ophthalmoscopy and colour photography only the larger microaneurysms, over about 20 μ in diameter, are visible. Fluorescence angiograms show up many more, since even the smaller ones can be seen. Capillary degeneration is the initial incident in diabetic retinopathy and may be part of the generalised microangiopathy which is so commonly present in diabetes. At first, the microaneurysms appear as capillary dilatations filled with blood, which may later thrombose or show reduplication of the basement membrane. Proliferation of endothelial cells may seen within the aneurysm. Hyalinisation, thrombosis or reduplication of the basement membrane may all lead to progressive obliteration of the lumen of the capillary. Dissecting microaneurysms may occur in which blood leaks and flows between the reduplicated layers of thickened basement membrane. The outstanding feature on electron microscopy is diffuse thickening of the basement membrane of the capillary which may precede the development of clinical diabetes.

4. *Haemorrhages* are characteristically deep in the retina, round and red, and, like the microaneurysms, are localised mainly in the posterior pole. In the early stages, it may be difficult to differentiate small haemorrhages from microaneurysms, but with progression of the retinopathy, haemorrhages increase in number and size and in the later stages superficial haemorrhages appear. They may resolve spontaneously, producing striking improvement in fundoscopic appearances. Late in the course of retinopathy, pre-retinal and sub-hyaloid haemorrhages may occur.

5. *Exudates* are typically hard, and white or yellowish. They usually develop later than microaneurysms.

6. *Cottonwool Spots* as a feature of diabetic retinopathy have only been recognised in the last 10 years, and are a feature of the retinopathy itself and not of associated hypertension (Kohner, 1972). They represent retinal infarcts, the result of arterial occlusion. The most important fact about these lesions is their prognostic significance. The presence of more than five in any one eye, in the absence of hypertension, indicates that the retinopathy has entered a more rapidly advancing stage and that proliferative retinopathy is likely to develop within the next 6 to 18 months (Kohner, 1972).

7. *Macular Disease* (maculopathy) is a major cause of blindness. The macula may be directly affected by hard exudates or by haemorrhage, but the main cause of visual loss is macular oedema, which can result from leakage from diseased local capillaries or may spread from oedema at a near-by focus of retinal hypoxia; rarely a group of new vessels can cause this condition. The ophthalmoscopic changes in patients with macular oedema may be slight, although

fluorescence angiography will commonly show abnormal or closed blood vessels, together with extensive leakage of dye from the diseased vessels.

8. *Vitreous Haemorrhages* from new vessels are usually sudden in onset and cause visual impairment of variable degree. Absorption is usually rapid, but may be delayed, and persisting haemorrhage is usually followed by fibrosis. Vitreous haemorrhages appear as a haze or simply as a red

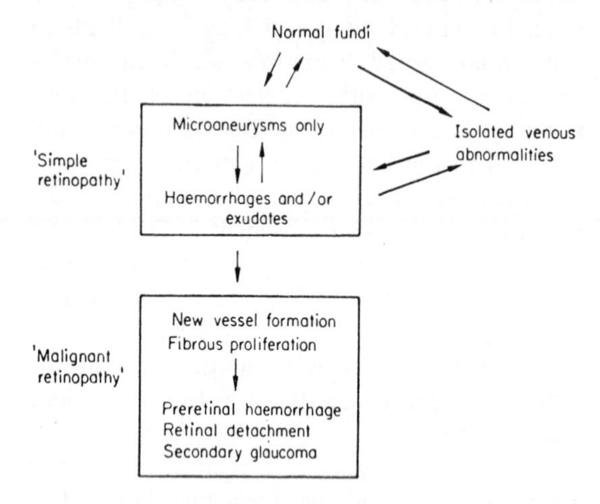

FIGURE 15.5 A classification of diabetic retinopathy (from Caird *et al.*, 1969. Reproduced by permission of the authors and publishers)

or black reflex on fundoscopy. As the haemorrhage absorbs vitreous 'floaters' may be formed.

9. *Proliferative Retinopathy*. Formation of new vessels is the most important of all retinal lesions, because their progression and complications frequently lead to blindness and since the appearance of new vessels immediately worsens the visual prognosis. New vessels may develop which lie flat on the disc or which extend forward into the vitreous; they may occur at any site on the retina and are of most sinister import when they arise on or adjacent to the optic disc or at the macula. Haemorrhage is frequent from new vessels and leads to fibrosis which may extend into the vitreous. As the tissue becomes organised and shrinks, retinal tearing and detachment may occur. Proliferative retinopathy may also be seen in Eale's disease and in the later states of venous thrombosis.

The Prevalence of Diabetic Retinopathy

Prior to the introduction of insulin, retinopathy seemed to appear only after the age of forty since juvenile diabetics did not survive long enough to develop it. However, it is now apparent that the lesions may develop in the great majority of subjects who have had diabetes for a sufficiently long time. After 15 years, about 50 per cent of diabetics show some evidence of retinopathy, and after 25 years more than 66 per cent have retinal changes. Vision is not affected in all cases; microaneurysms alone appear to have little effect on visual acuity. On the other hand, macular disease of all types may affect vision at an early stage, and once visual symptoms have developed the ultimate prognosis becomes much worse. The prognosis is also much poorer in those with new vessel proliferation. Diabetic retinopathy may precede the clinical onset of diabetes, and where retinopathy is present nephropathy and neuropathy are more likely to be found.

Classification and Progression of Retinopathy

Many of the earlier classifications of diabetic retinopathy were unsatisfactory since they were purely descriptive and not easily applied to individual cases, or since they implied a progression from stage to stage which did not always occur. A satisfactory classification which emphasises the dynamic aspects of retinopathy and which also indicates the features which mainly affect prognosis has been described by Burditt *et al.* (1968) and Caird *et al.* (1969). This classification is shown in Fig. 15.5. Patients are classified according to the changes present in the most severely affected eye. Those with preretinal haemorrhage, new vessel formation or fibrous proliferation are grouped together as having 'malignant retinopathy', while patients with only microaneurysms, retinal haemorrhage or exudates are grouped as having 'simple retinopathy'. The term 'simple' is preferred to benign since it does not necessarily imply a good prognosis. Patients with abnormalities of the retinal veins only are described as having 'isolated venous abnormalities'. The changes in the 'simple' group may regress to develop again later; those in the 'malignant' group are permanent and progressive leading ultimately to blindness. Another classification of retinopathy, which is basically descriptive, but which stresses the prognostic and therapeutic implications, has recently been described (Beaumont and Hollows, 1972).

The Natural History of Diabetic Retinopathy

This has been reviewed by Burditt *et al.* (1968) and by Kohner (1972). Retinal photography and, in particular, fluorescence angiography have made it possible to evaluate in a quantitative way the natural history of retinopathy. Prospective studies indicate that the rate of appearance of new lesions such as microaneurysms and cottonwool spots are more important than their disappearance. In particular the appearance of many cottonwool spots in the absence of hypertension indicates the early onset of new vessel proliferation. Patients with visual impairment when first seen are more prone to develop new vessel proliferation within the next five years than those whose vision is normal at initial assessment. In patients whose diabetes is diagnosed before the age of twenty who have proliferative retinopathy 11 per cent per year will show moderate visual deterioration and about 8 per cent will show gross deterioration. In patients without proliferative retinopathy the figures for rates of progression, are about one fourth of those for proliferative retinopathy. The five year prognosis for vision in patients without visual symptoms when first seen is good unless they develop new vessels arising from the optic disc.

The Pathogenesis of Diabetic Retinopathy

It is usually considered that retinopathy is only one manifestation of the generalised microangiopathy seen in diabetes, and it has been suggested—on slender evidence—that patients with with vascular lesion may have a constitutional or genetic tendency to small-vessel disease linked to the diabetic gene. It would seem more probable that some diffuse metabolic disturbance, not necessarily confined to carbohydrate metabolism, underlies this microangiopathy, which may precede the onset of overt diabetes. The chemical nature of the diabetic basement membrane is no different from normal, but it has been suggested that in microangiopathy there may be altered synthesis and turnover of the membrane constituents. It is also possible that immunological mechanisms may be involved in the production of basement membrane thickening. Whatever the mechanism, it appears that hypoxia is the factor responsible for most of the retinal lesions.

Treatment of Diabetic Retinopathy

Evaluation of therapy is difficult—the progression of retinopathy is variable, and stationary periods or remissions may occur. For proper evaluation of any form of treatment serial full-field retinal photographs, if possible using fluorescence angiography must be taken. The forms of therapy presently available and their efficacy as described in reliable studies include:

1. *Heparin Injections.* In a large trial described by Syllaba *et al.* (1967) intramuscular heparin 20–40,000 IU daily often appeared to produce visual improvement. In about 50 per cent of patients treated, new haemorrhages did not appear over a period of five years. These results have not always been reproduced by others.

2. *Clofibrate.* The compound Atromid-S has been shown to be beneficial in the treatment of exudative retinopathy. The results are sometimes striking, but after the first year or so of treatment lesions tend to recur. However, there is quite definite evidence that this drug may significantly improve both the number of exudates and the visual state in some patients, although even after exudates disappear many patients are left with areas of retinal ischaemia or degeneration which adversely affect vision.

3. *Photocoagulation.* In light coagulation a xenon arc light is focussed on the retina, and the light is converted into heat by the retinal and

choroidal pigment to produce a burn and later a scar. This technique can be used to occlude vascular lesions and new vessels, or a 'pattern-bombing' technique may be used to produce an iatrogenic choroidoretinitis—there is evidence that destruction of areas of retina in this way may lead to improved nutrition and oxygenation of the remainder of the retina. The results of the treatment of suitable cases of diabetic retinopathy by xenon arc photocoagulation are encouraging (Hill, 1972). A laser can also be used; this converts light into heat by contact with the pigment inside the eye. These two sources of photocoagulation are only effective in occluding those new blood vessels which lie in the plane of the retina; they are of no value when vessels have grown forward into the vitreous or are surrounded by extensive glial tissue. Nor can these methods be used when new vessels are on the disc or on its margin, at the macula or between the macula and the disc, since the resulting scars may produce marked visual loss. The argon laser is likely in such cases to prove an advance on earlier forms of light coagulation. The green argon light is absorbed by haemoglobin, and thus heat can be generated in the vessels themselves. This type of laser may provide considerable help in dealing with new blood vessels growing forward or those situated in the disc-macular region.

4. *Hypophysectomy and Yttrium Implantation.* Since a report that diabetic retinopathy in a young woman showed considerable amelioration after post-partum necrosis of the pituitary (Poulsen, 1953; 1966), various methods of pituitary ablation have been attempted and assessed. Reports of the efficacy of the procedures vary. There is general agreement that surgical hypophysectomy results in a reduction in insulin requirements and clearing of vitreous and retinal haemorrhages, although the operative mortality and subsequent morbidity is high.

In an attempt to reduce these complications, Fraser, Oakley, Joplin, and their associates (1967) pioneered the use of yttrium-90 pituitary implantation by the trans-nasal route. After assessment of 45 eyes in 30 patients by retinal photography 6 months to 5 years after treatment with yttrium implantation, they concluded:

(*a*) Microaneurysms, venous abnormalities, new vessels, and haemorrhages are reversible components.

(*b*) Hard exudates and retinitis proliferans are irreversible and commonly show progression.

The greater the degree of pituitary ablation, as shown by pituitary function tests, the greater the amount of improvement that occurred. These workers consider that the indication for implantation is the presence of reversible lesions of moderate extent in an eye that still has reasonable visual acuity and whose vision is not immediately threatened by irreversible lesions. Impairment of renal function is a contraindication, as is postural hypotension. There is of course greatly increased insulin sensitivity after pituitary ablation, and hypoglycaemia may be a serious and dangerous problem. Complete hormonal replacement therapy must be given and all the hazards of panhypopituitarism are present. Impotence is a troublesome sequel in the male, and postural hypotension may be incapacitating unless patients are carefully screened before the procedure is carried out. At present, it is probably best that the technique should be limited to those centres where both experience and facilities are available until the long-term benefits of the therapy can be assessed.

DERMATOLOGICAL

Dermatological lesions are common in the diabetic:

1. *Pyogenic Infections.* Furunculosis and recurrent staphylococcal boils are a common presenting feature of diabetes and tend to recur when the disease is poorly controlled. Extensive infection of this type increases insulin requirements and results in impairment of diabetic control.

2. *Candidiasis* is common in the maturity onset diabetic, particularly the female, either as a generalised infection or affecting the vulva and

perineum, or areas of intertrigo. Candidal balanitis is not uncommon in uncircumcised diabetic men. Specific anti-candidal therapy is indicated, but unless the diabetes is controlled there is a tendency to relapse.

3. *Pseudoxanthoma nigricans* occurs particularly in the obese diabetic. The lesions are dusky, pigmented and hyperkeratotic being most frequently seen in the axillae, groins and the skin folds around the neck. Although they are histologically identical with true acanthosis nigricans they do not indicate the presence of an occult neoplasm, and are benign. Improvement often occurs after weight loss.

4. *Diabetic dermopathy*. The lesion has also been named 'spotted leg' or 'pigmented pretibial patches'. In a survey of 300 diabetics carried out in New York, 14 per cent were affected (Alpert and Belson, 1967). The lesions are usually distributed over the anterior tibial region and vary in shape and size from small pigmented macules to oval pigmented scars. Histologically there is basilar hypermelanosis, slight proliferation of small blood vessels, and minimal non-specific inflammatory change. PAS staining of the tissues is within normal limits. Neuropathy is commonly associated, as are retinopathy and nephropathy though large vessel disease is rare. The majority of patients are insulin-dependent, and the lesion is specific for diabetes. It is probably precipitated by trauma in association with neuropathy and is unlikely to be microangiopathic in origin.

5. *Xanthoma diabeticorum* may occur as scattered papules or nodules in the skin of diabetics who have pronounced hyperlipaemia. The lesions, which are not specific for diabetes, consist of clusters of histiocytes loaded with lipids. They improve with treatment of the diabetes as the lipaemia returns towards normal.

6. *Necrobiosis lipoidica* is not confined to diabetics and is of unknown aetiology. The lesions are asymptomatic and occur chiefly on the legs. Beginning as small papules, they gradually increase in size to become large plaques appearing somewhat like localised scleroderma; ulceration is not uncommon. The histological appearance of the lesions is variable—some contain large amounts of lipid, others contain none. Microangiopathic changes are inconsistent, but glycogen deposition is usual and is found in the histiocytes in the lesion and in the surrounding tissue spaces. Elastic tissue is well preserved and foam cells may be found. The lesions are more common in females and below the age of forty, and may precede the onset of clinical diabetes. They tend to disappear with localised injections of hydrocortisone, but may recur. Fibrosis and involution may occur after many years.

7. *Granuloma annulare*. There is an increased incidence of diabetes in association with this unusual skin disorder.

CHRONIC INFECTIONS

Tuberculosis and chronic urinary infections are more frequent in the diabetic. Weight loss, despite satisfactory diet and diabetic control, demands urgent investigation, and routine yearly chest X-rays should be carried out in all diabetics.

THE FEET IN DIABETES AND DIABETIC OSTEOPATHY

Lesions on the feet are common, distressing to the patient, and if unattended may lead ultimately to the need for amputation. Infections between the toes, paronychia, and chronic ulcers are frequent, may lead to extensive cellulitis or gangrene, and are the result of trauma, poorly fitting shoes, or careless chiropody practised by the patient, in association with poor hygiene of the feet, poor blood supply, and neuropathy. A skilled chiropodist may save many limbs and significantly reduce the demand for hospital beds. All diabetic patients, particularly the elderly, should be educated in the proper care of the feet. The feet should be washed frequently, and after washing, the feet and toes should be patted dry and not rubbed vigorously. Talcum powder may be used on the feet after bathing. Trauma should obviously be avoided. Despite these precautions, ulcers of the feet and superficial infections are common, and the patient must be warned to seek professional advice as soon as possible.

Pogonowska and co-workers (1967) pointed out that radiographically detectable abnormalities are common in the feet of diabetics, having found abnormalities in 33 per cent of 242 random diabetic patients. The most common lesion, apart from arterial calcification, is 'osteopathy' consisting of diffuse or localised osteoporosis and, in more advanced cases, juxta-articular bone defects in the phalanges and metatarsals. At a later stage, osteolysis of the bone ends and apparent destruction of entire bones may occur. The lesions may occur in the distal or proximal part of the foot. In the former, it is presumed that the changes are due to a combination of neuropathy, chronic trauma, infection, and arterial insufficiency, whereas in the latter the osteopathy is usually neurogenic in origin.

PREGNANCY AND DIABETES

Glycosuria is found in the great majority of non-diabetic women at some time during pregnancy when sensitive and specific methods are used to detect glucose in the urine. In the majority of such patients glycosuria is due to a lowered renal threshold for glucose, but a small percentage have true gestational diabetes (latent diabetes) which usually disappears after delivery. In urine samples collected after meals from apparently normal women a single finding of glycosuria can be ignored in the absence of a family history of diabetes or of a history of previous abnormal glucose tolerance tests, stillbirths or large babies, but two or more tests showing glycosuria in excess of 'trace' on 'Clinitest' call for further investigation, even when there are no other pointers to the diagnosis of diabetes (Soler and Malins, 1971).

The maternal mortality rate is only slightly increased in diabetics, though fetal mortality rate remains high—in the region of 10 to 15 per cent. The value of continuous antenatal supervision of pregnancy complicated by diabetes by a single specialised team is generally accepted, and to ensure accurate control must start as early as possible. Throughout the greater part of pregnancy control is achieved by weekly or fortnightly visits to adjust insulin dosage and dietary needs (the diet may need to be supplemented to allow for carbohydrate lost in the urine), and even closer supervision is necessary after about the thirtieth week of pregnancy. It is recommended that all patients should be treated with soluble insulin twice daily, with or without isophane, and the use of soluble insulin is mandatory after the 30th to 32nd weeks. During pregnancy, the incidence of miscarriage, pre-eclampsia, polyhydramnios and accidental haemorrhage is increased. The birth weight of the child is increased and there is a higher incidence of congenital malformations. The major causes of stillbirth or neonatal death may be classified under the following headings:

Medical (in the mother): poor diabetic control.
Obstetric: pre-eclampsia, placental insufficiency, birth trauma and intrauterine infection.
Paediatric: respiratory distress syndrome, congenital defects.

The last group contributes most to the mortality. About one-quarter of all fetal deaths occur as stillbirths for which no obvious cause other than the presence of diabetes in the mother can be ascertained.

The Management of the Diabetic Pregnancy. Fetal mortality can be greatly improved if the management outlined below is followed.

1. Careful control of diabetes during pregnancy. There is no predictable pattern in the changes of insulin requirements during pregnancy—about 25 per cent of women can continue on an unaltered dose of insulin. The most common sequence is for insulin requirements to fall

slightly or remain unaltered during the first trimester, to be followed by a slight rise during the second trimester, which is accelerated during the third trimester. After delivery, requirements fall rapidly to normal. Because of the lowered renal threshold for glucose little reliance can be placed on urine tests during pregnancy and treatment must be based on the results of frequent blood sugars. Random blood sugars should not exceed 160 mg/100 ml, and at the first sign of anything more than mild and transient instability hospital admission must be arranged. Accurate control of the blood glucose during pregnancy results in a smaller baby, and may reduce the chances of polyhydramnios.

2. Excessive weight gain should be avoided; there is evidence that this reduces the incidence of pre-eclampsia.

3. Choice of time for delivery. It is now agreed that premature delivery is necessary and greatly improves fetal mortality, the optimum time being between the 37th and 38th week—earlier, the neonatal death-rate is high, and later, the stillbirth rate increases. Special reasons such as renal or cardiovascular disease, polyhydramnios or severe antepartum haemorrhage may modify this policy.

4. Mode of delivery. The patient should be admitted to hospital a few weeks before the intended delivery so that the diabetes may be more closely controlled and adequate time allowed to plan the delivery. The choice of the mode of delivery is less important than selection of the time, and the choice between Caesarean section and induction of labour will take into account obstetric factors, the personality of the patient, and the severity of the diabetes. To take extremes, a multiparous patient in her mid-thirties with mild or moderate diabetes will almost invariably undergo induction; a young primiparous diabetic will commonly have a Caesarean section. There is little difference in the results obtained between these two methods. Caesarean section has the advantage that it can be planned and timed more precisely, and also makes easier the management of the diabetes, which may be complicated by a prolonged vaginal delivery. Caesarean section should be performed if the infant is large-for-dates, if there is any indication that induction of labour will not proceed smoothly and rapidly, or if a delivery earlier than 37 weeks is planned, and many obstetricians would recommend that all primipara should be delivered by Caesarean section. The management of the patient's diabetes in the pre-operative, operative, and post-operative phases is outlined in the section dealing with planned operations in diabetics.

5. The child should be treated as a premature infant, and features of hypoglycaemia (the 'jittery baby') should be watched for.

DIABETES AND SURGERY

The following regimens are recommended for the care of the diabetic patient undergoing operation:

PLANNED OPERATIONS

In every case the patient should be admitted to hospital for observation and stabilisation a few days before the date of the operation.

(i) *Patients on diet alone.* The blood glucose levels should be checked frequently before and after operation, and soluble insulin may sometimes be required if control is unsatisfactory.

(ii) *Patients on oral drugs.* In all except minor operations, it is best to change to soluble insulin pre-operatively, returning to oral drugs when post-operative progress is satisfactory.

(iii) *Patients on insulin* should be controlled on soluble insulin in the pre-operative and post-operative phases. Ideally, the operation should take place shortly after the morning dose of insulin. A dextrose or dextrose-saline intravenous drip should be erected shortly before the insulin injection is given, and regulated (supplemented by intravenous boluses of 25 per cent or 50 per cent glucose injected slowly into the drip tubing as required) to provide the required daily amount of carbohydrate until an adequate oral intake can be re-established. It is not usually necessary to increase the insulin dosage on the day of operation, although an increase is usually required on the first three or four post-operative days.

EMERGENCY OPERATIONS

These will usually cause difficulties only in the insulin requiring diabetic or in the patient on oral agents who is poorly controlled. The degree of control will be checked on admission by estimation of blood glucose and routine electrolytes. The precise management thereafter depends on the nature of the operation and the surgeon's assessment of its urgency. Sometimes the regimen described for planned operations can be followed, at other times when the diabetic control has been upset it may be necessary to delay surgery for a few hours while ketosis, hyperglycaemia and dehydration are corrected. In these patients a graduated scale of insulin and intravenous glucose along the lines indicated in an earlier section should be started after initial measures have been undertaken and continued into the post-operative phase.

It is vital to remember that severe abdominal pain and vomiting are occasionally the outstanding initial features of diabetic ketosis, and these may mimic an acute intra-abdominal emergency. The response to preliminary treatment for ketosis will usually clarify the diagnosis.

LIPOATROPHIC DIABETES

This very rare syndrome is characterised by diabetes that tends to be insulin-resistant but which does not lead to ketosis, generalised atrophy of adipose tissue, severe hyperlipaemia with subcutaneous xanthomatosis, and hepatosplenomegaly. The basal metabolic rate is elevated, but this is not due to thyroid overactivity. At a later stage cirrhosis of the liver develops. The lipoatrophy usually precedes the diabetes, but the two may develop simultaneously. The cause of the syndrome is unknown. It has been suggested that the body may be unable to store excess calories as fat, and thus hyperglycaemia develops, although convincing experimental support for this hypothesis is lacking. Louis and his colleagues (1963; 1969) have isolated a diabetogenic polypeptide from the urine of patients with lipoatrophic diabetes, and have shown that this compound provokes insulin resistance and temporary impairment of glucose tolerance when given to dogs and to humans. Its physicochemical properties closely resemble those of a diabetogenic polypeptide isolated from the pituitary gland of some animals (Louis and Conn, 1968), and Louis and his co-workers have postulated that in lipoatrophic diabetes the polypeptide may act as a lipoprotein insulin antagonist, blocking glucose metabolism in adipose tissue but not in other tissues.

Not all patients with partial or total lipodystrophy show frank carbohydrate intolerance, although high fasting insulin levels, an abnormally elevated insulin response to glucose, insulin resistance and a failure of growth hormone levels to suppress after oral glucose seem to be constant features. It has been suggested that in lipodystrophy the primary lesion may be a widespread abnormality of β-adrenergic receptors in which their sensitivity is increased in affected areas and their specificity reduced (Boucher *et al.*, 1973).

Treatment of lipoatrophic diabetes consists of insulin and diet.

REFERENCES

Adnitt, P. I., and Taylor, E. (1970). *Lancet*, **i**, 652.

Alberti, K. G. M. M., Darley, J. H., Emerson, P. M., and Hockaday, T. D. R. (1972). *Lancet*, **ii**, 391.

Alberti, K. G. M. M., Hockaday, T. D. R., and Turner, R. C. (1973). *Lancet*, **ii**, 515.

Alpert, S., and Belson, M. A. (1967). In *Sixth Congress of the International Diabetes Federation.* London: Excerpta Medica Foundation, p. 2.

Antoniades, H. N. (1961). *Endocrinology*, **68**, 7.

Antoniades, H. N., Huber, A. M., Boshell, B. R., Saravis, C. A., and Gershoff, S. N. (1965). *Endocrinology*, **76**, 709.

Baird, J. D., Hunter, W. M., and Smith, A. W. M. (1973). *Postgrad. Med. J.*, **49**, 132.

Bajaj, J. S., and Vallance-Owen, J. (1971). *Lancet*, **i**, 16.

Banting, F. G., and Best, C. H. (1922). *J. lab. clin. Med.*, **7**, 251.

Beaumont, P., and Hollows, F. C. (1972). *Lancet*, **i**, 419.

Beaumont, P., Hollows, F. C., Schofield, P. J., Williams, J. F., and Steinbeck, A. W. (1971). *Lancet*, **i**, 579.

Bell, E. T. (1957. *Amer. J. Clin. Path.*, **33**, 499.

Billewicz, W. Z., Anderson, J., and Lind, T. (1973). *Brit. Med. J.*, **1**, 573.

Bloodworth, J. M. B. (1970). In *Advances in Metabolic Disorders*, Suppl. I: *Early Diabetes* (Ed. Camerini-Davalos, R. E., and Cole, H. S. New York: Academic Press, p. 260.

Bloom, A. (1972). *J. Roy. Coll. Phycns.* (Lond.), 7, 61.

Boucher, B. J., Cohen, R. D., Frankel, R. J., Stuart Mason, A., and Broadley, G. (1973). *Clin. Endoc.*, **2**, 111.

Boyle, D., Bhatia, S. K., Hadden, D. R., Montgomery, D. A. D., and Weaver, J. A. (1972). *Lancet*, **i**, 338.

Buchanan, K. D., and McCarroll, A. M. (1972). *Lancet*, **ii**, 1394.

Burditt, A. F., Caird, F. I., and Draper, G. J. (1968). *Quart. J. Med. N.S.*, **37**, 303.

Butterfield, W. J. H. (1964). *Proc. roy. Soc. Med.*, **57**, 196.

Caird, F. I., Pirie, A., and Ramsell, T. G. (1969). In *Diabetes and the Eye.* Oxford and Edinburgh: Blackwell Scientific Publications, p. 19.

Camerini-Davalos, R. A. (1964). In *Diabetes Mellitus: Diagnosis and Treatment* (Ed. T. S. Danowski). New York: American Diabetes Association Inc., p. 195.

Cerasi, E., Efendić, S., and Luft, R. (1973). *Lancet*, **i**, 794.

Cerasi, E., and Luft, R. (1967). *Acta endocr. Copenh.* **55**, 330

Chlouverakis, C., Jarrett, R. J., and Keen, H. (1967). *Lancet*, **i**, 806.

Clements, R. S., Jr., Blumenthal, S. A., Morrison, A.D., and Winegrad, A. I. (1971). *Lancet*, **ii**, 671.

Colwell, J. A. (1966). *Diabetes*, **15**, 497.

Conn, J. W. (1958). *Diabetes*, **7**, 347.

Cremer, G. M., Molnar, G. D., Taylor, W. F., Moxness, K. E., Service, F. J., Gatewood, L. C., Ackerman, E., and Rosevear, J. W. (1971). *Metabolism*, **20**, 1083.

Danowski, T. S., Fisher, E. R., Khurana, R. C., Nolan, S. and Stephen, T. (1972). *Metabolism*, **21**, 1125.

Davidson, M. B., and Poffenbarger, P. L. (1970). *Metabolism*, **19**, 668.

Diabetic Survey—Report of a Working Party (1962). *Brit. med. J.*, **i**, 1497.

Dixon, K., Exon, P. D., and Hughes, H. R. (1972). *Lancet*, **i**, 343.

Dollery, C. T., and Oakley, N. W. (1965). *Diabetes*, **14**, 121.

Downie, E., and Martin, F. I. R. (1959). *Diabetes*, **8**, 383.

Editorial (1971*a*). *Lancet*, **i**, 381.

Editorial (1971*b*). *Lancet*, **ii**, 804.

Editorial (1971*c*). *Lancet*, **ii**, 694.

Editorial (1972*a*). *Lancet*, **ii**, 637.

Editorial (1972*b*). *Lancet*, **ii**, 1071.

Editorial (1972*c*). *Lancet*, **ii**, 583.

Fajans, S. S. (1963). *J. Amer. med. Assn.*, **186**, 199.

Fajans, S. S., and Conn, J. W. (1954). *Diabetes*, **3**, 296.

Fitzgerald, M. G., and Keen, H. (1964). *Lancet*, **i**, 1325.

Forrest, J. M., Menser, M. A., and Burgess, J. A. (1971). *Lancet*, **ii**, 332.

Gamble, D. R., Kinsley, M. L., Fitzgerald, M. G., Bolton, R., and Taylor, K. W. (1969). *Brit. med. J.*, **3**, 627.

Gamble, D. R., and Taylor, K. W. (1969). *Brit. med. J.*, **3**, 631.

Garland, H. (1955). *Brit. med. J.*, **ii**, 1287.

Hadden, D. R., Montgomery, D. A. D., and Weaver, J. A. (1972). *Lancet*, **i**, 335.

Hales, C. N., Greenwood, F. C., Mitchell, F. L., and Strauss, W. T. (1968). *Diabetologia*, **4**, 73.

Hill, D. W. (1972). In *Clinics in Endocrinology and Metabolism*, **1:3** (Eds D. A. Pyke, W. B. Saunders, London), p. 789.

Hockaday, T. D. R., and Alberti, K. C. M. M. (1972). In *Clinics in Endocrinology and Metabolism*, **1:3** (Eds D. A. Pyke, W. B. Saunders). London, p. 751.

Jackson, W. P. U., van Mieghem, W., and Keller, P. (1972). *Lancet*, **i**, 1040.

Jenkins, D. J. A. (1967). *Lancet*, **ii**, 341.

Johansen, K. (1972). *Metabolism*, **21**, 1177.

Johansen, K., and Ørnsholt, J. (1972). *Metabolism*, **21**, 291.

Joplin, G. F., Fraser, R., and Keeley, K. J. (1961). *Lancet*, **ii**, 67.

Joplin, G. F., Oakley, N. W., Hill, D. W., Kohner, E. M., and Fraser, T. R. (1967). *Diabetologia*, **3**, 402.

Keen, H., and Jarrett. R. H. (1970). In *Proceedings of the Second Symposium on Atherosclerosis* (Ed. R. J. Jones). New York: Springer-Verlag, p. 435.

Khurana, R. C., Robin, J. A., Jung, Y., Corredor, D. G., Gonzalez, A., Sunder, J. H., and Danowski, T. S. (1971). *Horm. Metab. Res.*, **3**, 71.

Kipnis, D. M. (1968). *Ann. Intern. Med.*, **69**, 891.

Kohner, E. M. (1972). *J. Roy. Coll. Phycns.* (Lond.), **6**, 259.

Lawrence, R. D., and Oakley, W. (1944). *Brit. med. J.*, **i**, 422.

Lind, T., Van C. de Groot, H. A., Brown, G., and Cheyne, G. A. (1972). *Brit. med. J.*, **3**, 320.

Louis, L. H. (1969). *Metabolism*, **18**, 545.

Louis, L. H., Conn, J. W. and Minick, M. C. (1963). *Metabolism*, **12**, 867.

Louis, L. H., and Conn, J. W. (1968). *Metabolism*, **17**, 475.

Malins, J. M. (1971). *J. Roy. Coll. Phycns* (Lond.), **6**, 75.

Marks, V. (1971). *Ann. Clin. Biochem.*, **8**, 49.

Meade, R. C., Brush, J. S., and Klitgaard, H. M. (1968). *Diabetes*, **17**, 369.

Megyesi, C., Samols, E., and Marks, V. (1967). *Lancet*, **ii**, 1051.

Oakley, N., Hill, D. A., Joplin, G. F., Kohner, E. H., and Fraser, T. R. (1967). *Diabetologia*, **3**, 406.

Oakley, W., Hill, D. W., and Oakley, N. (1966). *Diabetes*, **15**, 1966.

Osuntokun, B. O. (1971). *The Neurology of Diabetes Mellitus in Nigerians*, M.D. Thesis, University of London.

Paasikivi, J. (1970). *Acta med. Scand.*, Suppl. 507.

Pogonowska, M. J., Collins, L. C., and Dobson, H. L. (1967). *Radiology*, **89**, 265.

Poulsen, J. E. (1953). *Diabetes*, **2**, 7.

Poulsen, J. E. (1966). *Diabetes*, **15**, 73.

Randle, P. J., Garland, P. B., Hales, C. N., and Newsholme, E. A. (1963). *Lancet*, **i**, 785.

Rubenstein, A., Cho, S., and Steiner, D. F. (1968). *Lancet*, **i**, 1353.

Seltzer, H. S., Allen, W. E., Herron, A. L., and Brennan, M. T. (1967). *J. clin. Invest.*, **46**, 323.

Soler, N. G., and Malins, J. M. (1971). *Lancet*, **ii**, 724.

Sönksen, P. H., Srivastava, M. C., Tompkins, Ch. V., and Nabarro, J. D. N. (1972). *Lancet*, **ii**, 155.

Stowers, J. M. (1970). In *Early Diabetes* (Ed. F. Hoffman). Excerpta Medica, New York, p. 54.

Stowers, J. D. (1972). *J. Roy. Coll. Phycns.* (Lond.), **7**, 69.

Syllaba, J., Lochar, M., and Kolín, V. (1967). In *Sixth Congress of the International Diabetes Federation*. London: Excerpta Medica Foundation, p. 21.

Tattersall, R. B., and Pyke, D. A. (1972). *Lancet*, **ii**, 1120.

Tomkins, A. M., and Bloom, A. (1972). *Brit. med. J.*, **1**, 649.

Tunbridge, R., and Wetherill, J. H. (1970). *Brit. med., J.*, **2**, 78.

Ungar, G., Freedman, L., and Shapiro, S. L. (1957). *Proc. Soc. exp. Biol.* (N.Y.), **95**, 190.

University Group Diabetes Program (1970). *Diabetes*, **19**, Suppl. 2, 747.

Vallance-Owen, J. (1966). In *Diabetes Mellitus* (Ed. L. J. P. Duncan). University of Edinburgh Pfizer Medical Monographs I, p. 21.

Wall, J. R., Pyke, D. A., and Oakley, W. G. (1973). *Brit. med. J.*, **1**, 577.

Warren, S., LeCompte, P. M., and Legg, M. A. (1966). In *The Pathology of Diabetes Mellitus*, 4th Edition. London: Henry Kimpton, p. 85.

Watkins, J. D., Roberts, D. E., Williams, T., Martin, D. A., and Coyle, V. (1967). *Diabetes*, **16**, 882.

Watkins, B. M., and Calder, J. S. (1971) *Diabetics*, **20**, 628.

Wieland, O. (1965). In *On the Nature and Treatment of Diabetes* (Eds B. S. Liebl, and G. A. Wrenshall). Amsterdam; Excerpta Medica.

Yalow, R. S., and Berson, S. A. (1961). *Diabetes*, **10**, 339.

Yalow, R. S., Glick, S. M., Roth, J., and Berson, S. A. (1965). *Ann. N. Y. Acad. Sci.*, **131**, 357.

16

HYPOGLYCAEMIA

The normal fasting level of blood glucose ranges from 50 to 90 mg/100 ml (Marks, 1959), when the specific glucose oxidase method is used to perform the estimation. However, slightly lower or higher figures may be obtained without any symptoms or without clinical evidence of disease, and in this country a venous blood glucose level of 40 mg per cent has been taken as being the absolute lower limit of normal (Griffiths, 1961). Levels lower than 40 mg per cent can be termed hypoglycaemia.

SYMPTOMS AND SIGNS

The symptoms and signs produced by hypoglycaemia fall into two groups:

1. Those due to adrenaline release.
2. Those due to neuroglycopoenia (Marks *et al.*, 1961).

These manifestations may occur at different blood glucose levels in different individuals. In some, particularly in diabetics, they may occur with concentrations above 40 mg/100 ml, while in others the level may fall lower than this before symptoms become evident.

Adrenaline Release

These are early symptoms and are most frequently seen when the fall in blood glucose occurs rapidly. They usually precede the symptoms due to neuroglycopoenia, and consist of *nervousness*, *weakness*, *hunger*, *sweating*, *pallor*, *apprehension*, *circumoral numbness*, and *tachycardia*. Headache is a common symptom and may be severe. The blood pressure may be slightly elevated. The same pattern of symptoms tends to recur in an individual patient. Sometimes the adrenaline response is sufficient to raise blood glucose levels by mobilising liver glycogen and, thus, neuroglycopoenic symptoms may be aborted.

Neuroglycopoenia

All tissues except the brain and kidney have readily available stores of glycogen which can support them during an episode of hypoglycaemia. Pyruvate, lactate, ketone bodies, and free fatty acids may also serve as metabolic substrates in muscle, liver, and fat. Few, if any, substances can replace glucose in maintaining cerebral function, although the brain can metabolise administered glutamate. This substance will increase the level of consciousness when given to a hypoglycaemic patient, but is much less effective than glucose in this situation. The symptoms and signs due to neuroglycopoenia fall into two clinical groups.

(*a*) *Psychiatric.* The highest centres in the brain suffer first and there is some overlap between the type of symptoms due to impaired nutrition of these centres, and those due to adrenaline release.

Thus, restlessness and mental instability may be present, as well as irritability, obstinacy, and agitation. Additional psychiatric symptoms that may occur include mental confusion, negativism, psychopathic behaviour, voluble and incoherent speech, retrograde amnesia, or delirium.

(*b*) *Neurological manifestations*. There may be diplopia, headache, and aphasia or dysphasia. Tremors may develop and the gait may become unsteady. As the condition progresses, unconsciousness may suddenly supervene, and convulsions are not uncommon. When first seen the patient may be deeply unconscious, with stertorous breathing, and he often has the appearance of one who has had a massive intracerebral haemorrhage. The physical signs are protean: there may be hyper-reflexia, signs of hemiplegia, monoplegia or paraplegia, but extensor plantar responses are invariable in the more severe cases. It is important to remember that one attack of severe neuroglycopoenia can lead to irreversible coma or a decerebrate state, even when treatment is instituted without apparent delay. The condition, therefore, should always be treated with great urgency.

PATHOLOGY

Deep coma may lead to death or permanent brain damage. The effects of hypoglycaemia on the brain are more severe in the elderly and atherosclerotic. Permanent myocardial damage may also occur following the mobilisation of glycogen from cardiac muscle, particularly if ischaemic heart disease is already present. Changes similar to those of hypokalaemia are reported to occur in the electrocardiogram, but they are not sufficiently frequent to be useful in diagnosis. Even after reversible hypoglycaemia of short duration, focal neurological signs may persist for some hours or days. There is definite evidence that recurrent episodes of hypoglycaemia, although promptly treated, can lead to mental and neurological deterioration, and to a reduction in the cortical cell population. Histologically, in patients dying as a result of neuroglycopoenia, there is widespread degeneration and necrosis of cerebral cortical cells, the appearance resembling that seen in anoxia.

CAUSES

Hypoglycaemia indicates that the body has been unable adequately to initiate or sustain the normal compensatory mechanisms brought into play when the blood glucose level falls. Normal subjects free from hepatic or endocrine disease may fast for at least forty-eight hours and then engage in violent exercise without becoming hypoglycaemic. Obese patients may be fasted for considerably longer periods without the blood sugar falling to hypoglycaemic levels, and in these cases glycogen breakdown and gluconeogenesis are sufficient to maintain the blood glucose level in the low normal range.

The main causes of hypoglycaemia are classified below:

1. *Iatrogenic:* insulin administration, sulphonylurea drugs.
2. *Factitious*
3. *Toxic:* Ackee poisoning, amanita phalloides, salicylates, antihistamines, mono-amine oxidase inhibitors.
4. *Spontaneous hypoglycaemia:*
   Fasting

   (*a*) *Islet cell hyperfunction*—benign or malignant neoplasms, islet cell adenomatosis, islet cell hyperplasia (as in infants of diabetic and prediabetic mothers)
   (*b*) *Idiopathic hypoglycaemia of childhood*
   (*c*) *Leucine and fructose* sensitivity
   (*d*) *Galactosaemia*
   (*e*) *Liver disease*—hepatocellular, hepatoma, chronic congestion
   (*f*) *Endocrine disease*—hypopituitarism, Addison's disease, adrenogenital syndrome
   (*g*) *Glycogen storage diseases*
   (*h*) *Non-pancreatic neoplasms*—typically retroperitoneal sarcoma, also rarely observed with bronchogenic and other carcinomas.

Reactive

(*a*) *to glucose*

(i) 'functional'

(ii) post-gastrectomy and post-gastro-enterostomy

(iii) in the prediabetic

(*b*) *to other substances*

(i) leucine, fructose, galactose sensitivity

(ii) alcohol (due to inhibition of gluco-neogenesis)

(iii) tobacco

5. *Due to excessive loss or utilisation of glucose with relative failure of compensatory mechanisms* (all very rare)

(*a*) Starvation

(*b*) Prolonged exercise

(*c*) Pregnancy and lactation

(*d*) Renal glycosuria.

It is not necessary to discuss all these causes at length. Many are exceedingly rare, and others should present no problem in diagnosis or management. Some will be discussed further in the section on hypoglycaemia in childhood below. It is, however, important to note that combinations of causes may be present in an individual case, e.g. alcohol and hepatocellular damage in a cirrhotic. *Factitious hypoglycaemia* must always be born in mind, particularly in those who may have easy access to insulin.

Islet cell tumours are probably the most important cause of spontaneous hypoglycaemia; there are now about 1,300 cases in the world literature (Laurent, Delry and Floquet, 1971). The clinical presentations are protean. The diagnosis may be delayed for years and may be made only after the patient has seen a succession of physicians and has had many diagnostic tests performed. The majority of cases present first either to the neurologist or the psychiatrist. The condition must be considered in all patients with unexplained psychiatric or neurological disease, particularly those with bizarre psychiatric symptoms, with intermittent or focal neurological signs and symptoms or with epileptic fits. A carefully taken history will usually establish the relationship of the symptoms to fasting or exertion, and the patient may himself have noticed relief after ingestion of glucose or other carbohydrate. However, it is important to remember that in the early stages hypoglycaemia may be reactive, and typically occurs at midday or during the early afternoon, although prolonged fasting will always produce hypoglycaemia in such patients. Difficulty in waking in the morning is a common later symptom, and features of hypoglycaemia may be present at this time. Hunger is not common, and weight gain is not so frequent as might be expected. Marks and Rose (1965) found that hunger was a symptom in only 14 per cent of cases and weight loss was almost as common as weight gain, although the majority of patients showed no weight change. Weight gain tends to occur only in those patients who notice that sugar or food will relieve their symptoms. Sweating is less prominent than with other causes of hypoglycaemia, perhaps because there are no sharp and sudden falls in blood sugar. Twenty to 25 per cent of patients with the condition have a family history of diabetes. In the large series described by Howard *et al.* (1950) 10 per cent of tumours were malignant, 10 per cent doubtful, and the remainder benign. It is often difficult to be certain whether malignancy is present from the histological picture alone. About 10 per cent of the benign tumours are multiple, and islet cell adenomas may occur in association with other endocrine adenomas (*see* Chapter 18).

Islet cell hyperplasia is commonly seen in the neonatal period in infants of diabetic mothers. Such children have hypersecretion of insulin, which may be responsible for the increased deposition of body fat so characteristic in these cases, and hypoglycaemic symptoms sometimes occur after birth. It is uncertain whether islet cell hyperplasia producing hypoglycaemia occurs as a distinct entity in the adult (Karlie and White, 1972).

Reactive hypoglycaemia in a patient who has had gastric surgery is well recognised. After partial gastrectomy, hypoglycaemia may occur several hours after a meal, i.e. later than the symptoms of the 'dumping' syndrome. A glucose tolerance test shows a typical lag curve with a high peak and a fall to hypoglycaemic levels 2 to 4 hours after glucose. Post-gastrectomy hypoglycaemia may possibly be caused by overactivity of the 'entero-insular axis' resulting in excessive release of intestinal glucagon-like activity and probably other hormones which augment insulin secretion after an oral glucose load (Vance, Stoll, Fariss and Williams, 1972; Rehfeld, Heding and Holst, 1973).

'Functional' hypoglycaemia, commonly diagnosed in the USA, is being recognised more frequently in the UK. Blood glucose falls to hypoglycaemic levels 2 to 4 hours after an oral carbohydrate load and there is a delay in the normal response of plasma insulin to ingested carbohydrate, often with an exaggerated peak. The delay in insulin secretion may possibly be due to relative insensitivity of the islets to the normal hyperglycaemic stimulus. Disturbance of the normal entero-humoral response to oral carbohydrate (Rehfeld *et al.*, 1973) or right vagal overactivity may also play a part. Many patients with reactive hypoglycaemia have a family history of diabetes, and many later develop this syndrome themselves. The symptoms usually (but not always) stop short of coma or convulsions, and are reported to occur particularly in emotionally labile individuals.

Leucine stimulates insulin secretion, and a significant number of patients with islet cell adenomas are *leucine sensitive*. Leucine sensitivity does not appear to exist as a specific entity in adults. In susceptible children, insulin levels rise after leucine administration but the raised levels do not necessarily coincide with the fasting hypoglycaemia which occurs in this condition. Idiopathic hypoglycaemia of childhood and inborn errors of metabolism are discussed in a later section.

DIAGNOSIS

If spontaneous hypoglycaemia is suspected, it is first necessary to demonstrate by blood glucose levels that hypoglycaemia does in fact exist, and this may necessitate provocative tests, since the patient may have no symptoms when seen. The possibility of hypoglycaemia is often not considered, since many of the symptoms and signs are entirely subjective or are non-specific.

In this country, when iatrogenic and factitious hypoglycaemia are excluded, the diagnosis of spontaneous hypoglycaemia in the adult is usually due to one of the following conditions

1. Islet cell tumour
2. 'Functional' or reactive hypoglycaemia
3. Addison's disease } rare
4. Hypopituitarism }
5. Liver disease } very rare
6. Sarcomas or carcinomatosis }

It may be necessary to exclude a number of conditions which present with some of the non-specific (i.e. adrenaline release) symptoms common to spontaneous hypoglycaemia, e.g. phaeochromocytoma, thyrotoxicosis, reactions to mono-amine oxidase inhibitors (which may rarely produce genuine hypoglycaemia), chronic anxiety states, and a wide gamut of psychiatric and neurological disease. Full physical examination is essential to exclude liver disease, hypofunction of the adrenals or pituitary, and extensive sarcoma or carcinoma.

The following tests may be of use in investigating a patient with suspected spontaneous hypoglycaemia (not necessarily in this sequence):

1. Oral glucose tolerance test over 4 hours (with standard preparation).
2. X-ray of skull, chest, and barium meal. Coeliac axis arteriogram.
3. 48- (72-) hour fast.
4. Tolbutamide test.
5. Glucagon test.
6. Plasma immunoreactive insulin assay.

More specific tests may be performed to exclude the less common causes of hypoglycaemia, such as hypoadrenalism or hypopituitarism, inborn errors of metabolism, and extensive liver disease.

1. *Glucose Tolerance Test.* The standard oral and intravenous glucose tolerance tests are not of great value in the diagnosis of islet cell tumour, and no consistent pattern of response is obtained. A test in which blood glucose samples are taken at half-hourly intervals for up to four hours after the oral dose may be helpful in the diagnosis of reactive hypoglycaemia, when very low blood glucose levels, sometimes associated with symptoms, are observed between two and four hours.

2. *X-ray of Skull, Chest, and Barium Meal. Coeliac Axis Arteriogram.* Radiology is of rather limited value in the diagnosis of the cause of spontaneous hypoglycaemia. Destructive tumours of the pituitary or adrenal and extensive bronchogenic carcinoma may rarely be diagnosed. The incidence of peptic ulceration in patients with islet cell tumours is twice that of the average population, though this finding cannot be considered diagnostic. Very rarely, deformity of the duodenum may be seen due to a large islet-cell tumour in the head of the pancreas. Coeliac axis arteriogram performed by retrograde catheterisation via the femoral artery may sometimes be of value in localising an islet cell tumour after the diagnosis has been made on other grounds (Dunn *et al.*, 1968). This procedure has a negligible mortality in experienced hands and can positively confirm the presence of a tumour in about 20 per cent of cases (McGarity and Braistley, 1970), although with greater radiological experience and more-certain biochemical diagnosis this figure rises. Negative angiography does not exclude the presence of a tumour.

3. *Forty-eight (seventy-two) hour Fast.* This is one of the most useful diagnostic tests. Its aim is to demonstrate Whipple's classical triad (1938, 1944): (1) symptoms induced by fasting, (2) hypoglycaemia demonstrated at the time of symptoms, (3) reversal of symptoms after administration of glucose. The test should be carried out only under close supervision in hospital. Unsweetened fluids are given and the blood glucose is estimated at three-hourly intervals. At the onset of symptoms the blood glucose level is estimated, blood is taken for insulin immunoassay and glucose given. Electroencephalograms recorded before and after glucose can be helpful. Most patients with islet cell tumours develop symptoms of neuroglycopoenia well within forty-eight hours, and the blood glucose level invariably falls to less than 30 mg per cent. Only rarely does the fast need to be prolonged to seventy-two hours, but this should be done if no neuroglycopoenic symptoms have occurred by forty-eight hours. If necessary, a period of exercise is given at the end of the fast, before its termination with glucose. If seventy-two hours of fasting and a period of exercise fail to induce hypoglycaemia and neuroglycopoenia, then islet cell tumour can be excluded with almost complete certainty. Normal subjects and patients with reactive hypoglycaemia remain normoglycaemic during a seventy-two-hour fast. It is suggested that this test is performed before the tolbutamide and glucagon tests.

4. *Tolbutamide Test* (Fajans and Conn, 1959). The intravenous injection of one gramme of sodium tolbutamide dissolved in 20 ml distilled water is followed in normal subjects, and in those with reactive hypoglycaemia, by a slight or moderate fall in blood glucose reaching its lowest level at about 30 minutes after injection. The level returns to at least 70 per cent and usually 80 per cent of the fasting level by 120–180 minutes. In patients with islet-cell tumours the initial fall may not exceed that seen in normal subjects, but the blood glucose level remains well below 70 per cent of the fasting level (if this was normal) up to three hours. Estimation of plasma immunoreactive insulin levels during the test are most useful, and are discussed further below. The test should not be performed if the fasting blood glucose test is at hypoglycaemic levels on the morning of the test, for severe neuroglycopoenia may occur, even with little further fall in the blood glucose. Spurious results using this test are comparatively rare but hepatic disease may produce a false positive. The test is not without danger in patients with islet cell tumours, and should not be performed without good reason.

5. *Glucagon Test* (Marks, 1960). The injection of 1 mg of glucagon intramuscularly in normal

patients produces a sharp and unsustained rise in blood sugar with a peak at or before 30 minutes, and this is followed by a return to the fasting level or slightly below within 1½–2 hours; the fall never reaches hypoglycaemic levels. Patients with islet-cell tumours show a similar sharp rise, but this is followed by a fall to hypoglycaemic levels within the next 1½–3 hours. It may be necessary to estimate blood glucose levels for up to three hours to demonstrate hypoglycaemia. The fall in blood glucose in these patients is due to stimulation of pancreatic insulin release by glucagon, and insulin levels rise sharply during the test. This test may be more useful and safer than the tolbutamide test in the diagnosis of islet cell tumour.

6. *Plasma Immunoreactive Insulin Assay*. The immunoassay of plasma insulin is most helpful in the diagnosis of islet cell tumour. A high fasting level of insulin in the absence of administered insulin or hypoglycaemic agents is almost pathognomonic of islet cell tumour, although not all cases show increased fasting levels. More important than the finding of an absolute increase in the insulin level is the demonstration that the level, although perhaps still within the normal range, is inappropriately high for the level of blood glucose observed at the time. There may in these patients be rapid spontaneous fluctuations in the plasma insulin level. Marked elevation of plasma insulin in such patients is much more frequent after tolbutamide or glucagon. Peak values may be found as early as two to five minutes after tolbutamide. Very high plasma insulin levels have rarely been found in some patients with extensive fibrosarcoma and spontaneous hypoglycaemia, but here the true diagnosis will rarely be in doubt. Such tumours more commonly secrete hypoglycaemic substances other than insulin (*see* Chapter 20). The fasting plasma insulin level is normal in idiopathic leucine-sensitive hypoglycaemia and 'functional' and reactive hypoglycaemia. Administration of leucine will produce a rise in plasma insulin in leucine-sensitive individuals, and about 50 per cent of patients with islet cell tumours are sensitive to this amino-acid.

TREATMENT

In patients with Addison's disease or hypopituitarism, therapy is clearly defined once the diagnosis is made. In patients with other conditions, such as some of the inborn errors of metabolism in childhood, non-pancreatic neoplasms, and advanced liver disease curative therapy is not possible and treatment must be symptomatic. When hypoglycaemia is a serious problem the hyperglycaemic substance diazoxide is helpful. Diazoxide is a non-diuretic benzothiadiazine originally introduced for the treatment of hypertension. The major action of this substance is to decrease pancreatic insulin secretion though it may also have a peripheral effect. It has been used to control the symptoms of hypoglycaemia in the post-gastrectomy syndrome, islet cell carcinoma, and idiopathic hypoglycaemia of infancy. The daily dose is 5 to 15 mg/kg body weight orally. It does not produce marked hypotension in this dosage although with doses in excess of 200 mg/day nausea and vomiting may occur. Excessive hair growth may be a troublesome complication. Its use should be limited to those cases where the hypoglycaemia cannot be controlled by other means and where neuroglycopoenia is frequent, incapacitating, and a potential danger to cerebral function or to life.

Where hypoglycaemia is truly reactive, as for instance to fructose, leucine or galactose, attempts should be made to remove the offending substance from the diet or to give very small amounts (e.g. the minimal daily requirement of leucine is 150–250 mg/kg body weight). In some cases diazoxide therapy may be considered. Such dietary treatment is not possible when hypoglycaemia is induced by carbohydrate, as in 'functional' hypoglycaemia, and here it is recommended that meals should be frequent and should be high in protein, high in fat and low in carbohydrate. The administration of tolbutamide 250–500 mg before each meal can often be of benefit in reactive hypoglycaemia, and presumably acts by accelerating the release of insulin, thus restoring the normal pattern of secretion. Diazoxide is ineffective in this group.

The treatment of islet cell tumours is surgical, but this simple statement belies the difficulties very commonly encountered by the surgeon. The tumours are almost always very small—rarely exceeding 3 cm in diameter and commonly measuring only a few millimetres. Ten per cent are multiple and at least 10 per cent malignant. The tumour may be extrapancreatic, and situated in the duodenal wall, the splenic hilum or in ectopic pancreatic tissue in a Meckel's diverticulum. Although tail islets contain more beta cells than those in the head, the tumours occur with equal frequency in all parts of the pancreas, and localisation of the suspected tumour is often difficult. Radioisotope scanning techniques that attempt to localise the tumour pre-operatively or at the time of operation have so far proved disappointing, although coeliac axis arteriograms will localise a percentage. If the tumour is not apparent on inspection or on palpation at laparotomy, then the tail and body of the pancreas must be mobilised and reflected anteriorly so that the posterior surface can be inspected. Duodenotomy and inspection of other ectopic sites may need to be carried out. Frozen sections should be examined when necessary, and islet cell adenomatosis may be diagnosed in this way. This condition is very uncommon and the most appropriate therapy is resection of the body and tail of the pancreas. If the most careful and detailed search fails to reveal a tumour the pancreas should be left intact and the patient's symptoms controlled by diazoxide with a view to a subsequent laparotomy when the tumour may be larger. The former practice of resection of the body and tail of the pancreas is not to be recommended (Mengoli and Le Quesne, 1967). Glucose should be infused intravenously before and during the operation and the rate of infusion adjusted to ensure a blood glucose level of 80–100 mg as the operation commences. Serial estimation of blood glucose levels to maintain this level during the preliminary exploration is mandatory. A sharp rise of blood glucose is observed, usually within 5–10 minutes, after removal of the tumour, although this rise may be delayed for as long as 20–30 minutes. Post-operative complications include transient glycosuria and hyperglycaemia, which may necessitate the temporary use of insulin, pancreatic fistula, and acute haemorrhagic pancreatitis. If a malignant islet cell tumour is found, radical surgery should be undertaken wherever possible. If distant metastases are present, conservative post-operative therapy with diazoxide (or very rarely alloxan) is the treatment of choice. Streptozotocin has been used in the treatment of inoperable islet cell carcinoma, but the drug is highly toxic and must be infused direct into the coeliac axis, and results are not encouraging.

Diabetes mellitus may supervene some years after successful removal of a benign islet cell tumour (Dunn, 1971).

HYPOGLYCAEMIA IN CHILDHOOD

The causes and manifestations of hypoglycaemia in the child differ somewhat from those observed in the adult. Some of the more common causes are discussed below.

Neonatal Hypoglycaemia. The blood sugar level usually falls after birth, reaching its lowest levels about 2 to 4 hours after delivery and returning to normal over the next 3 to 5 days. In some children this fall in blood glucose may be excessive and prolonged and symptoms of hypoglycaemia may develop, typically during the second and third days after birth. The symptoms observed include tremor (the 'jittery baby'), attacks of apnoea and cyanosis and, in more severe cases, convulsions and coma. Hypocalcaemia may occur. The cause of this syndrome in infants of non-diabetic mothers is unknown but it seems to be an exaggeration of the normal post-partum fall in blood sugar. Children of low birth-weight, particularly small-for-dates babies, and the smaller of twins are at particular risk of hypoglycaemia. Neonatal hypoglycaemia may be symptomatic or asymptomatic, but all babies with hypoglycaemia must be treated promptly, initially with intravenous glucose and later, if necessary, with hydrocortisone (*British Medical Journal*, 1971). The levels of blood glucose diagnostic of neonatal hypoglycaemia vary with the status at birth. In the full-term infant, two or more true blood glucose values of less than 30 mg/100 ml and in the low birth-weight infant (less than 2,500 g) a blood glucose of less than 20 mg/100 ml confirm the diagnosis (Cornblath and Schwartz, 1966).

Recovery occurs spontaneously within a few days, but may be delayed longer. If the condition is not recognised and treated, residual mental retardation may occur.

Hypoglycaemia in Children of Diabetic Mothers. These babies tend to be large and have a higher perinatal and neonatal mortality and morbidity than the normal child. Islet cell hypertrophy and hyperinsulinism are present. Symptoms begin a little earlier than in the neonatal hypoglycaemia described above, and usually appear within a few hours of birth. Glucose should be used for treatment; but since glucose may itself increase the hyperinsulinism, fructose (which does not stimulate insulin secretion) may also be used for treatment although it should not be employed during the first twenty-four hours of life: during this period there is transient fructose intolerance which may further lower blood glucose levels through unknown mechanisms. The condition of hypoglycaemia in children of diabetic mothers rarely persists for longer than a few days.

Idiopathic Hypoglycaemia of Childhood (*IHC*). This syndrome was first described by McQuarrie (1954). The symptoms may be present at birth, usually appear before the age of two, and almost always before the age of five, physical signs are absent and there is a tendency to spontaneous recovery. There is a familial tendency. The syndrome is heterogeneous, and a number of conditions are responsible for IHC including *leucine sensitivity*. The hypoglycaemia which follows the ingestion of leucine in sensitive patients is due to hyperinsulinism, but fasting hypoglycaemia also occurs in patients with leucine-sensitive and other types of IHC, and in these cases hyperinsulinism is not present. The cause of the fasting hypoglycaemia is therefore unknown, although it has been suggested that defective pituitary-adrenal function plays a part.

The symptoms of IHC are identical with those produced by other causes of spontaneous hypoglycaemia in childhood. Convulsions are present in virtually every case. The symptoms are seen most commonly after fasting, but in the leucine-sensitive cases they may also occur after feeding. The only certain means of distinguishing IHC from islet cell tumour is to measure the plasma insulin after fasting or after tolbutamide. In IHC, plasma insulin shows a normal response to these stimuli. The insulin response to leucine is of little value as it is positive in some patients with islet cell tumour as well as those with leucine sensitive IHC. Blood glucose levels alone after tolbutamide are also of no value in differentiating the two conditions.

IHC is treated with ACTH or hydrocortisone, and in many individuals symptoms will abate with only small doses. In leucine-sensitive cases attempts may also be made to reduce the leucine content of the diet, but this is difficult and often unsuccessful. In resistant cases, diazoxide (*see* above) has been used with good effect.

Islet Cell Tumour. This is exceedingly rare in childhood. Convulsions are almost invariable, and attacks of unconsciousness occur almost as frequently. Fasting plasma insulin levels are usually elevated, and immunoassay of insulin is most helpful in differentiating the condition from IHC.

Prediabetes. Symptoms of hypoglycaemia not uncommonly occur in children who are prediabetic or have latent diabetes, and may precede the onset of glycosuria and carbohydrate intolerance by a variable period of time. There is usually a strong family history of diabetes, and the symptoms commonly follow a carbohydrate meal.

They are usually mild, although loss of consciousness may occur. A low carbohydrate and high fat protein diet may be given, but frank diabetes mellitus often supervenes.

Hypoglycaemia may also occur in childhood in some types of *glycogen storage disease* where liver glycogen cannot be converted to glucose, and in the other rare *inborn errors of metabolism* galactosaemia, hereditary fructose intolerance, and familial fructose and galactose intolerance (Dormandy's syndrome). The mechanism of the hypoglycaemia in these latter conditions is not known. Neither fructose nor galactose stimulate insulin secretion in these patients and the hypoglycaemia may be due to excessive accumulation of galactose-1-phosphate and fructose-1-phosphate interfering with hepatic gluconeogenesis by inhibiting various enzyme systems.

THE MANAGEMENT OF HYPOGLYCAEMIA IN CHILDHOOD

Neonatal hypoglycaemia requires a high 'index of suspicion' for diagnosis and a sense of urgency in treatment. In the older child, reactive hypoglycaemia associated with early diabetes or prediabetes is usually mild, convulsions are rare, there is usually a strong family history of diabetes, and the age of onset will often exclude the possibility of IHC.

In practice, therefore, the differential diagnosis that may cause difficulty is between IHC and islet cell tumour. Plasma insulin assays, if available, will usually serve to differentiate the two. If these are not available, it is wise to regard a child under the age of four in whom no organic cause for spontaneous hypoglycaemia is found as suffering from IHC, and to treat with ACTH or hydrocortisone. In those children who fail to respond to this therapy, and particularly those in whom the symptoms begin after the age of four, laparotomy may be necessary, and should not be delayed if attacks of hypoglycaemia are frequent despite therapy. In those patients with IHC who fail to respond to steroids and in whom the diagnosis of islet cell tumour may be excluded with certainty, diazoxide (5–15 mg/kg/day) may be given.

GLUCAGON-SECRETING TUMOURS

There have been a number of isolated case reports of patients who have presented with apparent functioning α-cell tumours of the pancreas. In one such patient (Yoshinga *et al.*, 1966) the tumour was associated with severe diabetes mellitus and high levels of serum glucagon-like activity. However, the glucagon activity was measured only by a bioassay technique, and the tumour was detected clinically about six months before the onset of the diabetes. The increased serum glucagon-like activity may have precipitated diabetes in an already susceptible individual.

REFERENCES

Cornblath, M., and Schwartz, R. (1966). *Disorders of Carbohydrate Metabolism in Infancy*, Philadelphia, Saunders.

Dormandy, T. L., and Porter, R. J. (1961). *Lancet*, **i**, 1189.

Dunn, D. C. (1971). *Brit. med. J.*, **2**, 84.

Dunn, D. C., Birnstingl, M. A., and Leggett, H. A. (1968). *Proc. roy. Soc. Med.*, **61**, 957.

Editorial (1971). *Brit. med. J.*, **2**, 130.

Fajans, S. S., and Conn, J. W. (1959). *J. lab. clin. Med.*, **54**, 811.

Griffiths, W. J. (1961). *Modern Trends in Endocrinology*, second series (Ed. Gardiner-Hill, H.). London: Butterworth.

Howard, J. M., Moss, N. H., and Rhoades, J. E. (1950). *Surg. Gyn. Obst.*, **90**, 417.

Karlie, H., and White, T. T. (1972). *Ann. Surg.*, **175**, 326.
Laurent, J., Delry, G., and Floquet, J. (1970). *Hypoglycaemic Tumours.* Amsterdam: Excerpta Medica.
Marks, V. (1959). *Clin. Chim. Acta*, **4**, 395.
Marks, V. (1960). *Brit. med. J.*, **i**, 1539.
Marks, V., Marrack, D., and Rose, F. C. (1961). *Proc. roy. Soc. Med.*, **54**, 747.
Marks, V., and Rose, F. C. (1965). *Hypoglycaemia.* Oxford: Blackwell Scientific.
McGarity, W. C., and Braistley, J. W. (1970). *Amer. J. Surg.*, **119**, 705.
McQuarrie, I. (1954). *Amer. J. Dis. Child.*, **87**, 399.
Mengoli, L., and Le Quesne, L. P. (1967). *Brit. J. Surg.*, **54**, 749.
Rehfeld, J. F., Heding, L. G., and Holst, J. J. (1973). *Lancet*, **i**, 116.
Vance, J. E., Stoll, R. W., Fariss, B. L., and Williams, R. H. (1972). *Metabolism*, **21**, 405.
Whipple, A. O. (1938). *J. Internat. Chir.*, **3**, 237.
Whipple, A. O. (1944). *Surgery*, **16**, 289.
Yoshinaga, T., Okuno, G., Shinji, Y., Tsujii, T., and Nishikawa, M. (1966). *Diabetes*, **15**, 709.

17

OBESITY

The authors make no apology for including a chapter on obesity in a textbook of endocrinology. Although obesity is very rarely of endocrine origin, it is one of the most common reasons for referral to an endocrine clinic, and patients with the disease (and sometimes their physicians) are often convinced that there is 'something wrong with the glands'. This illusion must be dispelled. Nevertheless, in any discussion on obesity, reference to the endocrine system will be inevitable, if only to exclude endocrine abnormalities as a significant causative factor in the vast majority of cases.

In terms of the frequency with which it occurs, the mortality and morbidity associated with it and the mental distress it engenders, the syndrome of obesity is the most common form of malnutrition and, indeed, one of the most significant afflictions seen in the western world. While its pathogenesis is relatively simple to understand, we still lack knowledge about many of the factors normally concerned with the regulation of energy balance and appetite.

Subcutaneous fat is not present simply to provide pleasing cosmetic effects or insulation against the cold. If an organ is defined as that part of an animal adapted by its structure for a particular function, the cells comprising it being capable of reacting under normal conditions as a single unit, then there is little doubt that, as Kekwick (1960) has pointed out, the fat depots of the body may be regarded as an organ. The function of the adipose organ is to store surplus carbohydrate not metabolised immediately after ingestion, in the form of triglyceride or neutral fat, and when necessary to liberate free fatty acid to be oxidised in peripheral tissues to provide energy. Such a storage and releasing depot is essential, since the supply of carbohydrate and of calories is intermittent, while cellular metabolism must continue throughout the twenty-four hours and requires 'fuel'. In more primitive communities, a reserve of metabolic substrate is even more vital in order to provide for periods when food is not available. The adipose organ is, therefore, in a dynamic metabolic state and should not be regarded as an inert, non-functional mass.

DEFINITION

Obesity is best defined as an excessive accumulation of triglyceride fat in the adipose organ. In obesity of early onset there is an increase in the number as well as the size of fat cells—hyperplasia of the adipose organ. In obesity of later onset there is predominantly increased 'packing' of the fat cells with triglyceride (hypertrophy), although obese adults to appear to have more fat cells than the lean. Weight gain and loss in the adult, however, produces no change in adipose cell number, although fat cell size varies with weight change (Hirsch and Knittle, 1970). Perhaps those obese adults with increased numbers of fat cells have been 'potentially' obese since childhood, since it appears that the number of fat cells in any one individual alters little after the basic complement of cells is fixed in early childhood following a sensitive period in adipose cell replication (Brook, 1972). The increase in the size of fat cells in the obese is of more than academic interest, since the larger the fat cell the less sensitive it is to the effects of insulin (Salans, Knittle and Hirsch, 1968) and the higher the fasting immunoreactive insulin level (Stern, Batchelor, Hollander, Cohn and Hirsch, 1972). Both hyperinsulinism and insulin insensitivity are features of obesity. All available evidence indicates that this accumulation of body fat arises because the intake of calories exceeds the output, the balance being laid down as fat.

DIAGNOSIS AND MEASUREMENT

In the 'normal' lean adult male, 15 to 20 per cent of the total body weight is made up of adipose tissue, and in the 'normal' lean female this figure rises to 20 to 25 per cent. Higher percentages are observed in patients over the age of 60 (Lesser, Deutsch and Markofsky, 1971). In obesity, adipose tissue contributes a greater proportion of the total body weight, but there is also an increase in lean body tissue. Skin thickness, density and collagen content remain normal, despite the increase in skin surface (Black, Bottoms and Shuster, 1971). The terms 'lean body mass' and 'fat mass' as currently defined are unphysiological. 'Lean body mass' consists of cell solids, extra-cellular and intra-cellular water, and mineral mass; thus, 'fat mass' simply includes triglyceride fat without taking into account its water content or its cellular constituents. It is impossible to measure adipose tissue mass in the living organism with accuracy, but a rough approximation can be calculated on the basis of the estimated 'fat mass' by assuming the water content of adipose tissue to be approximately 15 per cent by weight. A number of methods have now replaced the original technique of under-water weighing which was used to estimate body specific gravity to give an indirect measure of body fat. Skin-fold thickness can be measured by constant-pressure calipers when the accumulation of subcutaneous adipose tissue is not gross, and such measurements appear to correlate well with estimates of fat mass obtained by other means (Durnin and Rahaman, 1967). A single measurement of the triceps skin-fold posteriorly at mid-humeral level has been used as a standard—a skin-fold of greater than 15 mm in the male or 25 mm in the female is taken to indicate an excess of adipose tissue. Considerable experience is required before reproducible results can be obtained. Other measurements of adipose tissue mass are essentially indirect and involve estimation of various body-water compartments, from which lean body mass and fat mass may be calculated (Hamwi and Urbach, 1953). The krypton space method (Hytten *et al.*, 1966) gives a more direct estimation of fat mass but is too complex for routine use. In practice, it is usual to rely largely on body configuration in association with body weight to give an indication of the presence or absence of excess adipose tissue. In the absence of any disturbance of body fluids, it has been suggested that an increase in weight of 15 per cent above desired or ideal weight (i.e. median weight for height and sex at age 25) may be regarded as obesity but there is not general agreement about this figure—such an arbitrary figure does not take into account variations in body build, bone size, and muscularity. The incidence of obesity rises progressively with increasing age, reaching a peak in the 40's in men and in the 50's in women, and thereafter falling slightly. No accurate figure can be given, but it is usually stated that both in the UK and in the USA at least 50 per cent of the population over 40 years of age are significantly overweight (*see* Appendix).

CALORIE BALANCE AND ENERGY METABOLISM

Energy is gained by the body almost exclusively in the form of calories taken in as food. Although at least 95 per cent of the total dietary calories, whatever the calorie content of the food, are absorbed into the body in the absence of intestinal malabsorption, there are small individual differences so that one individual may absorb 80–140 kcal more than another on a similar caloric intake (Durnin, 1971). These amounts are small but may in the long term lead to considerable amounts of energy being available and possibly deposited in the body as adipose tissue. Differences of this sort are not easily measured and are obviously variable. Nevertheless, from now on in this chapter the term 'energy intake' will refer to calories absorbed into the body and not to dietary calories, unless otherwise stated. There is little evidence that under normal circumstances absorption of heat from the environment plays a significant role in calorie intake.

The components of energy output are shown in Table 17.1. Energy output in the non-work

TABLE 17.1 *The Components of Energy Output*

1. Basal metabolism	via radiation, conduction and convection
2. Activity metabolism	
3. Specific dynamic action of food	

4. Non-work fraction—
   - evaporation of sweat and insensible perspiration (modified by climate and activity output)
   - heat content of excreta
   - heat value of shed portions of skin and hair, faeces, and urine
   - heat lost in expired gas
   - heat value of organic constituents in expired gas

fraction under normal circumstances accounts for only a very small proportion of the energy lost to the body and remains fairly constant. Heat and energy are lost mainly as a result of basal metabolism—the process of staying alive—and by physical activity during the waking hours. In childhood, of course, calories are also utilised in the process of normal growth and development. In the normal individual who follows the same pattern of life, energy-loss varies little from day to day. Fluctuations in energy balance may be expressed in terms of calories. Calorie balance may be positive, when intake exceeds output, or negative if the reverse applies. Excess of water or electrolytes can be excreted from the body, but there is no way in which excess energy (not utilised for normal metabolism or for growth) can be eliminated, nor is an increase in calorie intake compensated for by an increase in metabolic rate except in the case of calories taken in the form of protein where the specific dynamic action causes a small but probably insignificant increase in energy loss. When sudden and marked changes in energy output occur, there is a gradual readjustment of food intake to maintain balance. However, minor changes in energy expenditure within the physiological range are not necessarily accompanied by detectable changes in calorie intake. The evidence at present available suggests that day-to-day calorie balance under physiological conditions is maintained mainly by regulation of food intake.

It follows from the above considerations, that any excess of calories must be stored until the need for their utilisation arises. The excess cannot be stored in the form of carbohydrate or protein in more than small amounts and the major part is stored in the form of lipid in the adipose organ. There is virtually no limit to the amount of fat that can be stored in this way. In grossly obese patients, e.g. of 150 kg, there may be as much as 700,000 kcal present in depot fat. Theoretically, this is equivalent to seven to eight months supply of food.

The concept of calorie balance may therefore be summed-up in the statement: assuming lean body mass stays constant, then changes in adiposity are equal to the difference between calorie (food) intake and calorie (energy) output. An example of what this involves is given in Table 17.2, in which are expressed the approximate daily calorie requirements of a moderately active adult male. His daily intake averages 3,200 kcal/

TABLE 17.2 *Adult Male Aged 25, Weight 70 kg*

Daily energy expenditure (in kcal)

8 hours in bed at basal rate	= 500
8 hours recreation*	= 1,500
8 hours light occupation (2·5 kcal/min)	= 1,200
Total	= 3,200

Yearly energy output (on the basis of constant-activity level)

$= 365 \times 3{,}200 \simeq 1{,}000{,}000$ kcal

Presumed

excess = 100 kcal/day
= 36,500 kcal/year
$\simeq$ 3–4 per cent of total intake

If activity remains at constant level as above, net weight gain would be approximately 10 lb/year as adipose tissue.†

* Includes personal necessities, walking, eating, reading, active recreation, etc.

† 1 lb adipose tissue is approximately equivalent to 3,500 kcal.

day, approximately 1×10^6 kcal/year. If his weight were to remain steady over this time, he would expend 1×10^6 kcal. A daily intake of 100 kcal in excess of requirements (an excess calorie balance of about 3 per cent) would amount over a year to about 36,000 kcal, which is approximately equivalent to a gain of 10 lb in weight if the excess were to be laid down as adipose tissue. If this state of positive balance continued for five years, there would be a net weight gain of some 50 lb. The factors that normally control caloric balance and which can maintain weight at a constant level over long periods are not really understood, and there is, perhaps, cause for wonder that obesity is not even more common, and admiration for the precision with which the body controls energy balance. Passmore (1966) has estimated that over thirty-five years he has consumed 17 tons of food, and his weight has never fluctuated by more than 5 lb. This illustrates that obesity may not always arise from a gross disturbance of eating, but can result from a fractional offsetting of a regulatory mechanism of great precision. It must be stressed that calorie balance is a long-term matter—a normal person is not in balance from day to day, but more from week to week or even month to month. Thus, short-term studies of calorie balance must be interpreted with caution, and any study of less than one week's duration is likely to be of little value. Weight gain is not necessarily constant or progressive, although obviously the long-term trend must be towards positive balance as obesity develops.

ENERGY EXPENDITURE

Many fat people complain that they are 'small eaters' and the myth persists that such individuals may, in some mystical way, handle food more economically than the lean. The law of conservation of energy is not suspended for the convenience of the obese. Tied up with this myth is the oft-repeated observation that some people may eat vast quantities yet remain lean, while others who eat much less 'have a tendency to flesh'. Of course, such statements ignore the question of energy expenditure, and to overlook this is to imply acceptance of the physically impossible. The first step in resolving this apparent paradox is to study the diet and types of food eaten, bearing in mind that dietary histories in the obese are notoriously unreliable.

The next step is to consider energy expenditure. It is now universally accepted that outwardly similar people may expend very different quantities of energy, though their activities might not appear to be so very different. Such discrepancies may be only slight, and may be within the physiological range of 'normal', but they nevertheless occur, and over long periods of time may assume significant proportions. Thus, some individuals may expend less energy than others, either under basal conditions or under standard conditions of exercise. There is also considerable variation in overall activity levels between different individuals. If food intake is identical in the two groups, then the individual who uses less energy will tend to gain more weight than his lean colleague—thus, obesity is initiated. Many factors cause these variations in activity and in energy expenditure—physical stature, age, weight, physical condition, and personality are all of importance. The hyperkinetic lean individual who is always 'on the go' is well recognised; the placid lean individual is also seen, although he is less likely to remain lean. It has been observed that a group of 'large eaters' had natural rates of walking consistently faster than those classed as 'small eaters' (Rose and Williams, 1961). Of course, these observations are not meant to imply that *all* those individuals with a naturally low energy expenditure will become fat and all those with a naturally high expenditure will remain lean. Weight differences would be observed only if food intake was the same in all cases. In practice, most of these individuals will remain in calorie balance and at a constant weight as a result of differences in calorie intake.

Energy Expenditure in Obesity. It has been observed repeatedly that patients with *established* obesity expend more energy than the lean in performing standard physical acts and that as weight increases there is a progressive increase in the amount of energy expended. This could serve as a compensatory mechanism, the increased energy expenditure restricting weight gain until a new equilibrium is established when the increased energy output balances the excessive energy intake. However, this would be so only if the *overall physical activity level* remained constant. Unfortunately, the more energy needed to perform a physical act, the less likely it is to be carried out. Therefore, while basal energy output and energy expenditure in the performance of isolated physical acts increases as weight rises, so overall daily activity, which may have been low to begin with, falls even further. There is no doubt that under all circumstances obese individuals are very much less active than the lean (Mayer, 1965; Bloom and Eidex, 1967) and the latter workers have drawn attention to the significance of inactivity both in the initiation and the maintenance of obesity. No matter how high or low the daily energy output of the obese patient, if his weight is steady or is rising then he is not in negative calorie balance and his calorie intake must equal or exceed his expenditure.

THE CONTROL OF FEEDING AND THE AETIOLOGY OF OBESITY

Obesity can arise only in the presence of positive calorie balance. The only way by which the body can deal with an excess of calories is to lay them down as fat, and the visible manifestations of positive calorie balance will be the same in all cases. Obesity is, therefore, not a homogeneous and distinct disease process but may be the final manifestation of a number of different mechanisms that have resulted in a gain of calories to the body. In some, excessive intake is the primary event; in others, low energy output initiates obesity. In most patients, both factors play a part. Exactly the same considerations apply in obesity in childhood, and the underlying mechanisms in no way differ from those present in the adult.

The factors that control and modify feeding are diverse. While hunger contractions of the stomach in animals may increase the drive to obtain and eat food, in civilised man they are a crude and urgent mechanism that tends to set a lower limit to the food intake and that normally plays little part in the daily regulation of feeding. Animal studies have demonstrated the presence of medial satiety and lateral appetite centres in the hypothalamus but in man the automatic control exercised by the hypothalamic centres may be dominated by cortical factors and conditioned reflexes, even in what appears to be automatic feeding. This is particularly likely to be true of the appetite centre, although the satiety centre is probably still important in calling a stop to food ingestion. There is evidence suggesting that the satiety response is absent or is much diminished in many obese patients (Hollifield *et al.*, 1964). Obesity in man due to organic hypothalamic disease is very rare, and in addition to disturbances of feeding, apathy and inactivity may contribute to the development of the obese state in these patients.

A number of factors may modify appetite and feeding patterns by what is presumed to be an effect on the higher centres. Genetic factors are, in general, of little importance in the regulation of appetite or in the aetiology of obesity. Habits and patterns of feeding and of physical activity tend to be acquired during childhood, which is the time at which the number of fat cells in the adipose organ seems to be determined (Brook, 1972), and these environmental factors are of much greater importance than any genetically determined predisposition to excessive weight-gain. Palatability, habit, and socio-economic and cultural influences play a large part in determining the feeding pattern of an individual. Carbohydrate foods, and particularly those containing a high proportion of refined sugar, are palatable and cheap. They may be nibbled or eaten as snacks and provide a compact and immediate source of carbohydrate which the consumer is often seduced into thinking will not increase his weight. In times of financial depression, carbohydrate foods may be consumed in relatively large quantities because of their ready availability and their cheapness. Thus, eating patterns may be laid down in the young that may persist for a lifetime and, if calorie intake is maintained at a high level, obesity may result in middle life when activity levels fall. The pattern of meal-eating is also important. Many obese patients tend to be 'nibblers', and others fall into the group described as 'binge eaters', in that they consume the great majority of their daily calories in one meal, usually in the evening. If rats are trained to follow this eating pattern, they consume more food and become fatter than control animals that are allowed to feed freely. Modern civilisation predisposes to obesity, and the feeding habits that were essential for people who did manual work for many hours each day, who had no transport and who lived in poorly heated surroundings are quite out of place in the present affluent society. At the same time, food has become more freely available to all classes, and in particular carbohydrate foods have become popular items of diet and in some cases necessities of life.

Psychiatric disorders may result in overeating in response to emotional tensions or as a means of escape, and hyperphagia and obesity in childhood often begin after an emotional crisis. Others may develop anorexia under conditions of stress, and it is presumed that this difference in response reflects basic personality differences. While drug taking and excessive drinking are condemned by the community, and excessive smoking is felt by most to be undesirable, excessive eating, short of actual gluttony, is not necessarily considered abnormal or immoral. Eating is pleasant and passes the time, it is a pleasure that costs little, it can be indulged in at will, and it does not interfere with the lives of others. It is therefore 'acceptable' in a modern community. The obese patient is sometimes an object of amusement, very rarely one of scorn or revulsion as may be the drug addict or the alcoholic.

The influences that have resulted in overeating may in some patients be longstanding, while in others they are relatively more acute. The overweight patient is usually anxious to seek an explanation for obesity that does not include overeating, he hopes that he is the *one* individual who genuinely has a metabolic defect and who gains weight because his body, in some mystical way, utilises food more efficiently. Such a patient must be disabused of the idea that there is anything unique or complex about his disease.

METABOLISM IN OBESITY

A number of metabolic 'abnormalities' have been found in obese patients, all of which return towards normal as weight is lost. The cortisol production rate and urinary excretion of 17-hydroxycorticosteroids may be increased, particularly in younger patients where they may be related to a high protein intake. However, if these parameters are expressed on the basis of total weight or lean body mass they are usually within the normal range, although in some patients the results remain a little high, even after correction for these factors. The plasma total and free cortisol levels are normal or reduced in obese patients, urinary 11-hydroxycorticosteroids are within the normal range, and a normal rise of urinary 11-hydroxycorticosteroids is observed in response to injected insulin. The normal circadian rhythm of plasma cortisol is maintained. The urinary excretion of 17-oxosteroids may also be elevated in obesity, but usually to a lesser degree than the increase in 17-hydroxycorticosteroids. The excretion of both of these groups of steroids is reduced as weight is lost.

It has been suggested that some obese patients have a defect of fatty acid mobilisation since their plasma free fatty acid levels, while elevated after an overnight fast, show a smaller increase after more prolonged starvation than is seen in lean, individuals. However, the simple estimation of plasma free fatty acid levels may be misleading, and Issekutz *et al.* (1967) have shown that there is no impairment of fat mobilisation and that there is, in fact, a higher turnover rate of fatty acids in obese patients than in the lean. Galton and his colleagues (1966, 1970) have observed both enzyme defects and defects of glucose utilisation (the latter similar to a defect observed in adult diabetics) in the adipose tissue of obese patients. The significance of these findings, which may possibly be adaptive or which perhaps reflect the heterogeneous nature of obesity, remains uncertain.

Carbohydrate intolerance and frank diabetes are common in obese patients though in most cases these return to normal as weight is lost. In these patients, the pathogenesis and treatment of the obesity is the same as in those who show a normal response to ingested carbohydrate. A large proportion of obese individuals, both with normal and with mildly impaired carbohydrate tolerance, show increased fasting insulin levels and an increased response to a glucose load. These return to normal in most cases as weight is lost. It is tempting to speculate that in such individuals some form of insulin antagonism might be present (*see* Chapter 15), but an alternative explanation is that the raised insulin levels observed result from the insensitivity to insulin of the large fat cell (Salans *et al.*, 1968; Stern *et al.*, 1972). There is no evidence that an abnormality in glucose metabolism causes a disturbance in food intake that leads to obesity (Stunkard and Blumenthal, 1972).

Hyperlipoproteinaemia, particularly type IV and, less commonly, types IIa and IIb (Beaumont *et al.*, 1970), is a frequent accompaniment of obesity and predisposes to premature atherosclerosis. Type IV responds well to a low carbohydrate diet, with, if necessary, clofibrate orally. Type II hyperlipidaemia is more refractory to treatment. In these varieties, a low animal fat/low cholesterol diet, clofibrate and cholestyramine may be helpful.

ENDOCRINE DISEASE AND OBESITY

In Cushing's syndrome, gluconeogenesis may divert calories into fat while depleting lean body tissue and, in addition, cortisol stimulates the appetite, causing obesity with its characteristic distribution. Menstrual irregularities are common in obesity, but these should not be taken to indicate a primary endocrine abnormality since the patient's previous menstrual pattern is usually re-established with weight reduction. However, 40 per cent of patients with the polycystic ovary syndrome are obese and the condition should always be considered in overweight females with amenorrhoea or oligomenorrhoea and with hirsutism (p. 212). Each clinical feature of the syndrome requires separate treatment, and the obesity requires nothing more than a weight-reducing diet. Patients with obesity have normal thyroid function and the increase in weight which often occurs in hypothyroidism is due to deposition of myxoedematous tissue and to water retention. When true obesity is present in patients with hypothyroidism it is not a result of thyroid deficiency but of positive calorie balance brought about by the mechanisms previously described. Fröhlich's syndrome is exceedingly rare, and the overwhelming majority of young children in whom this diagnosis is suggested have 'simple' obesity with a physiological delay in the onset of puberty. Normal sexual maturation may be expected to occur in these children, and will develop earlier if weight is lost.

The endocrine secretions may have indirect influences on the intake and output of energy and may alter the distribution of body fat, but they cannot induce new mechanisms for the more efficient handling of food after absorption which might result *per se* in accumulation of adipose tissue.

THE COMPLICATIONS OF OBESITY

Obesity significantly shortens the life span, and is associated with an increased incidence of a multitude of major and minor diseases. Almost all common causes of death occur more frequently and at an earlier date in obese patients. The more severe the degree of obesity, the greater is the risk of an early demise. The statistics on which these conclusions are based are drawn from the reports of insurance companies, but even these underemphasise the dangers, since they refer only to cases that have *been selected* for insurance, albeit as sub-standard risks. We have no information on mortality trends in those individuals who are rejected for life insurance on the grounds of obesity alone, but it is assumed that in these patients the same trend continues, and thus, the mortality and morbidity associated with obesity in general are almost certainly greater than is apparent from published experience. Very roughly, the expectation of life decreases by one per cent below the normal for every pound of excess weight. Death from diabetes and its sequelae is about four times more common, from cirrhosis twice as common, and from coronary disease and cerebral haemorrhage about one and a-half times more common in the obese, and similarly, the morbidity from these diseases is more frequent. Of the most common causes of death, only suicide and tuberculosis are less frequent in the obese, and patients with tuberculosis would by the very nature of the disease be expected to be underweight. Other conditions more common in the obese include hypertension, generalised osteoarthrosis, biliary tract disease, and hiatal hernia. Obese patients are greater operative risks than are the lean, and in some cases elective or emergency surgery may be delayed because of the technical difficulties expected, adding further distress to the obese patient. Post-operative complications of all types are more frequent, particularly thromboembolism. Accidents, especially on the road, are common and the consequences more severe. Many minor but distressing conditions are associated with obesity—varicose veins, eczema and intertrigo, and moniliasis of the skin and genitalia, and here again the presence of obesity may of itself jeopardise the chances of cure and increase the rate of relapse.

THE PICKWICKIAN SYNDROME

The syndrome of alveolar hypoventilation and polycythaemia in the grossly obese was first described by Sieker *et al.* (1955). Burwell *et al.* (1956) introduced the term Pickwickian syndrome, after 'Fat Joe', the servant of Mr Wardle in *Pickwick Papers*. The main features are marked obesity with short stature, somnolence, twitching, cyanosis, secondary polycythaemia, right ventricular hypertrophy and failure. The excess of fat in and around the thorax leads to alveolar hypoventilation causing a rise in arterial pCO_2 and hypoxia. Respiratory acidaemia results, with further depression of the respiratory centre. There is no doubt that patients may recover from this serious syndrome if weight reduction is ensured, as shown in Table 17.3. The condition is almost inevitably fatal unless weight reduction is achieved.

TABLE 17.3 *Pulmonary Function Tests* in a Patient with the Pickwickian Syndrome Before and After Weight Reduction*

(Patient: N.M. male, date of birth 13th December, 1932)

Test	Normal value	17th January, Weight: 378 lb	28th November, Weight: 235 lb
Indirect arterial pCO_2:			
awake	40 mm Hg	53·7 mm Hg	39·4 mm Hg
asleep	—	61·6 mm Hg	
Physiological dead space	130 ml	253 ml	80 ml
Maximum voluntary ventilation	—	73 1/min (50% of predicted)	99 1/min (70% of predicted)
Ventilation equivalent for O_2	2·3–2·9 (litres of air for 100 ml O_2)	1·63	2·26
Pulmonary compliance	0·25–0·09 (1/cm H_2O)	0·43	0·19
Non-elastic work of breathing	less than 0·035 kg m/min.	0·168 kg m/min.	0·032 kg m/min.

* Performed by Dr G. L. Leathart.

THE TREATMENT OF OBESITY

The successful treatment of obesity is dependent upon interest and enthusiasm on the part of the physician, and co-operation coupled with a genuine desire to lose weight on the part of the patient. The physician should be firm but sympathetic, and accusations of downright gluttony at the first interview will damage, perhaps irreparably, his relationship with the patient. A feeling of mutual confidence should be established as early as possible, and whatever the details of the therapy recommended the patient should be seen frequently by the same physician. Where possible, the help of a dietitian should be sought.

The periodic fluctuations in water balance which normally occur are greatly aggravated by a reducing diet. In the first few days of strict dieting there is a sharp drop in weight due mainly to loss of water. Subsequently, marked fluctuations in water content may interfere with the expected trend of weight loss and the patient must be warned of this possibility. Diuretics may be prescribed to prevent excessive water retention though these alterations in water balance tend to correct themselves if weight reduction is carried on long enough.

DIET

In the long term, the only factor that causes weight loss is a reduction in the intake of calories below the level of energy expenditure—an induced negative calorie balance. When obese patients are admitted to hospital and given a normal diet without calorie restriction, which usually amounts to 2,400–2,800 kcal/day, weight loss is invariable, provided the patient remains ambulant and does not supplement the diet by his own resources. This will demonstrate to the patient how high his calorie intake must have been at home.

There are many weight-reducing diets, and the only effective regimens depend on a reduced calorie intake, although they differ in attractiveness and the ease with which they can be followed. The more restrictive a diet, the less likely is the patient to keep to it unless motivation is strong. The aim is to achieve dietary re-education rather than severe calorie restriction. Any abnormalities of eating pattern such as 'binge eating' or 'nibbling' should be corrected. The best diet is one that is attractive, that is simple for the patient to observe, that does not involve unnecessary expense, and does not disorganise the eating habits of the family. The intake of protein, minerals and vitamins should be sufficient to avoid deficiencies. A suitable diet was devised by Marriott (1949). This diet restricts milk to half a pint a day, and bread to three small slices. No sugars, sweets, alcohol, fats or fried foods are allowed, but the patient can eat normal portions of meat, eggs, fish, potatoes, vegetables and fresh fruit. It is psychologically good, because it does not lay down firm rules for the day's meals, and emphasises the wide variety of foods that may be eaten freely. The diet allows about 1,200 kcal daily, and the patient may be expected to lose at least two pounds a week. It is suggested that this diet should be used initially in the treatment of all cases of obesity, as it is the most attractive and realistic. At a later date, more severe calorie restriction may be needed if the patient becomes lax. Motivation is strong at the beginning of treatment, but will rapidly be lost if the initial diet is too strict since the patient may well feel that the sacrifice is not worth making. Patients often feel 'light-headed' during the early days of a reducing diet but they can be assured that this feeling will soon pass.

While the essential feature of any diet is that it should restrict calories, some physicians prefer diets that are relatively high in protein or fat. The theoretical advantages of high fat diets will be discussed later. High protein diets may increase energy loss due to their specific dynamic action effect, and they are very satisfying. However, their high cost is a distinct disadvantage. Proprietary slimming foods should be avoided: not only are they expensive but they may actually mislead the patient to suppose that he may consume them in addition to his diet and still lose weight.

FAT-MOBILISING SUBSTANCE

Studies by Kekwick and Pawan (1956, 1967) indicated that calorie or carbohydrate deficiency in man or in animals resulted in the excretion of a substance in the urine which they named fat-mobilizing substance (FMS). This material appears to act at a cellular level and causes release of fatty acids from the isolated fat pad, an increase in blood FFA and ketone bodies on injection into mice and, on repeated injection, a diminution in the carcase fat of the animals. It cannot be identified after starvation or carbohydrate deprivation in humans or animals with pituitary deficiency, and it appears to be distinct from ACTH.

It has been suggested for many years that high fat diets might be more effective in reducing weight than iso-caloric diets high in carbohydrate. One possible reason for this apparent difference was that a diet high in fat was less palatable and more satiating that one high in carbohydrate, and that patients on such diets consumed less calories since they were less likely to exceed their allowances than those receiving mainly carbohydrates. Kekwick and Pawan have suggested that the increased weight loss they observed in patients on isocaloric high fat as compared with high carbohydrate diets might be explicable by the greater production of fat-mobilising substance. If differences in weight loss with iso-caloric diets do genuinely occur, then the explanation can only be that there are differences in the absorption of the diet (of which there is no evidence), that metabolic rate is increased (which has not been observed to occur) or that there is an increase in the excretion of energy-containing molecules in the stools and urine, with consequent loss of this energy to the organism. Kekwick and Pawan favour the last explanation, and have produced some data that seem to support this. Kinsell *et al.* (1964) have shown that *in the long term*, under conditions of precise constancy of caloric intake, and essentially constant physical activity, qualitative modification of the diet as regards the amounts of protein, fat or carbohydrate allowed, makes little or no difference to the rate of weight loss, which is determined almost entirely by the caloric content of the diet, bearing no relationship to the proportions of the nutrients employed. They point out that, in view of the fluctuations that occur during the course of any reducing regimen, data from short-term studies should be interpreted with caution. FMS has been used therapeutically and Kekwick and Pawan (1968) showed that the substance appeared in man to have a similar effect to that observed in mice. Patients lost weight more rapidly when receiving injections of FMS than when they were given injections of saline. However, these results require confirmation, and the precise significance of FMS in long-term dieting is not certain, although the part that it plays (if any) is likely to be small.

TOTAL STARVATION

This is probably the oldest treatment used in obesity, but although very prolonged fasting was used extensively in the 1960s it seems to be practised less today. Patients should not be fasted for very prolonged periods for the simple purpose of 'burning up' endogenous fat, and such a regimen seems to miss the most important point in the treatment of obesity, which is to reverse the underlying hyperphagia by re-educating the patient in his dietary habits. Starvation is not re-education. Such prolonged fasting is not without danger: a number of deaths have been reported during total starvation, sometimes because the well-recognised contra-indications to the therapy were ignored. Many metabolic changes occur during prolonged fasting: an initial natriuresis, elevation of plasma uric acid levels, a negative nitrogen balance, abnormalities of liver function tests and, after very long periods of fasting, atrophy of the jejunal mucosa. It is uncertain whether all of these changes are completely reversible. A negative nitrogen balance is particularly undesirable, although it has been found that even after relatively prolonged starvation the participation of protein metabolism in energy expenditure on exercise is very small.

Many physicians feel that shorter periods of starvation restricted to from five to ten days are of value as an introduction to dietary therapy. Hollifield (1964) has shown that after such short periods of starvation there is temporary depression of appetite and increased satiety, for a variable period, on refeeding which thus enables the patient to keep more easily to his diet. During short periods of starvation the patient rarely feels hungry after the first 12 to 24 hours. He may feel a little 'light headed', but commonly has an almost exaggerated feeling of well-being. Ketonuria is invariable after the first two to three days.

The main purposes of such a short period of starvation are:

1. to demontrate to the patient that considerable weight loss is possible;
2. to make use of the temporary satiety effect on refeeding.

Weight loss averages 1·6 to 2 lb a day over the first seven to ten days of fasting, but much of this is due to loss of water. On refeeding, water retention ensues, and unless the patient is warned to expect this he may become very discouraged as he sees his weight rise, even on a strict diet. This tendency to fluid retention may be minimised by the judicious use of diuretics on refeeding. While some of the metabolic changes referred to above do tend to occur even during a short period of starvation, they appear in all cases to be rapidly and completely reversible. Fasting should always be carried out in hospital with the patient's activities restricted to a minimum. Complete bed rest should be advised if symptoms of postural hypotension occur. Adequate calorie-free fluids and supplementary vitamins should be given. The period of fasting should not exceed four days in the adolescent or ten days in the adult, and it is advisable not to use the regimen in those under fourteen or over sixty years of age. Patients with gout, atherosclerosis, ischaemic heart disease, heart failure, uncontrolled diabetes or peptic ulcer should *never* be subjected to starvation. Provided these precautions are taken, fasting for up to ten days seems to be without any danger. Recurrent short periods of starvation every four to eight weeks may be used, and it has been suggested that such regimens produce better long-term results than simple reducing diets, although it is possible that the interest and enthusiasm of the physician is as much responsible for this as the periods of fasting.

DRUGS IN THE TREATMENT OF OBESITY

Appetite suppressants have a small role in the treatment of obesity. Amphetamines and derivatives with amphetamine-like actions should never be used. All too often appetite suppressants are handed to the patient without adequate explanation, and the obese person then places more emphasis on taking his tablets than sticking to his diet, in the forlorn hope that his fat will magically be melted away. Clinical trials, even those in controlled situations, may be misleading in the circumstances of obesity, but there seems no doubt that fenfluramine and diethylpropion have significant anorectic effects. Some of the apparent benefit obtained from these drugs in routine clinical use may be due to a placebo effect. The initial dose of fenfluramine (Ponderax) is 20 mg at mid-morning and 40 mg in the evening. Fenfluramine appears to have a number of interesting metabolic effects (Butterfield and Whichelow, 1968; Bliss, Kirk and Newall, 1972); but it is difficult to separate many of these from metabolic effects due to weight loss as a result of the undoubted anorectic effect of the drug, and Garrow, Belton and Daniels (1972) have failed to demonstrate any mechanism whereby fenfluramine can promote weight loss other than by its effect in reducing appetite. As an alternative, diethylpropion (Apisate or Tenuate) may be used —the initial dose is one tablet taken before breakfast. Both fenfluramine in comparatively low dosage and diethylpropion fared equally in a trial conducted by Silverstone, Cooper and Begg (1970). Appetite suppressants should not be used in the initial treatment of obesity, as they may detract from the emphasis that must be placed on the reducing diet. At a later stage of therapy they may be given to patients who frankly admit to difficulty in keeping to their diets, but only after the reason for their use has been explained. If they are seen to be ineffective, their use should be discontinued.

Bulk preparations of methyl cellulose and guar gum are sometimes used to give a feeling of satiety. They often do not help, and the physiological basis for their use is dubious since if rats are given diets diluted with kaolin they rapidly consume a greater quantity of the diet to maintain weight. It seems, therefore, that animals, at least, eat for calories rather than bulk, and, according to Sebrell (1961), so too does man. It has already been mentioned that many obese individuals do not appear to experience the sensation of satiety.

Biguanides. Both phenformin and metformin have been reported to induce weight loss in obese non-diabetic patients without lowering the blood sugar. Part of the weight loss seems to be due to the anorectic effects of the dugs, although this does not fully explain their mode of action, and they also appear slightly to reduce the absorption of carbohydrate and produce a fall in high plasma insulin levels. The incidence of gastric irritation with these drugs is fairly high. The dose of metformin is 500 mg tds, that of phenformin sustained-release preparation 50 mg bd.

Diuretics are occasionally of use in the treatment of obesity and minimise the tendency to water-retention which so often occurs during a period of strict dieting. Frusemide or one of the thiazides may be used, but it should be remembered that the latter group may impair carbohydrate tolerance or induce frank diabetes in prediabetic individuals.

Thyroid hormones should *never* be used unless the patient has proven thyroid deficiency.

OTHER METHODS OF TREATMENT

Group therapy should not be derided and is probably one of the main reasons for the success of 'Weight-Watchers' clubs, although here the financial considerations involved are undoubtedly additional incentives which are shown to greatest effect in 'health farms'. An enthusiastic and dedicated general practitioner, with the help of a health visitor and if possible a dietitian, can achieve worthwhile results by starting a group obesity clinic.

Operations for obesity probably have a small place in the treatment of highly selected patients, although their use may be extended as experience increases. The purpose of the commonest operation, jejunoileostomy, is to produce a carefully controlled state of malabsorption, and it is a formidable procedure with a significant mortality and morbidity, which is still largely experimental. Its use (if it is used at all) should at present be restricted to very carefully selected obese patients (*British Medical Journal*, 1971).

'Apronectomy' has little or no place in the effective treatment of obesity. The amount of fat which can be removed by this procedure is comparatively trivial, there is a high incidence of postoperative complications, and the weight lost is usually rapidly regained. Removal of redundant folds of abdominal skin after successful and sustained weight reduction is rarely necessary, but is sometimes performed for cosmetic reasons.

THE BENEFITS OF WEIGHT LOSS

The obese patient may be assured that he will feel much fitter and be much healthier if successful weight loss is achieved. There are no symptoms or complications referrable to obesity that are not improved or cured by weight loss. Glycosuria and its associated symptoms will be improved in the diabetic, exercise tolerance will be greater, all grades of elevated blood pressure will fall, the pains of osteoarthrosis will be improved, and angina may vanish. In the younger patient, the benefits due to increased appeal to the opposite sex are not to be overlooked.

REFERENCES

Beaumont, J. L., Carlson, L. A., Cooper, G. R., Fejfar, Z., Fredrickson, D. S., and Strasser, T. (1970). *Bull. Wld. Hlth. Org.*, **43**, 891.

Bliss, B. P., Kirk, C. J. C., and Newall, R. G. (1972). *Postgrad. Med. J.*, **48**, 413.

Bloom, W. L., and Eidex, M. F. (1967). *Metabolism*, **16**, 679.

Brook, C. G. D. (1972). *Lancet*, **ii**, 624.

Burwell, C. S., Robin, E. D., Whaley, R. D., and Bickelmann, A. G. (1956). *Amer. J. Med.*, **21**, 811.

Butterfield, W. J. H., and Whichelow, M. J. (1968). *Lancet*, **ii**, 109.
Davison, Sir S., and Passmore, R. (1966). In *Human Nutrition and Dietetics*, 3rd Edition. Edinburgh and London: Livingstone.
Durnin, J. V. G. A. (1971). *Brit. J. Hosp. Med.*, **5**, 649.
Durnin, J. V. G. A. and Rahaman, M. M. (1967). *Brit J. Nutr.*, **21**, 681.
Editorial (1971). *Brit. med. J.*, **4**, 247.
Galton, D. J. (1966). *Brit. med. J.*, **2**, 1948.
Galton, D. J., and Wilson, J. P. D. (1970). *Clin. Sci.*, **38**, 661.
Garrow, J. S., Belton, E. A., and Daniels, A. (1972). *Lancet*, **ii**, 559.
Hamwi, G. J., and Urbach, S. (1953). *Metabolism*, **2**, 391.
Hirsch, J., and Knittle, J. (1970). *Fedn. Proc.*, **29**, 1516.
Hollifield, G., Owen, J. A., Jr., Lindsay, R. W., and Parson, W. (1964). *Southern Med. J.*, **57**, 1012.
Hytten, F. E., Taylor, K., and Taggart, N. (1966). *Clin. Sci.*, **31**, 111.
Issekutz, B., Jr., Bortz, W. M., Miller, H. I., and Paul, P. (1967). *Metabolism*, **16**, 1001.
Kekwick, A. (1960). *Brit. med. J.*, **ii**, 407.
Kekwick, A., and Pawan, G. L. S. (1956). *Lancet*, **ii**, 155.
Kekwick, A., and Pawan, G. L. S. (1967). *Metabolism*, **16**, 787.
Kekwick, A., and Pawan, G. L. S. (1968). *Lancet*, **ii**, 198.
Kinsell, L. W., Gunning, B., Michaels, G. D., Richardson, J., Cox, S. E., and Lemon, C. (1964). *Metabolism*, **13**, 195.
Lesser, G. T., Deutsch, S., and Markofsky, J. (1971). *Metabolism*, **20**, 792.
Marriott, H. L. (1949). *Brit. med. J.*, **2**, 18.
Mayer, J. (1965). *Ann. N.Y. Acad. Sci.*, **131**, 502.
Rose, G. A., and Williams, R. T. (1961). *Britl J. Nutrit.*, **15, 1.**
Salans, L. B., Knittle, J., and Hirsch, J. (1968). *J. clin. Invest.*, **47**, 153.
Sebrell, W. H. (1961). *Fedn. Proc.*, **20**, 393.
Sieker, H. O., Estes, E. H., Kelser, G. A., and McIntosh, H. D. (1955). *Amer. J. clin. Invest.*, **34**, 916.
Silverstone, J. T., Cooper, R. M., and Begg, R. R. (1970). *Brit. J. Clin. Pract.*, **24**, 423.
Stern, J., Batchelor, B. R., Hollander, N., Cohn, C. K., and Hirsch, J. (1972). *Lancet*, **ii**, 948.
Stunkard, A. J., and Blumenthal, S. A. (1972). *Metabolism*, **21**, 599.

18

PARATHYROID GLANDS AND CALCIUM METABOLISM

THE PARATHYROID GLANDS

EMBRYOLOGY

The superior parathyroids arise from the dorsal portion of the fourth branchial pouch, and migrate caudally together with the thyroid to reach their final position on its posterior surface. Aberrant superior glands may be found between the thyroid and oesophagus, within the carotid sheath, behind the innominate vein and, rarely, in the posterior mediastinum. The inferior pair arise with the thymus from the third branchial pouch and must, therefore, cross the superior pair during their migration. The position of the inferior glands is less constant than that of the superior pair, and ectopic inferior parathyroids may lie anywhere from the site of origin of the thymus in the neck to its final resting place in the anterior mediastinum. Widely displaced glands are relatively rare and 95 per cent of the inferior parathyroids are found in the immediate vicinity of the lower pole of the thyroid.

ANATOMY

The normal glands vary in size, shape, and location. In 88 per cent of individuals four glands are present. They are usually small brown bodies, situated along the posterior surface of the thyroid gland and measuring about 6 mm in length, 3 to 4 mm in breadth, and 0·5 to 2 mm in thickness. The superior glands are usually situated at the level of the lower border of the cricoid cartilage, behind the junction of the pharynx and oesophagus. The inferior pair may be situated below the thyroid gland, or in relation to one of the inferior thyroid veins. In man, the parathyroid glands are always outside the capsule of the thyroid gland, and on the occasions when a parathyroid gland is found apparently embedded within the substance of the thyroid, it will always be found to be separated from the thyroid by the capsule. The average weight of one superior gland varies between 20 and 40 mg, and of one inferior gland between 30 and 50 mg; the total weight of parathyroid tissue in one individual being about 120 mg.

Blood and Nerve Supply. The parathyroid glands receive a rich blood supply from the inferior thyroid arteries or from the anastomoses between the superior and inferior thyroid vessels. Identification of the inferior thyroid artery helps to localise the glands. Their nerve supply is derived from the sympathetic nervous system, either directly from the superior or middle cervical ganglia, or indirectly via a plexus in the fascia on the posterior surface of the thyroid gland.

HISTOLOGY

With increasing age, the colour of the glands changes from brown to yellow, due to the deposition of fat, and the compact epithelial cell complexes are divided even more by connective tissue stroma. The characteristics of the four types of cell present in the gland are shown in Table 18.1.

TABLE 18.1 *The Cells of the Parathyroid Glands*

Cell type (and synonyms)	Appearance	Function	Other details
Chief cell (principal cell, light chief cell)	Rich in glycogen Small Golgi apparatus. Scanty endoplasmic reticulum. Few secretory granules. Dark nuclei, definite chromatin network.	Secrete parathyroid hormone.	May rarely become hyperplastic and assume secretory function.
Transitional cell (dark chief cell)	Poor in glycogen. Prominent Golgi apparatus and endoplasmic reticulum. Many secretory granules.	Main source of parathyroid hormone.	Derived from chief cells.
Oxyphil cell (eosinophil cell)	No glycogen. Granular cytoplasm. Smaller denser nuclei. Vary in size but larger than chief cells.	Secrete parathyroid hormone.	Appear after puberty. Derived from chief cells.
Water clear cell	Large polygonal cells up to 40 μ Cytoplasm inconspicuous, vacuolated.	None assigned but capable of secreting parathyroid hormone.	Appear after puberty. Derived from chief cells.

PARATHYROID HORMONE

Parathyroid hormone is an 84 amino-acid straight chain polypeptide without disulphide bridges. The complete sequences of the bovine and porcine hormones have been established (Parsons and Potts, 1972). The sequence of the first 37 amino-acids of human parathyroid hormone has also been determined. They differ from those of bovine and porcine parathyroid hormone, but in man, as in the pig, the amino terminal residue is serine. Biological activity resides in the amino terminal part of the molecule. A peptide consisting of the first 34 amino-acids has been synthesized and shown to have both phosphaturic and calcium-mobilising activity. A 90 amino-acid prohormone is believed to be present within the parathyroid glands akin to proinsulin in the islet cells.

ACTIONS OF PARATHYROID HORMONE

The biochemical changes that result from an excess of parathyroid hormone are:

1. hypercalcaemia,
2. hypophosphataemia,
3. hyperphosphaturia,
4. hypercalcuria,
5. increased urinary hydroxyproline excretion.

The main function of parathyroid hormone is to regulate the concentration of ionised calcium in body fluids, by its actions on bone, the small intestine and the kidneys. The relative importance of the osseous and renal regulatory mechanisms is still controversial. Rapid regulation of serum calcium levels probably depends on simple buffering by the large exchangeable calcium pool in bone. Intermediate regulation probably involves both bone and kidney, whereas long-term regulation is probably mediated by renal and intestinal mechanisms.

Action on Bone. Parathyroid hormone acts directly on bone to accelerate its metabolic destruction. This action is a complex one, involving effects of parathyroid hormone on virtually all of the constituents of bone (Rasmussen, 1971).

Calcium mobilisation is enhanced with resultant hypercalcaemia, an action opposed by calcitonin. Parathyroid hormone activates adenyl cyclase in both bone and kidney and also increases uptake of calcium by these cells which may be revealed by a transient hypocalcaemia after an injection of the hormone. The rise in intracellular cyclic AMP concentration which results from stimulation of the adenyl cyclase system leads to activation of one or more protein kinases with the resultant phosphorylation of specific proteins which mediate the cellular response. Cyclic AMP also alters the distribution of calcium within the cell, causing a shift from the mitochondrial pool to the cell cytosol. Thus parathyroid hormone increases the calcium concentration within the cell cytosol by a direct action on the cell membrane, increasing its permeability to calcium and indirectly via cyclic AMP which causes a shift in calcium to the cytosol. Calcium enhances some of the cyclic AMP effects since it is in itself an activator of some of the phosphoprotein products of the cyclic AMP-dependent protein kinases. In addition calcium acts as a negative feedback inhibitor of adenyl cyclase and may enhance destruction of cyclic AMP by activating the phosphodiesterase system. The magnitude of the effect of parathyroid hormone on bone appears to depend on the serum calcium level, possibly because in hypocalcaemia less calcium enters bone as second messenger. The hypercalcaemia induced by parathyroid hormone is probably complex, involving fast and slow components, the latter involving new enzyme synthesis.

Bone matrix is also affected by parathyroid hormone which enhances its destruction. This action is mirrored by an increase in plasma and urinary levels of hydroxyproline.

Cellular effects of parathyroid hormone are also important. It stimulates synthesis of cytoplasmic RNA in osteoclasts and increases secretion of collagenase and a variety of other lysosomal enzymes concerned with matrix destruction, including an acid phosphatase. Cyclic AMP and increased cell cytosol calcium may both be involved in this increased enzyme production. Complex effects of parathyroid hormone on osteocytes and osteoblasts are also involved in its actions on bone.

Action on Kidneys. Parathyroid hormone has two apparently independent actions. It inhibits proximal renal tubular reabsorption of phosphate which leads to phosphaturia and hypophosphataemia. This action may be related in some way to a parallel inhibition of sodium reabsorption and is probably mediated by the adenyl cyclase system. Parathyroid hormone also decreases calcium excretion by a different mechanism at a different site. This action tends to be obscured by the effect of parathyroid hormone on bone, whereby enhanced calcium mobilisation increases serum calcium concentrations and provides a greater filtered load with resultant hypercalcuria.

Action on Small Intestine. Calcium absorption is increased by parathyroid hormone, possibly by a direct action on membrane permeability to calcium. There is as yet no firm evidence that vitamin D is involved in the action of the hormone on calcium absorption. The action of parathyroid hormone on the intestine may be important in the long-term adaptation to a low calcium intake. Phosphate and magnesium absorption by the intestine are also increased by the action of parathyroid hormone.

CONTROL OF PARATHYROID HORMONE SECRETION

The concentration of ionised calcium in the blood regulates the secretion of parathyroid hormone, a low level of calcium leading to increased output of the hormone. If the serum ionised calcium is raised by mechanisms other than hyperparathyroidism, parathyroid hormone secretion is reduced, though the immediate lowering of serum calcium is probably mediated by calcitonin (*see* below). Hypermagnesaemia has also been shown to lower parathyroid hormone output but this probably has no physiological significance. There is no evidence that elevations in serum phosphate levels stimulate hormone output, and the parathyroid hyperplasia seen in chronic renal failure is probably due to mechanisms other than the hyperphosphataemia.

Distribution and Fate of Parathyroid Hormone

Parathyroid hormone has a very short half-life in the circulation—mean values of about 20 minutes have been reported—and changes in secretion rate in response to fluctuations in the blood calcium are rapid. It has been postulated that the liver destroys part of the circulating hormone and fragments of the hormone can be detected in the bloodstream and the urine.

ASSAY OF PARATHYROID HORMONE

Various bioassay techniques have been developed to measure the hormone in blood. One of these, in rats, was based exclusively on phosphate excretion and was too insensitive to detect activity in the blood of normal rats. Another more widely used technique is based upon the calcium mobilising action of the hormone and employs thyroparathyroidectomised rats. More recently, parathyroid hormone has been assayed by a method based on the action of the hormone in increasing phosphate uptake by isolated mitochondria. The most sensitive technique for assaying parathyroid hormone in biological fluids is the radioimmunoassay. There are many technical difficulties to overcome when human plasma is used and most assays have utilised an antibody to bovine parathyroid hormone which shows partial cross reaction with the human hormone. Few assays have so far been capable of detecting the small amounts of hormone in normal plasma but the raised levels seen in chronic renal failure and primary hyperparathyroidism are usually detectable. The situation is further complicated by the rapid appearance of hormone fragments, which may affect the results. Normal values found by O'Riordan *et al.* (1972) using both a standard radioimmunoassay and an immunoradiometric assay (which uses labelled antibody as tracer rather than labelled hormone) range from 0·15–1·2 ng/ml with a mean of 0·4 ng/ml.

CALCITONIN

It was demonstrated some years ago that thyroparathyroidectomised dogs could not respond normally to an acute calcium load, and from 1957 onwards Copp carried out a series of experiments that indicated the presence of a circulating hypocalcaemic factor which he named calcitonin. He considered that this hormone was secreted by the parathyroid glands, but later work demonstrated that calcitonin originates in the thyroid. A comprehensive review on the subject of calcitonin has been provided by Foster *et al.* (1972).

Source of Calcitonin

Foster *et al.* (1964) were the first to suggest that the parafollicular or C cells of the thyroid were the site of origin of the hormone. The parafollicular cells are distinct from the follicular cells of the thyroid, being derived from the neural crest, from which they migrate to the last branchial pouch. This explains why medullary carcinomas and phaeochromocytomas, both of neuroectodermal origin, contain a variety of amines and are sometimes associated in the familial medullary carcinoma of the thyroid syndrome. The C cells are members of the APUD cell series. The term APUD is derived from the initial letters of the three most reliable characteristics *A*mine content, amine-*P*recursor *U*ptake, and amino-acid *D*ecarboxylase content. The series includes the medullary carcinoma, bronchial and intestinal carcinoids and phaeochromocytomas. The common origin also explains why C cell tumours can secrete ACTH and carcinoid cells on occasion produce calcitonin. In non-mammalian vertebrates such as fish, reptiles, and birds the ultimobranchial glands which also arise from the neural crest, remain separate—the thyroid gland of the chicken does not contain any detectable calcitonin, whereas the ultimobranchial gland contains a large amount. Calcitonin should not, therefore, be regarded as an exclusively thyroid hormone, and the original name calcitonin is preferable to thyrocalcitonin.

In man calcitonin is also present in the parathyroids and thymus as well as in the thyroid. This could explain why no striking changes in bone metabolism are seen in totally thyroidectomised patients adequately maintained on thyroxine. If C cells are present outside the thyroid, then tumours of these cells (medullary carcinomas) might be expected to arise outside the thyroid.

H - Cys - Gly - Asn - Leu - Ser - Thr - Cys - Met - Leu - Gly -
1 2 3 4 5 6 7 8 9 10

- Thr - Tyr - Thr - Gln - Asp - Phe - Asn - Lys - Phe - His - Thr -
11 12 13 14 15 16 17 18 19 20 21

- Phe - Pro - Gln - Thr - Ala - Ile - Gly - Val - Gly - Ala - Pro* - NH_2
22 23 24 25 26 27 28 29 30 31 32

* (Prolinamide)

FIGURE 18.1 Structure of human calcitonin.

Structure of Calcitonin

Human calcitonin has been purified, sequenced and synthesized. It is a single chain, 32 amino-acid polypeptide (Fig. 18.1) with a molecular weight near 3,000. There are 18 amino-acid substitutions when compared with porcine calcitonin, a surprisingly high number of changes. As well as the calcitonin monomer (calcitonin M), a dimer (calcitonin D) has also been isolated from human medullary carcinoma tissue. This is composed of two monomers covalently linked in anti-parallel fashion by rearrangement of the disulphide bond. The complete 32 amino-acid peptide is essential for full biological activity and integrity of the first nine amino-acids is probably of major importance. Salmon calcitonin which differs in amino-acid sequence from human calcitonin, has a longer half-life and is a more potent calcium-lowering agent on a weight basis.

Factors Affecting Secretion of Calcitonin (Foster *et al.*, 1972)

The major stimulus for calcitonin secretion is a rise in the serum calcium level, but other factors, including magnesium, some hormones e.g. glucagon, and antibiotics may also be involved. Hypercalcaemia has a direct action on the C cells, increasing both the synthesis and secretion of calcitonin. Hypermagnesaemia also stimulates calcitonin secretion but at levels higher than are seen under physiological or pathological conditions. Glucagon, pancreozymin and streptomycin stimulate calcitonin secretion but the significance of these observations is unknown.

Sites and Mechanisms of Action and Distribution of Calcitonin.

Calcitonin inhibits bone resorption but has no effect on bone formation, an action reflected by a reduced urinary excretion of hydroxyproline. Unlike parathyroid hormone, calcitonin has no significant actions on the gut. Urinary excretion of phosphate and sodium is increased but the physiological significance of the renal effects is unknown.

The mechanism of action of calcitonin is also unknown. It acts on bone cells to lower the calcium concentration in the cytosol by increasing calcium efflux from the cell and enhancing calcium uptake into the mitochondrial compartment. Although cyclic AMP concentrations within the cell are increased by the calcitonin-induced fall in cytosol calcium concentration which activates adenyl cyclase, bone resorption is inhibited because of the lowered cytosol calcium which inactivates some of the phosphoprotein products of the cyclic AMP-dependent protein kinases.

Calcitonin is mainly concentrated in the liver and kidney and the latter is the main site of its degradation. The half-life of human calcitonin is less than 15 minutes.

Assay of Calcitonin

Calcitonin can be assayed by its effect on the serum calcium of rats. The sensitivity of the assay can be greatly increased by the use of a high phosphate diet or by giving injections of phosphate at the time that the animals are given calcitonin. Radioimmunoassays for calcitonin capable of detecting the amounts present in the circulation in normal man have now been developed.

Physiological Significance of Calcitonin

The physiological role of calcitonin remains uncertain. It may be a factor involved in the regulation of the serum calcium concentration, acting along with parathyroid hormone to dampen oscillations in the serum calcium level. Evidence for this action of calcitonin has been obtained in totally thyroidectomised subjects infused with calcium. The rate at which their serum calcium level falls at the end of infusion is slower than normal suggesting the absence of a hypocalcaemic factor. It may protect bone and promote calcium storage in the skeleton. This action has been demonstrated in pregnant animals (Lewis *et al.*, 1971). Thirdly, it may influence calcium concentrations in the cell cytosol, thereby modifying the action of parathyroid hormone on bone and kidney.

Pathological Significance of Calcitonin

While no definite clinical syndromes are associated with calcitonin deficiency, increased calcitonin secretion has been demonstrated in certain situations. The medullary carcinoma of the thyroid is a tumour of the parafollicular cells and contains high levels of calcitonin (*see* Chapter 5). In the majority of cases, serum calcitonin levels are also raised or can be inappropriately raised by calcium infusions. Hence measurements of calcitonin are of value in the diagnosis of medullary carcinoma of the thyroid and in detecting its recurrence. No clinical sequelae result from the increased levels of calcitonin in the circulation but parathyroid hyperplasia and raised levels of parathyroid hormone can sometimes be demonstrated. Calcitonin can also be demonstrated in some carcinoid tumours, but rarely enters the circulation in this condition.

Clinical Applications of Calcitonin

Calcitonin is of value in the treatment of hypercalcaemia due to disseminated malignant disease, parathyroid adenomas, idiopathic hypercalcaemia of infancy and Vitamin D intoxication (*Brit. Med. J.*, 1973). Its major clinical role, however, is in the treatment of Paget's disease of bone. It is indicated if bone pain is troublesome and does not respond to simple analgesics, if there is extensive bone deformity or high-output cardiac failure, if there is evidence of compression of nerves or the spinal cord or if there is a fracture through a weight-bearing limb. Bone pain is relieved by calcitonin and there is a progressive fall in the numbers of osteoclasts and in the alkaline phosphatase and the urinary excretion of hydroxyproline. Calcium balance returns to normal and the bone formed during treatment has a normal lamellar structure. The hormone must be given by injection, initially once or twice daily and then possibly once or twice a week. At present porcine calcitonin is available for clinical use. Side-effects are minor and transient and include a feeling of warmth, flushing of the face and transient nausea and tingling in the pharynx and abdomen. Antibodies have not developed after treatment with the human hormone but could possibly pose problems with animal preparations.

There is as yet no good evidence that calcitonin has a place in the treatment of osteoporosis.

OTHER HORMONAL EFFECTS ON CALCIUM METABOLISM

1. *Adrenocortical Hormones.* The glucocorticoids cause:

(*a*) increased rate of gluconeogenesis and, thus, catabolism of protein, which will involve osteoid tissue;
(*b*) reduction in osteoblastic activity;
(*c*) decrease in the rate of bone formation;
(*d*) increased bone resorption;
(*e*) decreased calcium absorption from the gastrointestinal tract;
(*f*) increased calcium excretion by the kidneys.

In man, the glucocorticoids produce hypercalcuria, which is mainly due to a reduction in the amount of calcium removed from body fluids for deposition in bone, but serum calcium levels are not altered. In a number of conditions in which hypercalcaemia occurs, e.g. hypervitaminosis D, sarcoidosis, and in some patients with metastatic carcinoma, the administration of cortisol results in a fall in serum calcium concentrations due mainly to a reduction in the absorption of calcium, a test that can be used to differentiate these diseases from primary hyperparathyroidism.

Pharmacological doses of corticosteroids acting on calcium metabolism and on bone cause osteoporosis with thinning of both cortical bone and trabeculae. In the spine, compression of the weakened bone leads to relative prominence of the end plates of the vertebrae. Wedging and collapse of vertebrae result, with attacks of severe pain in the affected areas and ultimate reduction in height. Fractures of ribs, which are often spontaneous may occur, and are made obvious by the surrounding callus.

In children endochondral calcification is affected and as a result of this and other factors such as antagonism to the metabolic effects of growth hormone, there is a reduction in the rate of linear growth and shortness of stature.

2. *Thyroxine.* In the hypoparathyroid animal, parathyroid hormone and vitamin D are less effective in raising the serum calcium if there is an associated thyroid hormone deficiency. Thyroxine tends to produce hypercalcuria in association with increased bone resorption, but except

in the most severe cases of hyperthyroidism there is usually a reduction in the production of parathyroid hormone, so that normocalcaemia is maintained. Hypercalcaemia occasionally occurs in thyrotoxicosis but the reason for this is unknown. It does not appear to be related to any abnormalities of calcitonin production.

Hypothyroidism in infancy causes shortness of stature with retention of infantile proportions. There is failure of development of the nasal and orbital contours and retardation of bone age. As well as delay in ossification, there may be abnormal epiphyseal calcification termed epiphyseal dysgenesis. The cortex of the long bones may be greatly thickened. Hypothyroidism in adults has no striking effects on the skeleton, although occasional patients show hypercalcaemia.

3. *Glucagon* can cause hypocalcaemia in man both directly by inhibiting bone resorption and indirectly by causing release of calcitonin.

4. *Growth Hormone*. The effects of growth hormone on the rate of bone growth are discussed elsewhere. The hypercalcuria and increase in plasma inorganic phosphate seen in some cases of acromegaly are probably due to increased secretion of growth hormone. Most, if not all, of the metabolic actions of growth hormone on bone and cartilage may be mediated by sulphation factor produced in the liver.

5. *Sex Hormones*. (*a*) *Androgens*. These have a protein anabolic action and they also accelerate the rate of bone growth and stimulate osteogenesis. There is no direct effect on the serum calcium level, but urinary and faecal calcium excretion are reduced.

(*b*) *Oestrogens*. These also have a general protein anabolic effect, and are thought to have a specific stimulatory effect on the osteoblasts. Oestrogens cause more calcium retention than androgens. Early castration may result in osteoporosis whereas oestrogen administration causes a fall in urinary calcium excretion possibly due to the slight fall in serum calcium which results from inhibition of bone resorption.

EFFECTS OF VITAMIN D ON CALCIUM METABOLISM

VITAMIN D

Vitamin D is the generic name for a group of sterol compounds that possess a significant antirachitic effect. Vitamin D_2, also known as calciferol, ergocalciferol and irradiated ergosterol, is of plant origin. Vitamin D_3, also known as cholecalciferol and activated 7-dehydrocholesterol, is found in animals and may be produced by radiation of 7-dehydrocholesterol in the skin. Antitetanic substance No. 10 (AT10) is a mixture, the main component of which is dihydrotachysterol. The structures of vitamin D_2, vitamin D_3 and dihydrotachysterol are shown in Fig. 18.2.

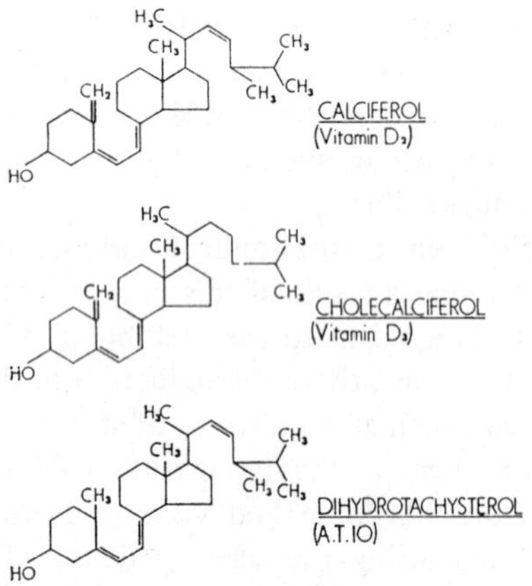

FIGURE 18.2 Structure of calciferol (vitamin D_2), cholecalciferol (vitamin D_3) and dihydrotachysterol (AT 10)

The major action of vitamin D is to ensure the calcification of newly formed bone. In the absence of vitamin D, osteoid remains uncalcified and rickets or osteomalacia results. Vitamin D also has a direct but complex action on the kidney, increasing renal excretion of calcium out of proportion to the changes in serum calcium and in certain circumstances reducing the rate of phosphate excretion.

CALCIFEROL

Dose. In the prevention of rickets—20 μg (800 units) daily; in the treatment of rickets and osteomalacia—0·125–1·25 mg (5,000 to 50,000 units) daily; in the treatment of hypoparathyroidism, 1·25–5 mg (50,000 to 200,000 units) daily.

Toxic Effects. These usually result from prolonged high doses, but occasional patients are sensitive to relatively low doses and tolerance may vary. Symptoms of overdosage are anorexia, nausea, vomiting, diarrhoea, polyuria, thirst, headache, lassitude and muscular weakness, drowsiness and mental symptoms. Most of these are manifestations of hypercalcaemia. Calcium may be deposited in many tissues, including arteries and the kidneys, and hypertension and renal failure may ensue. All patients receiving high doses of calciferol should be kept under outpatient observation with checks of the serum calcium and phosphate levels.

Treatment of calciferol toxicity is similar to that for hypercalcaemia. Obviously, the drug should be withdrawn and only re-introduced if necessary at a much lower dosage level with careful monitoring.

Human Requirements. The recommended daily dietary intake for infants, children and adults including females during pregnancy and lactation is 400 units (10 μg).

Uses. Calciferol is necessary for the absorption of calcium and phosphorus from the gut, and deficiency is associated with rickets in children and osteomalacia in adults and may play a part in dental caries. Poor absorption may occur in chronic diarrhoea, steatorrhoea and biliary obstruction when the dose must be increased. Calciferol may also assist in the healing of bone disease associated with hyperparathyroidism. In this situation, only small doses should be used and the complication of hypercalcaemia should be borne in mind.

Preparations

Calciferol capsules (*Univ. Coll. Hosp.*) contain calciferol 0·25 or 1 mg in arachis oil.

Calciferol injection (*BPC, BNF*) contain calciferol 7·5 mg (300,000 units) per ml.

Strong calciferol tablets (*BP, BNF*) contain 1·25 mg (50,000 units).

Calcium with vitamin D tablets (*BPC, BNF*) contain calcium sodium lactate 450 mg, calcium phosphate 150 mg (total calcium content not less than 79 mg) and calciferol 12·5 μg (500 units).

Calcium-vitamin D mixture for infants contains calcium gluconate 50 mg, calcium lactate 50 mg, calcium hypophosphite 25 mg and calciferol 15 μg (600 units) with syrup to 5 ml.

CHOLECALCIFEROL

Dose. This is the same as for calciferol. Cholecalciferol is the chief form of vitamin D present in fish-liver oils. Like calciferol it contains 40,000 units of antirachitic activity per mg.

Toxic Effects, Requirements and Uses are the same as for calciferol. Some patients who have become resistant to calciferol may still respond to cholecalciferol. Cholecalciferol has been used as a test for Vitamin D deficiency. After giving a dose of 1 mg intravenously (mixing the solution with venous blood immediately prior to injection), a significant increase in the serum phosphate on the fourth or fifth days after injection indicates Vitamin D deficiency.

Preparations

Cholecalciferol capsules (*Univ. Coll. Hosp.*) contain 0·25 or 1 mg in arachis oil.

Cholecalciferol injection contains 100 mg of the vitamin, 10 ml dehydrated alcohol and propylene glycol to 100 ml, 1 ml doses being used as a test for vitamin D deficiency.

DIHYDROTACHYSTEROL

Dose. 0·125 to 1·25 mg daily.

Toxic Effects and Uses are similar to those of calciferol. It is given by mouth in an oily solution containing 250 μg per ml. In the acute treatment of the hypocalcaemia of hypoparathyroidism, daily doses of 0·25–2·5 mg raise the serum calcium to normal in five to ten days. The dose is then reduced to a maintenance dose of 0·25-2·5 mg weekly.

Preparations

Dihydrotachysterol capsules (*Ind. NF*) contain 625 μg of the compound.

Dihydrotachysterol capsules (*Univ. Coll. Hosp.*) contain 0·1, 0·25 or 1 mg of the compound in arachis oil.

AT10 (*Winthrop*) contains 250 μg of dihydrotachysterol in each ml of oily solution.

1,25-DIHYDROXY-CHOLECALCIFEROL (1,25-DHCC)

This is the most potent form of vitamin D yet known and can be regarded as a hormone secreted by the kidney according to the needs of the body, which acts on gut and bone (Lawson *et al.*, 1971; Kodicek, 1972). It is produced in the kidney by further hydroxylation of 25-hydroxycholecalciferol (25-HCC), itself formed by hydroxylation of cholecalciferol in the liver. 25-HCC is the main circulating form of vitamin D being carried bound to an alpha$_2$ globulin. In the kidney 25-HCC can also be converted to an inactive or less active compound 21,25-DHCC. The delay in action of cholecalciferol can now be accounted for by the time required for its transformation to its active form, 1,25-DHCC.

In states of calcium depletion more 1,25-DHCC is formed in the kidney whereas when calcium supplies are abundant, inactive forms of vitamin D such as 21,25-DHCC are formed. Intracellular calcium concentrations may modify these processes. Parathyroid hormone may suppress the conversion of 25-HCC to 1,25-DHCC and enhance its conversion to 21,25-DHCC (Galante *et al.*, 1972), actions possibly mediated by changes in intracellular calcium concentrations. These findings could explain the occurrence of vitamin D deficiency (manifested as osteomalacia) in patients with primary hyperparathyroidism. Similarly, such an action of parathyroid hormone could contribute to the vitamin D resistance seen in chronic renal failure.

Cholecalciferol is inactive *in vitro* but both 25-HCC and 1,25-DHCC act on bone *in vitro* to increase calcium mobilisation. The effects of vitamin D can be abolished by giving actinomycin D which affects transcription of messenger RNA from DNA within the nucleus. It is likely that 1,25-DHCC causes production of a calcium-binding and transport protein within the cells of the intestinal mucosa, thereby enhancing calcium absorption.

SYNDROMES RESULTING FROM VITAMIN D DEFICIENCY OR RESISTANCE

Rickets and Osteomalacia

Children present with knock knees or bow legs shortly after they are able to stand and thickening of the wrists, prominence of the costochondral junctions and bossing of the skull may also be seen. The osteomalacia of adults presents with focal or diffuse pain particularly in the legs, ribs and spine. Walking may be difficult and the gait waddling. Proximal muscle weakness may cause difficulty in climbing stairs.

In this country rickets is now very rare in children because of the use of vitamin D supplements. Dietary vitamin D deficiency is seen more often in the elderly. Immigrants from India and Pakistan have a much higher incidence of these disorders, which is probably multifactorial in origin. Dietary vitamin D deficiency, pigmentation of the skin resulting in the synthesis of less endogenous vitamin D and calcium-binding by phytate from chapatis may all contribute to the development of osteomalacia. Certainly the level of 25-HCC is lower than normal in Asians especially those with a raised alkaline phosphatase or clinical osteomalacia.

The important diagnostic features of rickets and osteomalacia are:

1. Serum calcium low (or normal)
2. Serum phosphate low
3. Alkaline phosphatase high
4. Pseudofractures visible on X-ray
5. Bone biopsy shows excess osteoid.

Not all of these features may be present in an individual patient and the diagnosis may sometimes depend on the response to vitamin D treatment. In all cases the underlying cause for vitamin D deficiency should be sought.

Vitamin D-Resistant Rickets

Azotaemic Osteodystrophy is present in the majority of patients with long-standing severe renal failure (*see* section on secondary hyperparathyroidism, p. 409). It may show components of osteomalacia and osteitis fibrosa cystica and also osteoporosis and osteosclerosis. Large doses of vitamin D (50,000–150,000 units a day) or of dihydrotachysterol are required to treat the condition. The relative resistance to vitamin D may be due at least in part to the reduction in functional renal mass causing a decrease in synthesis of 1,25-DHCC. Such patients respond markedly to very small doses of 1,25-DHCC (Brickman *et al.*, 1972). The situation is different in the acute uraemic state where formation of 1,25-DHCC is not abnormal and some factor blocking the action of 1,25-DHCC after its entry into the intestinal mucosal cell has been postulated.

Malabsorption Syndromes may cause osteomalacia or rickets which respond to large doses of Vitamin D.

Renal Tubular Rickets may result from a variety of renal tubular disorders characterised by a renal leak of phosphate causing hypophosphataemia and hyperphosphaturia. The means by which hypophosphataemia leads to failure of calcification of newly formed bone is uncertain. Other renal tubular defects may also be present leading to glycosuria, amino-aciduria, hypokalaemia and renal tubular acidosis. In children the commonest form of the condition is inherited as a dominant sex-linked disorder with weaker penetrance in females. Similar cases can occur in adults without obvious cause, although very rarely bony tumours of the haemangiopericytoma type may be responsible and the disease can then be cured by excision of the tumour (Evans and Azzopardi, 1972). It is postulated that the tumour produces some factor which interferes with Vitamin D action.

Other Causes of Vitamin D-Resistant Rickets include chronic ingestion of aluminium hydroxide causing phosphate depletion and treatment with anti-convulsant drugs, especially barbiturates and phenytoin (Dent *et al.*, 1970). These drugs act largely by the induction of liver enzymes which accelerate the metabolism of vitamin D_3, increasing its conversion to 25-HCC and possibly its further metabolism and excretion in the bile.

CALCIUM AND PHOSPHATE HOMEOSTASIS AND THE DYNAMICS OF BONE

CALCIUM

The body of the adult contains about 1,000 g of calcium (25 moles), of which about 99 per cent is in the skeleton.

The Absorption of Calcium

The daily intake of calcium in the form of inorganic and organic salts is about 1 g. The faecal excretion of calcium represents not only unabsorbed calcium, but also calcium secreted from the upper gastrointestinal tract. There does not appear to be any significant excretion of calcium from the large bowel. The faecal excretion of calcium usually amounts to between 20 and 40 per cent of the intake, but may rarely exceed the intake. Calcium is absorbed in the upper small bowel, especially the duodenum. The absorption of calcium is an active process, the mineral being transported from the mucosal to the serosal fluid against an electrochemical gradient. Active absorption of calcium is more marked in the young. Vitamin D facilitates the absorption of calcium by acting directly upon the transport mechanism, and other factors that increase or decrease absorption are listed below

Increase	*Decrease*
1. Acid environment (increases solubility of calcium).	1. Alkali.
2. Parathyroid hormone (dependent on presence of vitamin D).	2. Excessive fat in the intestinal contents.
3. High-protein diet.	3. Excess oxalates.
4. Pregnancy.	4. Excess phosphate, particularly in the form of insoluble phytates.
5. Low calcium diet or prolonged calcium deprivation.	5. Glucocorticoids.
6. Certain disease states associated with increased sensitivity to vitamin D, e.g. sarcoidosis.	6. Vitamin D resistance (as in chronic renal failure).

Distribution of Calcium (Fig. 18.3)

After absorption, calcium enters the calcium pool in the plasma and extracellular fluid (approximately 900 mg).

This calcium pool is constantly being exchanged by:

1. gastrointestinal absorption and secretion
2. glomerular filtration and tubular reabsorption
3. bone deposition and resorption
4. ion exchange with the calcium in the crystals of the bone mineral.

This last process is very rapid, and the entire extracellular calcium pool exchanges several times each day without there being any net gain or loss in the pool of extracellular calcium. There is no turnover of calcium in the teeth, although if calcium metabolism is abnormal in childhood the teeth may fail to calcify.

The normal uncorrected fasting serum calcium level ranges from 8·2–10·2 mg per cent, but values differ from laboratory to laboratory. Some of the calcium in the circulation is loosely bound to protein, mainly albumin (about 0·8 mg is bound per gram of albumin) and is non-diffusible. A small amount (less than 5 per cent) is diffusible but non-ionised, being complexed for example to

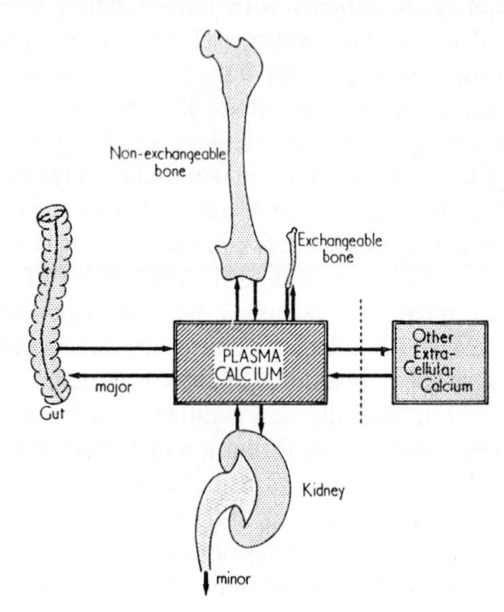

FIGURE 18.3 Distribution of calcium

citrate, and the remainder (about 50 per cent) is ionised. The ionised calcium is the only fraction which has been shown to have physiological and pathological importance.

The rather wide normal range for serum calcium is largely due to the wide variations in serum protein concentrations, especially of serum albumin. The serum albumin, and hence the total calcium, but not the ionised calcium, falls with age, in liver disease and often in the presence of systemic disease, whereas it increases with venous stasis. It is necessary to make allowances for the protein-bound calcium fraction, usually on the basis of a simultaneous serum albumin measurement. It is assumed that: albumin binds 100 per cent of the bound calcium (in fact 80 per cent is bound to albumin and 20 per cent to globulins); the binding factor is not affected by the concentration of albumin; the serum pH remains constant. On the basis of these assumptions, each gram of albumin is considered to bind 0·8 mg of calcium and a nominal mean albumin of 4·7 g/100 ml is used. For each 0·1 g of albumin above the nominal mean of 4·7 g/100 ml, 0·08 mg/100 ml of calcium is subtracted from the estimated total serum calcium. Conversely, for each 0·1 g of albumin below the nominal mean, 0·08 mg of calcium is added to the total serum calcium. Using these corrections, the upper limit of normal for the serum calcium is 10·5 mg/100 ml. In the presence of wide deviations of plasma protein levels from normal, the results of such corrections must be interpreted with caution.

The total serum calcium level may be altered considerably in hyper- and hypoproteinaemic states. The fraction of prime biological importance is the ionised calcium, which appears to be concerned with the various metabolic functions of calcium and is maintained by efficient homeostatic mechanisms in which parathyroid hormone and possibly calcitonin play a major part. An increase in bicarbonate (as in non-respiratory alkalosis), phosphate, citrate (as in massive blood transfusions), or other organic ions will result in an increase in complexed calcium and a reduction in ionised calcium levels, thus producing tetany in the presence of a normal total calcium concentration. Respiratory alkalosis produced by hyperventilation will also produce tetany by reducing the proportion of ionised calcium. Acidosis, non-respiratory or respiratory, increases the ionisation of calcium. The concentration of calcium in the extracellular fluid is about 70 per cent of that in the plasma. In intracellular fluid the calcium concentration is very low, and most appears to be in a bound form.

Calcium in Urine. The situation here is more complex than in plasma. The phosphate concentration may be high, and the solubility product of calcium phosphate may be exceeded in normal urine. However, the high concentration of anions such as nitrate, lactate, and glucuronate is usually sufficient to keep the calcium ions in solution. The high concentration of urea serves also to increase the solubility of the calcium salts.

Excretion of Calcium

Calcium may leave the body by several routes:

1. In faeces as a constituent of the intestinal secretions (major route).
2. In urine.
3. To the fetus during pregnancy.
4. In milk during lactation.

Although nearly 10 g of calcium are filtered each day by the glomeruli, only 1 to 2 per cent of this (100–200 mg) is excreted in the urine. The process of tubular reabsorption of calcium, like that of absorption of calcium from the gut, is an active one. There does not seem to be a well-established maximum tubular capacity for calcium, and even in hypercalcaemia, with consequent hypercalcuria, only a small part of the calcium filtered at the glomeruli appears in the urine. Urinary excretion of calcium becomes negligible when the total serum calcium level falls below 7·5 mg per cent. At the other extreme, any increase in serum calcium concentration is reflected by hypercalcuria. The main factor controlling the excretion of calcium is the filtered load—the product of the serum ionisable calcium concentration and the glomerular filtration rate. The urinary excretion of calcium may, therefore, be profoundly influenced by disturbances in the glomerular filtration rate.

PHOSPHATE

The bulk of phosphate in the body is present within the bone and only 10–20 per cent is situated in the plasma and in tissue cells.

Absorption

The normal adult requires an intake of about 0·8 g of phosphate (calculated as phosphorus) per day, while larger amounts are necessary in the growing child, and the pregnant or lactating woman. Phosphate is present in food in either organic or inorganic forms and any ingested in the organic form must be hydrolysed before absorption. The proportion of ingested phosphate absorbed is high, although certain organic phosphates such as phytates resist hydrolysis, and hence are not absorbed. There does not seem to be any very effective mechanism for controlling phosphate absorption, a process that is not well understood. Since most of the dietary phosphate is absorbed from the gut, there is virtually no phosphorus in the faeces. Renal phosphorus excretion must therefore equal the dietary intake, and the prime site of regulation of phosphorus balance is in the kidney. Neither vitamin D nor parathyroid hormone appear to affect phosphate absorption directly. Factors that do influence the process include:

Increase	*Decrease*
1. Low calcium diet.	1. High calcium diet.
2. Excess of fat.	2. Alkali.
3. Acids.	3. Divalent or trivalent anions such as calcium, strontium, magnesium, barium and aluminium, which form insoluble salts with phosphate.

Distribution of Phosphate

After absorption phosphate may be stored in bone, utilised in metabolic processes, incorporated into intracellular fluid, or excreted. In normal plasma, about one-third of the phosphorus is in inorganic form, and the other two-thirds are present as phospholipids. A small fraction is present in the form of phosphate esters. About 90 per cent of the inorganic phosphate is ultrafilterable, suggesting that only a small proportion is protein bound. The normal range for plasma inorganic phosphate varies much more than that of calcium, and is affected principally by age, diet, and metabolic status. The normal adult range is 3–4·5 mg/100 ml in the fasting state; in growing children, it ranges from about 4·5–6 mg per cent. When the phospholipids and phosphate esters are taken into account, the total phosphate content of the plasma is about 12·5 mg per cent. Serum phosphate levels are raised in uraemia and hypoparathyroidism and low in phosphaturic rickets or after ingestion of aluminium hydroxide.

The inorganic phosphate level is influenced by parathyroid hormone, and by vitamin D, glucocorticoids, insulin, and the gonadal and growth

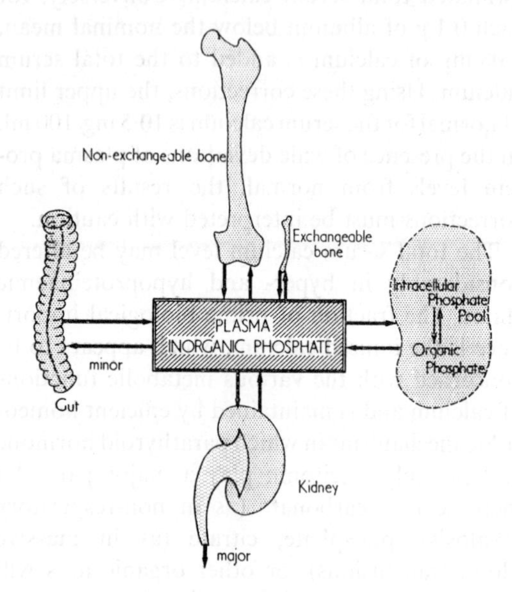

FIGURE 18.4 Distribution of phosphate

hormones. It may also be altered as a result of renal disease. The level of phosphate in the plasma at any one time is the result of a balance between uptake and excretion from the gut, excretion via the kidney, deposition into and release from bone, and intracellular uptake and release (Fig. 18.4). The concentration of inorganic phosphate in extracellular fluid approximates to that found in plasma.

Phosphate is one of the major intracellular anions, and the pool of inorganic phosphate ions is in rapid equilibrium with that of the many organic phosphate constituents of the cell. Transport mechanisms bring about the entry of phosphate into the cell, which is increased along with glucose under the influence of insulin.

Phosphate in Urine. The majority of ingested phosphate is excreted in the urine. The ionic form of phosphate in the urine depends on pH. At pH 4·5 the predominant form is $H_2PO_4^-$ and at pH 7·8 the main form is $HPO_4^=$. This shift in the phosphate ions provides an important buffer system in the urine.

Excretion of Phosphate

The routes by which phosphate leaves the body are the same as those for calcium, although renal excretion plays the major role. Phosphate is reabsorbed mainly in the proximal convoluted tubule. There is a definite maximum tubular capacity (Tm) for phosphate reabsorption, and changes in this reabsorptive process account for the alterations in phosphate excretion observed in clinical conditions where there is excess or deficiency of vitamin D or parathyroid hormone. There is still disagreement as to whether secretion of phosphate by the distal tubule, which some have held to be the process stimulated by parathyroid hormone, occurs to any significant degree. The renal excretion of phosphate is also influenced by vitamin D, by growth hormone, and thyroxine and may be considerably modified either by renal tubular defects or chronic renal disease.

BONE

Bone is a mass of organic tissue in which there is deposited a crystalloid calcium phosphate salt. Among this mineral material are other ions such as magnesium, sodium, citrate, and bicarbonate, and heavy metal impurities.

Organic Tissue. Although the protein matrix amounts for only 30–35 per cent of the total dry weight of bone, it is this matrix that determines its shape and size. The matrix (osteoid tissue) is composed mainly of collagen (95–99 per cent), which is a fibrous protein rich in proline, hydroxyproline, and glycine. The collagen is apparently synthesised by osteoblasts, and is embedded in a ground substance of acid mucopolysaccharides and mucoproteins. Collagen assumes a fibrillary pattern, and a single fibril is made up of units—tropocollagens (MW 360,000)—which, in turn, are composed of 3 amino-acid chains twined around each other.

Inorganic Tissue. The bone mineral exists in crystalloid form and gives the X-ray diffraction pattern characteristic of hydroxyapatites. The hydroxyapatite crystals are extremely small and are orientated, perhaps through electrostatic charges, to fairly precise regions in the long axes of bone collagen. The inorganic crystals of hydroxyapatite account for 65–70 per cent of the dry weight of bone.

Bone Formation

Bone is in a dynamic metabolic state and is continually being formed and resorbed. The formation of bone proceeds in two stages.

The *first stage* involves the laying down of the organic matrix. The rate of bone formation is determined by the osteoblasts, whose role is concerned with the laying down of the collagen fibrils in their ground substance. This function is probably carried out through the mediation of a series of enzymes. One of these, alkaline phosphatase, is produced inside osteoblasts, but the part played by this enzyme in the production of the matrix is rather obscure, and it seems unlikely that its essential function is to produce inorganic phosphate locally from organic phosphates. Bone alkaline phosphatase is probably not the major constituent of the total alkaline phosphatase in normal serum. The factors controlling osteoblastic activity are rather poorly understood, but one very important stimulus to activity is mechanical stress. Many other substances, including protein, ascorbic acid, growth hormone, and the gonadal hormones are necessary for normal osteoblastic activity. The gross dimensions and shape of bone are determined by the rate of osteoid formation, whereas bone remodelling, i.e. the formation of a bone that is strong but not bulky, is controlled mainly by the rate of bone resorption.

The *second stage of bone formation*, mineral accretion, consists of the deposition of calcium salt in the organic matrix. This process is generally considered to be determined by physicochemical rather than biological means, although recent work suggests that the osteoblastic cells play an important part in regulating mineral accretion as well as controlling the synthesis of the collagenous matrix. Calcification of bone involves, first, the nucleation of hydroxyapatite crystals at specific sites within the hollow collagen fibrils and the subsequent growth of these crystals as a result of the deposition of additional mineral ions.

The classical view is that mineral accretion depends principally on the product of the concentrations of calcium and phosphate ions in the extracellular fluid, but while this explanation is valid *in vitro*, in the intact animal the bone cells are mainly responsible for regulating the exchange of ions into and out of bone.

Mineral Mobilisation

Only about 1 per cent of bone calcium equilibrates rapidly with extracellular fluid, and bone mineral may leave the partially calcified exchangeable compartment by a process of ion exchange. This process of mineral mobilisation is distinct from bone resorption and is the means by which minor and rapid adjustments may be made in the circulating mineral levels in the body, the exchangeable bone mineral serving a 'buffering' function without involving other processes.

Bone Resorption

The release of calcium and phosphate from the fully calcified non-exchangeable compartment of bone involves two processes:

1. the removal of the matrix;
2. the release of the calcium phosphate salt.

These events appear to take place simultaneously, but in fact the matrix may actually be the first to be removed. Bone resorption is mediated through the action of the osteoclasts and other osteolytic cells. Osteoclasts are large multinuclear cells, but these and the mononuclear osteoblasts have a common origin and may be converted from one to the other under the influence of environmental and other factors. The cellular activity of the osteoclasts is controlled by parathyroid hormone, vitamin D, and thyroxine. Calcitonin may also reduce osteoclastic activity and, hence, bone resorption. Bone resorption is not only a function of the osteoclasts—osteoclastic osteolysis—but also of the osteocytes, which are metabolically active and capable of osteolytic activity. This process of osteocytic osteolysis is also stimulated by parathyroid hormone. The calcium and phosphate removed from the non-exchangeable bone are returned to the extracellular fluid and, thus, will increase the ionic product of calcium and phosphate, although this process is considerably slower than the changes that occur as a result of mineral mobilisation.

Each day, about 500 mg of calcium is removed from extracellular fluid and laid down as new bone, and as much is removed by resorption and is returned to the ECF. Thus, a dynamic balance of bone formation and bone resorption is maintained in the normal adult, and imbalance between these two processes leads to the various types of metabolic bone disease.

THE SYNDROMES RELATED TO THE PARATHYROID GLANDS

HYPERPARATHYROIDISM

Hyperparathyroidism arises as a result of increased secretion of parathyroid hormone, which may occur in three situations:

1. Primary hyperparathyroidism.
2. Secondary hyperparathyroidism—due to reactive hyperplasia of the glands as a result of chronic renal failure, osteomalacia, or rickets.
3. Tertiary hyperparathyroidism—this term has been used to describe a further stage in the development of the secondary type, where autonomy of the parathyroids occurs.

PRIMARY HYPERPARATHYROIDISM

Causes. The syndrome may result from adenoma, diffuse hyperplasia or carcinoma. Solitary adenomas outnumber all other causes, and occur in about 85 per cent of patients. The adenomas are multiple in 6 per cent of cases, and diffuse hyperplasia occurs in a similar proportion (Nordin, 1973). Carcinoma of the parathyroid glands is rare, accounting for 1 to 2 per cent of all cases of hyperparathyroidism. The parathyroid overactivity seen in association with an adenoma is not necessarily completely autonomous (Murray *et al.*, 1972).

Pathology. Adenomas may consist of chief cells, oxyphil cells or water clear cells (*see* Table 18.1). Even though chief and oxyphil cells are normally in a resting state, they may still be the components of hyperfunctioning adenomas, and in a recent review of primary hyperparathyroidism (Lloyd, 1968) chief cell adenoma was by far the commonest histological type encountered. Adenomas range in size from 0·5–100 g. Any gland larger than 60 mg is suspected of being abnormal. Hyperplasia usually involves the water clear cells, although generalised hyperplasia of the chief cells with hyperfunction is a distinct, although uncommon, clinical entity which was first described by Cope *et al.* (1958). In 4 of his 10 cases there were associated adenomas of other endocrine organs and the condition showed the same dominant inheritance seen in patients with the multiple endocrine adenomatosis syndrome.

It may be very difficult to differentiate between benign adenoma and carcinoma on purely histological grounds for giant and multiple nuclei and even invasion of vessels may be seen in benign adenomas. Parathyroid carcinoma should be diagnosed only if there is local invasion beyond the capsule, which is said to be thicker and more fibrous in malignant glands, if distant metastases are present, or if there is local recurrence of the neoplasm. Metastases are relatively rare, and tend to occur in bone marrow. Malignant glands are hard and whitish, whereas benign adenomas are soft and brown.

The bone changes in primary hyperparathyroidism fall into four main groups:

1. osteitis fibrosa;
2. bone cysts;
3. giant cell tumours (osteoclastomas);
4. osteomalacia.

In *osteitis fibrosa* there is *osteoclastic resorption* of both cortical and cancellous bone, which is replaced by vascular connective tissue, the changes predominantly affecting the long bones and spine. Although bone resorption is usually predominant, osteoblastic activity may be manifest by osteoid zones lining the surface of the bone trabeculae. Rarely, osteoblastic activity may be greater than osteoclastic resorption, leading to the hyperostotic forms of the syndrome of von Recklinghausen.

Generalised osteitis fibrosa is not specific for primary hyperparathyroidism—similar histological changes also occur in hyperparathyroidism secondary to chronic renal disease or osteomalacia. Fibrous osteitis may also be seen in other bone diseases such as Paget's disease and polyostotic fibrous dysplasia.

Bone cysts vary in size and may be multiple or single. They are lined by connective tissue and are filled with brownish fluid or mucoid material. They are most likely to be the result of intraosseous haemorrhage. Spontaneous fracture through a bone cyst may occur, and the cysts usually persist after parathyroidectomy.

The giant cell tumours are brownish in colour, due to the presence of haemoglobin derivatives, and vary from microscopic nodules to large tumours the size of a coconut. In some cases, osteoclastomas may be the only skeletal manifestation of hyperparathyroidism. Solitary osteoclastomas located in one of the skull bones are very strongly suggestive of hyperparathyroidism, and the great majority of giant cell tumours unrelated to hyperparathyroidism are situated in the long bones, although giant cell tumours in hyperparathyroidism also occur in these sites. Many pathologists consider that a distinction cannot be made on histological grounds between osteoclastomas due to hyperparathyroidism and true neoplastic osteoclastomas.

Histologically, the giant cell tumours are composed of large osteoclasts. Since the normal function of osteoclasts is to infiltrate and dissolve bone trabeculae, infiltration of bone by a giant-cell tumour cannot be taken as proof of malignancy. All giant-cell tumours in hyperparathyroidism, regardless of situation or number, are biologically benign, and all recalcify rapidly after parathyroidectomy. It is therefore important to determine whether a giant-cell tumour is an accompaniment of hyperparathyroidism, treatment of which will prevent what might be a major and, possibly, a mutilating operation for the removal of an osteoclastoma.

It is becoming increasingly recognised that true *osteomalacia* may sometimes occur in primary hyperparathyroidism, and this picture may be mixed with the classical features of osteitis fibrosa (Stanbury, 1972a). In such cases the accompanying biochemical changes may be atypical. The most reasonable explanation for this syndrome is that the osseous expression of primary hyperparathyroidism has been modified by vitamin D deficiency, although in most patients the possibility that the parathyroid autonomy has arisen on the basis of secondary hyperparathyroidism cannot be excluded. However, in some cases there is evidence that the factor responsible for the vitamin D deficiency has arisen as a consequence of primary hyperparathyroidism (Keynes and Caird, 1970, and *see* p. 390).

Prevalence. The prevalence of primary hyperparathyroidism is about one per 1,000 in the population (Boonstra and Jackson, 1971). The condition is approximately twice as common in females as in males, and presents most commonly in postmenopausal women, although it may be seen at any age. Primary hyperparathyroidism is rarely familial (Marsden *et al*., 1971) and in these cases multiple gland involvement is usually found. The histological appearances in these cases are variable and familial hyperparathyroidism is likely to be a manifestation of the syndrome of multiple endocrine adenomatosis. 5–10 per cent of patients with renal calcium phosphate stones are shown to have hyperparathyroidism but as many as 20–30 per cent of all cases of nephrocalcinosis suffer from the syndrome. However, only 5–10 per cent of patients with primary hyperparathyroidism have nephrocalcinosis (Nordin, 1973).

CLINICAL FEATURES

The clinical features of primary hyperparathyroidism are variable but occur irrespective of the nature of the glandular lesion. They may be divided into four groups:

1. *Due to hypercalcaemia and hypercalcuria*

   Anorexia, nausea, vomiting, constipation and weight loss.
   Fatigue and muscular weakness.
   Polydipsia and polyuria (diabetes insipidus-like syndrome).
   Mental changes ('neurosis', stupor, personality changes, coma, convulsions)

2. *Due to visceral calcification*

   Renal: calculi, nephrocalcinosis.
   Ocular: conjunctival and eyelid deposits, band keratopathy.

3. *Due to increased bone resorption*

   Bone pain and deformity.
   Pathological fractures.
   Osteoclastomas.
   Radiological changes (*see* below).

4. *Rare presentations*

Renal insufficiency (particularly with calculi or nephrocalcinosis).
Peptic ulcer (particularly with renal changes or any of the symptoms described above).
Zollinger-Ellison syndrome.
Acute pancreatitis.
Chronic pancreatitis and pancreatic calculi.
Tetany in the neonate (suggests hyperparathyroidism in the mother).
Mass in neck (palpable or on barium swallow).
Multiple endocrine adenomatosis syndrome.
Hyperuricaemia, gout.
Pseudo-gout (may also follow parathyroidectomy; Bilezikian *et al.*, 1973.)

Any of these presenting features should alert the physician to the possibility of hyperparathyroidism.

Physical Signs. There are few physical signs related to hyperparathyroidism except for those that can be deduced from the above list of presenting features, such as renal calculi, bone deformity or fracture, or band keratopathy. The presence of a palpable parathyroid tumour is rare, and most palpable lumps in the neck turn out to be thyroid adenomas. The physician may, in very rare cases, be able to elicit the so-called 'watermelon plunk' sound on percussion of the skull involved by osteitis fibrosa, but bone infiltrations such as myelomatosis and metastatic carcinoma give the same sign.

Rarely, acute *hypercalcaemic crisis* may occur. This is associated with headache, muscular weakness, anorexia, thirst and polyuria, dehydration, nausea, persistent vomiting, abdominal pain, and constipation. The patient is hypotensive, lethargic, and may be delirious. Acute psychiatric syndromes such as catatonic stupor or confusional psychosis may occur. Myocardial necrosis, acute calcium infarction and necrosis of the renal tubules, oliguria, and renal failure may supervene. In patients with neurological or psychiatric symptoms an EEG may be helpful, but the changes are non-specific. The condition is dangerous, and emergency parathyroidectomy may be life-saving. The administration of phosphate, sodium sulphate, or calcitonin is recommended by some authors (*see* below).

ECG Changes. As the serum calcium level rises, the Q-Tc duration is shortened, although with serum calcium levels above 16 mg per cent, prolongation of the T wave also occurs and, thus, the Q-Tc interval becomes disproportionately long. There do not appear to be any effects on cardiac rhythm, the P wave, the QRS complex, the ST segment or the polarity of the T wave but there is a tendency towards prolongation of the PR interval.

Radiological Features of Hyperparathyroidism

Today overt bone disease is relatively uncommon, although biochemical and histological evidence of some increase in bone resorption can usually be found. Skeletal involvement is not often apparent on radiological grounds since at least 25 per cent of bone calcium must be resorbed before X-ray changes are seen. In more advanced cases, generalised demineralisation is observed. No difference in the dietary intake of calcium has been observed between patients with and without radiological bone disease although there is evidence that some individuals are able to compensate for increased renal loss of calcium by an increased utilisation of dietary calcium. In general, the incidence of bone involvement appears to be largely related to the duration and severity of the syndrome, although additional factors may be involved, as has been suggested by Lloyd (1968). He was able to classify 138 cases of primary hyperparathyroidism into three groups: one in which there was overt bone disease without kidney stones, one with kidney stones without overt bone disease, and one in which neither occurred. After studying these groups, Lloyd put forward the hypothesis that there are two main types of parathyroid tumour: one growing rapidly, highly active, and causing more severe hypercalcaemia with overt bone disease, and the other growing slowly, of low activity, and causing kidney stones. Those patients with bone disease tend to have larger tumours. Tumour histology bore no relationship to the clinical variety of the disease. It is tempting to speculate that differences in calcitonin secretion might contribute to the differences between the three groups described.

The radiological appearances which may be seen are:

Changes in Long Bones. 1. *Subperiosteal resorption of bone* is the earliest and most specific skeletal change, and it is seen, characteristically, in the phalanges of the hands. A lace-like pattern is observed beneath the periosteum of the phalanx, giving the 'rotten wooden gatepost' appearance, and similar changes may also occur in other long bones, particularly in the distal end of the ulna and the inferior surface of the femoral neck. Subperiosteal erosion may be seen in the lower surface of the outer third of the clavicle.

2. *Generalised demineralisation* varies in degree and will be apparent only when a considerable proportion of the bone calcium has been resorbed. Skeletal rarefaction is a non-specific radiological appearance but in some patients with hyperparathyroidism localised zones of osteitis fibrosa superimposed on the generalised rarefaction will be seen.

3. *Bone cysts and giant-cell tumours* may present singly as a first abnormality or may be seen in large numbers in patients with advanced skeletal rarefaction. A cyst or an osteoclastoma may expand the bone and present as a palpable swelling. The commonest site for bone cysts in the long bones is the central medullary part of the shaft; cysts are also common in the metacarpals, ribs, and pelvis. Giant-cell tumours usually have a septate structure which may present a honeycomb appearance on X-ray, but frequently this is not discernible, and then a giant-cell tumour cannot be differentiated from a bone cyst until after the condition is treated; the giant-cell tumour will then rapidly re-calcify whereas the bone cyst will remain unchanged. The radiological appearances of the cysts and giant-cell tumours of hyperparathyroidism are not specific, and plasma cell tumours, lipoid granulomas, and, sometimes, metastatic malignancies, may produce identical radiological changes.

4. *Osteosclerosis* may very rarely be seen in primary hyperparathyroidism. It is a more common finding, although still infrequent, in secondary hyperparathyroidism.

Changes in the Skull. The same changes occur in the skull as have been described in the long bones, i.e. subperiosteal erosion, generalised demineralisation, bone cysts, and osteoclastomas. Subperiosteal erosion is seen in the skull as loss of the lamina dura, but this is now generally regarded as being a rather non-specific appearance and it is often unhelpful, for many of the patients investigated are endentulous. The decalcified skull on X-ray shows, typically, a finely mottled or ground-glass appearance, which may occasionally resemble that seen in Paget's disease. Bone cysts or osteoclastomas of the jaw may be the first symptom of hyperparathyroidism, and similar lesions may occur in the other facial bones.

Changes in the Spine and Pelvis. As in the long bones and skull, generalised demineralisation may occur, and vertebral collapse is not infrequent. Central compression by the nucleus pulposus may produce the appearance of codfish vertebrae, and spinal deformities such as kyphosis are not uncommon. In the pelvis, all of the bone changes previously described may be seen.

THE BIOCHEMICAL FEATURES OF PRIMARY HYPERPARATHYROIDISM

(*a*) *Plasma or serum calcium* is the most useful single estimation. Hypercalcaemia is almost invariable in primary hyperparathyroidism, and Dent (1962) has suggested that a single normal estimation with the correct technique makes a diagnosis of primary hyperparathyroidism most unlikely, although, very rarely, proven cases have been reported in which the serum calcium was normal in the absence of renal failure (Wills, 1971). Normocalcaemic hyperparathyroidism is rare, and difficult to explain unless it is attributable to vitamin D deficiency (Woodhouse *et al.*, 1971a).

(*b*) *Urinary calcium.* The 24-hour urine calcium is frequently elevated. In the fasting state the urine calcium, although usually raised, is not as high as would be expected from the plasma level due to the high tubular reabsorption of calcium (Nordin and Peacock, 1969). There are many other causes of hypercalcuria and, thus, while it may support the diagnosis of hyperparathyroidism, the urinary calcium concentration alone is not of very great diagnostic value.

(*c*) *Plasma inorganic phosphate.* This is suggestive of primary hyperparathyroidism if low, but normal or raised levels may be seen, especially when renal damage supervenes. Like the urinary calcium, the plasma inorganic phosphate is supportive rather than diagnostic.

(*d*) *Urinary inorganic phosphate.* This estimation is not usually very helpful unless the dietary intake is rigorously controlled. Persistent hyperphosphaturia while the patient is on a low phosphate diet is suggestive of hyperparathyroidism. A number of tests of parathyroid function, discussed briefly on page 403, have been devised that depend on the renal handling of phosphate.

(*e*) *Plasma chloride.* The plasma chloride was reported by Wills and McGowan (1964) to be elevated in primary hyperparathyroidism. These authors state that hyperparathyroidism is unlikely if the level is below 102 mEq/litre. Similar findings have been reported by others (Pyrah *et al.*, 1966), and the accurate measurement of plasma chloride and an assessment of the patient's hydrogen ion status (metabolic acidosis of some degree is usual in primary hyperparathyroidism) would seem to be very worthwhile diagnostic procedures.

(*f*) *Plasma alkaline phosphatase.* This is usually raised only in the presence of radiological bone disease.

(*g*) *Urinary hydroxyproline.* An increase in the urinary hydroxyproline excretion has usually been observed in patients with radiological bone disease and an elevated alkaline phosphatase level. Increased excretion has also been reported in patients who show no radiological or clinical evidence of bone involvement.

(*h*) *Serum magnesium.* This is low in a small proportion of patients with hyperparathyroidism. There is a significant inverse relationship between serum levels of calcium and of magnesium (King and Stanbury, 1970).

THE DIAGNOSIS OF PRIMARY HYPERPARATHYROIDISM

When there is suspicion of primary hyperparathyroidism, investigation should proceed in four stages:

1. to establish that unequivocal hypercalcaemia exists;
2. to exclude other causes of hypercalcaemia and, if possible, to prove the presence of primary hyperparathyroidism on biochemical grounds;
3. to establish the nature and localisation of the parathyroid lesion;
4. to search for any complications and associations of primary hyperparathyroidism.

1. *To Establish that Unequivocal Hypercalcaemia Exists*

The serum calcium concentration is the most helpful and important single investigation in the diagnosis of hyperparathyroidism, and the hypercalcaemia may be of any degree. It is necessary that the patient should be fasting when blood is taken, which should be done with a minimum of venous occlusion. Serum proteins should be estimated on the same specimen, for each one gram of albumin adsorbs about 0·8 mg of calcium, a point to be noted when interpreting the serum calcium concentration. Another, and probably preferable method of correcting for changes in serum albumin is based on the specific gravity of the serum of plasma, correcting to a specific gravity of 1·026. For every deviation of 0·001 a correction of 0·25 mg per cent is made, i.e. if the observed value for the serum calcium is 9·5 mg per 100 ml and the specific gravity 1·024, the corrected figure is 10 mg per 100 ml; if the specific gravity were 1·028 the corrected value would be 9 mg per 100 ml. Minor fluctuations in the serum calcium level occur in normal individuals and in patients with primary hyperparathyroidism—after meals the serum calcium may rise by 0·5 mg per 100 ml—and the normal range for serum calcium concentration varies slightly from laboratory to labortory; the mean and standard deviation of the estimation in the laboratory concerned should thus be known. A single normal fasting calcium does not exclude primary hyperparathyroidism and the investigation should be repeated on several occasions.

2. *To Exclude Other Causes of Hypercalcaemia and, if possible, to Make a Positive Diagnosis of Hyperparathyroidism*

The most frequent causes of hypercalcaemia are:

(*a*) Primary hyperparathyroidism
(*b*) Sarcoidosis
(*c*) Metastatic carcinoma of bone
(*d*) Myelomatosis
(*e*) Carcinomas not involving bone
(*f*) Milk-alkali syndrome
(*g*) Vitamin D intoxication
(*h*) Thyrotoxicosis
(*i*) Untreated Addison's disease
(*j*) Idiopathic hypercalcaemia of childhood
(*k*) Extensive Paget's disease with immobilisation.

Often, the diagnosis will be apparent after a careful history is obtained and physical examination carried out; sometimes, however, more specific investigations may be necessary. Hypercalcaemia in Addison's disease occurs only when it is untreated and when an Addisonian crisis is either present or imminent. Difficulties may arise with non-metastic carcinoma where hypercalcaemia may be due to the elaboration of a parathyroid hormone-like substance by the tumour (*see* Chapter 20). A test of value in the differential diagnosis of hypercalcaemia is the hydrocortisone suppression test. The oral administration of 120 mg of hydrocortisone daily for ten days has been found to suppress the serum calcium concentration significantly in patients with vitamin D intoxication or sarcoidosis, whereas the hypercalcaemia of hyperparathyroidism usually remains unaffected (Dent, 1956). The effect of steroids on the serum calcium concentration in myelomatosis, secondary carcinomatosis, and the milk-alkali syndrome is inconsistent. This test will be valid only when unequivocal hypercalcaemia is present; the pre- and post-steroid blood samples must be obtained under identical conditions.

Idiopathic hypercalcuria should not give rise to difficulty for, although there may be recurrent renal calculi, the serum calcium concentration is always normal.

More refined tests have been devised to confirm the diagnosis of primary hyperparathyroidism but in practice none is as useful as repeated fasting serum calcium estimations.

Serum Ionisable Calcium. Some workers consider that, regardless of the total calcium concentration in the serum, an increase in the ionisable calcium is diagnostic of primary hyperparathyroidism. Unfortunately, the position does not seem to be as clear cut as this, and the actual estimation technique is fraught with difficulties and possible sources of error. In special laboratories, where the method is critically standardised, it may give useful confirmation of hypercalcaemia when the total calcium is only marginally raised.

Calcium Deprivation. A low calcium diet is given for five to seven days. A reduction in existing hypercalcuria is evidence against a diagnosis of hyperparathyroidism, but persistence of hypercalcuria is by no means specific for the condition.

Phosphate Deprivation. A diet containing less than 500 mg of phosphate and 200 mg of calcium is given for thirteen days. During the last three days 45 ml of aluminium hydroxide gel is given before each meal. If hyperparathyroidism is present, more than 250 mg of calcium is excreted in the 24-hour urine specimen collected at the end of the test. Normal persons excrete less than 230 mg/day (Pronove *et al.*, 1961). Other authors have found the test of little value (Pyrah *et al.*, 1966).

Calcium Absorption and Turnover. In hyperparathyroidism there is increased absorption of calcium from the bowel, although this finding is not specific. Evidence of increased turnover of calcium after an intravenous injection of ^{47}Ca may be of value in making a diagnosis of hyperparathyroidism but, again, results are inconsistent. More sophisticated techniques, while perhaps more valid, would appear to have little place in the routine diagnosis of hyperparathyroidism.

Phosphate Clearance and Phosphate Excretion Index. The estimation of phosphate clearance (C_p) is by itself inadequate although it has been suggested that if clearance is expressed as a fraction of the endogenous creatinine clearance (C_p/C_{cr}) or as the percentage tubular reabsorption of phosphate (TRP) then more valid results might be obtained. However, studies have shown that these indices are of little value in distinguishing primary hyperparathyroidism from many other diseases. Phosphate clearance is, of course, dependent on the plasma phosphate level, and in an attempt to improve the specificity of the test, Nordin and Fraser (1960) described the phosphate excretion index (PEI) by relating the clearance ratio C_p/C_{cr} to the plasma phosphate level. Subsequently, Nordin and Bulusu (1968) confirmed the general validity of the PEI but also pointed out that a better index would be one which derived from the phosphorus excretion per 100 ml of glomerular filtration rather than from the phosphate/creatinine clearance ratio. They devised a modified formula for the index of phosphate excretion (IPE):

$$\text{IPE} = P_E - \frac{P_p - 2{\cdot}5}{2}$$

P_p is the plasma inorganic phosphorus and P_E is the phosphate excretion per 100 ml of GFR:

$$P_E = \frac{U_p \times P_{cr}}{U_{cr}}$$

where U_p and U_{cr} are the urinary concentrations of phosphate and of creatinine in mg per 100 ml and P_{cr} is the plasma concentration of creatinine. The normal range for the IPE is $\pm$ 0·5 and levels over 0·5 are obtained in hyperparathyroidism. While this test, if carefully carried out, may be of more value than many of the other tests, false positives and negatives are not infrequent and Bijvoet *et al.* (1969) have stated that such indices of phosphate excretion can have no physiological meaning. These workers have expressed phosphate as an estimated Tm/GFR and have published a nomogram of this relationship. This provides the same degree of discrimination between normal and abnormal cases as the index of phosphate excretion (Nordin, 1973).

Estimation of Maximal Tubular Reabsorptive Capacity for Phosphate (TmP). Estimation of the TmP during an infusion of phosphate is a time-consuming and difficult test and, even when a technically acceptable result has been achieved, false positives and false negatives are not infrequent, and the 'doubtful' range is wide. More sophisticated procedures have been devised to measure TmP but these seem to be of little practical value in the diagnosis of hyperparathyroidism.

Calcium Infusion Tests. The intravenous infusion of calcium might indicate whether or not parathyroid function can be inhibited by a rise in serum calcium. It has also been reported (Keiser *et al.*, 1964) that intravenous infusion of calcium causes a rapid fall in urinary hydroxyproline excretion in normal subjects, but no change in patients with hyperparathyroidism. Earlier calcium infusion tests were of questionable value. However, Pak *et al.* (1972) have proposed a modified calcium infusion which appears to provide more diagnostic accuracy. Patients with primary hyperparathyroidism showed a significantly smaller decrease in urinary phosphate excretion following a four-hour infusion of calcium (15 mg/kg body weight given as calcium gluconate) after equilibration on a constant calcium, phosphate and sodium diet. There was in this study complete separation between the control individuals and the patients with primary hyperparathyroidism. This test may prove of particular value in normocalcaemic primary hyperparathyroidism.

Assay of Parathyroid Hormone. Both bioassay

and radioimmunoassay techniques are available. There are many difficulties attached to the bio-assay, and while the radioimmunoassay is specific and sensitive, it is still of limited diagnostic value. O'Riordan *et al.* (1972) estimated circulating parathyroid hormone (PTH) using an immuno-radiometric assay in 69 patients with primary hyperparathyroidism. In those patients without radiological evidence of osteitis fibrosa, the mean concentration of circulating PTH was higher than in a group of normal subjects, but there was great overlap with the normal range. Much higher concentrations were, however, found in patients with osteitis fibrosa. Massage of the neck before venesection has not improved discrimination, but selective venous catheterisation with estimation of PTH is of considerable value in the localisation of tumours (*see* below).

Urinary Cyclic Adenosine Monophosphate. Twenty-four-hour urinary excretion of 3′,5′-cAMP in patients with primary hyperparathyroidism does not differ from that of normal controls. Correction for urinary creatinine excretion improves discrimination, but best segregation of the two groups results from calculation of a discriminant function:

$$\psi = 3{\cdot}37\,(\mu\text{mole cAMP/G creatinine}) - (\mu\text{mole cAMP/24 hours})$$

(Neelon *et al.*, 1973). No hyperparathyroid subjects and 91 per cent of controls had values of ψ less than 11·0 in this series; 91 per cent of hyperparathyroid patients and only 4 per cent of controls had ψ values greater than 12.0.

3. *To Establish the Nature and Localisation of the Parathyroid Lesion*

Parathyroid adenomas are very rarely palpable. Current methods used to help in the localisation of adenomas are:

(*a*) *Straight X-ray Neck, with and without Barium Swallow.* Plain X-rays of the neck and mediastinum are usually of no value, but rarely they may demonstrate the presence of an adenoma. Barium swallow occasionally reveals tracheal displacement but this is more commonly due to thyroid lesions. Very occasionally, an irregularity or filling defect may be seen in the oesophagus, which later proves to be of parathyroid origin.

(*b*) *Arteriography.* Percutaneous catheterisation of the brachial artery is used to obtain filling of the inferior thyroid artery, the catheter being slowly moved, under screening control, until its tip lies in the subclavian artery a little distal to the thyroid axis. The adenomas themselves cannot be visualised after injection of contrast medium, but displacement of the inferior thyroid artery may be seen. This technique may be helpful in localising a tumour, but experience is somewhat limited and the procedure is not without risk. Arch aortography has rarely been performed and sometimes reveals a tumour blush (Taylor, 1972). This procedure also is not one which should be entered upon lightly.

(*c*) *^{75}Se Selenomethionine Scan.* Selenomethionine is normally taken up by the thyroid and parathyroid glands. After the uptake by the thyroid gland has been blocked by the administration of tri-iodothyronine, the administration of ^{75}Se selenomethionine, followed by scintillation scanning over the neck, may demonstrate areas of increased activity, indicating the site of adenomatous or hyperplastic parathyroid glands. It is not of major value since only large tumours can be detected.

(*d*) *Selective Venous Catheterisation and Immunoassay.* This technique was introduced by Reitz *et al.* (1969). A catheter is introduced into the femoral vein and passed through the inferior and superior vena cava to the neck. It is directed by means of localisation with injections of radio-opaque fluid until samples of venous blood can be taken from the jugular veins and the innominate vein at a number of different levels. The presence of a high concentration of PTH at any site indicates that the point in the vein where it was obtained must be near the tumour. This technique has proved of great value in the localisation of adenomas, particularly when previous negative neck exploration has been performed or where tumours are multiple. In 75 per cent of patients, it is possible to predict either the side of the tumour or generally the actual gland involved. By sampling from the small superior, middle and inferior thyroid veins further diagnostic accuracy may be achieved.

4. *To Search for any Complications and Associations of Primary Hyperparathyroidism*
Rare presentations of hyperparathyroidism have already been mentioned, and only the renal complications will be considered here.

The most frequent and important complications of primary hyperparathyroidism are those related to the kidneys. In all patients, and particularly those in whom a presenting feature is a renal calculus or nephrocalcinosis, it is vitally important to assess the state of renal function. Renal calculi are present in some two-thirds or more of patients with hyperparathyroidism. Hypertension is also common, and in some this is related to renal damage, although in others there is no evidence of impaired renal function. Five main factors appear to contribute to the production of the renal lesions and eventual renal failure:

(*a*) Calcium deposits, fibrosis and scarring of the renal parenchyma.
(*b*) Renal calculi in the pelvi-calyceal system.
(*c*) Obstructive uropathy.
(*d*) Urinary infection.
(*e*) Lack of tubular responsiveness to antidiuretic hormone.

Proteinuria, isosthenuria and other signs of impaired renal function are not uncommon in hyperparathyroidism even in the absence of renal calculi or obvious nephrocalcinosis. The initial lesion seems to be tubular, with loss of concentrating ability. With continuing hypercalcaemia further renal damage and fibrosis develop, leading inevitably to azotaemia, despite treatment of the primary condition. When hyperparathyroidism and renal failure coexist it is often difficult and may be impossible to determine which is the primary condition. The syndrome of severe polyuria and polydipsia, which resembles diabetes insipidus, is not due simply to the increased solute load of calcium nor can changes in glomerular filtration rate be incriminated. The condition remits after parathyroidectomy, and it is presumed that loss of distal tubular responsiveness to ADH caused by hypercalcaemia is mainly responsible.

THE TREATMENT OF PRIMARY HYPERPARATHYROIDISM

When the diagnosis is made, early operation is normally indicated. However, if the tumour is small and the hypercalcaemia slight a prolonged and sometimes fruitless search may be necessary. In such mild cases there does not appear to be any urgency for surgery, since stone-formation can generally be controlled by means of a restricted calcium diet and such patients appear to maintain normal health for many years without complications. However, this procedure is unwise in post-menopausal women in whom bone resorption leads to accelerated osteoporosis. In such patients, administration of oestrogens reduces plasma and urine calcium and urine hydroxyproline (Gallagher and Nordin, 1972), and this might be expected to prevent bone disease by inhibiting bone resorption and stone disease by reducing urine calcium. In mild cases, this treatment appears to offer an alternative to surgery. The only contra-indications to operation are terminal anuric renal failure, when it is felt that death is imminent and recovery impossible, and other medical conditions that would render operation hazardous. Impairment of renal function, unless terminal, and advanced skeletal deformities are not absolute contra-indications, and in making a decision in patients with severe renal failure much depends on the available facilities for treatment and rehabilitation pre- and post-operatively.

The exploratory operation may be tedious, and great skill and care is necessary. The tumours occur most frequently in one of the inferior glands (75 per cent of total) and 5 to 6 per cent are situated in the mediastinum. Primary hyperplasia is much less frequent than an adenoma. If an adenoma is identified it is removed, and histological confirmation should be sought by examination of a frozen section. The firm diagnosis of an adenoma practically excludes the possibility of hyperplasia of all four glands, although the combination may be found in tertiary hyperparathyroidism (*see* below). After an adenoma is removed, the other three glands must be identified and shown to be normal so that multiple tumours may be excluded. If all four glands are found to be hyperplastic, then three are removed and a sub-total removal of the fourth carried out. There is less certainty of a complete cure and, likewise, a greater possibility of post-operative hypoparathyroidism in patients with generalised hyperplasia of the glands. The ideal treatment for carcinoma is the removal of the tumour, together with a radical clearance of the fat and areolar tissue around the tumour. Sometimes infiltration of surrounding tissues will have occurred, and radical surgery may not be possible. Histological diagnosis is commonly difficult, and the surgeon may have to rely on the gross morphological appearance to make the diagnosis. If the tumour is hard, fixed, and infiltrates surrounding tissues, it is likely to be malignant.

At the time of the cervical operation, it should be possible to search in the fat of the upper mediastinum for tumours or hyperplastic glands, if it is necessary to do so. A formal sternum-splitting anterior mediastinotomy will rarely be necessary but may need to be performed if a meticulous dissection of the neck has proved the existence of three normal glands, if an intrathyroidal adenoma has been excluded and if exploration of the anterior mediastinum at the time of the cervical operation has been negative. Most surgeons prefer to perform mediastinotomy as a separate operation at a later date.

Acute Hypercalcaemic Crisis. In some patients with hypercalcaemia early operation is necessary to save life. However, in the most gravely ill patients, temporary therapeutic measures are occasionally necessary to improve the patient's condition prior to operation. A high fluid intake is given along with a low-calcium, high-phosphate diet. Intravenous infusion of phosphate may be used in the emergency treatment of hypercalcaemia in order to reduce the serum calcium level but it should be given with great caution and is best reserved for those patients in whom it is deemed that hypercalcaemia is an immediate threat to life. A suitable regime was described by Goldsmith and Ingbar (1966). 500 ml of 0·1 M phosphate buffer made up of disodium phosphate (0·081 M) and monopotassium phosphate (0·019 M) is given by slow intravenous infusion. This supplies 50 mM of phosphorus (1·55 g). Depending on the response of the serum calcium, a further 500 ml may be given. With single infusions in excess of 50 mM severe hypocalcaemia and tetany may result. Intravenous sodium phosphate lowers the serum calcium concentration without increasing urine calcium excretion and there is a risk of extraskeletal deposition of calcium as $CaHPO_4$ which may, among other complications cause acute renal damage with failure, particularly if there is significant pre-existing renal disease. Chakmakjian and Bethune (1966) have described the use of intravenous sodium sulphate infusions in patients with severe hypercalcaemia. Three litres of an isotonic solution of sodium sulphate in water given intravenously over a period of nine hours resulted in a prompt fall in serum calcium levels, a rise in urinary calcium, and definite clinical improvement. The infusions seem to be well tolerated but a major disadvantage of sulphate infusions is the large volume of fluid which is given and which in the presence of impaired renal or cardiac function may be hazardous. Fulmer *et al.* (1972) have recently reviewed the efficacy of intravenous infusions of phosphate, sulphate and hydrocortisone in the treatment of hypercalcaemia due to malignant disease. Hydrocortisone produced only minor changes in serum calcium, and maximum reduction was noted in those patients who received 100 mM of disodium and monopotassium phosphate (81 mM of Na_2HPO_4 and 19 mM of KH_2PO_4 in 1,000 ml of 5 per cent dextrose in water, infused over 6–8 hours) and Fulmer and his colleagues concluded that although phosphate infusions are potentially hazardous, they are of value in the emergency treatment of hypercalcaemia, although the dose of phosphate given should depend on the magnitude of reduction in serum calcium required as well as on the initial serum phosphate concentration and the adequacy of renal function. Chelating agents have been used with good effect but may lower the serum magnesium. Haemodialysis has occasionally been attempted but, as yet, experience is limited and it is unlikely that dialysis is any more effective than phosphate infusion. Porcine calcitonin is of some value in the treatment of hypercalcaemia, and intravenous infusion of 8 MRC units per kg per hour reduces the serum calcium by as much as 3·5 mg/100 ml in patients with hyperparathyroidism and with vitamin D intoxication (West *et al.*, 1971), although the effect is short-lived. The preparation may also be given by intramuscular or subcutaneous injection in a dose of at least 8 MRC units per kg, six-hourly.

Postoperative Course

Following successful removal of an adenoma or of hyperplastic glands, the serum calcium almost invariably falls within the first 24 to 48 hours to normal or subnormal levels. This fall occurs because the removal of the excess parathyroid hormone rapidly diminishes the efflux of calcium from bone, whereas there is rapid deposition of calcium in the large amount of osteoid tissue. It is unusual for the hypocalcaemia to persist for more than a few days, although sometimes it may persist for weeks or even months. The situation may be aggravated by functional parathyroid deficiency due to atrophy of the remaining glands. Rarely, true hypoparathyroidism may have been produced by faulty surgical technique. Tetany resulting from functional hypoparathyroidism is usually only transient and will promptly be relieved by intravenous calcium gluconate. When tetany persists, oral and intravenous calcium and magnesium and vitamin D may be needed. Patients with early renal complications usually do well, and the incidence of recurrent stone formation is reduced although sometimes hypertension or other manifestations of renal insufficiency may supervene. However, severe impairment of renal function and/or development of hypertension will be delayed, if not prevented, by the removal of the adenoma or hyperplastic glands.

The rate of recurrence of hyperparathyroidism over the five years following operation is 15 per cent (Marsden and Day, 1973). In this series recurrences were limited to cases with involvement of other endocrine glands, a family history of hyperparathyroidism or multiple parathyroid gland involvement found at operation. One or more of these three factors is found in 39 per cent of all cases of primary hyperparathyroidism, and they serve as prognostic indices of a high recurrence rate.

THE SYNDROME OF MULTIPLE ENDOCRINE ADENOMATOSIS

The syndrome of multiple endocrine adenomatosis was first referred to in 1903, but the first detailed observations were made by Underdahl *et al.* in 1953. It is now apparent that a number of clinical entities may be interrelated and fall into this general group.

In the 'classical' syndrome, adenomas or hyperplasia may be present in the pancreas, the parathyroids, the anterior pituitary or the adrenals. Adenomas may be active in all four of these sites, or in any combination. The following combinations were reported by Schmid *et al.* (1961):

Pituitary, parathyroids and islet cells	34 per cent
Pituitary and parathyroids	25 per cent
Parathyroids and islet cells	22 per cent
Pituitary and islet cells	19 per cent

The syndrome is inherited as an autosomal

dominant, and it will be obvious that the clinical presentations are protean. In one series (Moldower *et al.*, 1954), 25 per cent of the patients had peptic ulcers which tended to be large, multiple, and resistant to therapy, and this syndrome may be identical to that described by Zollinger and Ellison (*see* below).

The pathological changes that may occur in the endocrine glands and their sequelae are shown in Table 18.3.

The patient may present initially with any of the endocrine syndromes listed, the other adenomas and their manifestations being discovered incidentally.

The *Zollinger-Ellison syndrome* of recurrent and resistant peptic ulceration with massive gastric oversecretion is associated with gastrin-producing islet-cell tumours of the pancreas, and there may be, in addition, adenomas or hyperplasia affecting other endocrine glands.

TABLE 18.3

Gland	Lesion	Manifestation
Parathyroids	Adenoma or hyperplasia (usually chief cell)	Hyperparathyroidism
Pituitary:		
(*a*) acidophil	Adenoma or hyperplasia	Acromegaly
(*b*) basophil	Adenoma or hyperplasia	Usually no endocrine syndrome
(*c*) chromophobe	Adenoma or hyperplasia	Usually pressure effects only; perhaps hypopituitarism
Pancreas:		
Islet cells	Functioning adenoma (producing insulin)	Spontaneous hypoglycaemia
	Functioning adenoma (producing gastrin)	Zollinger-Ellison syndrome
Adrenals:		
Cortex	Adenoma or hyperplasia	Cushing's syndrome (rare)

The syndrome of *primary parathyroid chief-cell hyperplasia* with hyperparathyroidism was first described by Cope *et al.*, in 1958. In 4 out of 10 cases in this series, which shows autosomal dominant inheritance, there were associated adenomas of other endocrine organs.

Peptic ulceration is a common association of primary hyperparathyroidism and if severe or recurrent should raise the possibility of an islet-cell adenoma.

SECONDARY HYPERPARATHYROIDISM

Secondary hyperparathyroidism is a well-recognised entity defined by Albright and Reifenstein (1948) as 'a condition when more parathyroid hormone is manufactured than is normal but where this hormone is needed for some compensatory purpose'. There is generalised hyperplasia of all four glands, the predominant histological feature being hyperplasia of the chief cells, although in some cases transitional and oxyphil cells are also present.

Aetiology. The commonest cause of secondary hyperparathyroidism in the western world is chronic renal failure, particularly chronic pyelonephritis or glomerulonephritis. A number of factors seem to contribute to the genesis of the elevated blood phosphate and the hypocalcaemia which stimulate the parathyroid hyperfunction and hyperplasia, but the role of phosphate retention appears particularly important. It has been shown both in experimental and clinical renal failure that the phosphaturic effect of secondary hyperparathyroidism limited the rise in serum phosphate resulting from reduction in glomerular filtration (Slatopolsky *et al.*, 1969) and from these observations these workers extrapolated to suggest that this compensatory mechanism must come into operation from the earliest stages of renal disease. Any reduction in glomerular filtration would tend to produce a rise in serum phosphate and reciprocal reduction in serum calcium, if constant entry of phosphate into the extracellular fluid is assumed. The resulting parathyroid response would tend to correct both abnormalities in the serum, and normal or near normal concentrations of calcium and phosphate would be sustained by increasing parathyroid secretion as renal failure progressed, until the phosphaturic effect of parathyroid hormone was inadequate to compensate for reduced glomerular filtration (Bricker, 1969).

Secondary hyperparathyroidism would thus seem to be an early development in renal failure. Confirmation for this hypothesis has recently been published (Slatopolsky *et al.*, 1971). In dogs with experimental renal failure it was possible to prevent the development of secondary hyperparathyroidism by gross restriction of the dietary intake of phosphorus. Thus, when a patient with chronic renal failure is found to have hypocalcaemia without hyperphosphataemia, this must imply the presence of a second factor in addition to secondary hyperparathyroidism, and the obvious candidate for this role is acquired resistance to vitamin D. Secondary hyperparathyroidism may also occur in association with other hypocalcaemic states such as osteomalacia (usually, in the UK, as a result of malabsorption syndrome) and rickets. Vitamin D resistance may play an important role in contributing to the hypocalcaemia of chronic renal failure (which may be due at least in part to a reduction in functional renal mass causing a decrease in synthesis of 1,25-DHCC—*see* p. 391) and some forms of rickets.

Biochemical Findings. The serum calcium level is usually low but may occasionally be normal. In patients with chronic renal failure, the plasma inorganic phosphate is almost invariably raised, often to a very high level, although when vitamin D resistance is present the concentration may be low normal. In the earliest stages of renal impairment, before the glomerular filtration rate falls below 40 ml/min, serum phosphorus levels may also be low, even though increased serum concentrations of parathyroid hormone may be detected when the GFR is as high as 70–80 ml/min. In osteomalacia or rickets the phosphate concentration is reduced. In secondary hyperparathyroidism the intestinal absorption of calcium is reduced, in contrast to primary hyperparathyroidism.

Radiological Findings. The findings in secondary hyperparathyroidism are indistinguishable from those of the primary disease although the typical appearances of osteomalacia or rickets are usually also present. In chronic renal failure, features of hyperparathyroidism, osteomalacia, and osteosclerosis may co-exist and the radiological findings can be complex. Soft tissue and metastatic calcification can be seen in any form of hyperparathyroidism.

DIAGNOSIS AND TREATMENT

The differentiation between primary and secondary hyperparathyroidism can cause difficulty and may be almost impossible. Renal impairment with its concomitant biochemical features may occur in primary hyperparathyroidism caused by an adenoma, and in these cases secondary hyperplasia of the normal glands may develop. In some cases of secondary hyperparathyroidism an autonomous adenoma may develop in one of the hyperplastic glands (tertiary hyperparathyroidism). Histology of the glands is of no help, as primary chief-cell hyperplasia is now a recognised entity. It can usually be assumed that if, in the presence of chronic renal failure, the serum calcium concentration is considerably lowered, then any radiological evidence of hyperparathyroidism is due to secondary hyperplasia, and parathyroidectomy is not normally indicated. If the serum calcium is elevated in the presence of chronic renal failure the possibility of the presence of an autonomous or partially autonomous adenoma should be considered, although hypercalcaemia may develop in the course of primary renal failure even when the structural changes in the parathyroid glands are those of secondary hyperplasia (Stanbury, 1972b). It is in those patients with chronic renal failure and a normal serum calcium that difficulty arises, and sometimes it is impossible to resolve the issue. In such patients, exploration of the neck may sometimes be justified, on the grounds that an adenoma (either primary or arising in a hyperplastic gland) cannot be excluded and that if 'overcompensation' has occurred as a result of secondary hyperparathyroidism, then subtotal parathyroidectomy may be carried out with benefit to the patient. The features of secondary hyperparathyroidism in chronic renal failure can sometimes be improved by haemodialysis, and in these instances an exploratory operation can be avoided. The use of gut phosphate binders such as Aludrox may also be very helpful, and in patients treated by this means healing of the bone lesions on bone biopsy may be observed, even after relatively short periods of treatment. In patients with osteomalacia or rickets, supplements of calcium and vitamin D or dihydrotachysterol are required and some recommend that these may also be given to those patients with chronic renal failure who have severe hypocalcaemia. In such patients, the physician should watch for evidence of soft tissue calcification.

TERTIARY HYPERPARATHYROIDISM

This syndrome has been described and documented by Davies *et al.* (1968). In their first 200 cases of primary hyperparathyroidism proved at operation they found 12 patients with parathyroid adenomas which probably developed on the basis of longstanding hyperplasia due to malabsorption or chronic renal failure. They accept the term *tertiary hyperparathyroidism*, first suggested by Dr Walter St Goar (1963), to describe patients who develop parathyroid adenomas causing hypercalcaemia on the background of reactive or secondary parathyroid hyperplasia.

As in primary hyperparathyroidism, women are more often affected with the tertiary condition. The ages of the patients described by Davies *et al.* (1968) ranged from 28 to 72 years, and more cases were associated with malabsorption than with chronic renal failure. The syndrome has also been described after renal transplantation, when parathyroid overactivity has continued despite correction of renal failure. In some of these last cases the autonomous overactivity subsides with time. Tertiary hyperparathyroidism should be suspected in any patient with malabsorption or renal failure who develops hypercalcaemia. This is occasionally observed during treatment with vitamin D, but its persistence after this is withdrawn should raise the possibility of an adenoma. When total plasma calcium levels are only marginally raised, estimation of the ionised calcium may give useful confirmation. In about three-quarters of the patients, bone X-rays or biopsies show signs of osteomalacia, and in a similar number there is evidence of increased parathyroid action on bone—osteitis fibrosa cystica. While it might be argued that some patients with tertiary hyperparathyroidism might have suffered from the primary condition which was initially undiagnosed, or masked by vitamin D deficiency this seems unlikely in all reported cases, since the evolution of the syndrome from the secondary variety has been observed in several patients.

Like primary hyperparathyroidism, the tertiary form requires surgical treatment to remove an adenoma unless renal failure is too advanced to allow operation, when haemodialysis can sometimes be helpful. After removal of the adenoma, treatment with Vitamin D may sometimes be required to prevent hypocalcaemia.

HYPOPARATHYROIDISM

There are three main types of hypoparathyroidism:

1. Idiopathic
2. Postoperative
3. Neonatal

IDIOPATHIC HYPOPARATHYROIDISM

In this condition there may be imperfect intrauterine development of the parathyroid glands. In autopsied cases, only one or two atrophic glands have been found, in which most of the parenchyma has been replaced by fat and fibrous tissue. Congenital absence of the parathyroids is rare and is associated with malformation or absence of the thymus. Such children rarely survive.

Blizzard *et al.* (1966) have demonstrated parathyroid antibodies in 38 per cent of 74 patients with idiopathic hypoparathyroidism. A significant number of these patients also had adrenal, thyroid and/or gastric parietal cell antibodies, even in the absence of adrenal or thyroid disease or pernicious anaemia. Conversely, 26 per cent of 92 patients with idiopathic Addison's disease, 12 per cent of 49 patients with Hashimoto's disease, and only 6 per cent of 245 control patients showed the presence of parathyroid antibodies. The presence of antibodies to parathyroid tissue in a proportion of patients has been confirmed by Irvine and Scarth (1969). Whether these circulating parathyroid antibodies play any causative role in idiopathic hypoparathyroidism remains to be determined, but it is possible that some cases of acquired idiopathic hypoparathyroidism may result from autoimmune processes.

POSTOPERATIVE HYPOPARATHYROIDISM

This may occur as a result of thyroid or parathyroid gland surgery, or after radical surgery for laryngeal or oesophageal carcinoma. The damage during thyroid surgery generally results from interference with the blood supply to the parathyroid glands, e.g. ligation of the inferior thyroid artery. Resulting hypoparathyroidism can be either transient or permanent, and sometimes it may not develop for a considerable time after operation. With modern techniques it is a much rarer complication of partial thyroidectomy. Transient hypoparathyroidism is common after removal of a functioning parathyroid adenoma or excision of hyperplastic glands.

NEONATAL HYPOPARATHYROIDISM

The serum calcium concentration falls shortly after birth, and many normal infants have total serum calcium levels below 8 mg per cent at some time during the first three weeks of life. Transient hypoparathyroidism with symptoms due to hypocalcaemia may occur in the neonatal period in several situations. In normal children, it may rarely be precipitated by a high phosphate diet and appears to occur particularly in those children who are fed with artificial foods such as cow's milk, which have a high phosphate content.

Symptoms are seen after the fourth day of life. Symptomatic hypocalcaemia is sometimes seen in children of low birth weight, particularly small-for-dates babies, and may be associated with hypoglycaemia. Although the condition is usually transient, such children have a high mortality. Transient hypoparathyroidism may also occur in children born to hyperparathyroid mothers, parathyroid activity presumably having been suppressed *in utero* by maternal hypercalcaemia.

Incidence

Up to about 1955, the incidence of hypoparathyroidism following thyroidectomy was 0·5 to 3 per cent. Since that time the incidence has fallen considerably. Hyperthyroidism is more common in females than males, and, thus, post-operative hypoparathyroidism shows a similar sex incidence. Idiopathic hypoparathyroidism is considerably less common and the sex incidence is equal. The great majority of cases occur sporadically, although a rare sex-linked recessive variety which tends to be mild has been reported. Idiopathic hypoparathyroidism may present at any age, but generally does so in infancy with tetany, epilepsy or mental disturbance.

CLINICAL FEATURES

The dominant clinical features of hypoparathyroidism are due to hypocalcaemia. The decrease in serum ionised calcium causes increased neuro-muscular excitability. Symptoms of tetany are the rule, consisting of paraesthesiae, numbness and tingling in the extremities or circumoral region, and muscle cramps and stiffness. Chvostek's and Trousseau's signs are usually positive. Chvostek's sign is obtained by tapping over the branches of the facial nerve in the parotid gland above the angle of the jaw, or just in front of the gland below the zygomatic arch, and the authors recognise three grades: (1) when only the lips show twitching; (2) when the lips and alae nasi twitch; (3) when the whole of that side of the face tested twitches. Grade one can occur in normal individuals; grades two and three are almost certainly abnormal. In the overt tetanic attack there is hyper-reflexia and carpal spasm and, in children particularly, laryngeal stridor and convulsions. Tetany is not confined to hypoparathyroidism and may occur in all hypocalcaemic states. It may also occur when the serum ionised calcium concentration is reduced because of alkalosis in the presence of a normal total serum calcium level. Tetany may also be seen in association with hypokalaemia and hypomagnesaemia.

Peripheral cataracts can result from prolonged hypocalcaemia from any cause and occur in 50 per cent of patients with idiopathic hypoparathyroidism.

In addition to these symptoms of hypocalcaemia other clinical features are present in the idiopathic form of hypoparathyroidism, which is characterised by a number of developmental defects. The condition is congenital but, although signs and symptoms usually appear in childhood, the diagnosis is sometimes not made until adult life. Mental development may be retarded, and intelligence is subnormal in 20 per cent of cases. Dentition is poor, and there are a number of more general ectodermal defects such as dry scaly skin and sparse hair growth. The nails are usually deformed, brittle and ridged, and moniliasis is a common complication that may result in loss or deformity of finger and toe nails. Occasionally, eczema or exfoliative dermatitis is seen, and these appear to fluctuate in intensity with changes in the calcium levels. Central nervous system abnormalities are frequent and include, in addition to mental retardation, papilloedema, calcification of the basal ganglia, and extra-pyramidal dyskinesis. The combination of papilloedema and convulsions may lead to the mistaken diagnosis of cerebral tumour, and fits in association with mental retardation may similarly suggest cerebral birth trauma or longstanding idiopathic epilepsy. As with hyperparathyroidism, other endocrine gland abnormalities may be present. Adrenocortical hypofunction may be associated, although it is almost entirely confined to juvenile cases. Thyroid disease or pernicious anaemia may also occur in association with idiopathic hypoparathyroidism.

ELECTROCARDIOGRAPHY AND RADIOLOGY

The electrocardiogram in hypoparathyroidism of all types reflects the hypocalcaemia, showing prolongation of the QTc interval and sometimes T wave changes.

Skeletal changes in hypoparathyroidism are uncommon. There is no consistent appearance on X-ray of the bones and although demineralisation or generalised or localised osteosclerosis may be seen the appearances are more commonly normal. Soft tissue calcification, usually in the basal ganglia, can be seen radiologically in about one-third of patients with the idiopathic form.

THE BIOCHEMICAL ABNORMALITIES AND DIAGNOSIS OF HYPOPARATHYROIDISM

The serum findings in both surgical and idiopathic hypoparathyroidism are the reverse of those found in hyperparathyroidism, namely hypocalcaemia and hyperphosphataemia. Hypocalcuria is often found, but the urine calcium excretion may be normal (Nordin, 1973). There is relative hypophosphaturia. The absorption of calcium from the gut is diminished and the serum alkaline phosphatase level is usually normal, although infrequently may be elevated. Urinary hydroxyproline is low and bone formation and resorption are also low. Hyperuricaemia is common and unexplained.

Estimation of the serum calcium concentration is the most valuable test. Hypocalcaemia is also found in: (1) osteomalacia or rickets, (2) chronic renal failure, (3) hypoproteinaemia, (4) acute pancreatitis, (5) after administration of chelating agents such as EDTA, (6) pseudohypoparathyroidism, and (7) hypercalcitoninaemia. In *osteomalacia and rickets* the cause of the hypocalcaemia is usually apparent, and in these conditions the serum inorganic phosphate is normal or low, the serum alkaline phosphatase is raised, and typical X-ray changes are often present. In *renal insufficiency*, due to chronic renal disease or to tubular defects, hypocalcaemia and hyperphosphataemia are frequently seen, and the combination may suggest hypoparathyroidism. There is a further possible source of confusion in that in some patients with chronic renal failure, particularly those maintained on intermittent haemodialysis, corneal calcification may occur. However, associated evidence of renal failure will serve to differentiate the two conditions. It is not expected that *acute pancreatitis* or the administration of *chelating agents* will ever give any difficulty in diagnosis. The urinary excretion of phosphate increases in normal patients and in those with hypoparathyroidism after administration of parathyroid extract. This can be used as a diagnostic test to differentiate between hypoparathyroidism and *pseudohypoparathyroidism* but each batch of parathyroid extract used diagnostically must be tested first in a normal subject and shown to have phosphaturic effect. *Pseudohypoparathyroidism*, and *hypercalcitoninaemia* are discussed further in later sections.

THE TREATMENT OF HYPOPARATHYROIDISM

At present, preparations of parathyroid extract are expensive and must be given by parenteral injection. Antibodies that render the preparation ineffective may also develop. Most patients respond to vitamin D preparations by mouth, with large oral calcium supplements. While this therapy will usually restore the serum calcium to normal there is little phosphaturic effect with normal doses and, thus, a degree of hyperphosphataemia may persist. Although large daily doses of vitamin D may be needed, it is wise to begin therapy with moderate amounts, e.g. 0·25–1 mg (10,000–40,000 IU) daily, increasing cautiously and slowly by increments of 0·25 mg every two weeks until the plasma calcium has reached 8 mg/100 ml, to avoid the danger of hypercalcaemia. Thereafter, a maintenance dose of from 1 mg–5 mg (40,000–200,000 IU) daily is usually adequate, although some patients require less. As an alternative, dihydrotachysterol may be used for initial and for maintenance therapy. The initial dose is 0·25–2·5 mg daily, and its action more closely resembles that of parathyroid hormone. Both vitamin D and dihydrotachysterol seem equally effective in the treatment of hypoparathyroidism. In patients with hypoparathyroidism which appears resistant to vitamin D therapy the possibility of magnesium deficiency should be considered—correction of magnesium depletion will in such cases lead to an adequate response to vitamin D. Supplementary calcium may be given as calcium lactate, gluconate, or citrate orally. 'Calcium Sandoz' (calcium gluconogalactogluconate) is a useful preparation—each effervescent tablet contains the equivalent of 380 mg of elemental calcium, and two to eight tablets may be given daily, depending on requirements. Milk should not be used as a source of calcium due to its high phosphorus/calcium ratio. The acute attack of tetany is best treated by slow intravenous injection of 10–20 ml of a 10 per cent solution of calcium gluconate.

It must be noted that while vitamin D and calcium correct the neuromuscular symptoms of hypoparathyroidism, it is less certain that they benefit the ectopic calcification, cataracts, mental disturbances, and skin manifestations of the idiopathic variety. During the treatment of hypoparathyroidism the physician must be on the alert for hypercalcaemia. If this occurs, cortisol is effective in lowering serum calcium concentrations. Vitamin D therapy should be withdrawn and re-established in lower dose after the hypercalcaemia has been corrected.

PSEUDOHYPOPARATHYROIDISM

Albright *et al.* (1942) described a number of patients who exhibited all the biochemical and most of the clinical features of idiopathic hypoparathyroidism, while manifesting additional somatic anomalies. They did not, however, respond to parathyroid hormone, and parathyroid glands that were explored or biopsied were found to be normal or hyperplastic.

Aetiology. A strong hereditary tendency is present in pseudohypoparathyroidism. The condition is twice as common in females, and it has been suggested that it is transmitted as a sex-linked dominant. It appears likely that the somatic anomalies are genetically related to the metabolic abnormalities but that they are not interdependent.

Kolb and Steinbach (1962) noted evidence of osteitis fibrosa in the hand X-rays of patients with pseudohypoparathyroidism and postulated that the essential disorder was a high obligatory renal tubular reabsorption of phosphorus with secondary hyperphosphataemia, hypocalcaemia and hyperparathyroidism. It is now thought that the essential defect is a lack of adenyl cyclase in the renal tubules and consequent absence of the phosphaturic response to parathyroid hormone (Chase *et al.*, 1969). The term 'pseudohypoparathyroidism' is therefore rather misleading and refers only to the biochemical features observed. The condition does in fact appear to be a form of secondary hyperparathyroidism. Observations have indicated that in patients with pseudohypoparathyroidism the calcitonin content of the thyroid gland is greatly increased (Aliopoulios *et al.*, 1966; Tashjian *et al.*, 1966) but the significance of this is unknown.

Clinical Features. The condition is more common in girls than boys, and the presentation is always in early childhood. All the clinical features of idiopathic hypoparathyroidism, with the possible exception of papilloedema, may be seen in pseudohypoparathyroidism, although their relative frequency differs. Cataracts are rather less common but calcification of the basal ganglia is more frequent than in idiopathic hypoparathyroidism. Subcutaneous soft tissue calcification, which is almost unknown in idiopathic hypoparathyroidism, occurs in more than 50 per cent of patients, and subnormal intelligence is much more common. The following additional features also occur in pseudohypoparathyroidism: (1) a round face, often with a perpetual smile, (2) short and stocky stature, (3) metacarpal and/or metatarsal dyschondroplasias which result in shortening of one or more of these bones. This anomaly is seen most often in the fourth and fifth metacarpals, producing a characteristic dimpling which appears when a fist is made. (4) Subcutaneous bone formation and exostoses.

Biochemical Features. Hypocalcaemia and hyperphosphataemia are present, although the abnormalities are not usually as extreme as in idiopathic hypoparathyroidism. Tubular reabsorption of phosphate is high. The plasma alkaline phosphatase is sometimes raised. The condition is occasionally associated with hypothyroidism due to selective TSH deficiency (Zisman *et al.*, 1969).

Diagnosis. Pseudohypoparathyroidism can usually be differentiated from hypoparathyroidism on clinical and radiological grounds. Parathyroid hormone can be detected in the plasma and administration of a parathyroid hormone preparation which has been shown to have a phosphaturic effect in a normal individual does not produce the normal rise in renal excretion of cyclic AMP or any phosphaturic response.

A number of other skeletal and developmental defects may simulate the somatic features of pseudohypoparathyroidism. These include: (1) pseudo-pseudohypoparathyroidism, (2) myositis ossificans progressiva, (3) familial brachydactyly, (4) Turner's syndrome, (5) epiphyseal dysplasia of various types, (6) hereditary multiple exostoses.

The superficial physical resemblance of patients with pseudohypoparathyroidism and those with hypothyroidism has initiated studies of thyroid function in the former condition. The two diseases have occasionally been shown to coexist (*see* above).

THE TREATMENT OF PSEUDOHYPOPARATHYROIDISM

Although patients with the syndrome appear refractory to endogenous and oxogenous parathyroid hormone, vitamin D given in sufficiently large amounts is effective in correcting the biochemical abnormality. Doses up to several hundred thousand units daily may be necessary and dihydrotachysterol in doses up to 2·5 mg daily or even higher may be used as an alternative. Considerable care must be exercised in the initial stages of therapy, until the patient's response to small or moderate doses of vitamin D has been assessed. Calcium supplements should be given. In some patients with persistent hypophosphaturia and hyperphosphataemia, probenecid 1·5 g/day may be used to enhance renal excretion, and aluminium hydroxide gel by mouth may reduce the intestinal absorption of phosphate.

PSEUDO-PSEUDOHYPOPARATHYROIDISM

Albright and his colleagues (1952) described a patient who showed many of the somatic but none of the biochemical features of pseudohypoparathyroidism. This syndrome was named by them pseudo-pseudohypoparathyroidism.

Aetiology and Genetics. The syndrome has been described as a distinct entity and as a result of the work of Mann *et al.* (1962), it is now believed that pseudohypoparathyroidism and pseudo-pseudohypoparathyroidism are closely linked and are distinct from other syndromes in which developmental and bony defects occur. There have been several reports in which both syndromes appeared in the same family; in one family a pair of twins was described where one had pseudohypoparathyroidism and the other pseudo-pseudohypoparathyroidism. Several patients have been reported who, while presenting with pseudo-pseudohypoparathyroidism, later developed hypocalcaemia and hyperphosphataemia. The condition is twice as frequent in females, and inheritance appears to be as a sex-linked dominant. It has been suggested that pseudo-pseudohypoparathyroidism is a mild or incomplete form of the pseudohypoparathyroidism syndrome.

Clinical Features. Since the serum calcium is normal there are no neuromuscular symptoms. The somatic features that occur are identical with those seen in pseudohypoparathyroidism. Calcification of the basal ganglia is, however, not seen although soft tissue calcification elsewhere is frequent. Mental subnormality is common.

Diagnosis. The condition may be differentiated from other syndromes with brachydactyly and/or dwarfism on clinical and radiological grounds. The predilection for shortening of the 4th and 5th and other metacarpals differs from the pattern seen in most other diseases, although this may also occur in Turner's syndrome. The diagnosis is complicated by the observations of Van der Werff Ten Bosch (1959) who has described a series of eight patients who appeared clinically to have pseudo-pseudohypoparathyroidism, three of whom showed in addition stigmata of Turner's syndrome and had chromatin-negative buccal smears. The connection, if any, is not yet apparent.

Shortening of the metacarpals and metatarsals also occurs in myositis ossificans progressiva, but here the thumbs and great toes are also involved, whereas in pseudo-pseudohypoparathyroidism the abnormality is more frequently present in the digits.

No therapy is available.

Syndromes Related to Disturbance of Calcitonin Secretion

The discovery of a new hormone is of great interest in itself, but the clinician is also concerned to known whether alterations in its secretion may give rise to manifestations of disease. Since the discovery of calcitonin, a number of clinical situations have been described in which a disturbance of its secretion may be present, although in most cases the significance of this is unknown. No bone syndrome that might be due to hypercalcitoninaemia has yet been reported.

AFTER TOTAL THYROIDECTOMY

There is some evidence that calcium homeostasis is impaired by removal of the major source of calcitonin.

Patients maintained on l-thyroxine after total thyroidectomy have normal fasting serum calcium concentrations but show an impaired ability to restore the calcium level to normal after infusion of calcium gluconate (Williams *et al.*, 1966). Similarly, thyroidectomy augments hypercalcaemia induced by either vitamin D or parathyroid hormone. However, the precise significance of these observations in terms of normal physiology is uncertain, because of the alternative sites of production of calcitonin.

PSEUDOHYPOPARATHYROIDISM

In some patients with pseudohypoparathyroidism the calcitonin content of the thyroid gland is greatly increased, although the significance of this is unknown (Aliapoulios *et al.*, 1966; Tashjian *et al.*, 1966). These results must be interpreted with caution in view of the imperfections still present in the immunoassay for calcitonin.

MEDULLARY CARCINOMA OF THYROID

This condition is discussed earlier and in the chapter dealing with the thyroid gland. The tumour arises from the parafollicular or C cells of the thyroid, which are the site of production of calcitonin. Milhaud and his colleagues first demonstrated that tumours from patients with this condition contained calcium-lowering activity and it has since been confirmed that this neoplasm is rich in calcitonin and that the plasma calcitonin concentration is high in this syndrome (Cunliffe *et al.*, 1968; Dubé *et al.*, 1969). The hormone has been isolated from tumour tissue (Riniker *et al.*, 1968). Since plasma calcitonin is greatly increased in most patients with medullary carcinoma, its estimation is a valuable diagnostic test and may also be used to evaluate the success of surgical removal of a tumour, and to detect possible recurrence. There are no overt skeletal abnormalities in medullary carcinoma, and disturbances in serum calcium are rare.

CARCINOID SYNDROME

Calcium-lowering activity has been demonstrated in a small number of cases in both plasma from patients with this disease and in their tumours (Milhaud, 1972). Tumour extracts have also been shown to contain a substance which is immunologically similar to calcitonin (Foster *et al.*, 1972). However, abnormal amounts of calcitonin are not found in all patients, and hypersecretion of the hormone is probably not a primary characteristic of the disease. It may be that argentaffinoma cells have the potential to elaborate the hormone, but only rarely manifest this ability.

OSTEOPOROSIS

Calcitonin inhibits bone resorption, and it has been suggested that some varieties of idiopathic osteoporosis, where bone resorption is increased, may be associated with calcitonin deficiency, although convincing evidence for this is lacking. Experimental conditions similar to osteoporosis produced in rats or cats are prevented by concurrent administration of calcitonin. In man, reports on short-term studies also suggest that calcitonin may have beneficial effects when given to patients with osteoporosis (Milhaud, 1972), although final assessment of its use cannot be made until long-term clinical trials have been carried out (Foster, *et al.*, 1972). Long-term treatment with porcine calcitonin induces circulating antibodies, although this development has not been observed in patients treated with the human hormone. To date, the greatest therapeutic success with calcitonin has been achieved in patients with Paget's disease of bone (Woodhouse *et al.*, 1971b) (*see* p. 387).

OSTEOPOROSIS

Osteoporosis has been defined as a reduction in bone mass per unit volume, without any known change in chemical composition (Nordin, 1961; 1973). It represents, therefore, atrophy of bone. It is generally accepted that the condition is the end result of a number of different disorders of skeletal homeostasis, and the term osteoporosis may be considered analogous to the equally non-specific term 'anaemia'. Osteogenesis imperfecta is a form of osteoporosis due to a congenital defect in the bone matrix. The reduction in bone mass, which is the essential feature of osteoporosis, must be the result of an imbalance between the rates of bone formation and bone destruction. Albright *et al.* (1940) suggested that the essential lesion in osteoporosis was a failure in the synthesis of the collagenous bone matrix. This failure could be due to: lack of anabolic hormones which normally stimulates this process (e.g. oestrogens, androgens), increase of hormonal activity (e.g. due to adrenocortical steroids), and/or failure of osteoblastic activity due to disuse. It was presumed that in osteoporosis both the calcification of the bone matrix, and bone resorption (under the influence of parathyroid hormone) were normal. It is now accepted that the classical concept is probably incorrect, and that in all forms of osteoporosis bone formation rates are normal but bone resorption rates are increased (Jowsey, 1966), although bone formation rate may be reduced in crush fracture cases. The imbalance between bone formation and bone resorption responsible for osteoporosis may occur at all levels of bone turnover rate—low, normal or high—but the cause of the increased bone resorption is unknown.

CLASSIFICATION OF OSTEOPOROSIS (modified after Nordin, 1964)

Osteoporosis is seen in the following situations:

1. *Generalised Osteoporosis*
   (*a*) Idiopathic (Primary)
      (i) Juvenile
      (ii) Post-menopausal
      (iii) Senile
   (*b*) Secondary
      (i) Hyperthyroidism
      (ii) Acromegaly
      (iii) Excess of adrenocorticosteroids either exogenous or endogenous.
      (iv) Hypovitaminosis C
      (v) Heparin osteoporosis
      (vi) Malabsorption syndromes.
   (*c*) Congenital—osteogenesis imperfecta
2. *Localised Osteoporosis*
   (*a*) Disuse and immobilisation
   (*b*) Sudeck's atrophy
   (c) Rheumatoid arthritis.

Clinical Biochemical and Radiological Features. The incidence of osteoporosis rises considerably with age and at all ages is more common in the female. The essential clinical manifestation of osteoporosis is fracture, and osteoporosis may present clinically because of involvement of the spine or of the peripheral bones. In the first case, the presenting symptom is usually backache, which usually (but not always) indicates vertebral collapse; in the second, bone fractures. Osteoporosis contributes to three characteristic fracture syndromes: The Colles' fracture, which occurs in post-menopausal women; the fracture of the proximal femur which occurs in the elderly of either sex; and crush fractures of vertebrae, which occur in association with severe spinal osteoporosis.

The blood calcium, phosphate, and alkaline phosphatase concentrations are normal, although there is a clear tendency for the fasting plasma and urinary calcium to rise after the menopause, particularly after an artificial menopause. The fasting plasma and urine calcium concentrations and the 24-hour urinary calcium excretion are often low in old persons, presumably reflecting incipient osteomalacia. Some young patients with rapidly progressive osteoporosis may show slight hypercalcaemia and hypercalcuria.

The diagnosis is made principally on radiological grounds and loss of bone density is the prominent feature. Very early changes are not detectable on X-ray, and even in the later stages it may be necessary to compare the X-rays with control radiographs to be certain that density is diminished. In the spine, lack of bone density and accentuation of the vertical trabeculae are observed, to be followed, in more advanced instances, by vertebral biconcavity and collapse.

Iliac crest biopsy may assist in the diagnosis of osteoporosis, when a decrease in the number of vertical and horizontal trabeculae is seen. Sometimes, evidence of increased bone resorption (osteolysis) is observed histologically.

AETIOLOGY OF OSTEOPOROSIS

Idiopathic Osteoporosis. The studies of Nordin (1961, 1964, 1971) suggest that negative calcium balance might be a significant factor in the aetiology of oesteoporosis, although others feel that the calcium intake has little relationship to the condition. Nordin (1973) has pointed out that the negative calcium balance required to produce primary osteoporosis is very small indeed, since the total amount of bone lost with age is only about 15 per cent of the skeleton, or 150 g of calcium. These small quantities would not necessarily be detected by conventional balance techniques. However, although some relief of symptoms may follow the correction of negative calcium balance, the long-term improvement with such treatment as shown by increases in bone density on X-ray are, to date, disappointing. Age-related loss of bone starts at the age of 40–50 in women, and rather later in men. Oophorectomised women have significantly less bone than controls, and the post-menopausal loss of bone can be prevented or delayed by oestrogens. These observations imply that bone status is related to gonadal function. It has been suggested that declining calcium absorption is an important contributant to the progressive bone loss that normally occurs in old age.These seems to be an inverse relation between osteoporosis and the fluoride content of the local water, and in some very rare cases, vitamin C deficiency may be associated with osteoporosis. Some consider that a deficiency in bone matrix may be causally related to the increased bone resorption, while others regard vertebral osteoporosis, at least, as due to diminished vascularity of bone. It has been suggested (Pak *et al.*, 1969, Jowsey *et al.*, 1969) that osteoporosis arises from an imbalance between the secretion of parathyroid hormone and the secretion of calcitonin, but the conclusions of these workers has been questioned (*Lancet*, 1970) and the possible role played by a disturbance of calcitonin secretion in the pathogenesis of osteoporosis must remain undefined. Idiopathic juvenile osteoporosis may be a separate condition from so-called post-menopausal or senile osteoporosis, possibly with different aetiological factors involved.

Osteoporosis in Association with Endocrine Disease. Osteoporosis is common in Cushing's syndrome and also occurs, although much more rarely, in acromegaly and thyrotoxicosis. In Cushing's syndrome there is increased bone resorption, which may be partly compensated for by increased bone formation. Reduced absorption of calcium from the gut may also contribute to loss of bone. At a later stage, a low turnover rate of bone probably occurs. The catabolic effect of cortisol together with the negative calcium balance commonly found may contribute to the aetiology of the condition. The bone disease of acromegaly differs in some respects from other forms of osteoporosis. Vertebral collapse rarely, if ever, occurs and the increased bone resorption involves principally cortical bone. Periosteal new bone is common, and a characteristic feature is increased concavity of the posterior surfaces of the vertebral bodies. The cause of the 'osteoporosis' in acromegaly is unknown; negative calcium balance and hypogonadism may contribute. In thyrotoxicosis both bone resorption and bone formation are increased although the former predominates. Although the findings on bone biopsy sometimes resemble osteitis fibrosa rather than typical osteoporosis, there is no evidence that parathyroid overactivity or deficiency of calcitonin is involved. The bone changes appear to result from the catabolic effects of excess thyroid hormone.

Osteoporosis has been reported in patients treated for long periods with *heparin* (Griffith *et al.*, 1965) and this appears to be due to increased bone resorption produced by the drug. *Malabsorption of calcium* can lead to or aggravate osteoporosis, and is frequently seen in the crush fracture cases. This malabsorption may be part of a more generalised malabsorption syndrome, or may be due to mild vitamin D deficiency insufficient to produce osteomalacia.

THE TREATMENT OF OSTEOPOROSIS

Calcium Supplements. These are easily given, but while there are some reports of symptomatic improvement following their use, the long-term results are not striking and no convincing radiological improvement has yet been obtained, even after fairly prolonged periods. Supplements are best given in the form of calcium glycerophosphate 3–6 g daily (Nordin, 1973).

Intravenous calcium infusions (15 mg/kg body weight as calcium gluconate-glucoheptonate given on 12 occasions over a period of two to three weeks) may strikingly improve bone pain in some patients, and may also improve calcium balance, decrease bone resorption and increase bone formation (Bartter, 1970). These effects may result from simultaneous suppression of parathyroid function and stimulation of calcitonin secretion during the period of the infusion; however, the effects may persist for weeks or even months. Further confirmation of these results is required before calcium infusions can be recommended for general use.

Vitamin D. There is some evidence (Munck, 1963; Dent and Friedman, 1965) that vitamin D, given alone or with androgenic hormones, causes improvement in some cases of juvenile osteoporosis. Vitamin D may be useful in patients in whom malabsorption of calcium can be demonstrated.

Oestrogens, Androgens, Anabolic Steroids. Although there is evidence that post-menopausal osteoporosis may be retarded by administration of oestrogens, there is no objective evidence that these steroids given alone or in conjunction with calcium and/or vitamin D are of use in osteoporosis except in these cases and in the rare juvenile cases mentioned above.

Sodium Fluoride. It has been reported that sodium fluoride improves calcium balance in osteoporosis and causes relief of symptoms. However, the long-term results seem disappointing and the toxicity of fluoride is an added disadvantage.

Calcitonin. It has been shown that calcitonin has a profound effect in suppressing bone resorption in experimental animals, although there is a striking decrease in its effectiveness in animals of increasing age. Short-term studies suggest that calcitonin may have beneficial effects in osteoporosis (Milhaud, 1972), but this experience has not been general when porcine calcitonin is used (Brown *et al.*, 1970) and the results of long-term trials using human hormone are awaited.

POLYOSTOTIC FIBROUS DYSPLASIA
(Albright's Syndrome)

The syndromes of fibrous dysplasia result from the replacement of normal bone by patchy and asymmetrical areas of vascular fibrous tissue. Such fibrous dysplasia may affect only one bone, the monostotic type, or may be scattered throughout the skeleton, resulting in the polyostotic form.

Albright *et al.* (1937) drew attention to cases, usually of the polyostotic type, in whom there was associated skin pigmentation and sexual precocity. Females were more often affected. More recent reports have described similar cases in which sexual retardation has been seen, but these seem to occur much less frequently than the cases showing sexual precocity. It is unlikely that the abnormalities of sexual development result from compression of the hypothalamus due to deformity in the base of the skull. In none of the reported cases of sexual retardation has there been any evidence of deficiency of anterior pituitary hormones other than the gonadotrophins.

Both goitre and hyperthyroidism have been reported in association with Albright's syndrome, and rarer endocrine associations include Cushing's disease, acromegaly, accelerated skeletal growth and maturation and gynaecomastia. Hall and Warrick (1972) have suggested that the endocrine sequelae of the syndrome may be the result of a congenital hypothalamic abnormality causing overproduction of a variety of releasing hormones which are responsible for pituitary overactivity and increased function of the target organs.

REFERENCES

Parathyroid Hormone

O'Riordan, J. L. H., Watson, L., and Woodhead, J. S. (1972). *Clinical Endocrinology*, **1**, 149.

Parsons, J. A., and Potts, J. T. (1972). In *Clinics in Endocrinology and Metabolism* (Ed. Iain MacIntyre), "Physiology and Chemistry of Parathyroid Hormone". London: Saunders Ltd., p. 33.

Rasmussen, H. (1972). In *Clinics in Endocrinology and Metabolism* (Ed. Iain MacIntyre), "The cellular basis of mammalian calcium homeostasis". London: London: Saunders Ltd., p. 3.

Roth, S. I. (1971). *Amer. J. Med.*, **50**, 612.

Calcitonin

Foster, G. V., MacIntyre, I., and Pearse, A. G. E. (1964). *Nature* (*Lond.*), **203**, 1029.

Foster, G. V., Byfield, P. G. H., and Gudmundsson, T. V. (1972). In *Clinics in Endocrinology and Metabolism* (Ed. Iain MacIntyre), "Calcitonin". London: Saunders Ltd. p. 93.

Leading article (1973). *British Med. J.*, **1**, 371.

Lewis, P., Rafferty, B., Shelley, M., and Robinson, C. J. (1971). *J. Endocrinology*, **49**, ix-x.

Woodhouse, N. J. Y. (1972). In *Clinics in Endocrinology and Metabolism* (Ed. Iain MacIntyre), "Paget's disease of bone". London: Saunders Ltd., p. 125.

Vitamin D

Brickman, A. S., Coburn, J. W., and Norman, A. W. (1972). *New Engl. J. Med.*, **287**, 891.

Dent, C. E., Richens, A., Rowe, D. J. F., and Stamp, T. C. B. (1970). *British Med. J.*, **4**, 69.

Evans, D. J., and Azzopardi, J. G. (1972). *Lancet*, **i**, 353.

Galante, L., Colston, K., MacAuley, S., and MacIntyre, I. (1972). *Lancet*, **i**, 985.

Kodicek, E. (1972). In *Clinics in Endocrinology and Metabolism* (Ed. Iain MacIntyre), "Recent advances in Vitamin D metabolism". London: Saunders Ltd., p. 305.

Lawson, D. E. M., Fraser, D. R., Kodicek, E., Morris, H. R., and Williams, D. H. (1971). *Nature*, **230**, 228.

Primary Hyperathyroidism, Hypercalcaemia

Bijvoet, O. L. M., Morgan, D. B., and Fourman, P. (1969). *Clin. Chim. Acta.*, **26**, 15.

Bilezikian, J. P., Aurbach, G. D., Connor, T. B., Pachas, W. N., Aptekar, R., Wells, S. A., Freijanes, J., and Decker, J. L. (1973). *Lancet*, **i**, 445.

Boonstra, C. A., and Jackson, C. E. (1971). *Amer. J. Clin. Path.*, **55**, 523.

Chakmakjian, Z. H., and Bethune, J. E. (1966). *New Eng. J. Med.*, **275**, 862.

Cope, O., Keynes, W. M., Roth, S. I., and Castleman, B. (1958). *Ann. Surg.*, **148**, 375.

Dent, C. E. (1956). *Brit. med. J.*, **i**, 230.

Dent, C. E. (1962). *Brit. Med. J.*, **ii**, 1419, 1495.

Fulmer, D. H., Dimick, A. B., Rothschild, E. O., and Mayer, W. P. L. (1972). *Archs. Intern. Med.*, **129**, 923.

Gallacher, J. C., and Nordin, B. E. C. (1972). *Lancet*, **i**, 503.

Goldsmith, R. S., and Ingbar, S. H. (1966). *New Eng. J. Med.*, **274**, 1.

Keiser, H. R., Gill, J. R., Sjoerdsma, A., and Bartter, F. C. (1964). *J. clin. Invest.*, **43**, 1073.

Keynes, W. M., and Caird, F. I. (1970). *Brit. Med. J.*, **1**, 208.

King, R. G., and Stanbury, S. W. (1970). *Clin. Sci.*, **39**, 281.

Lloyd, H. M. (1968). *Medicine*, **47**, 53.

Marsden, P., Anderson, J., Doyle, R., Morris, B. A., and Burns, D. A. (1971). *Brit. med. J.*, **3**, 87.

Marsden, P., and Day, J. L. (1973). *Clin. Endocrinol.*, **2**, 9.

Murray, T. H., Peacock, M., Powell, D., Monchik, J. M., and Potts, J. T. Jr. (1971). *Clin. Endocrinol.*, **1**, 235.

Neelon, F. A., Drezner, M., Birch, B. M., and Lebovitz, H. E. (1973). *Lancet*, **i**, 631.

Nordin, B. E. C. (1973). In *Metabolic Bone and Stone Disease*. Edinburgh and London: Churchill Livingstone.

Nordin, B. E. C., and Bulusu, L. (1968). *Postgrad. Med. J.*, **44**, 93.

Nordin, B. E. C., and Fraser, R. (1960). *Lancet*, **i**, 947.

Nordin, B. E. C., and Peacock, M. (1969). *Lancet*, **ii**, 1280.

O'Riordan, J. L. H., Watson, L., and Woodhead, J.S. (1972). *Clin. Endocrinol.*, **1**, 149.

Pak, C. Y. C., East, D., Sanzenbacher, L., Ruskin, B., and Cox, J. (1972). *Archs. intern. Med.*, **129**, 48.

Pronove, P., Bell, M. H., and Barter, F. C. (1961). *Metabolism*, **10**, 364.

Pyrah, L. N., Hodgkinson, A., and Anderson, C. K. (1966). *Brit. J. Surg.*, **53**, 245.

Reitz, R. *et al.* (1969). *New Eng. J. Med.* **281**, 348.

Stanbury, S. W. (1972a). In *Clinics in Endocrinology and Metabolism* (Ed. I. MacIntyre). London: Saunders, p. 239.

Taylor, S. 1972). In *Clinics in Endocrinology and Metabolism* (Ed. I. MacIntyre). London: Saunders, p. 79.

West, T. E. T., Joffe, M., Sinclair, L., and O'Riordan, J. L. H. (1971). *Lancet*, **i**, 675.

Wills, M. R. (1971). *Lancet*, **i**, 849.

Wills, M. R., and McGowan, G. K. (1964). *Brit. med. J.*, **1**, 1153.

Woodhouse, N. J. Y., Doyle, F. H., and Joplin, G. F. (1971*a*). *Lancet*, **ii**, 283.

Secondary and Tertiary Hyperparathyroidism

Albright, F., and Reifenstein, E. C., Jr (1948). In *The Parathyroid Glands and Metabolic Bone Disease: Selected Studies*. Baltimore: Williams & Wilkins Co.
Bricker, N. S. (1969). *Archs. Intern. Med.*, **124**, 292.
Davies, D. R., Dent, C. E., and Watson, L. (1968). *Brit. med. J.*, **iii**, 395.
St Goar, W. (1963). In 'Case records of Massachisetts General Hospital,' *New Eng. J. Med.*, **268**, 943.
Slatopolsky, E., Caglar, S., Pennell, J. P., Taggart, D. D., Canterbury, J. M., Reiss, E., and Bricker, N. S. (1971). *J. clin. Invest.*, **50**, 492.
Slatopolsky, E., Robson, A. M., Elkan, I., and Bricker, N. S. (1969). *J. clin. Invest.*, **47**, 1865.
Stanbury, S. W. (1972b). In *Clinics in Endocrinology and Metabolism* (Ed. I. MacIntyre). London: Saunders, p. 267.

Multiple Endocrine Adenomatosis

Cope, C., Keynes, W. M., Roth, S. I., and Castleman, B. (1958). *Ann. Surg.*, **148**, 375.
Moldower, M. P., Nardi, G. I., and Baker, J. W. (1954). *Amer. J, med. Sci.*, **228**, 190.
Schmid, J. R., Labbart, A., and Rossier, P. H. (1961. *Amer. J. Med.*, **31**, 343.
Underdahl, L. O., Woolner, L. B., and Black, B. M. (1953). *J. clin. Endocrinol.*, **13**, 20.

Hypoparathyroidism

Blizzard, R. M., Chee, D., and Davis, W. (1966). *Clin. exp. Immunol.*, **1**, 119.
Irvine, W. J., and Scarth, L. (1969). *Clin. exper. Immunol.*, **4**, 505.
Nordin, B. E. C. (1973). In *Metabolic Bone and Stone Disease*. Edinburgh and London: Churchill Livingstone.

Pseudo- and Pseudo-pseudohypoparathyroidism

Albright, F., Burnett, C., Smith, P., and Parson, W. (1942). *Endocrinology*, **30**, 922.
Albright, F., Forbes, A. P., and Henneman, P. H. (1952). *Trans. Amer. Physicians*, **65**, 337.
Aliapoulios, M. A., Voekel, E. F., and Munson, P. L. (1966). *J. clin. Endocrinol.*, **26**, 897.
Chase, L. R., Melson, G. L., and Aurbach, G. D. (1969). *J. Clin. Invest.*, **48**, 1832.
Kolb, F. O., and Steinbach, H. L. (1962). *J. clin. Endocr.*, **22**, 59.
Mann, J. B., Alterman, S., and Hills, A. G. (1962). *Ann. Int. Med.*, **56**, 315.
Tashjian, A. H., Frantz, A. G., and Lee, J. B. (1966). *Proc. nat. Acad. Sci.* (Wash.), **56**, 1138.
Van der Werff Ten Bosch, J. J. (1959). *Lancet*, **i**, 69.
Zisman, E., Lotz, M., Jenkins, M. E., and Barter, F. C. (1969). *Amer. J. Med.*, **46**, 464.

Syndromes Related to Disturbance of Calcitonin Secretion

Aliapoulios, M. A., Voekel, E. F., and Munson, P. L. (1966). *J. clin. Endocrinol.*, **26**, 897.
Cunliffe, W. J., Black, M. M., Hall, R. Johnston, I. D. A., Hudgson, P., Shuster, S., Gudmondsson, T. V., Joplin, G. F., Williams, E. D., Woodhouse, N. J. Y., Galante, L., and MacIntyre, I. (1968). *Lancet*, **ii**, 63.
Dubé, W. J., Bell, G. O., and Aliapoulios, M. A. (1969). *Archs. Intern. Med.*, **123**, 423.
Foster, G. V., Byfield, P. G. H., and Gudmundson, T. V. (1972). In *Clinics in Endocrinology and Metabolism*, **1:1** (Ed. I. MacIntyre). London: Saunders, p. 93.
Milhaud, G. (1972). In *Proceedings of the Fourth Parathyroid Conference* (Eds R. V. Talmadge and P. L. Munson). Excerpta Medica: Amsterdam.
Tashjian, A. H., Frantz, A. G., and Lee, J. B. (1966). *Proc. nat. Acad. Sci* (Wash.), **56**, 1138.
Williams, G. A., Hargis, G. K., Galloway, W. B., and Henderson, W. J. (1966). *Proc. Soc. exp. Biol.* (*N.Y.*), **122**, 1273.
Woodhouse, N. J. Y., Reiner, M., Bordier, P., Kalu, D. N., Fisher, M., Foster, G. V., Joplin, G. F., and MacIntyre, I. (1971*b*). *Lancet*, **i**, 1139.

Osteoporosis

Albright, F., Bloomberg, E., and Smith, P. H. (1940). *Trans. Amer. Physicians*, **55**, 298.
Bartter, F. (1970). *Proc. roy. Soc. Med.*, **63**, 339.
Brown, P., Thin, C. G., Malone, D. N. S., Roscoe, P., and Strong, J. A. (1970). *Scot. Med. J.*, **15**, 207.
Dent, C. E., and Friedman, M. (1965). *Quart. J. Med.* (N.S.), **34**, 177.
Editorial (1970). *Lancet*, **i**, 180.
Griffith, C. G., Nichols, G. Jr, Asher, J. D., and Flanagan, B. (1965). *J. Amer. med. Ass.*, **193**, 91.
Jowsey, J. (1966). *Amer. J. Med.*, **40**, 485.
Jowsey, J., Hoye, R. C., Pak, C. Y. C., and Bartter, F. C. (1969). *Amer. J. Med.*, **47**, 17.
Munck, O. (1963). *Acta Orthop. scandinav.*, **33**, 407.
Nordin, B. E. C. (1961). *Lancet*, **i**, 1011.
Nordin, B. E. C. (1964). In *Advances in Metabolic Dis-Orders*, Vol. 1 (Eds R. Levine and R. Luft). London: Academic Press, p. 126.
Nordin, B. E. C. (1971). *Brit. med. J.*, **1**, 571.
Nordin, B. E. C. (1973). In *Metabolic Bone and Stone Disease*. Edinburgh, London: Churchill Livingstone.
Pak, C. Y. C., Zizman, E., Evens, R., Jowsey, J., Delea, C. S., and Bartter, F. C. (1969). *Amer. J. Med.*, **47**, 7.

Polyostotic Fibrous Dysplasia

Albright, F., Butler, A. M., Hampton, A. O., and Smith, P. (1937). *New Eng. J. Med.*, **216**, 727.
Hall, R., and Warrick, C. K. (1972). *Lancet*, **i**, 1313.

19

CARCINOID SYNDROME

The term 'carcinoid' was first proposed early this century, in order to emphasise the malignant appearance of these tumours in association with their apparently benign course. The tumours arise from the argentaffin cells (Kultschitzky's cells) of the intestinal mucosa near the bases of the crypts of Lieberkuhn, and they often contain granules that have an affinity for silver or chromium compounds—argentaffinomas. They seem principally to be connected with structures of the embryological midgut. About 90 per cent are situated in the ileocaecal region, either in the terminal ileum or in the appendix, but they may also be found anywhere in the gut from the stomach to the rectum or in the gallbladder and biliary system. Rarely, an argentaffinoma may be present in an ovarian or testicular teratoma, and bronchial adenomas may assume a carcinoid appearance. It would seem that bronchial carcinoids and oat cell carcinomas might be variants of the same disease spectrum, originating from a common type of cell. The argentaffin reaction is less frequently seen in bronchial carcinoids (foregut) than in those arising from the embryonic midgut. In some 20 to 25 per cent of cases multiple tumours are present. The relationships between carcinoid tumour and medullary carcinoma of the thyroid are discussed below.

While the tumours (particularly the bronchial carcinoids) tend to be locally invasive, distant metastases are, in general, rare. They are very uncommon with appendicular carcinoids, but occur more frequently with those arising in the ileum, caecum, colon or stomach. Metastases are particularly prone to occur from those bronchial adenomas that are associated with the classical carcinoid syndrome (*see* below). The usual sites of metastatic involvement are the regional lymph nodes and the liver, and, less frequently, the ovaries, lungs, and bone. The tumours may occur at any age, but metastasising argentaffinomas are commoner in the older age groups. The sex incidence is equal.

CLINICAL FEATURES OF THE CARCINOID SYNDROME

A clinical syndrome that may occur in association with carcinoid tumours has been well recognised for over twenty years (Biörck *et al.*, 1952; Rosenbaum *et al.*, 1953). In most cases, the presence of this syndrome indicates widespread metastatic deposits in the liver. The syndrome is caused by the liberation into the circulation of large quantities of 5-hydroxyindoles and vasoreactive peptides. Since one passage of these substances through the liver inactivates them, tumour deposits producing the syndrome must have direct venous drainage into the systemic circulation. Such tumours may be situated in the liver in sites allowing them to secrete their products directly into the inferior vena cava or its tributaries, but may also occur less frequently elsewhere in the abdomen where venous drainage is directly into the inferior vena cava or azygos systems. Bronchial adenomas may also secrete directly into the systemic circulation. In such cases primary tumours may produce the syndrome without metastases to the liver. The clinical features of the carcinoid syndrome are due to the effects of the humoral agents on the gastro-intestinal tract and on the cardiovascular and respiratory systems. Due to the slow growth of the tumour the symptoms may extend over many years despite the presence of extensive metastases.

The manifestations of the syndrome will be described under the main systems affected.

Gastro-intestinal. Abdominal discomfort is common, and hyperperistalsis with recurrent or persistent diarrhoea also occurs. Nausea and vomiting may be present, and colicky abdominal pain and loud borborygmi occur in association with the diarrhoea. Hepatomegaly is common and indicates carcinoid metastases. Occasionally, tumours in the appendix may obstruct the lumen of the organ, and symptoms indistinguishable from those of acute appendicitis may occur. More rarely, distal small bowel obstruction may be a presenting or a late feature.

Cardiovascular: (a) Vasomotor. The commonest and often the most striking feature of the syndrome is facial flushing. This may be periodic or continuous. The reddish or violaceous flush begins in the face and neck, characteristically spares the area round the eyes and mouth, and spreads to involve the upper chest and shoulders. Spread may occur to involve other parts of the body. Flushing is often accompanied by a feeling of dizziness and a transient fall in blood pressure. In the later stages there may be permanent and marked dilatation of the small blood vessels of the cheeks.

The attacks of flushing begin acutely and usually last only a few minutes, but may be much more persistent and may recur frequently. The severity, frequency and duration of the flushes increase as the disease progresses. Flushing attacks may be provoked by emotional stimuli, eating, alcohol ingestion, and pressure over the tumour tissue. They may also be produced by injection of adrenaline, noradrenaline, or histamine.

(b) Cardiac Involvement. Involvement of the right side of the heart, particularly pulmonary stenosis, appears fairly late in the course of the disease and occurs in about half of all advanced cases. The characteristic appearance of the valves is of a pearly grey fibrosis of the endocardium, with rigidity and thickening. Right-sided heart failure may develop. It is presumed that the predominance of right-sided cardiac lesions is due to the fact that the substances responsible for the cardiac lesions are inactivated in the lungs (Goble *et al.*, 1955). The precise pathogenesis of the valvular lesions is not understood. Nevertheless, left-sided lesions, involving most frequently the mitral valve, are seen. Communication between the right and left sides of the heart is not necessary for the development of such lesions, although there are several reports of patients with the carcinoid syndrome who have such communication and who show lesions involving both sides of the heart. There has been only one report of a patient with lesions confined to the left heart, and this occurred with a bronchial tumour.

Respiratory. The respiratory symptoms in the carcinoid syndrome consist of episodic changes in the depth and rate of respiration, and reversible airways obstruction, producing a wheeze. The former may occur without the latter and are probably mediated by 5-hydroxytryptamine release. Airways obstruction occurs in 20–30 per cent of patients and seems unlikely to be due to 5-hydroxytryptamine or bradykinin release; histamine may be the precipitating factor in these cases (Turck, Zeithin, Smith, and Grant, 1972).

Other Features. Other clinical features, rarely observed, include abnormal skin pigmentation with pellagra-like lesions, arthropathy, and oedema of the face, hands or ankles. Hypoglycaemia has rarely been reported.

THE BIOCHEMICAL FEATURES OF THE CARCINOID SYNDROME

Tryptophan is the principal precursor of the 5-hydroxyindoles, and an outline scheme of the metabolic pathways involved is given in Fig. 19.1. It has been known for twenty years that an increased urinary excretion of 5-hydroxytryptamine (5-HT, serotonin) and of its breakdown product 5-hydroxyindole acetic acid (5-HIAA) is present in the carcinoid syndrome, as well as an increase in urinary histamine. It has also been demonstrated that the majority of argentaffinomas secrete an excess of 5-HT or of other 5-hydroxyindoles. In patients with the syndrome the tryptophan—5-HT pathway becomes the metabolic route of as much as 50 per cent of the dietary tryptophan, in contrast to the one per cent normally metabolised by this route. As a result, much less tryptophan is available for protein and nicotinic acid production, which is the normal metabolic pathway, and thus protein deficiency and pellagra may result. The excess production of histamine may arise as a result of the local tissue effects of 5-HT, but work in recent years has suggested that there are biochemically different types of carcinoid and that excessive histamine production may be characteristic of some of them. Foregut argentaffinomas produce mainly 5-hydroxytryptophan and histamine; those derived from the embryological midgut produce mainly 5-hydroxytryptamine (Ross, 1972). While increased circulating levels of 5-HT and/or histamine are presumed to be largely responsible for the gastro-intestinal and respiratory symptoms, it is now apparent that these substances cannot wholly account for the facial flushing (*Lancet*, 1966). Another group of hypotensive peptides, the kinins, appear to play a major role in producing the carcinoid flush and probably some of the other symptoms. One representative of the group of kinin-forming enzymes, the kallikreins, has been detected in high concentration in argentaffinoma tissue.

These enzymes act on a plasma alpha-2 globulin, kallidinogen, to produce the decapeptide lysyl-bradykinin (kallidin), and it has been shown that kallikrein from carcinoid tissue will liberate kallidin *in vitro*. An aminopeptidase in plasma brings about the prompt conversion of lysyl-bradykinin to bradykinin, and this nonapeptide is the circulating kinin found in patients with the carcinoid syndrome. It seems, therefore, that argentaffinomas that are associated with the carcinoid syndrome may secrete a number of different vaso-reactive compounds—5-hydroxytryptamine and other 5-hydroxyindoles including 5-hydroxytryptophan and tryptamine, histamine, and bradykinin. It is apparent that a

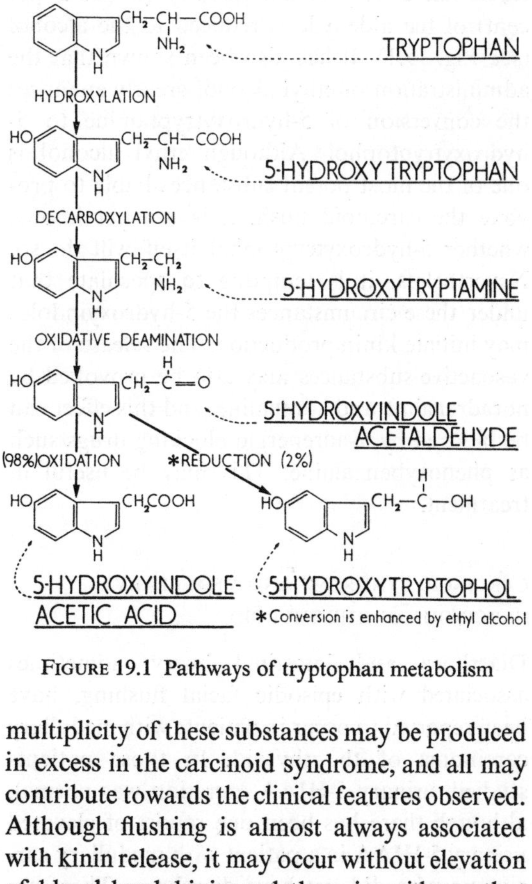

TRYPTOPHAN
HYDROXYLATION
5-HYDROXY TRYPTOPHAN
DECARBOXYLATION
5-HYDROXYTRYPTAMINE
OXIDATIVE DEAMINATION
5-HYDROXYINDOLE ACETALDEHYDE
(98%)OXIDATION
*REDUCTION (2%)
5-HYDROXYINDOLE-ACETIC ACID
5-HYDROXYTRYPTOPHOL
*Conversion is enhanced by ethyl alcohol

FIGURE 19.1 Pathways of tryptophan metabolism

multiplicity of these substances may be produced in excess in the carcinoid syndrome, and all may contribute towards the clinical features observed. Although flushing is almost always associated with kinin release, it may occur without elevation of blood bradykinin and there is evidence that vasodilator substances other than the kinins and those others mentioned above, but as yet unidentified, are also involved in the carcinoid syndrome. The prostaglandins may be included among these substances—high tissue levels of prostaglandin $F_2\alpha$ have been reported in bronchial carcinoids.

Another recent advance in our knowledge of tryptophan metabolism has been the identification of both tryptophan 5-hydroxylase and

5-hydroxytryptophol. Tryptophan 5-hydroxylase is the enzyme involved in the first and rate-limiting step in the conversion of tryptophan to 5-hydroxytryptamine, which is in turn oxidatively deaminated to 5-hydroxyindole acetaldehyde. This compound is oxidised further to 5-hydroxy-indole acetic acid. However, it has been shown that both in normal patients and in patients with carcinoid, a very small quantity (about 2 per cent) of the aldehyde is reduced to the alcohol (*see* Fig. 19.1). It has also been shown that the administration of ethyl alcohol greatly enhances the conversion of 5-hydroxytryptamine to 5-hydroxytryptophol. Although ethyl alcohol is one of the most potent substances liable to provoke the carcinoid flush, it is not yet known whether 5-hydroxytryptophol itself will do so. Nevertheless, it is tempting to speculate that under these circumstances the 5-hydroxyindoles may initiate kinin production. The release of the vasoactive substances may also be provoked by noradrenaline and adrenaline, and this effect can be blocked by α-adrenergic blocking drugs such as phenoxybenzamine. This may be useful in treatment.

CARCINOID SYNDROME AND MEDULLARY CARCINOMA OF THE THYROID

Diarrhoea and intestinal hurry, sometimes associated with episodic facial flushing, have been reported to occur in patients with medullary carcinoma of the thyroid. In those patients studied, urinary 5-HIAA excretion was normal, although there has been one report of elevated urinary 5-HIAA in a patient with medullary carcinoma who did *not* have diarrhoea. There are other similarities between argentaffinoma and medullary carcinoma of the thyroid (Williams, 1966). There is first a histological resemblance between the two tumours. The medullary carcinoma arises from the parafollicular or C cells in the thyroid gland, which lie between the follicular epithelium and the basement membrane in a similar situation to that of the kultschitzky cells in the gut from which the carcinoid tumour arises. Medullary carcinoma of the thyroid may elaborate prostaglandins, serotonin, and kinin-forming enzyme (Williams *et al.*, 1968). It seems quite likely therefore that this carcinoma is a tumour allied to the carcinoid group of neoplasms, and that it may on occasion produce a similar range of vaso-reactive substances to those elaborated by the argentaffinoma. In addition, both carcinoid tumours of lung or gut and medullary carcinomas may be associated with 'ectopic' production of ACTH (*see* Chapter 20), and there is evidence that some carcinoids might secrete calcitonin (Milhaud, 1972), although this is not observed in all cases.

DIAGNOSIS OF CARCINOID SYNDROME

The clinical features of the carcinoid syndrome are variable. The most constant feature is the liability to attacks of facial flushing. The association of intermittent diarrhoea or bronchospasm with flushing attacks is strongly suggestive of the diagnosis, particularly if hepatomegaly, right-sided valvular lesions or congestive heart failure are also present. A number of clinical conditions may possibly give rise to confusion in diagnosis—these include medullary carcinoma of the thyroid, phaeochromocytoma, spontaneous hypoglycaemia (where flushing during the attacks is not usually seen), and simple panic attacks.

Confirmation of the diagnosis of carcinoid syndrome may be obtained by estimating the urinary excretion of 5-hydroxyindole acetic acid, which is invariably elevated. However, urinary 5-HIAA may also be slightly elevated in a number of other situations, and it is necessary to exclude these before making a confident diagnosis of carcinoid. These include idiopathic steatorrhoea, ingestion of glycocollates (as in cough syrups), ingestion of foods containing significant amounts of serotonin such as bananas, tomatoes or walnuts, and transiently after administration of reserpine. Phenothiazine drugs and mephanesin carbamate interfere with the colour reaction in the estimation. Normal excretion of 5-HIAA is 2–10 mg in 24 hours; urinary levels in the carcinoid syndrome almost invariably exceed 50 mg/24 hr and as much as 1 g/day may be excreted in some cases. A rapid screening test involves the use of Ehrlich's aldehyde reagent—a purple coloration indicates an excretion of 40 mg/24 hr, or more, of 5HIAA. If facilities are available, blood serotonin levels may also be diagnostic. The normal range is 0·1–0·3 μg/ml of whole blood, while patients with the carcinoid syndrome have been reported to show concentrations ranging from 0·5–3 μg/ml. The carcinoid flush may be provoked by the intravenous administration of adrenaline, 1 to 10 μg (Peart *et al.*, 1959), and this can be most helpful in diagnosis. This test seems very reliable, but should be used with caution in the presence of severe cardiac or respiratory symptoms.

THE TREATMENT OF CARCINOID SYNDROME

Surgical removal of the tumour is the only satisfactory therapy. Unfortunately, by the very nature of the disease, metastases are almost invariably present when the syndrome becomes clinically apparent. Nevertheless, the primary tumour and any accessible metastases, including if possible liver deposits, should be removed when feasible, since the tumours progress remarkably slowly and quite marked amelioration of symptoms may be obtained. Medical treatment on the whole is most disappointing, and this is not at all surprising when it is realised that such therapy has been directed towards antagonising or inhibiting the 5-hyproxyindoles, which are now known to be only one of the factors involved in the pathogenesis of the syndrome. Serotonin antagonists such as lysergic acid diethylamide, cyproheptadine, and chloropromazine are relatively ineffective, although the latter may produce some improvement in the diarrhoea. Methysergide, another serotonin antagonist, in a dose of 2 mg tds is often effective in controlling bowel symptoms but it is not devoid of side effects. The drug ρ-chlorophenylalanine, an inhibitor of tryptophan 5-hydroxylase, is effective in depleting serotonin and relieves gastrointestinal symptoms in most patients, although mental changes may occur during treatment (Shani and Sheba, 1970). Antihistamines are completely without effect. In some patients with the gastric type of tumour, which predominantly secretes 5-hydroxytryptophan, good results have been obtained by the use of α-methyldopa, which reduces the rate of decarboxylation of 5-hydroxytryptophan to 5-hydroxytryptamine in peripheral target organs. Local perfusion of metastatic deposits in the liver with cytotoxic drugs infused via an hepatic artery cannula has been attempted, but results of this form of treatment are variable and the dangers great.

There is no specific treatment for the airways obstruction. However, Turck and his colleagues (1972) found that inhaled adrenaline and isoprenaline aerosols were of value in the patient they described, and did not have the disadvantages of intravenous adrenaline, which, as mentioned above, provokes the carcinoid flush.

The frequency of the attacks of flushing may be substantially reduced and the patient made more comfortable by treatment with α-adrenergic blocking drugs (Adamson *et al.*, 1969). Phenoxybenzamine may be given orally in a dose of 10 mg three or four times daily.

REFERENCES

Adamson, A. R., Graham-Smith, D. G., Peart, W. S., and Star, M. (1969). *Lancet*, **ii**, 293.

Biörck, G., Axén, O., and Thörson, A. (1952). *Amer. Heart J.*, **44**, 143.

Editorial (1966). *Lancet*, **ii**, 1013.

Goble, A. J., Hay, D. R., and Sandler, M. (1955). *Lancet*, **ii**, 1016.

Milhaud, G. (1972). In *Proceedings of the Fourth Parathyroid Conference* (Ed. Talmage, R. V. and Munson, P. L.). Amsterdam: Excerpta Medica.

Peart, W. S., Robertson, J. I. S., and Andrews, T. M. (1959). *Lancet*, **ii**, 715.
Rosenbaum, F. F., Santer, D. G., and Claudon, D. B. (1953). *J. lab. clin. Med.*, **42**, 941.
Ross, E. J. (1972). *Brit. Med. J.*, **1**, 735.
Shani, M., and Sheba, Ch. (1970). *Brit. Med. J.*, **4**, 784.
Turck, W. P. G., Grant, I. W. B., Zeitlin, I. J., and Smith, A. N. (1972). *Scot. Med. J.*, **17**, 244.
Turck, W. P. G., Zeitlin, I. J., Smith, A. N., and Grant, I. W. B. (1972). *Scot. Med. J.*, **17**, 237.
Williams, E. D. (1966). *Proc. roy. Soc. Med.*, **59**, 602.
Williams, E. D., Karim, S. M. M., and Sandler, M. (1968). *Lancet*, **i**, 22.

20

ECTOPIC HORMONE PRODUCTION BY NON-ENDOCRINE TUMOURS

Many different hormones can be secreted by tumours of tissues other than those normally responsible for their synthesis, so called 'ectopic' hormone production by tumours (Liddle *et al.*, 1965). Although these syndromes have been thought to be rare, they are being recognised with increasing frequency. Their development may precede other manifestations of the neoplasm, sometimes by many years, especially when the associated tumour is not malignant, e.g. a bronchial carcinoid. Some syndromes are so unusual that they immediately suggest the possibility of a tumour at a particular site, e.g. the syndrome of inappropriate secretion of vasopressin associated with a bronchogenic carcinoma. Awareness of these syndromes sometimes allows the underlying neoplasm to be diagnosed at an early stage. Improvement of the endocrine manifestations after removal of the neoplasm may be followed by their recurrence, along with recurrence of the tumour.

What then is the explanation for the synthesis of hormones by various tumours? Three theories have been put forward. The first suggests that hormones are synthesised by chance as a result of random or chaotic protein synthesis characteristic of neoplastic growth. Mutations of the DNA of malignant cells would allow coding of peptides with endocrine activity. On the basis of this theory, a tumour might synthesise active peptides with structures similar to the part of the naturally occurring hormone required for biological activity. Since the peptide sequences which constitute an immunoreactive site of a hormone are not necessarily the same as those needed for its biochemical function, the hormone secreted by a tumour might not be immunologically identical with the natural hormone. Thyroid stimulating hormone and insulin produced by tumours usually appear to be immunologically different from normal TSH and insulin, a finding consistent with the random synthesis theory, but other tumour hormones are both immunologically and biologically similar, e.g. ACTH, MSH, and vasopressin. It is not uncommon for a tumour to secrete more than one hormone, and this would be rather unlikely if random synthesis of peptides were occurring.

The second possibility is that certain tumours may have a high avidity for hormones, acting as 'hormone sponges' which concentrate the hormone from the circulation. Rapid breakdown of malignant cells in an enlarging tumour would allow release of the stored hormone or hormones. There does not seem to be any good evidence in support of this theory.

The demonstration that neoplastic tissues can continue to release hormones into the medium when they are maintained in organ culture clearly demonstrates that 'ectopic' synthesis as well as release of hormones may occur in non-endocrine tumours and provides strong evidence against the 'sponge' theory and strong support for the third, 'de-repression' theory. Furthermore, the 'sponge' concept cannot apply to the situation where the ectopically produced hormone would never normally be found in the patient, for example the ectopic production of placental lactogen in men with bronchial carcinomas. Clearly, in these cases, synthesis of the hormone must have occurred *de novo* within the tumour. The de-repression theory holds that tumour cells, like all other cells except the gamete cells, inherit an identical complement of DNA and, therefore, all the coded information requisite for synthesis of all normal proteins. Normal differentiation of cells involves reversible repression of specific segments of the DNA molecule, possibly by combination of DNA with histones, and much of the genetic potential of a normal cell is masked in this way. The malignant cell would revert to synthesis of various peptides, either by inactivation of the histone repressor, or by deletion of a regulator gene. This is normally thought to produce the repressor which combines with the operon normally slowing the manufacture of the messenger RNA molecules (Hobbs and Miller, 1966; *Lancet*, 1967). If de-repression is involved in tumour hormone synthesis, the hormone produced by the tumour would be likely to be identical with the natural hormone as seems to be the case for ACTH, MSH, vasopressin and parathormone, although final proof awaits chemical analysis of the hormones produced by tumours.

The explanation for the synthesis of hormones by tumours is therefore still uncertain, current evidence suggesting that some tumours might produce hormones because of random peptide synthesis, whereas most synthesise hormones apparently identical with natural hormones because of 'de-repression'.

Before it can be accepted that a tumour is responsible for an endocrine syndrome, certain criteria should be fulfilled:

1. The tumour should be shown to be able to synthesise the hormone. Usually, this has been assumed by finding a high tumour content of the hormone, improvement of the syndrome after removal of the tumour, and recurrence of the syndrome along with recurrence of the tumour. Incorporation of labelled precursors of the hormone by the tumour *in vivo* or *in vitro* would also be useful evidence. Demonstration of a higher concentration of the hormone in the venous blood draining the tumour than in the arterial supply is good evidence for release of hormone by the tumour and indirect evidence for its synthesis.
2. The hormonal material should be demonstrable in the circulation, and sometimes in the urine.
3. The hormone in the circulation should be capable of producing the endocrine syndrome affecting the patient.
4. Removal of the tumour or its treatment by radiation or other means should be followed by disappearance or fall in the level of the hormone in the circulation and improvement of the endocrine syndrome.

The endocrine syndromes associated with non-endocrine tumours are listed in Table 20.1, together with some examples of the ectopic production of hormones without associated clinical syndromes. Published accounts derived from isolated case reports are not helpful in determining the frequency of the syndromes. Certainly, these conditions are not rare although they are frequently overlooked.

THE SIGNIFICANCE OF ECTOPIC HORMONE PRODUCTION

This far outweighs that suggested by the actual incidence of the clinical syndromes. Firstly, if we understood the mechanisms whereby the malignant cell produces a hormone apparently quite foreign to the tissues from which the tumour was derived, we might gain some understanding of the nature of the biochemical or genetic changes

TABLE 20.1 *Hormones Produced 'Ectopically' by Non-Endocrine Tumours and their Associated Clinical Syndromes*

Hormone	Clinical Syndrome
ACTH* and MSH; occasionally with CRF or CLIP**	Cushing's syndrome.
Vasopressin	Inappropriate vasopressin secretion with water-retention.
Parathormone (or occasionally calciferol-like sterols)	Hypercalcaemia.
Growth hormone*	Hypertrophic pulmonary osteoarthropathy
Gonadotrophins*	Gynaecomastia or precocious puberty
Prolactin*	Galactorrhoea.
Insulin-like*	Hypoglycaemia.
TSH-like	Hyperthyroidism.
Enteroglucagon	Constipation.
Erythropoietin-like	Polycythaemia.
Prostaglandins, 5-hydroxytryptamine, 5-hydroxytryptophan	Atypical carcinoid.
Placental lactogen	None recognised.
Oxytocin	Found sometimes within appropriate vasopressin secretion.
Neurophysin	
Glucagon	Found sometimes in association with insulin.

* Also sometimes found in tumours without obvious clinical sequelae.
**CLIP—'corticotrophin-like intermediate lobe peptide'—*see* ectopic ACTH syndrome in text.

associated with malignancy. Furthermore, the identification of the hormonal products released by these tumours has allowed us to develop some insight into the reasons that tumours actually make people ill even though the lesions are often small and do not involve vital structures. Clearly they produce toxic chemicals, and this concept of 'biochemical malignancy' includes production not only of hormones but also enzymes and other abnormal proteins such as fetal proteins and immunoglobulins. Treatment can be directed at the effects of the toxic products; but in addition, by following the concentration of these 'biochemical markers of malignancy' the effects of any therapy directed at the tumour may be assessed. The blood or urine levels of the substance may be related to the mass of active tumour tissue and may indicate whether the tumour has been eradicated, or may suggest recurrence well before this is clinically obvious (Fig. 20.1).

The concept of endocrine markers of malignancy is already well established in association with non-'ectopic' secretion from functioning malignant tumours of endocrine tissues in which the blood or urine levels of the hormone are used to follow the progress of the disease. Such tumours include adrenocortical carcinomas (cortisol, androgen or oestrogen markers), phaeochromocytomas (catecholamines), medullary carcinoma of thyroid (calcitonin), parathyroid carcinoma (parathormone), carcinoid tumours (5-hydroxytryptamine and 5-hydroxytryptophan), islet-cell tumours of pancreas (insulin or gastrin), chorioncarcinoma of uterus or testis (HCG), interstitialcell tumours of testis (oestrogen), arrhenoblastomas or granulosa cell tumours of the ovary (testosterone or oestrogen). These conditions will not be considered further in this chapter.

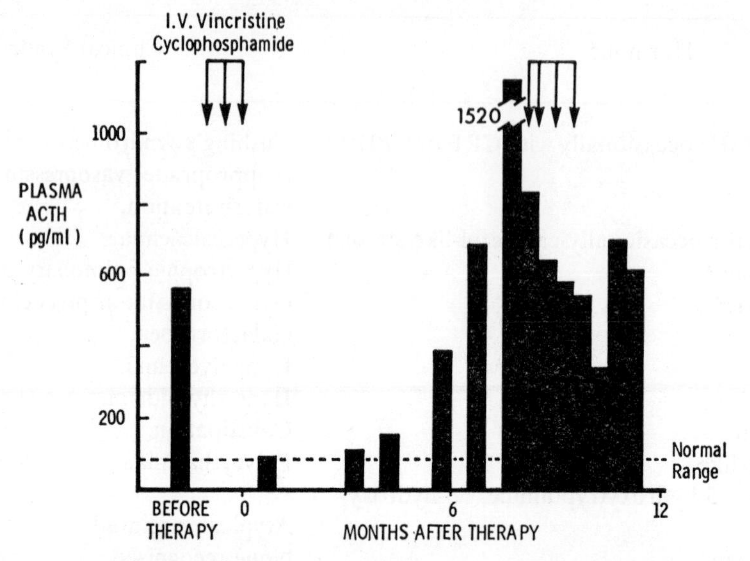

FIGURE 20.1 Plasma immunoreactive ACTH response to chemotherapy in a patient with the ectopic ACTH syndrome. The second rise in ACTH antedated the clinical recurrence by many weeks (data of Professor D. M. Wolff and Dr. J. G. Ratcliffe, from Besser, G. M., and Edwards, C. R. W. (1972), *Clinics in Endocrinology and Metabolism*, **1**, 451, by permission of the Editor).

THE ECTOPIC ACTH SYNDROME

The first of this group of diseases to become recognised was Cushing's syndrome resulting from overproduction of ACTH-like peptides from tumours, and was described by Liddle in 1962. It was later termed the ectopic ACTH syndrome by him. The first case appears to be that of Brown who, in 1928, described a patient with Cushing's syndrome due to bilateral adrenal hyperplasia who at post mortem was found to have an oat cell carcinoma of the bronchus. Although most cases of the ectopic ACTH syndrome are associated with bronchogenic carcinoma, particularly of this histological type, a wide variety of other tumours has been implicated (Table 20.2). β-MSH is almost always also secreted in excess in the ectopic ACTH syndrome and is responsible for the pigmentation.

CLINICAL FEATURES

Only a minority of patients show the typical features of Cushing's syndrome despite the high levels of cortisol production. When corticosteroids are given to a normal person it takes about two months for the stigmata of Cushing's syndrome to develop, and most patients with the ectopic ACTH syndrome do not live this long. The rapid weight loss due to the carcinoma may also mask the clinical picture. Many of the patients present with ankle oedema or with pigmentation, others complain of muscle weakness or of thirst and polyuria due to diabetes mellitus. Unlike other causes of Cushing's syndrome, the majority of the patients are men because of the male predominance of bronchogenic carcinoma,

TABLE 20.2 *Tumours Responsible for Ectopic ACTH Syndrome*

Tumour Site	Approximate Frequency
Lung (oat cell carcinoma of bronchus and bronchial adenoma)	+++
Thymus	++
Pancreas	++
Prostate	+
Breast	+
Phaeochromocytoma	+
Ganglioneuroma	+
Oesophagus	+
Stomach	+
Liver	+
Parotid	+
Thyroid (medullary carcinoma)	+
Ovary	+
Testis	+
Kidney	+
Central nervous system	+

TABLE 20.3 *Non-ectopic Cushing's Syndrome Compared with the Ectopic ACTH Syndrome: Clinical Features*

	Cushing's syndrome	Ectopic ACTH syndrome
Sex incidence	Predominantly female	Predominantly male
Speed of onset	Slow	Rapid
Increased pigmentation	Uncommon	Common
Oedema	Rare	Common
Weight loss	Uncommon	Common
Clinical course	Months to years	Days to weeks
Cause of death	Hypertension, infection	Carcinoma

and the ectopic ACTH syndrome should be suspected in any man presenting with Cushing's syndrome. A comparison of the clinical features of Cushing's syndrome and the ectopic ACTH syndrome is shown in Table 20.3. Ectopic ACTH production from benign bronchial adenomas (carcinoids) sometimes becomes confused with pituitary-dependent Cushing's disease. These tumours are often small and difficult to find and, as the tumour is benign, the patient lives on to become truly Cushingoid, unlike most other patients with ectopic ACTH production. Often the bronchial tumour is only discovered some years after a total adrenalectomy has been performed.

INVESTIGATIONS

The most important clue to the diagnosis is the presence of hypokalaemic alkalosis, the result of the very high cortisol production rate, and this is unusual in other types of Cushing's syndrome (Table 20.4). Plasma and urinary corticosteroid and ACTH concentrations are elevated to levels higher than in most other patients with Cushing's syndrome and are usually unaffected by dexamethasone, or metyrapone (Table 20.4) (Ratcliffe *et al.*, 1972). The plasma corticosteroids and ACTH levels show no circadian fluctuation.

A chest X-ray is a routine investigation in any patient presenting with Cushing's syndrome, and where clinical clues indicate, lung tomography, sputum cytology, bronchoscopy, barium studies of gut, IVP, etc. to find the primary carcinoma should be performed.

PATHOGENESIS

High concentrations of ACTH have been found in the plasma of patients with the syndrome and a large amount of the hormone has been found in the carcinoma at operation or autopsy (Meador *et al.*, 1962). Because of the limited amount of tumour ACTH available for analysis, its amino-acid composition has not yet been fully established. However, tumour ACTH has proved

TABLE 20.4 *Cushing's Syndrome Compared with the Ectopic ACTH Syndrome: Investigations*

	Cushing's Syndrome	Ectopic ACTH Syndrome
Hypokalaemic alkalosis	Uncommon	Usual
Hyperglycaemia	Common	Usual
Plasma cortisol above 40 μg/100 ml	Rare	Common
Plasma ACTH greater than 200 pg/ml (*see* Fig. 6.10)	Rare	Common
Cortisol production rate	1·5–2 × normal	2–10 × normal
Response of urinary 17-OHCS to		
(*a*) metyrapone	Increase*	No change**
(*b*) 8 mg/day dexamethasone	Decrease*	No change**

* Unless due to adrenocortical tumour.
** Exceptions have been described, particularly with bronchial carcinoids.

identical with natural ACTH in a wide variety of biological and immunological procedures (Liddle *et al.*, 1965). The pituitary glands of patients with the syndrome have a low ACTH content (Meador *et al.*, 1962). Carcinoid tumours responsible for ectopic ACTH production have been shown to produce, in addition to ACTH and MSH, large amounts of a peptide provisionally called the corticotrophin-like intermediate lobe peptide (CLIP). This material appears to be part of the ACTH molecule (amino-acids 18 to 39) but is devoid of corticosteroidogenic or other known actions. Its name derives from the fact that it is otherwise only found in the intermediate lobes of the pituitaries of mammals such as rats and pigs, in association with α-MSH. CLIP can be measured by radioimmunoassay using appropriate antibodies to ACTH. Carcinoid tumours may be suspected in Cushingoid patients when the ACTH levels, using these antisera, appear to be out of proportion to the results of assays using antisera reacting with the first 16 amino-acids of ACTH. This may be the only clue to the true diagnosis (Ratcliffe *et al.*, 1972). Corticotrophin-releasing hormone (CRH)-like activity has also been reported to occur in 2 tumours from patients with the ectopic ACTH syndrome (Upton *et al.*, 1971).

TREATMENT

Patients with carcinoma who develop this syndrome usually have a very poor prognosis, the cortisol overproduction contributing to the short survival, but patients with bronchial carcinoid tumours usually do well. If the patient is fit enough for operation, and operation is feasible, then the tumour producing the ACTH should be removed. If removal is complete, the clinical and biochemical features of the syndrome remit (Liddle *et al.*, 1965). The patient may require large amounts of potassium pre-operatively to correct the hypokalaemia. Unfortunately, such tumours are usually inoperable, and only a small proportion are sensitive to radiotherapy or chemotherapy (Fig. 20.1). In the absence of adequate surgical treatment, or in preparation for it, cortisol production can be reduced using adrenocortical enzyme inhibitors such as metyrapone (750 mg, 6–8-hourly) with or without aminoglutethimide (250–500 mg, 8-hourly). As it is possible to produce an acute Addisonian crisis by overtreatment using these drugs it is wise to give prednisolone 5 mg, 12-hourly, while the dose is adjusted and the plasma corticosteroid levels monitored. Once the plasma cortisol level is reduced to between 15 and 20 $\mu g/100$ ml throughout the day, the prednisolone cover may be stopped. Unfortunately the patients often do badly however they are managed since the underlying tumour is frequently very malignant.

POLYCYTHAEMIA

More than 200 patients have been reported with polycythaemia associated with neoplastic disease. Table 20.5 shows the various neoplasms known to cause polycythaemia. Three of the tumours listed, the cerebellar haemangioblastoma, the hypernephroma, and the phaeochromocytoma may occur together in the Von-Hippel-Lindau syndrome.

TABLE 20.5 *Tumours Responsible for Polycythaemia*

Tumour	Approximate Frequency
Renal carcinoma	+++
Benign renal lesions including cysts, adenomas, hydronephrosis	++
Cerebellar haemangioblastoma	++
Uterine fibroma	+
Adrenocortical carcinoma or hyperplasia	+
Ovarian tumours	+
Hepatoma	+
Phaeochromocytoma	+

CLINICAL FEATURES AND INVESTIGATIONS

The patients show erythrocytosis with an elevated haemoglobin concentration and haematocrit. Unlike polycythaemia rubra vera there is no enlargement of the spleen and usually no alteration in white cell or platelet count. The red cell count returns to normal after complete removal of the tumour.

PATHOGENESIS

Many theories have been proposed to explain the association of erythrocytosis and tumours. It is unlikely to represent the chance occurrence of polycythaemia rubra vera with such a tumour since there is no leucocytosis, thrombocythaemia, or splenomegaly and the condition can be cured by resection of the tumour. Nor does anoxia appear to be a major factor since the arterial oxygen saturation has been reported to be normal in several patients.

As in other endocrine syndromes associated with tumours, the most likely explanation is that the tumour produces some humoral agent, which in this case is capable of stimulating erythropoiesis. Bioassays of renal tumour extracts or renal or cerebellar cyst fluid have confirmed the presence of an erythropoietin-like material which, like the natural hormone, was inactivated by the proteolytic enzymes trypsin and sialidase and moved identically on zone electrophoresis. The molecular weight of the tumour hormone, as determined by the radiation inactivation technique, was about 30,000, similar to that of erythropoietin. Again, the tumour hormone was inactivated by incubation with an antibody prepared against partially purified human erythropoietin (Lipsett *et al.*, 1964).

However, the polycythaemia observed in patients with hepatomas, uterine fibromas, and virilising tumours of the adrenal and ovary may have another explanation since it has not always been possible to demonstrate erythropoietin-like material in the serum of such patients or in their neoplasms. It is possible that other humoral agents are produced by these tumours.

HYPOGLYCAEMIA

More than 100 patients have been reported with hypoglycaemia in association with non-pancreatic neoplasms, usually a connective-tissue tumour of low grade malignancy, or a primary carcinoma of the liver. The first case was reported by Doege (1930) in a patient with a mediastinal fibrosarcoma. Although no blood sugar estimations were made, the patient suffered from episodes of irrational and maniacal behaviour which disappeared after removal of a tumour weighing 4½ lb. The tumours responsible for the syndrome are shown in Table 20.6. All the mesenchymal tumours causing hypoglycaemia have been large, weights ranging from 800–10,000 G, and all have been located in the abdomen or, less often, in the thorax. Many of the neoplasms have been benign, and at least twenty patients have been relieved of symptoms by resection of the tumour. The sex incidence of the tumours is about equal, most occurring in patients aged between forty and seventy years.

TABLE 20.6 *Tumours Responsible for Hypoglycaemia*

Tumour	Approximate Frequency
Mesenchymal including fibrosarcomas, mesotheliomas, neurofibromas, neurofibrosarcomas, spindle-cell sarcomas, leiomyosarcomas, and rhabdomyosarcomas	+++
Hepatic	++
Adrenal carcinoma	+
Miscellaneous, including bronchogenic carcinoma, other anaplastic carcinomas, adenocarcinomas, cholangiomas and pseudomyxomas	+

CLINICAL FEATURES

Hypoglycaemic attacks may occur spontaneously, or may be provoked only by prolonged fasting, sometimes antedating the clinical diagnosis of the tumour. The hypoglycaemia can be very severe and may not be preventable even with frequent feeding; it differs in no way from the hypoglycaemia resultings from islet cell tumours (*see* Chapter 16).

INVESTIGATIONS

The blood glucose level is low during hypoglycaemic episodes but the fasting plasma insulin level (as determined by immunoassay) is not raised. To distinguish the condition from an insulinoma, the intravenous tolbutamide test can be applied; patients with tumours outside the pancreas have a normal or depressed plasma-insulin response. The blood glucose response to tolbutamide is not helpful since patients may be sensitive or insensitive to this drug. Hypoglycaemia cannot usually be induced by administration of leucine.

PATHOGENESIS

The hypoglycaemia is unlikely to result from excessive utilisation of glucose by the tumour since the difference in arterial and venous glucose in vessels supplying these tumours is not great, nor does tumour tissue *in vitro* have a high rate of glucose consumption. Again, the hypoglycaemia associated with hepatomas is not adequately explained on the basis of decreased glucose output by the liver. Even in advanced cases there is usually a large amount of normal liver tissue, and other liver functions may be little deranged in the presence of severe hypoglycaemia.

It has been suggested that tumours cause hypoglycaemia by stimulating pancreatic insulin release, but failure to cure the syndrome by pancreatectomy (Miller *et al.*, 1959) makes this possibility unlikely.

There seems little doubt that the hypoglycaemia is usually due to the elaboration of a hypoglycaemic agent by the tumour. Insulin-like material extracted from many of the tumours is active on bioassays utilising the rat epididymal fat pad or the rat diaphragm. Variability in reports probably depend on methodological differences, particularly in the extraction procedure used. However, immunoassay procedures have usually failed to demonstrate material with the immunological properties of insulin in these tumours. An exception to this finding is the report by Unger *et al.* (1964) who detected insulin by a highly specific radioimmunoassay in a hepatic metastasis of a patient with an undifferentiated bronchogenic carcinoma. This tumour also contained a high concentration of glucagon-like material, and the patient had no clinical evidence of hypoglycaemia. Few workers have been able to demonstrate insulin-like material in the plasma of these patients. Further evidence that the hypoglycaemic agent is usually distinct from insulin is the report by Hayes *et al.* (1961) that free fatty acid levels were high during hypoglycaemia, whereas after insulin, fatty acid levels are low. Again, serum phosphorus levels did not fall during hypoglycaemia, as is usual with insulin.

The bulk of the evidence suggests that hypoglycaemia is in most cases due to some humoral agent, usually distinct from insulin, though the mechanism of action of this compound is still unknown.

TREATMENT

Removal of the tumour is obviously indicated, and is followed by relief of the hypoglycaemia. Since some of the tumours are benign or of low-grade malignancy, their size is no contraindication to operation. Symptomatic treatment of the hypoglycaemia by frequent high carbohydrate meals may be helpful if the tumour is inoperable.

HYPERCALCAEMIA

Hypercalcaemia is a frequent and potentially hazardous complication of malignant tumours. In many instances the hypercalcaemia is the result of osseous metastases, destruction of bone by the tumour releasing calcium at a faster rate than the kidneys, gut, or normal bone can excrete or take up the additional load. It has been estimated that dissolution of one gramme of bone liberates 100 mg of calcium.

Hypercalcaemia may also be found in patients with cancer who have no demonstrable bony metastases. Albright and Reifenstein (1948) first suggested that hypercalcaemia might result from the secretion of a parathyoid hormone-like material from a tumour. Their patient had a renal carcinoma with a solitary secondary deposit in the bony pelvis and hypercalcaemia. Irradiation of the metastasis caused a transient improvement in the hypercalcaemia. In 1956, Plimpton and Gellhorn reported ten cases of hypercalcaemia without radiological evidence of bony metastases, confirmed at autopsy in seven. In three of their patients, removal of the primary tumour was associated with a fall in the serum calcium with, in one case, a recurrence of the hypercalcaemia associated with recurrence of the tumour.

Various carcinomas have been reported to cause hypercalcaemia without bony metastases and these are listed in Table 20.7. The condition must often be overlooked, since Carey (1966) in a series of 100 consecutive patients with bronchogenic carcinoma found six patients with hypercalcaemia without bony metastes, in whom there was no alternative explanation for the elevation of the serum calcium.

TABLE 20.7 *Tumours Responsible for Hypercalcaemia without Bony Metastases*

Tumour site	Approximate Frequency
Lung (usually squamous carcinoma)	+++
Kidney	+++
Ovary	++
Uterus	++
Pancreas	++
Vagina	+
Bladder	+
Prostate	+
Penis	+
Liver	+
Colon	+
Oesophagus	+
Prostate	+

CLINICAL FEATURES

The clinical features are those of hypercalcaemia—thirst, polyuria, lassitude, muscular weakness, nausea, vomiting, cardiac arrhythmias, drowsiness, depression, mental confusion, and coma. They may simulate the picture of cerebral metastases. Milder degrees of hypercalcaemia may be asymptomatic and found only on the routine investigation, which should be undertaken on all patients with bronchial or renal malignancy. In 11 of 20 cases reviewed by Rosenberg the neoplasm was removed, and in 10 the serum calcium fell to normal within a few days of operation, Lipsett *et al.* (1964). In 3 of these 10 cases hypercalcaemia returned with recurrence of the neoplasm. In inoperable patients, the hypercalcaemia can usually be successfully treated and the symptoms alleviated with medical treatment. Patients with malignant disease should not be regarded as being untreatable simply because of symptomatic hypercalcaemia.

INVESTIGATIONS

Patients with the syndrome show elevation of the plasma ionised as well as total calcium, with a tendency for lower values in association with renal tumours. In the majority of patients the serum phosphorous levels are lowered and alkaline phosphatase concentration raised, but without isoenzyme studies the latter could as well have resulted from hepatic metastases as from the action of a parathyroid hormone-like material on bone. Hypercalciuria is common unless renal function is impaired. Nephrocalcinosis, ectopic calcification, and the radiological features of hyperparathyroidism are not found, although bone taken from such patients shows an increase in oxidative metabolism similar to that seen in experimental hyperparathyroidism (Goldberg *et al.*, 1964). The absence of radiological features of hyperparathyroidism is probably explained by the shorter duration of the disease.

DIFFERENTIAL DIAGNOSIS

The clinical picture is very similar to that of primary hyperparathyroidism though the hypercalcaemia of malignancy is usually of more rapid onset and is not associated with radiological changes of hyperparathyroidism. A marked fall in serum calcium after corticosteroids has been stated to distinguish the condition from primary hyperparathyroidism. Other causes of hypercalcaemia should be ruled out, and X-rays taken to show that there are no visible bony metastases and no subperiosteal erosions of simple hyperparathyroidism.

PATHOGENESIS

Several theories have been put forward to explain the hypercalcaemia associated with malignant disease in the absence of bony metastases. Without serial sections of the whole skeleton, it would be difficult to rule out small osseous metastases which could possible have a destructive effect out of proportion to their size. However, the dramatic fall in serum calcium after removal of the primary tumour virtually rules out this possibility in many of the cases, and supports the theory that some humoral factor produced by the tumour is responsible.

Several authors have suggested that the hypercalcaemia might result from increased protein binding, increased complex formation, or chelation of calcium by some factor produced by the tumour. Walser (1962) showed that there was no abnormality of ionised calcium or protein binding in several patients in whom the rise in ionised calcium was proportional to the increase in total serum calcium so this theory seems unlikely.

Gordon *et al.* (1966, 1967) have reported on a series of patients with metastatic carcinoma of the breast and hypercalcaemia with normal or elevated serum phosphorus levels. These patients were found to have large amounts of the vitamin D-like sterols stigmasterol acetate and 17-hydroxysitosterol acetate in their plasma and breast tissue, whereas these sterols were absent from the plasma or breast of normal patients. Stigmasterol acetate is a powerful hypercalcaemic agent but, in man, it does not decrease the renal tubular reabsorption of phosphate. Parathormone-like activity has only rarely been found in breast tumour tissue.

Rarely, hyperplasia of the parathyroids has been described in patients with hypercalcaemia and malignant disease and it has been postulated that in these cases at least the tumour is producing a humoral agent capable of stimulating the parathyroids. A trophic hormone for the parathyroids has not so far been demonstrated, and it is possible that the parathyroid hyperplasia in these cases was due to renal failure or a malabsorption syndrome induced by the neoplasm.

The most convincing evidence suggests that the syndrome is due to the production of a material with parathyroid hormone-like activity by the tumour. Munson *et al.* (1965) reported a parathyroid hormone-like substance in tumour extracts which specifically inhibited the immunological reaction between bovine parathyroid hormone and its specific antiserum. Sherwood *et al.* (1967) have also demonstrated a substance identical to parathyroid hormone in tumour extracts by its chemical, physical, and immunological characteristics.

TREATMENT

Hypercalcaemia warrants therapy unless the patient is moribund with extensive malignant disease. An increased intake of fluids and saline infusions may sometimes suffice, whereas other patients require treatment with subcutaneous porcine calcitonin 60–120 MRC units 12-hourly, oral or intravenous phosphate, intravenous sodium sulphate or high doses of corticosteroids. In most patients with malignant hypercalcaemia the calcium can be lowered with prednisolone although sometimes doses as high as 80–100 mg/day) must be used in the first instance. When possible, the primary tumour should be resected or irradiated. If inoperable, the hypercalcaemia can often be controlled over long period of time, sometimes several years, with small doses of prednisolone (10–15 mg/day). Oral phosphate (effervescent phosphate tablets, 3–6 daily) and a high fluid intake may be required in addition.

INAPPROPRIATE SECRETION OF VASOPRESSIN (water retention)

In 1938, Winkler and Crankshaw reported a patient with carcinoma of the bronchus who had hyponatraemia and a high rate of sodium excretion in the urine. Schwartz *et al.* (1957) described two similar patients, who excreted hypertonic urine despite having hypotonic plasma and an expanded extracellular fluid volume. They pointed out that the only known cause for secretion of hypertonic urine in the presence of hypotonic plasma is an excess of vasopressin. They showed that the hyponatraemia in these cases was largely dilutional and suggested that it was due to overproduction of vasopressin which was *inappropriate* because, in normal circumstances, the low plasma osmolality should have switched-off vasopressin secretion. Since then many patients have been described with this syndrome, mostly associated with oat cell carcinoma of the bronchus.

This dilutional hyponatraemia may also occur in a wide variety of non-malignant conditions, e.g. after head injury, in cerebro-vascular disease, in brain and pituitary tumours, in encephalitis, poliomyelitis, the Guillain–Barré syndrome, and tuberculous meningitis, in a variety of chest conditions, including pulmonary tuberculosis and staphylococcal pneumonia, in myxoedema, and in acute intermittent porphyria. In these conditions the hyponatraemia disappears when the primary disorder improves.

CLINICAL FEATURES

The clinical features specific to dilutional hyponatraemia are largely those of *water intoxication* with depression, lethargy, mental confusion, irritability, anorexia, nausea, and generalised muscular weakness, but no oedema. The patient may show marked personality changes, becoming aggressive and uncooperative. If the plasma sodium falls below 110 mEq/litre, neurological abnormalities such as areflexia, pseudo-bulbar palsy and extensor plantar responses may be noted. With further reduction stupor, coma convulsions and death may occur. As the condition is usually easily remediable, the possibility of hyponatraemia should always be borne in mind in appropriate circumstances. Hyponatraemia may precede other clinical evidence of a bronchogenic carcinoma, and should always alert the physician to the possibility of this diagnosis. Care must be taken not to incorrectly ascribe the symptoms to the underlying disease, e.g. to the presence of hidden cerebral or hepatic metastases.

INVESTIGATIONS

The abnormalities found are the result of the inappropriate secretion of vasopressin, causing overhydration. Plasma sodium is low, usually less than 125 mEq/litre and, occasionally, as low as 100 mEq/litre. Plasma chloride and urea are also low, and plasma potassium is low or normal. The plasma volume is normal or increased, the extra-cellular volume and the total body water are increased, and the haematocrit is low or normal. Plasma osmolality is low, almost always less than 270 m Osmol/kg and the urine osmolality is higher than that of the plasma. The glomerular filtration rate measured by inulin or creatinine clearance is normal. There is excessive urinary loss of sodium despite the low plasma sodium level. This is sometimes due to reduction in aldosterone secretion consequent upon the expanded plasma volume, but in many patients aldosterone secretion is normal. In these patients it seems that there is inhibition of the normal sodium reabsorption at the proximal tubule. However, although there is usually a state of mild negative overall sodium balance, the principal abnormality is the vasopressin secretion and water overload. The cardinal feature in the laboratory investigations, therefore, is the simultaneous occurrence of hypotonic plasma, and urine which is more concentrated than the plasma.

Patients with dilutional hyponatraemia are unable to excrete a water load, and a test based on this abnormality can provide useful confirmation of the condition.

DIFFERENTIAL DIAGNOSIS

Hyponatraemia *per se* gives little information as to the sodium balance of an individual patient; it may be present when the total body sodium is low or normal, and in various diseases associated with oedema such as congestive heart failure, cirrhosis of the liver, and the nephrotic syndrome, total body sodium may be increased in the presence of hyponatraemia. Oedema is not usually a feature of the syndrome of inappropriate secretion of vasopressin. Depletion of total body sodium due to gastro-intestinal loss, adrenocortical insufficiency, and 'salt-losing nephritis' may also be associated with hyponatraemia. These conditions usually result in haemoconcentration, hypertonic plasma, extra-renal uraemia, and hypotension—a raised blood urea concentration and haematocrit, and a lowered plasma volume all suggest sodium depletion. Patients with dilutional hyponatraemia do not show these features and are not usually hypotensive.

Adrenocortical insufficiency causes most problems in diagnosis and this may also be the result of a bronchogenic carcinoma. Skin pigmentation may also occur with the vasopressin excess syndrome because of simultaneous overproduction of ACTH or MSH-like peptides by the tumour or as a result of the skin pigmentation commonly associated with malignant tumours. Tests of adrenocortical function easily distinguish the two disorders, plasma corticosteroids showing a prompt rise after ACTH in patients with dilutional hyponatraemia.

The hyponatraemia of inappropriate vasopressin secretion must not be confused with *pseudohyponatraemia* resulting from hyperlipidaemia or hyperproteinaemia. In these conditions, the amount of water per unit volume of plasma is reduced by the high fat or protein content. As the sodium is confined to the water phase of the plasma, it appears to be low only because it is diluted out by the fat or protein, but in reality its concentration within the plasma water is normal. In this situation, the plasma osmolality is normal despite the apparent hyponatraemia.

PATHOGENESIS

There is little doubt that the cause of the hyponatraemia is vasopressin produced by the tumour. Large amounts of this material have been extracted from several tumours, and the elevated blood and urinary vasopressin levels in the patients with the syndrome do not fall normally during a water load test. The vasopressin levels are too high for the plasma tonicity and the secretion is autonomous. The syndrome has been reported to improve after removal of the tumour, or following radiotherapy (Ivy, 1961). After radiation of a primary tumour, it was found to contain smaller amounts of vasopressin than the non-irradiated secondary deposits (Bower *et al.*, 1964).

Bioassay and radioimmunoassay procedures suggest that the material produced by the tumour is the natural antidiuretic hormone, arginine vasopressin, but final proof awaits chemical analysis of the tumour hormone. In patients with inappropriate vasopressin secretion associated with non-malignant disease, the excess vasopressin appears to be secreted from the hypothalamic-posterior pituitary system but there is an abnormality of the control mechanisms which is not understood.

Oxytocin and neurophysin have also been extracted from tumours of patients with inappropriate vasopressin secretion. No known sequelae of the production of these hormones are recognised.

TREATMENT

Patients with inappropriate vasopressin secretion and dilutional hyponatraemia respond well to simple limitation of water intake. It is necessary initially to induce a negative water balance and this usually requires a fluid intake of no more than ½–1 litre/day. The patients frequently exhibit a most remarkable response to fluid restriction within 24 hours and the clinical improvement continues until the serum sodium has become normal. Administration of mineralocorticoids is not indicated since there is no evidence of adrenocortical insufficiency, but simply of excessive water retention. When corticosteroids are given, large doses are required to alter the serum sodium and they usually result in oedema. In most cases, the patient's clinical state, plasma electrolytes and osmolality can be controlled in the long term on less severe fluid restriction but the intake must be titrated against the plasma osmolality and sodium. Treatment should be directed to the tumour wherever possible, and dramatic improvement may follow resection, chemotherapy or radiation.

Infusion of hypertonic saline solution is not indicated except in emergencies, since sodium administration merely results in prompt excretion of the electrolyte load in the urine. However, occasionally when water intoxication is marked with severe neurological abnormalities such as coma or convulsions, infusion of 500 ml of hypertonic (3 per cent) saline will rapidly, but temporarily improve the situation. Fluid restriction should be commenced simultaneously.

HYPERTHYROIDISM

In 1962, De Gennes *et al.* reviewed 41 cases of hyperthroidism in patients with malignant disease, most commonly of the gastro-intestinal tract, although six of the patients had bronchogenic carcinomas. The diagnosis was confirmed by a raised BMR and by thyroid radioiodine studies. There was a higher incidence in men, the age group was higher than in other hyperthyroid patients, and there was a low frequency of exophthalmos and goitre. It is likely that many of these cases represent a chance association of two not uncommon conditions. However, a critical study by Hennen (1967) demonstrated a high concentration of a thyroid stimulating factor in a bronchogenic carcinoma which was, on histology, a poorly differentiated epidermoid epithelioma. This factor was similar to human pituitary TSH both in its biological activity in test animals and in its immunological properties. No clinical evidence of thyroid disorder was noted in this patient.

Odell (1968) described 14 patients with neoplasms containing trophoblastic cells and an unusual form of hyperthyroidism. Thirteen of the patients were women with choriocarcinomas or hydatidiform moles, and one was a man with metastatic testicular teratocarcinoma.

These patients had no convincing clinical evidence of hyperthyroidism but investigations revealed definite abnormalities. In all the patients, both the PBI and the 24-hour thyroid ^{131}I uptake were raised. Plasma TSH was elevated on bioassay in four patients. In one patient, both bioassay and radioimmunoassay of TSH were performed—the bioassay gave a high value whereas the radioimmunoassay gave a normal value. In all patients, urinary gonadotrophin excretion was very high but this material did not have an intrinsic TSH-like activity. Treatment of the neoplasms caused the abnormal tests to revert to normal. It should be noted that in the absence of clinical evidence of hyperthyroidism, abnormal thyroid function tests should be interpreted with caution. There are many sources of error in laboratory tests; oestrogens can increase thyroxine binding globulin, raising the PBI, and other drugs might effect renal clearance of iodide or have an antithyroid action.

However, current evidence is suggestive that trophoblastic tumours can produce a TSH-like material though they should not necessarily be considered as truly ectopic sites for production of this hormone since normal human chorionic tissue contains a thyroid stimulating agent (Henman, 1965; Hersham and Starnes, 1969). In view of the similarities in structure between TSH, FSH, LH, and HCG, it might be expected that trophoblastic tumours could secrete materials with TSH-like activity. Apart from the single case of Hennen (1967), TSH-like material has not been convincingly demonstrated, as yet, in non-trophoblastic tumours.

ATYPICAL CARCINOID SYNDROME

A variety of tumours derived from the primitive gut have been associated with the carcinoid syndrome (Table 20.8).

Clinical Features. These features are described fully in Chapter 19. They consist of episodic facial flushing and oedema, nausea, vomiting, and diarrhoea, bronchospasm, and sweating.

TABLE 20.8. *Tumours Responsible for Carcinoid Syndrome*

Tumour	Approximate Frequency
Bronchial adenoma	+++
Pancreatic duct-cell carcinoma	++
Bronchial carcinoma (oat cell)	+
Islet cell carcinoma	+
Gastric carcinoma	+
Neuroblastoma	+
Medullary carcinoma of the thyroid	+

Investigations. In typical cases of the carcinoid syndrome the tumour secretes 5-hydroxytryptamine (5-HT) which is metabolised to 5-hydroxyindole acetic acid (5-HIAA) and excreted in the urine. In the syndrome associated with neoplasms other than the small intestinal carcinoid, 5-hydroxytryptophan (5-HTP) is also produced and excreted in the urine. Urinary histamine excretion may also be increased and it has been suggested that excessive prostaglandin secretion may contribute to the symptoms.

Pathogenesis. Since removal of the tumour is followed by remission of the syndrome, it seems likely that the tumour is secreting these humoral agents. Assays of the tumours for 5-hydroxytryptamine and other tryptophan derivatives has been negative but this may have been due to lability of the compounds or the extraction procedures used.

Treatment. Removal of the tumour is indicated unless there are extensive metastases. Alphamethyldopa inhibits amino-acid decarboxylase and inhibits conversion of 5-HTP to 5-HT; it may thus prevent diarrhoea and bronchial constriction although it does not always prevent flushing. This compound has little effect in the typical carcinoid syndrome. The decarboxylation process requires pyridoxal phosphate as cofactor, and improvement has been reported in one patient treated with a low pyridoxine diet and 4-deoxypyridoxine, a pyridoxine antagonist (Gailani *et al.*, 1966).

GONADOTROPHINS

Overproduction of gonadotrophins by tumours may cause precocious puberty in children, and gynaecomastia in adult males.

PRECOCIOUS PUBERTY

Several cases of precocious puberty associated with hepatoblastomas have been reported. The patients, all boys, ranged from one to eight years in age. Serum and urine contained a substance with the properties of chorionic gonadotrophin, but there were no trophoblastic elements in the tumour. As a result of the gonadotrophin excess there was hyperplasia of the interstitial cells of the testes, and the urinary excretion of 17-oxosteroids, testosterone, and oestrogens was increased. In one patient, removal of the tumour and therapy with methotrexate and radiation caused the gonadotrophins to disappear from the plasma, and the signs of puberty to regress (Hung *et al.*, 1963). In another patient, material with the properties of a gonadotrophin was extracted from the hepatic tumour (Reeves *et al.*, 1959).

GYNAECOMASTIA

Gynaecomastia is a not uncommon occurrence in patients with bronchogenic carcinoma and it may improve after pneumonectomy. Ginsberg and Brown (1961) found increased urinary and blood oestrogen levels in 11 patients with hypertrophic pulmonary osteoarthropathy, 10 being due to bronchogenic carcinoma. Gynaecomastia was present in 2 of these patients. Conjugation of oestrogens was normal and there was no impairment of oestrogen degradation to account for the raised levels. However, since the raised urinary oestrogen levels persisted for several weeks after removal of the tumour it seems the tumour did not itself secrete the oestrogens.

This discrepancy has been resolved in a classical study by Faiman *et al.* (1967) who directly demonstrated gonadotrophin production by a bronchogenic carcinoma in a patient with gynaecomastia. The patient, a 49-year-old Negro presented with aching pains of the knees, ankles, and elbows, and painful swelling of both breasts. He was found to have hypertrophic pulmonary osteoarthropathy and a bronchogenic carcinoma. Resection of the tumour showed it to be mostly well differentiated, with adenomatous characteristics; in other areas, it was pleomorphic and epidermoid in character. After operation, the arthropathy and the gynaecomastia improved. Both serum FSH and LH levels were raised at the time of operation when determined by a sensitive and specific radioimmunoassay technique. There were higher levels of FSH, but not LH, in pulmonary venous than in arterial blood, indicating that the tumour was secreting FSH. Immunologically reactive FSH and LH were present in the tumour, and within forty days of operation serum levels of both FSH and LH fell to normal. Total urinary oestrogen excretion was moderately increased prior to operation and fell somewhat afterwards. The preoperative excretion of oestradiol was greatly increased and fell to normal afterwards when, for reasons that were not apparent, the oestriol excretion increased.

There seems little doubt from this study that the tumour secreted FSH, and possibly LH, which stimulated the interstitial cells of the testes to produce oestrogens which may have been the cause of the gynaecomastia. Whether the gonadotrophins or other humoral factors were responsible for the hypertrophic pulmonary osteoarthropathy remains uncertain.

GROWTH HORMONE

Steiner *et al.* (1968) have reported a patient with pulmonary osteoarthropathy who had a raised fasting level of growth hormone. After operation, the growth hormone level fell to normal. These authors suggested that growth hormone production by a tumour may be a factor in the development of hypertrophic osteoarthropathy and there have since been a number of other patients described with growth hormone secretion in association with bronchial carcinoma and pulmonary osteoarthropathy, although growth hormone production without clinically obvious sequelae has been described in patients with poorly differentiated lung or stomach tumours (Beck and Burger, 1972). The relevance of the osteoarthropathy to the growth hormone production is entirely uncertain.

MULTIPLE ECTOPIC HORMONES

A number of patients whose neoplasms produced two or more hormones have been described. This tendency for multiple hormone production seems particularly marked in the oat cell variety of bronchogenic carcinoma and tumours of the carcinoid type and has been quoted as evidence for the 'derepression' theory of tumour hormone synthesis (see before). When an active search is made for hormones in malignant tissues, a great variety may be found, frequently without clinical sequelae, (*see* Table 20.1). The reasons for the lack of clinical effects are not clear. In one recent series of 31 tumours studied for their ACTH content, biologically active and immunoreactive ACTH was found in significant quantities in every one, although the clinical ectopic ACTH syndrome had occurred in only 17 of the patients (Ratcliffe *et al.*, 1973). In one of these tumours calcitonin was also found, in 3 other patients hypercalcaemia had occurred, and in a further one the urinary SHIAA was elevated. It may be that hormone production by tumours is indeed very common, but that clinical effects are encountered in only a small proportion of patients, since secretion of the hormone would have to be much greater than the normal production before adverse effects would be seen.

REFERENCES

Review Articles

Editorial (1967). *Lancet*, **i,** 86.

Hobbs, C. B., and Miller, A. L. (1966). *J. clin. Path.*, **19,** 119.

Liddle, G. W., Nicholson, W. E., Island, D. P., Orth, D. N., Abe, K., and Londer, S. C. (1969). *Rec. Prog. Horm. Res.*, **25,** 283.

Lipsett, M. B. (1965). *Cancer Res.*, **25,** 1068.

Ectopic ACTH Syndrome

Besser, G. M., and Edwards, C. R. W. (1972). *Clinics in Endocrinology and Metabolism*, **1,** 451.

Brown, W. H. (1928). *Lancet*, **ii,** 1022.

Liddle, G. W., Givens, J. R., Nicholson, W. E., and Island, D. P. (1965). *Cancer Res.*, **25,** 1057.

Meador, C. F., Liddle, G. W., Island, D. P., Nicholson, W. E., Lucas, C. P., Nuckton, J. G., and Luetscher, J. A. (1962). *J. clin. Endocrinol.*, **22,** 693.

Ratcliffe, J. G., Knight, R. A., Besser, G. M., Landon, J., and Stansfeld, A. G. (1972). *Clin. Endocrinol.*, **1,** 27.

Upton, G. V., and Amatruda, T. T. (1971). *New Eng. J. Med.*, **285,** 419.

Hypoglycaemia

Doege, K. W. (1930). *Ann. Surg.*, **92,** 955.

Hayes, D. M., Spurr, C. L., Felts, J. H., and Miller, E. C. (1961). *Metabolism*, **10,** 182.

Miller, D. R., Bolinger, R. E., Janigan, D., Crockett, J. E., and Friesen, S. R. (1959). *Ann. Surg.*, **150,** 684.

Hypercalcaemia

Albright, F., and Reifenstein, E. C. (Eds) (1948). *The Parathyroid Glands and Metabolic Bone Disease.* Baltimore: Williams & Wilkins.

Carey, V. C. (1966). *Amer. Rev. resp. Dis.*, **93,** 584.

Goldberg, M. F., Tashjian, A. H., Order, S. E., and Dammin, G. J. (1964). *Amer. J. Med.*, **36,** 805.

Gordan, G. C., Cantino, T., Erhardt, L., Hansen, J., and Lubich, W. (1966). *Science*, **151,** 1226.

Gordan, G. C., Fitzpatrick, M., and Lubich, W. (1967). *Proc. Amer. Coll. Phys.*

Munson, P. L., Tashjian, A. H., and Levine, L. (1965). *Cancer Res.*, **25,** 1062.

Plimpton, C. H., and Gellhorn, A. (1956). *Amer. J. Med.*, **21,** 750.

Sherwood, L. M., O'Riorden, J. L. H., Aurbach, G. D., and Potts, J. T. (1967). *J. clin. Endocrinol.*, **27,** 140.

Walser, M. (1962). *J. clin. Invest.*, **41,** 1454.

Inappropriate Secretion of Vasopressin

Bartter, F. C., and Schwartz, W. B. (1967). *Amer. J. Med.*, **42,** 790.

Bower, B. F., Mason, D. M., and Forsham, P. H., (1964). *New Engl. J. Med.*, **271,** 934.

Ivy, H. K. (1961). *Arch. intern. Med.*, **108,** 47.

Schwartz, W. B., Bennett, W., Curelop, S., and Bartter, F. C. (1957). *Amer. J. Med.*, **23,** 529.

Hyperthyroidism

De Gennes, L., Briccaire, H., and Leprat, J. (1962). *Pr. Med*, **70,** 2137.

Hennen, G. (1965). *Arch. int. Physiol.*, **73,** 689.

Hennen, G. (1967). *J. clin. Endocrinol.*, **27,** 610.

Hershman, J. M., and Starnes, W. R. (1969). *J. Clin. Invest.*, **48,** 923.

Atypical Carcinoid Syndrome

Gailani, S., Rogue, A. L., and Holland, J. F. (1966). *Ann. intern. Med.*, **65,** 1044.

Gonadotrophins

Faiman, C., Colwell, J. A., Ryan, R. J., Hershman, J. M., and Shields, T. W. (1967). *New Eng. J. Med.*, **277**, 1395.

Hardy, J. D. (1960). *J. Amer. med. Assn.*, **173**, 1462.

Hung, W., Blizzard, R. M., Migeon, C. J., Camacho, A. M., and Nyhan, W. L. (1963). *J. Pediat.*, **63**, 895.

Reeves, R. L., Tesluk, H., and Harrison, C. E. (1959). *J. clin. Endocrinol.*, **19**, 1651.

Growth Hormone

Beck, C., and Burger, H. G. (1972). *Cancer*, **30**, 75.

Steiner, H., Dahlbäck, O., and Waldenström, J. (1968). *Lancet*, **i**, 783.

APPENDICES

APPENDIX A. TESTS OF HYPOTHALAMIC-PITUITARY FUNCTION

INSULIN TOLERANCE TEST—for assessment of GH, ACTH and prolactin reserve.

A reproducible and standardised hypoglycaemic stress is produced when the patient's blood glucose concentration falls to less than 40 mg/100 ml *and* the patient is seen to sweat. Sweating is usually mild and only lasts 10 to 15 minutes. In response to this stimulus, growth hormone, ACTH, corticosteroids, prolactin and catecholamines should be secreted. Growth hormone, prolactin, ACTH and corticosteroid secretion will be impaired in the presence of hypopituitarism (a normally responsive adrenal cortex is assumed); in partial hypopituitarism growth hormone secretion alone may be impaired. Failure to obtain an ACTH/corticosteroid response to hypoglycaemia, accompanied by the subsequent demonstration of a normal ACTH/corticosteroid response to vasopressin suggests the lesion is at the hypothalamic level rather than at the pituitary level since vasopressin appears to cause release of any ACTH present in the adenohypophysis, probably by a direct action, whereas the hypoglycaemic response requires an intact hypothalamic-pituitary-adrenal axis.

Proceedure

1. The patient is weighed before the test and an E.C.G. recorded, (myocardial ischaemia is a contraindication) and is
2. fasted from midnight (water allowed).
3. At a convenient time prior to 8.30 a.m., an intravenous cannula is inserted (Braunula and stylet), or use a heparinised cannula such as a Butterfly.
4. 30 minutes later 12 ml of venous blood is obtained and the time noted.
5. A graded dose of soluble insulin is then given via the cannula (the dose depends upon the suspected diagnosis—*see* below) and is washed into the vein by withdrawing and expelling blood into and from the insulin syringe three times.
6. 12 ml of blood are drawn, 30, 45, 60 and 90 minutes after the insulin injection.
7. If the patient does not show evidence of adequate hypoglycaemia by 45 minutes, i.e. does not sweat, the insulin dose may be repeated and blood sampling restarted as above.
8. After the 90-minute blood sample a 20 g glucose drink plus breakfast is given and the test is terminated. A doctor should supervise the drinking of the glucose.

Blood Samples. Venous blood is collected at each time interval for:

(*a*) blood glucose;

(*b*) plasma fluorogenic corticosteroids (10 ml) in heparin or EDTA tube.

(*c*) growth hormone and prolactin (1 ml) in heparinised tube (if indicated).

Precautions

This test is perfectly safe providing there is adequate supervision. A medical attendant should be with the patient at all times and i.v. 25 per cent and 5 per cent dextrose should be in the room. It is very rarely necessary to terminate the test prematurely (in one centre, this has been required on only 6 occasions in over 1,000 tests), but is indicated for severe and prolonged sweating (over 20 minutes) or impending or actual loss of consciousness or fits. Sweating is usually mild and transient. If necessary give 25 ml of 25 per cent dextrose i.v. followed by a drip of 5 per cent dextrose, but continue sampling and administer 100 mg hydrocortisone i.v. at the end of the test.

Heparinisation of cannula. This is only required when a Braunula stylet is not used. Dilute 1 ml of 10,000-unit/ml heparin in 10 ml with saline and use 0·25 ml after each blood sample to heparinise the cannula. Withdraw 1 ml blood as deadspace before sampling.

Insulin Dose. Insulin sensitivity will vary with the endocrine status of the patient:

(*a*) Suspected hypopituitary patients; the most sensitive, dose 0·10 unit/kg.

(*b*) Probably normal patients; dose 0·15 unit/kg (for example in obese patients or to test the responsiveness to stress of patients who have been treated with corticosteroids in the past).

(*c*) Suspected Cushing's syndrome or acromegaly; the most resistant, start with 0·30 unit/kg.

Criteria for Adequate Hypoglycaemia

The patient should sweat *and* the blood glucose should fall to less than 40 mg/100 ml. While a hormonal response may occur after smaller degrees of hypoglycaemia, absence of an elevation of plasma growth hormone, prolactin or corticosteroid concentration cannot be interpreted in the absence of these 'adequate criteria' being fulfilled. It is convenient to note whether sweating has occurred by 45 minutes. If not, then the i.v. insulin dose may be repeated and the test procedure recommenced. This may save repetition of the test on another day.

Contraindications

1. Ischaemic heart disease, epilepsy. If there is only ECG evidence of heart disease, the potential value of the test must be weighed against the possible increased risks.
2. Severe unequivocal panhypopituitarism.

Normal Responses

Plasma Fluorogenic Corticosteroids should rise by at least 6 μg/100 ml and to a maximum of over 20 μg/100 ml.

Growth Hormone levels should rise to over 20 ng/ml (MRC Standard A). Levels between 10 and 20 ng/ml should be considered equivocal.

Prolactin levels rise, but the exact range of responses in normal patients has not yet been defined.

Note. In the USA, regular heparin may contain benzyl alcohol as preservative; this is a very fluorescent substance and therefore cannot be used to heparinise the i.v. cannula. Alternative preparations which do not contain benzyl alcohol should be used (such as Abbot's single-dose ampoules of 'Panheparin').

References

Greenwood, F. C., *et al.* (1966). *J. clin. Invest.*, **45**, 429.
Landon, J., *et al.* (1963). *J. Endocrinol.* **27**, 183.
Plumpton, F. S., and Besser, G. M. (1969). *Brit. J. Surg.*, **56**, 216.
Plumpton, F. S., *et al.* (1969). *Anaesthesia*, **24**, 3.

ARGININE TEST—for assessment of GH reserve.

Insert 2 forearm venous cannulae into fasting subject under local anaesthesia between 8 and 9 a.m. After 30 minutes, infuse 30 g arginine in 100 ml sterile water (in children 0·5 g/kg up to 30 g) over 30 minutes into one cannula. Sample blood for growth hormone each 30 minutes for 2 hours. Normal response (the maximum increment in growth hormone should be at least 7 ng/ml) excludes growth hormone deficiency. Adult males should be pretreated with stilboestrol 1 mg b.d. for 48 hours. Occasional normal subjects do not respond.

Reference

Merimee *et al.* (1969), *New Eng. J. Med.* **280**, 1434.

GLUCAGON TEST—for assessment of GH and ACTH reserve.

Forearm venous cannula inserted into fasting patient, between 8 and 9 a.m. After 30 minutes 1 mg glucagon is given subcutaneously (1·5 mg if patient weighs more than 90 kg). Sample 10 ml heparinised blood for plasma corticosteroids and growth hormone before, and 60, 90, 120, 150 and 180 minutes after glucagon. Nausea and vomiting sometimes occurs towards the end of the test. The maximum increase in growth hormone in a normal male subject should be at least 7 ng/ml and in females 10 ng/ml. Most subjects also show a rise in plasma corticosteroids towards the end of the test. Rarely normal subjects fail to show a growth hormone response and the test is unreliable in diabetes mellitus.

References

Mitchell, *et al.* (1970). *New Eng. J. Med.*, **282**, 539.
Mitchell, *et al.* (1973). Editorial: *Brit. med. J.* **1**, 188.

BOVRIL TEST—screening test for GH deficiency in children.

Bovril, 20 g per 1·5 sqm body surface is given by mouth in 100 ml warm water. Blood samples for growth hormone taken half-hourly for 2 hours. A rise in plasma growth hormone to more than 10 ng/ml is probably normal. This test should be regarded as a screening test. Non-responders should be checked with an insulin tolerance test.

Reference

Jackson *et al.* (1968). *Lancet*, **2**, 373.

ORAL GLUCOSE TOLERANCE TEST—for diagnosis of acromegaly and gigantism.

Forearm venous cannula inserted into resting, fasting patient. After 30 minutes give a solution of 50 g glucose in water (should be iced and flavoured to prevent nausea). Take blood samples before and each 30 minutes for 150 minutes. In normal subjects growth hormone levels will usually start at less than 10 ng/ml, but always suppress to less than 5 ng/ml at some time during the test. Failure of suppression suggests acromegaly or gigantism but may also be seen in severe liver or renal disease, in heroin addicts or in patients taking laevodopa.

CLOMIPHENE STIMULATION TEST—for assessment of gonadotrophin reserve.

This procedure has only been assessed provisionally as a test of LH reserve in hypogonadal males although the principles probably also apply to FSH, and to the assessment of both hormones in women with amenorrhoea. Clomiphene appears to compete with the gonadal steroids for receptors in the hypothalamus, and to result in LH and FSH secretion. This effect takes two to four days to begin to appear.

Procedure: Clomiphene is given in a dose of 3 mg/kg body weight per day in divided doses up to a maximum of 200 mg daily, for seven to ten days. Blood is sampled for LH and FSH before and on days, four, seven and ten.

Contraindications. The use of clomiphene should be avoided in patients with liver disease or a history of recent severe depression.

Side-effects. Patients should be warned that they may experience flickering visual phenomena at the periphery of vision or central haloes. These do not preclude continuation of the test. Occasional patients become depressed during the test and in these circumstances discontinuation should be considered.

Normal Response. At the present it would appear that a normal response is indicated by a rise in LH and FSH outside the normal range for the laboratory. In amenorrhoeic women, this rise is frequently followed by a secondary peak 14 days after the start of clomiphene and this may precede ovulation. Lack of response suggests hypogonadotrophism due to hypothalamic or pituitary disease. The response may be absent in severe anorexia nervosa, but often returns to normal as the patient gains weight even before the onset of menstruation.

Reference

Anderson *et al.* (1972), *Clin. Endocr.*, **1**, 127.

WATER DEPRIVATION TEST—for diagnosis of diabetes insipidus (after Dashe, 1963).

The essential step in establishing a diagnosis of diabetes insipidus is to show that the patient cannot elaborate a concentrated urine in response to a rise in plasma solute concentration. A satisfactory procedure for this is the 8 hour water deprivation test, which should be carried out only in a well hydrated patient who is under careful supervision because those with severe ADH deficiency may become dangerously dehydrated, whereas compulsive water drinkers may steal water or other fluids during this test, which is therefore best carried out during the daytime.

Preparation of Patient. If the patient is being treated with pitressin tannate in oil, this should be stopped 72 hours before the test. During this period any polyuria may be controlled with lysine vasopressin nasal spray. This should be stopped 8 hours before the test is begun and a high fluid intake is encouraged until the start of the test at 8.30 a.m. A light breakfast is allowed, but no tea, coffee or smoking should be permitted during the test. It is essential to ensure that circulating levels of corticosteroids are normal before the test is performed.

Procedure

No fluids for 8 hours: supervision essential: dry food permitted. Weigh patient before test and after 4, 6, 7 and 8 hours. Consider stopping test if more than 3 per cent body weight lost.
Samples:

Urine is passed hourly and volume recorded.
Keep urine for osmolality measurements:

U_1 first hour	8.30–9.30
U_2 third to fourth hour	11.30–12.30
U_3 sixth to seventh hour	2.30–3.30
U_4 seventh to eighth hour	3.30–4.30

Plasma for osmolality at mid point of each saved urine sample.
P_1 9 a.m., P_2 12 noon, P_3 3 p.m., P_4 4 p.m.

Interpretation

Under the conditions of this test, a normal subject will elaborate urine with an osmolality of 600 mOsm/kg or more and the plasma osmolality will not rise above 300 mOsm/kg because water will be retained to prevent dehydration. The urine flow rate falls to less than 0·5 ml per minute.

In diabetes insipidus, the plasma becomes abnormally concentrated with an osmolality in excess of 300 mOsm/kg whereas the urine remains dilute with an osmolality of less than 270 mOsm/kg and the urine volume is not reduced to the expected degree. No reliance can be placed on urine flow volumes without measurement of concentration because in severe diabetes insipidus dehydration may be marked and the glomerular filtration rate may fall with a reduction in urine flow. The ratio of the osmolality of the urine to that of the plasma in the third or fourth specimens (U_3P_3 or U_4P_4) does not rise above 1·9 in contrast to a normal subject who can produce urine that is at least twice as concentrated as the plasma.

Failure to elaborate a concentrated urine during water deprivation, but ability to do so after vasopressin administration (5–10 units of well warmed and shaken pitressin tannate), confirms the diagnosis of cranial diabetes insipidus. Failure to concentrate after pitressin suggests nephrogenic diabetes insipidus.

Compulsive water drinking can usually be differentiated from true diabetes insipidus without much difficulty provided the patient is prevented from drinking during the test. This may be difficult because the patients may go to considerable lengths to obtain water illicitly. The results in such patients usually fall within the normal range although a minor degree of impaired concentration, not as severe as in true diabetes insipidus, may occur. Unlike patients with diabetes insipidus, the plasma osmolality at the start of the test is usually normal (between 273 and 293 mOsm/kg) or low. The results of the test, together with the clinical evaluation of the patient and the relative dominance of thirst rather than polyuria, usually leave no doubt as to the diagnosis of psychogenic polydipsia.

Reference

Dashe *et al.* (1963). *J. Amer. med. Assoc.* **185,** 699.

APPENDIX B. GROWTH AND DEVELOPMENT

Data after Tanner *et al.*, *Arch. Dis. Childh.* (1966), Vol. 41, and *Growth at Adolescence*, 2nd ed. 1962, Blackwell, Oxford. Figures reproduced by kind permission of Professor J. M. Tanner.

BOTH SEXES, PUBIC HAIR

STAGE 1: Pre-adolescent. The vellus over the pubis is not further developed than that over the abdominal wall, i.e. no pubic hair.

STAGE 2: Sparse growth of long, slightly pigmented downy hair, straight or slightly curled, chiefly at the base of the penis or along labia.

STAGE 3: Considerably darker, coarser and more curled. The hair spreads sparsely over the junction of the pubis.

STAGE 4: Hair now adult in type, but area covered is still considerably smaller than in the adult. No spread to the medial surface of thighs.

STAGE 5: Adult in quantity and type, with distribution of the horizontal (or classically 'feminine') pattern. Spread to medial surface of thighs but not up linea alba or elsewhere above the base of the inverse triangle (spread up linea alba occurs late and is rated stage 6).

The changes in pubic hair development during puberty are shown in Fig. A.1 for girls and Fig. A.2 for males.

GIRLS, BREAST DEVELOPMENT

STAGE 1: Pre-adolescent elevation of papilla only.

STAGE 2: Breast bud stage: elevation of breast and papilla as small mound. Enlargement of areola diameter.

STAGE 3: Further enlargement and elevation of breast and areola, with no separation of their contours.

STAGE 4: Projection of areola and papilla to form a secondary mound above the level of the breast.

STAGE 5: Mature stage: projections of papilla only, due to recession of the areola to the general contour of the breast.

The changes in breast development during puberty in girls are shown in Fig. A.3.

BOYS, GENITAL DEVELOPMENT

STAGE 1: Pre-adolescent. Testes, scrotum and penis are of about the same size and proportion as in early childhood.

STAGE 2: Enlargement of scrotum and testes. Skin of scrotum reddens and changes in texture. Little or no enlargement of penis at this stage.

STAGE 3: Enlargement of penis, which occurs at first mainly in length. Further growth of testes and scrotum.

STAGE 4: Increased size of penis with growth in breadth and development of glands. Testes and scrotum larger, scrotal skin darkened.

STAGE 5: Genitalia adult in size and shape.

The changes in male genital development are shown in Fig. A.4.

MEASURING TECHNIQUE

Standing Height (recommended from 2 onwards) should be taken without shoes, the child standing with his heels and back in contact with an upright wall. His head is held so that he looks straight forward with the lower borders of the eye sockets in the same horizontal plane as the external auditory meati (i.e. head not with nose tipped upwards). A right-angled block (preferably counterweighted) is then slid down the wall until its bottom surface touches the child's head, and a scale fixed to the wall to read. During the measurements the child should be told to stretch his neck to be as tall as possible, though care must be taken to prevent his heels coming off the ground. Gentle but firm traction upwards should be applied by the measurer under the mastoid processes to help the child stretch. In this way the variation in height from morning to evening is

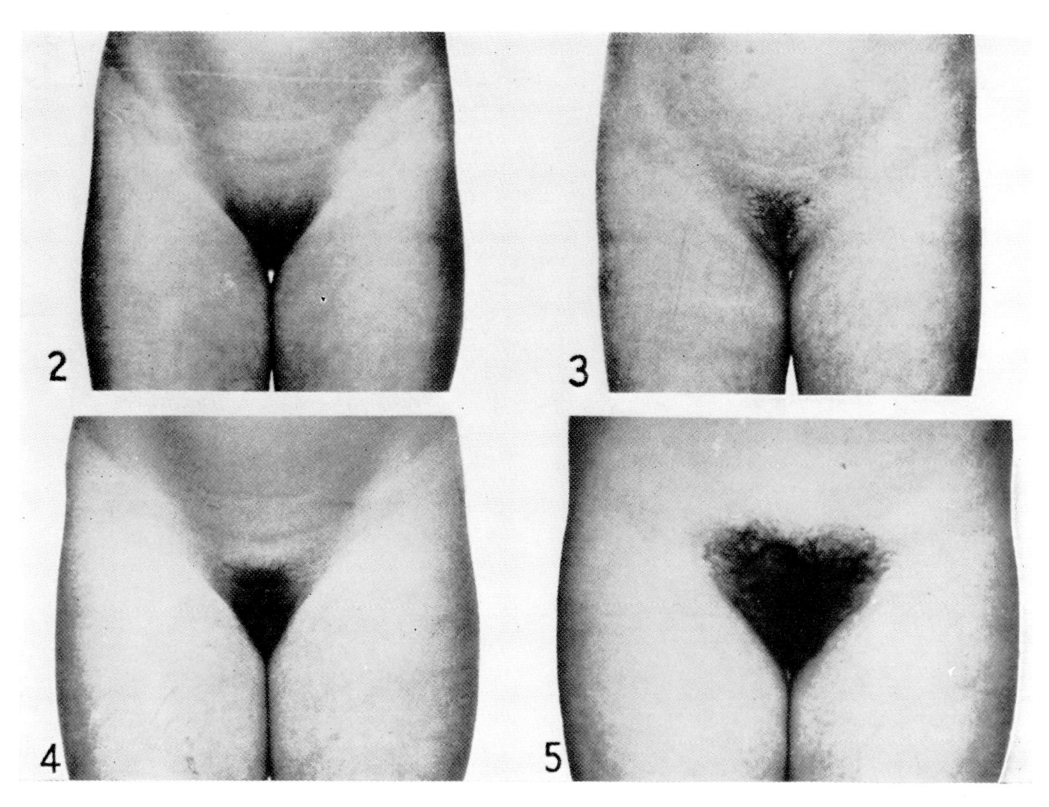

FIGURE A.1 Stages 2–5 in normal female pubic hair development

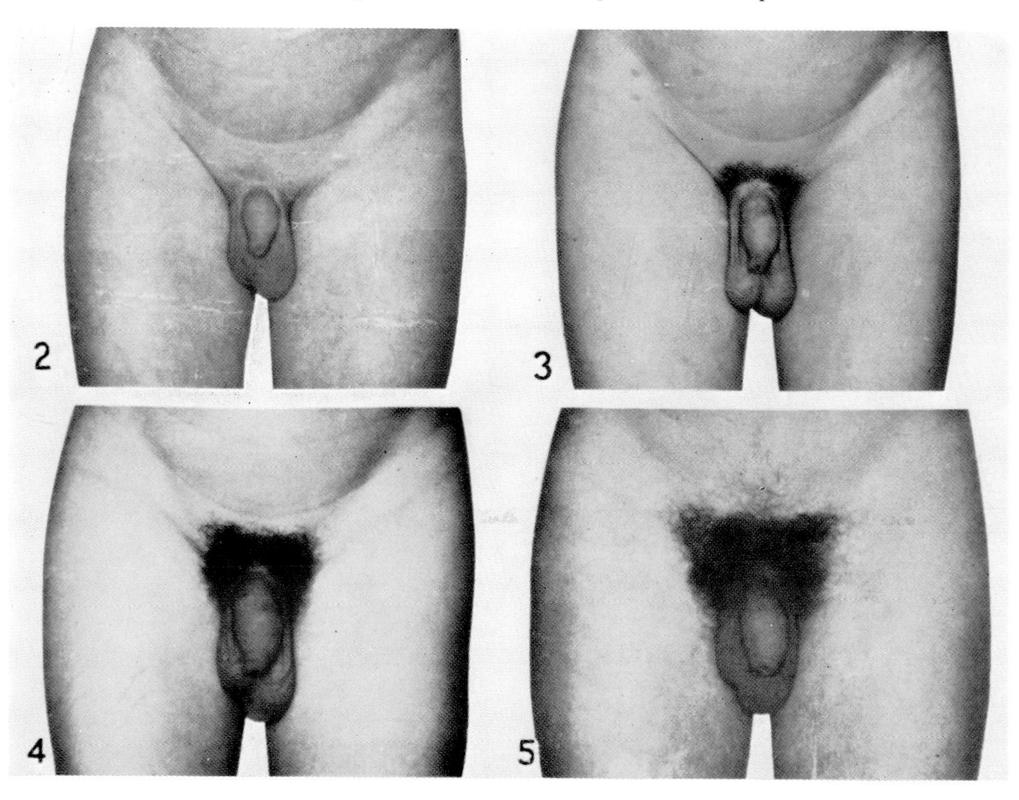

FIGURE A.2 Stages 2–5 in normal male pubic hair development

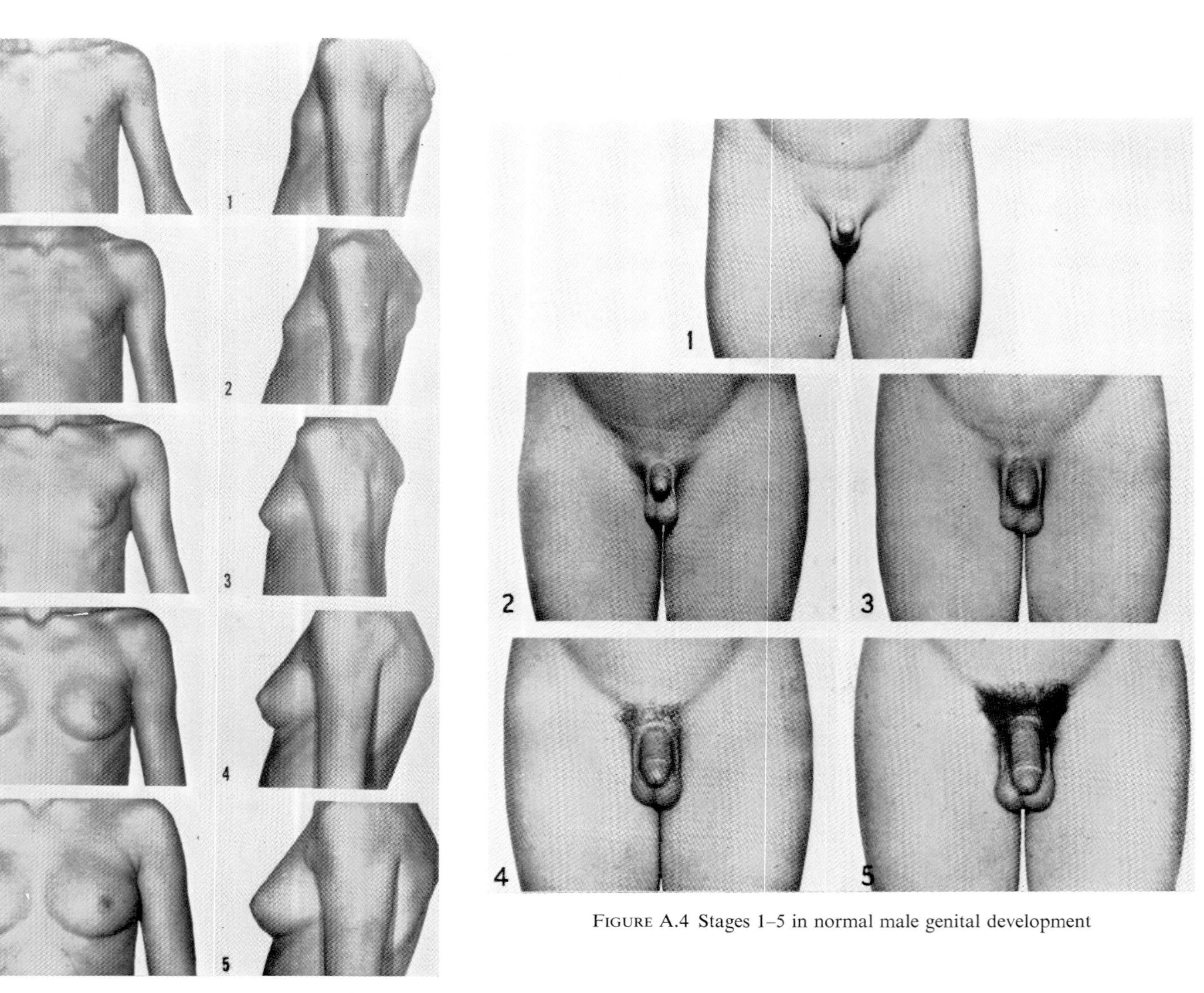

FIGURE A.3 Stages 1–5 in normal female breast development

FIGURE A.4 Stages 1–5 in normal male genital development

minimised. Standing height should be recorded to the nearest 0·1 cm.

Supine Length (recommended up to the age of 3 so that there is overlap with standing height at 2 to 3) is taken on a flat surface, with the child lying on his back. One observer holds his head in contact with a board at the top of the table and another straightens the legs, turns the feet at right-angles to the legs and brings a sliding board in contact with the child's heels.

Weight should be taken in the nude, or as near thereto as possible. If a surgical gown or minimum underclothing (vest and pants) is worn, then its estimated weight (about 0·1 kg) must be subtracted before weight is recorded. Weights are conveniently recorded to the nearest 0·1 kg over the age of six months. The bladder should be emptied.

APPENDIX C. TESTS OF THYROID FUNCTION

TRIIODOTHYRONINE SUPPRESSION TEST

The thyroid iodine uptake is normally under the control of TSH. When circulating thyroid hormone levels rise, the secretion of TSH falls. This forms the basis of the T3 suppression test. Thyroid uptake is measured using ^{132}I at 20 minutes or 4 hours, ^{99m}Tc at 20 minutes or ^{131}I at 6 hours. Triiodothyronine is then given for 7 days in a daily divided dose of 100 μg and the uptake measurement repeated. Total or partial failure of suppression of uptake indicates that thyroid function is wholly or partly independent of pituitary control. Similar information can be obtained by means of the TRH test (p. 81).

Risks. Triiodothyronine should not be given to patients with ischaemic heart disease or heart failure and any elderly patient should be considered to be at risk for the development of acute thyrotoxic heart disease.

Normal Response. The second uptake falls to less than 50 per cent of the first or is less than 10 per cent of the administered dose.

TSH STIMULATION TEST

Early measurements with ^{132}I, ^{99m}Tc or later measurements with ^{131}I can be used. A standard thyroid ^{131}I uptake at 24 hours, ^{132}I uptake at 4 hours, or ^{99m}Tc at 20 minutes is determined. Three injections each of 10 i.u. of Thyrotropar (Armour TSH) are given intra-muscularly on consecutive days. On the third day, a further tracer dose is given, and a second uptake determined. If ^{131}I has been used, either one week must be allowed to elapse between tests or the residual neck uptake must be counted before the second tracer dose.

Normal response is indicated by doubling of the control value or an increase in uptake of 15 per cent, whichever is greater. A normal response may be seen in some patients with mild hypothyroidism. Measurements of serum TSH levels have now replaced the TSH stimulation test in the diagnosis of primary thyroid failure.

PERCHLORATE DISCHARGE TEST

A tracer dose of ^{132}I or ^{131}I is given by mouth to the fasting patient. The thyroid uptake is measured at 60 min and then 600 mg potassium perchlorate in powder form is given with a drink of water. Further thyroid uptake measurements are made at 90 and 120 min after the dose.

Normal response $<$ 10 per cent fall of thyroid uptake at 90 or 120 min.

THYROTROPHIN-RELEASING HORMONE TEST

For details, *see* p. 81.

FACTORS AFFECTING THYROID FUNCTION TESTS

(From *Symposium on the Thyroid Gland*, by permission of Dr. G. K. McGowan and the Editors of *J. clin. Path.* (1967))

Factors (other than thyroid disease) that affect serum protein-bound iodine, thyroxine and other thyroid function tests based on a review by Davis, P. J. (*Amer. J. Med.* (1966), **40**, 918).

A. NATURAL VARIATIONS IN PBI LEVEL

1. *Age*. In the newborn PBI levels rise quickly to a mean of 12 μg/100 ml (SD ± 2·4) with a fall to 7·4 (SD ± 1·8) at 1–5 weeks, 6·9 (SD ± 1·8) at 6–12 weeks, and 6·3 (SD ± 1·0) at 3–12 months (Danowski *et al.* (1951) *Paediatrics*, **7**, 240).

In old age there may be a slight fall.

2. *Sex*. Females show a slight rise before and a fall after menstruation. In pregnancy there may be a marked rise, associated with a rise in binding proteins.

3. *Circadian variation* is negligible.

4. *Stress*, emotional or physical (including heat and cold), has little effect, though it may increase thyroxine turnover.

B. ERRORS IN BLOOD COLLECTION AFFECTING PBI LEVEL

1. The use of iodine or iodine containing antiseptics to clean the skin.

2. Haemostasis resulting in concentration of the plasma proteins.

3. Contamination of syringe or container with substances containing iodine or mercury (*see* D.3).

C. DIETARY FACTORS

1. Iodide intake, which is dependent on the variable content of local food, in particular on rich sources such as sea-foods and iodized salt. Variation of intake has little effect on the PBI level but may affect the thyroidal ^{131}I uptake by altering the plasma inorganic iodide.

2. Organic iodine compounds, such as the food dye erythrosine BS which gives high PBI levels (Keiding, R., *Lancet*, **ii**, 586).

3. Foods which impair iodide absorption by the gut; this is said to occur on soya bean diets and those with a high calcium content, causing the plasma inorganic iodide to fall (*see* C.1).

4. Natural vegetable goitrogens in the diet; these are rare and do not appear to affect man directly, but in certain areas such as the Congo may play a part in the pathogenesis of endemic goitre. They are believed to impair the synthesis of hormone by the gland.

D. DRUGS

1. Iodine containing, which by their presence raise the PBI.*

(*a*) Iodides, when given in large doses, especially in cough mixtures; they act partly by free iodide being to a small extent estimated with the PBI and partly by the formation of iodinated proteins. Some drugs, e.g. iodopyrine, liberate iodine in the gut (*see* C.1).

(*b*) Organic iodine compounds, especially X-ray contrast media whose duration of action varies according to the drug and its mode of use; thus those used for intravenous pyelography are rapidly excreted by the kidneys so that Hypaque, for example, lasts in the blood for only a few days, and Diodrast for a few weeks, whereas media used for myelography or bronchography, such as Lipiodol, last for years. A few of these drugs cross the placenta and may affect PBI levels in the next generation. A widely used drug containing iodine is the diarrhoea remedy Enterovioform used by travellers. Some organic iodine compounds, such a Rybarex and Flaxedil, may act by liberating iodine within the body.

2. Interfering with the synthesis of thyroxine:

(*a*) by interfering with the trapping of iodide, e.g. thiocyanate, chlorate, nitrate;

(*b*) by interfering with the incorporation of iodine into tyrosine and the formation of thyroxine; commonly used drugs in this group, apart from those used to treat hyperthyroidism, are sulphonylureas and p-aminosalicylic acid.

3. Interfering with the chemical analysis of PBI, especially mercurials, but also gold and silver compounds; low PBI levels result.*

4. Affecting the thyroxine binding capacity of the plasma:

(*a*) increased binding protein, especially due to oestrogens (e.g. pregnancy, oral contraceptives), etc., resulting in raised PBI, T_4 but hypothyroid T_3-uptake tests;

* Error avoided by checking the levels in such patients with a specific thyroxine assay.

(*b*) decreased binding protein, especially due to androgens or adrenal corticosteroids; resulting ing low PBI, T_4 but hyperthyroid T_3-uptake tests;

(*c*) competition for binding sites, especially by diphenylhydantoin and salicylates, with the same results as (*b*).

5. Thyroid replacement drugs; normally plasma contains both thyroxine and triiodothyronine, of which the latter is biologically more potent; if hypothyroid patients are maintained on the former, the PBI level may be slightly raised; if on the latter, the PBI is likely to be low.

E. NON-THYROID DISEASES

1. Affecting thyroxine binding capacity (*see* D.4), which tends to be lowered in hypoproteinaemic states such as the nephrotic syndrome and chronic debilitating diseases, and to be raised in acute hepatitis. In severe non-thyroid disease, it is reported that the PBI may be normal, the TBPA low, and the free T_4 high while the patient remains euthyroid.

2. Intestinal disorders, resulting in failure to reabsorb the thyroxine secreted in the bile, and producing an iodide deficiency (*see* C.1).

3. For unknown reasons, e.g. the raised PBI in acute porphyria.

4. Rarely due to familial increase or decrease in plasma level of thyroxine-binding globulin.

DRUGS AFFECTING THYROID FUNCTION TESTS

(From *Symposium on the Thyroid Gland*, by permission of Dr. G. K. McGowan and the Editors of *J. clin. Path.* (1967).

List of drugs that affect thyroid function tests.* The letters and figures refer to the paragraphs on pp. 454, 455 and indicate the manner in which the drugs interfere.

Adrenal suppressant	Amphenone, ? D.2. (*b*)
Amoebicides and enteritis remedies	containing iodochlorhydroxyquin or diiodohydroxyquin (Enterovioform etc.), D.1 (*b*)
Anabolic hormone	D.4 (*b*)
Analgesics	aspirin, salicylates, D.2 (*b*), D.4. (*c*)
Androgens	testosterone, methyl testosterone etc., D.4 (*b*)
Antibiotics	iodopenicillin, D.1 (*b*)
Anticholinergics	isopropamide iodide (Darbid), D.1 (*a*)
Anticonvulsants	diphenylhydantoin, D.4 (*c*)
Antihistamines	*p*-promdylamine maleate (brompheniramine, Dimotane), D.2 (*b*)
Antiseptics	iodine, B.1, D.1. (*a*) iodinated compounds (iodoform, Betadine), B.1
Arthritis remedies	phenylbutazone (Butazolidin), oxyphenbutazone (Tanderil) D.2 (*b*) gold compounds, D.3
Asthma remedies	Felsol and iodopyrine, D.1 (*a*), D.2 (*b*)
Chelating drugs	dimercaprol (BAL), D.2 (*b*), D.4 (*c*)
Contraceptives	oral, D.4 (*a*)
Contrast media	used for various purposes in radiology, D.1 (*b*)
Corticosteroids	glucocorticoids (hydrocortisone, prednisone, dexamethasone, etc.), D.4 (*b*)
Cough medicine and lozenges.	containing iodides, D.1 (*a*)
Diabetes remedies	sulphonylureas, especially tolbutamide, D.2 (*b*)
Diagnostic agents	bromsulphthalein, ? D.2 (*a*) ? D.1 (*b*) due to impurities containing iodine *see also* 'Contrast media'

[*continued on* p. 458]

* See also *Clinical Aspects of Iodine Metabolism*, Appendices II and III, by Wayne, E. J., Koutras, D. A., and Alexander, W. D. (1964). Oxford: Blackwell Sci.

RESULTS OF THYROID FUNCTION TESTS

(Modified from *Symposium on the Thyroid Gland*, by permission of Dr. G. K. McGowan and the Editors of *J. clin. Path.* (1967))

Diagnosis		PBI (Protein-bound Iodine)	Radioiodine Uptake Early[1] (20 min–6 hr)	Radioiodine Uptake Late (24–48 hr)	$PB^{131}I$ (48 hr)
Hyperthyroid	Graves' disease / Toxic adenoma	+	+	N to +	+
Hypothyroid goitrous	Iodine-deficient	−	+	+	
	Autoimmune (Hashimoto)	N to −	+ to −	N to −	N to +[10]
	Dyshormonogenetic[3]—				
	1 Trapping defect	−	−	−	−
	2 Other forms	+[11] to −	+	+[11] to −	+[11] to −
Hypothyroid non-goitrous	Primary (dysgenesis or auto-immune)	−	N to −	N to −	N, +, −
	Secondary (hypopituitary)	−	N to −	N to −	N to −
Euthyroid goitrous	Iodine-deficient[4]	N	+	+	N
	'Hot nodule'[5]	N	N to +	N to +	N to +
Euthyroid (treated hyper-thyroidism)	Thyroidectomy	N	N	N	N to +[10]
	^{131}I therapy	N to −	N	N	N to +[10]
	Antithyroid drugs[6]	N to −	N to +	N to +	N
Other euthyroid states	T_4-binding proteins high	+	N	N	N
	T_4-binding proteins low[7]	−	N	N	N
	Iodide intake high	N to +[8]	−	−	N
	Iodide intake low	N	+	+	N
	Pregnancy	N to +[12]	N to +	N to +	N

[1] Short-lived ^{99m} Tc or ^{132}I may be used.
[2] Measured directly or derived from PBI and residual binding capacity.
[3] In 'trapping defect', salivary glands fail to concentrate radioiodine.
In 'organification defect', perchlorate causes excessive discharge of radioiodine from gland.
In 'coupling defect', thyroid biopsy contains much iodotyrosine but little iodothyronine.
In 'deiodinase defect', excessive urinary excretion of injected labelled iodotyrosines.
In 'iodoprotein defect', an abnormal iodinated protein in plasma.
[4] May be nodular or diffuse (colloid).
[5] Autonomous hyperactive nodule, but patient still euthyroid because rest of gland is suppressed. Thyroid 'scintigram' may be useful.

RESULTS OF THYROID FUNCTION TESTS (*continued*)

Key: N = in normal range
+ = in hyperthyroid range
− = in hypothyroid range

xs = exaggerated response
abs = absent response
imp = impaired response

TSH	TRH Test	Triiodo-thyronine Uptake (*in vitro*)	Plasma-free Thyroxine[2]	TSH Stimulation Test	T_3 Suppression Test	Thyroid Auto-antibodies
N	abs	+	+		+	Positive Negative
−	xs	−	−		N	Negative
−	xs	−	−	N to −	N	Positive
−	xs	−	−	−		Negative
−	xs	−	−		N	Negative
−	xs	−	−	−		Positive
N	abs	−	−	N[9]		Negative
N to −	N to xs	N	N	N	N	Negative
N	N, imp, abs	N	N	N[9]	+	Negative
N to −	N, abs, imp, xs	N	N	N to −	N to +	Pos. or neg.
N to −	N, abs, imp, xs	N	N	N to −	N to +	Pos. or neg.
N to −	N, abs, imp, xs	N	N	N	N to +	Pos. or neg.
N	N	−	N	N	N	Negative
N	N	+	N	N	N	Negative
N	N to xs	N to −	N	N		Negative
N to −	N to −	N to −	N	N	N	Negative
N to −	N	−[12]	N	N	N	Negative

[6] For few weeks after cessation of anti-thyroid drugs, when some tests are modified by low level of intra- and extra-thyroidal iodine pools.
[7] Similar effect also produced by drugs which compete with T_4 for binding sites.
[8] Due to iodoalbumin.
[9] May be positive only after repeated TSH administration.
[10] Due to small intrathyroidal iodine pool.
[11] High when there is an 'idoprotein defect'.
[12] Due to high T_4-binding proteins in plasma.

Drugs affecting thyroid function tests (*continued from* p. 455)

Diuretics	mercurials, D.3 acetazolamide (Diamox), D.2 (*b*)	Suppositories	rectal—Anusol, Proctoids, D.1 (*b*) vaginal—Floraquin, Viozol, D.1 (*b*)
Gout remedies	phenylbutazone (Butazolidin), D.2 (*b*)	Throat gargles, lozenges	chlorate, hypochlorite, D.2 (*a*) Faringets, D.1 (*b*)
Haematinics	cobalt salts, D.2 (*b*)	Thyroid hormones	thyroxine and triiodothyronine, D.5; if given to patients who are euthyroid they suppress TSH secretion and produce low ^{131}I uptake and PB ^{131}I
Inhalants	Rybarex, D.1 (*b*)		
Neuromuscular blocking agents	gallamine triethiodide (Flaxedil), D.1 (*b*)		
Oestrogens	including contraceptive pill, D.4 (*a*)		
Ointments, lotions	resorcinol, D.2 (*b*) Vioform, Locorten-vioform, D.1 (*b*) Synalar C, D.1 (*b*) silver compounds, D.3	Thyroid suppressants	especially thionamides (thiourea, thiouracil, methimazole, carbimazole etc.), D.2 (*b*)
		Tranquillisers	chlorpromazine (Largactil), ? D.2 (*b*)
Sedatives	bromide, D.2 (*a*)	Tuberculosis therapy	p-aminosalicylic acid (PAS), D.2 (*b*), D.4 (*c*)
Steroids	*see* 'Anabolic Hormones', 'Androgens', 'Corticosteroids', and 'Oestrogens'	Vitamin preparations	vitamin A in excess, D.2 (*b*) iodinated preparations, (Naiodine, Thionaiodine) D.A (*b*)
Sulphonamides	as a group, D.2 (*b*)		

APPENDIX D. TESTS OF ADRENOCORTICAL FUNCTION

DEXAMETHASONE SUPPRESSION TEST—for diagnosis and differential diagnosis of Cushing's syndrome.

Dexamethasone suppresses pituitary ACTH output by operation of the negative feedback effect of corticosteroids on the hypothalamus and pituitary. Since dexamethasone does not interfere with the routine methods for measuring blood or urinary corticosteroids, a reduction of ACTH output can be assessed by following the fall in these corticosteroids.

Procedure and Interpretation

1. *Low-dose dexamethasone:* 0·5 mg 6-hourly for 48 hours (e.g. 9 a.m., 3 p.m., 9 p.m., 3 a.m.; blood sampling at 9 a.m., urine collections 9 a.m. to 9 a.m.). Normal response: 24-hour urinary 17-oxogenic corticosteroid excretion less than 5 mg/day. At 48 hours, plasma fluorogenic corticosteroids are normally less than 6 μg/100 ml.

2. *Single* (*low dose*) *dexamethasone:* 1 or 1·5 mg at 11 p.m. to midnight (less reliable than full test). At 9 a.m. plasma fluorogenic corticosteroids normally less than 7 μg/100 ml. Lack of suppression on low dose indicates Cushing's syndrome or a stressed patient.

3. *High-dose dexamethasone:* 2 mg 6-hourly for 48 hours. Suppression of plasma or urinary corticosteroids by 50 per cent usually indicates Cushing's disease rather than ectopic ACTH syndrome, adrenal adenoma or carcinoma.

The low-dose test may be used to differentiate

Cushing's syndrome from normality, whereas the high-dose test usually distinguishes the different causes. However, stressed patients without Cushing's syndrome may not suppress cortisol production on 2 mg/day of dexamethasone, e.g. in depression, and many exceptions to the interpretation of the high dose test have been described.

References

Liddle (1960). *J. clin. Endocr.* **20**, 1539.
Besser and Edwards (1972). *Clinics in Endocrinology and Metabolism*, **1**, 451.

METYRAPONE TEST for differential diagnosis of Cushing's syndrome.

Metyrapone is principally the drug used as an 11β-hydroxylase inhibitor which blocks the final step in the synthesis of cortisol, leading to an accumulation of 11-deoxycortisol and other cortisol precursors. The reduced plasma cortisol concentration stimulates a rise in plasma ACTH via the negative feedback which further stimulates the adrenal cortex to produce cortisol precursors which are excreted as urinary 17-oxogenic steroids; these are the metabolites of the corticosteroids which accumulate in the presence of metyrapone. Since metyrapone has only a brief circulating half-time and is a relatively weak enzyme blocker, it is important to give large doses frequently and to show that effective blood levels of metyrapone have been achieved by measuring the fall in plasma cortisol. Since 11-deoxycortisol does not fluoresce, the usual plasma fluorogenic corticosteroid assay of Mattingly can be used to follow the course of the enzyme blockade after the first dose.

Procedure

The normal dose of metyrapone is 750 mg given by mouth every four hours for 24 hours in patients weighing 70 kg or more. Even this dose produces no more than 90 per cent inhibition of the enzyme and smaller doses or failure to give the drug at the correct times may well vitiate the test, but this may be detected if there is no fall in plasma fluorogenic corticosteroids. Urine should be collected for 17-oxogenic corticosteroids for two days before the test, the day of metyrapone administration and the following day. Plasma for fluorogenic corticosteroids should be collected immediately before and hourly for four hours after the first dose of metyrapone to check that adequate enzyme blockade is being achieved.

INTERPRETATION

In patients with Cushing's disease there is an exaggerated or augmented ACTH and urinary 17-oxogenic steroid response to metyrapone. This contrasts with the responses in patients with adrenal adenomas or carcinomas who show no such rise since pituitary ACTH secretion is suppressed.

The normal 24-hour urinary 17-oxogenic steroid response to metyrapone 750 mg four-hourly for 24 hours is a maximum level (on the day of administration or day after metyrapone) of 24–36 mg/day. Impaired or absent response indicates adenoma or carcinoma of adrenal cortex in patients with established Cushing's syndrome; exaggerated response indicates Cushing's disease.

Side-effects. Dizziness and nausea may occasionally occur but this can usually be obviated by keeping the patient in bed.

Metyrapone as a Test for Impaired ACTH Reserve. This test has in the past been used to diagnose secondary adrenocortical insufficiency. It has been found to be inadequate for this purpose and has been replaced by the insulin tolerance test.

References

Liddle *et al.* (1959). *J. clin. Endocr.*, **19**, 875.
Hypothalamic-Pituitary-Adrenal Function Tests. Ciba Laboratories Ltd., 1971.

ACTH STIMULATION TESTS for adrenocortical insufficiency.

Low plasma corticosteroids which do not rise after brief ACTH administration confirm impaired adrenocortical reserve. If the impaired response persists after prolonged ACTH administration, primary adrenocortical insufficiency is indicated rather than secondary adrenocortical atrophy due to impaired ACTH secretion, the latter resulting either from prolonged corticosteroid therapy or hypothalamic-pituitary disease. Tetracosactrin (Synacthen or Cortrosyn) is the synthetic analogue of ACTH which is now most commonly used for the ACTH stimulation test.

Procedure

Short Test. Patient does not require to fast nor be at rest; 250 μg of tetracosactrin (plain) is administered intramuscularly between 8 and 9 a.m., and blood is taken for plasma corticosteroids before, 30 and 60 minutes after the injection.

Normal Response. Basal 9 a.m. plasma fluorogenic corticosteroid level 6–25 μg/100 ml, maximum increment during the test of more than 11 μg/100 ml, maximum value greater than 20 μg/100 ml.

Long Test. This should be carried out in patients who have failed to respond to the short test, and two alternative procedures are available.

(*a*) 1 mg depot tetracosactrin (Synacthen Depot) intramuscularly at 9 a.m., with blood samples for plasma fluorogenic corticosteroids before and at 1, 4, 6, 8 and 24 hours.

Interpretation. In secondary adrenocortical atrophy there is a delayed rise in corticosteroids, values remaining below 25 μg/100 ml for the first 4 hours of the test. In primary adrenocortical atrophy corticosteroid levels usually remain below 10 μg/100 ml throughout the procedure.

(*b*) 1 mg depot tetracosactrin intramuscularly daily for 3 days, and the short tetracosactrin test is performed on the fourth day. In secondary adrenal atrophy plasma corticosteroids will rise above 25 μg/100 ml, but in primary adrenal atrophy corticosteroid levels usually remain below 10 μg/100 ml.

Precautions. Once the initial short tetracosactrin test has been performed it is unnecessary to withhold treatment in patients suspected of adrenocortical insufficiency. Prednisolone in a dose of 5 mg b.d. should be given and a long ACTH stimulation test performed (prednisolone does not interfere in plasma corticosteroid estimations). Normal test does not exclude ACTH deficiency.

APPENDIX E. TESTS OF GONADAL FUNCTION

HCG STIMULATION TEST for primary testicular insufficiency.

Human chorionic gonadotrophin has interstitial cell stimulating activity (ICSH) and can therefore be used to test the ability of the interstitial cells of the testis to secrete testosterone.

Procedure. 2,000 i.u. of HCG is injected intramuscularly at 9 a.m., on days 1 and 4. Blood samples are obtained for testosterone measurement before each injection and 48 hours after the second injection.

Normal Response. The precise values obtained will depend on the particular testosterone assay used. If 17 βOH-androgens are measured (mainly testosterone and dihydrotestosterone) normal adult men show a peak response above 11 ng/ml at some stage during the test. In adults with primary testicular disease the response is reduced or absent, but in hypogonadotrophism a normal response may be obtained. In cryptorchidism, the response is often impaired and delayed.

For clomiphene test, *see* Appendix A.

APPENDIX F. BODY WEIGHTS

DESIRABLE WEIGHTS OF ADULTS[1]

Height (in shoes)			Desirable weight in pounds and *kilogrammes* (in indoor clothing), ages 25 and over					
			Small frame		Medium frame		Large frame	
ft	in	*cm*	lb	*kg*	lb	*kg*	lb	*kg*
				Men				
5	2	*157·5*	112–120	*50·8–54·4*	118–129	*53·5–58·5*	126–141	*57·2–64*
5	3	*160*	115–123	*52·2–55·8*	121–133	*54·9–60·3*	129–144	*58·5–65·3*
5	4	*162·6*	118–126	*53·5–57·2*	124–136	*56·2–61·7*	132–148	*59·9–67·1*
5	5	*165·1*	121–129	*54·9–58·5*	127–139	*57·6–63*	135–152	*61·2–68·9*
5	6	*167·6*	124–133	*56·2–60·3*	130–143	*59 –64·9*	138–156	*62·6–70·8*
5	7	*170·2*	128–137	*58·1–62·1*	134–147	*60·8–66·7*	142–161	*64·4–73*
5	8	*172·7*	132–141	*59·9–64*	138–152	*62·6–68·9*	147–166	*66·7–75·3*
5	9	*175·3*	136–145	*61·7–65·8*	142–156	*64·4–70·8*	151–170	*68·5–77·1*
5	10	*177·8*	140–150	*63·5–68*	146–160	*66·2–72·6*	155–174	*70·3–78·9*
5	11	*180·3*	144–154	*65·3–69·9*	150–165	*68 –74·8*	159–179	*72·1–81·2*
6	0	*182·9*	148–158	*67·1–71·7*	154–170	*69·9–77·1*	164–184	*74·4–83·5*
6	1	*185·4*	152–162	*68·9–73·5*	158–175	*71·7–79·4*	168–189	*76·2–85·7*
6	2	*188*	156–167	*70·8–75·7*	162–180	*73·5–81·6*	173–194	*78·5–88*
6	3	*190·5*	160–171	*72·6–77·6*	167–185	*75·7–83·5*	178–199	*80·7–90·3*
6	4	*193*	164–175	*74·4–79·4*	172–190	*78·1–86·2*	182–204	*82·7–92·5*
				Women				
4	10	*147·3*	92– 98	*41·7–44·5*	96–107	*43·5–48·5*	104–119	*47·2–54*
4	11	*149·9*	94–101	*42·6–45·8*	98–110	*44·5–49·9*	106–122	*48·1–55·3*
5	0	*152·4*	96–104	*43·5–47·2*	101–113	*45·8–51·3*	109–125	*49·4–56·7*
5	1	*154·9*	99–107	*44·9–48·5*	104–116	*47·2–52·6*	112–128	*50·8–58·1*
5	2	*157·5*	102–110	*46·3–49·9*	107–119	*48·5–54*	115–131	*52·2–59·4*
5	3	*160*	105–113	*47·6–51·3*	110–122	*49·9–55·3*	118–134	*53·5–60·8*
5	4	*162·6*	108–116	*49 –52·6*	113–126	*51·3–57·2*	121–138	*54·9–62·6*
5	5	*165·1*	111–119	*50·3–54*	116–130	*49 –59*	125–142	*49·4–64·4*
5	6	*167·6*	114–123	*51·7–55·8*	120–135	*54·4–61·2*	129–146	*58·5–66·2*
5	7	*170·2*	118–127	*53·5–57·6*	124–139	*56·2–63*	133–150	*60·3–68*
5	8	*172·7*	122–131	*55·3–59·4*	128–143	*58·1–64·9*	137–154	*62·1–69·9*
5	9	*175·3*	126–135	*57·2–61·2*	132–147	*59·9–66·7*	141–158	*64 –71·7*
5	10	*177·8*	130–140	*59 –63·5*	136–151	*61·7–68·5*	145–163	*65·8–73·9*
5	11	*180·3*	134–144	*60·8–65·3*	140–155	*63·5–70·3*	149–168	*67·6–76·2*
6	0	*182·9*	138–148	*62·6–67·1*	144–159	*65·3–72·1*	153–173	*69·4–78·5*

[1] Weights of insured persons in the United States associated with lowest mortality (*Statist. Bull. Metrop. Life Insur. Co., 40*, Nov.–Dec. 1959).

[From *Documenta Geigy Scientific Tables*, 7th edn., Basle, 1970. Based on data of the Metropolitan Life Insurance Company, New York (*Statistical Bulletin of the Metropolitan Life Insurance Company*, vol. 40. 1959). Table reproduced by permission of CIBA-GEIGY Limited, Basle, Switzerland.]

APPENDIX G. MISCELLANEOUS

UNITAGE

1 milligram = 1 mg = 10^{-3} g
1 microgram = 1 μg = 10^{-6} g
1 nanogram = 1 ng = 10^{-9} g
1 picogram = 1 pg = 10^{-12} g
1 femtogram = 1 fg = 10^{-15} g
1 attogram = 1 ag = 10^{-18} g

MEDIC-ALERT bracelets or necklace

We suggest that these bracelets or necklaces are worn by patients who suffer from adrenocortical insufficiency. They show the patient's diagnosis (hypopituitarism, Addison's disease, etc.), a code number referring to the patient and the telephone number of the Medic-Alert Foundation. The Foundation maintains a central file containing relevant information, including the doctor's name and address, which is released to authorised persons in emergencies. Application forms may be obtained from:

Medic-Alert Foundation,
9 Hanover Street,
London, W1R 9HF.

There are associated organisations in many parts of the world.

INSERTION OF AN INDWELLING CANNULA into a forearm vein.

(Modified from *Hypothalamic-Pituitary-Adrenal Function Tests*, 1971, Ciba Laboratories Ltd., Horsham.)

The needle should be inserted at least 30 minutes before starting any test. Otherwise, although painless, the apprehension occasioned by preparation and insertion of the needle may cause a temporary elevation of circulating corticosteroid, prolactin and GH levels which could influence the results obtained.

There are a number of points which, if followed, help ensure success and a minimum of discomfort to the patient. He should be lying comfortably on a bed with his arm supported firmly on a pillow; everything required should be immediately to hand, and the patient's veins should be fully distended. The latter is most important in facilitating the procedure and is best achieved by ensuring that the patient is kept warm and that his hands are kept hot (for example, by an electric heating pad), together with applying pressure at about 70 mm Hg using a cuff inflated around the upper arm.

A tray or trolley should be placed by the bedside containing the following:

1. Spirit soaked or cotton wool swabs.
2. Local anaesthetic (such as 1% lignocaine), together with a small syringe (1–2·5 ml) and small needle (size 19) for subcutaneous injection. This syringe is used subsequently to take waste samples.
3. Isotonic saline, to which is added heparin (10,000 units/10 ml). Sterile sodium citrate or some other anticoagulant should be used in place of heparinised saline if it is also intended to determine plasma-free fatty acid levels. This obviates the risk of small amounts of heparin entering the circulation and activating tissue lipases. A 20 ml syringe is also required to inject the anticoagulant into the indwelling needle between sampling. Heparinised saline is not required if a stylet is used to maintain patency of the cannula.
4. An indwelling needle. A disposable 'Braunula' pre-sterilised, size 1 Luer-fitting cannula and stylet ('Mandrin') (both distributed by Armour Pharmaceutical Company Ltd., Eastbourne) or a number 19 disposable Butterfly needle (distributed by Abbot Laboratories, Queenborough, Kent) are both suitable. These are preferred to non-disposable metal needles, which become blunt and require careful cleaning and sterilisation and which may get cut and dislodged into the vein.

5. A series of 10 ml syringes and lithium heparin-containing tubes, one for each sample, labelled with the patient's name and time of sampling.

6. A roll of sticking-plaster and a pair of scissors.

After cleaning the skin with spirit, about 0·1 ml of local anaesthetic is injected subcutaneously over the most suitable vein. For tests lasting only one or two hours, a vein in the antecubital fossa is satisfactory. However, for procedures requiring several hours, it it better to use a forearm vein so that the subject has more mobility and can, therefore, bend his elbow to prevent it becoming uncomfortable. The needle is introduced until about $\frac{1}{4}$ inch has entered the vein, the central sharp metal needle is then withdrawn slightly and the outer plastic part inserted up the vein a further inch. Cuff pressure is released, the metal component of the needle removed and the stylet inserted. A strip of sticking-plaster is used to hold it in position and another to keep a sterile swab over the point of entry through the skin.

In children or adults with difficult veins, it is often better to use a number 19 'Butterfly' disposable needle instead of a cannula. Patency of this is maintained by injecting 0·5 ml heparinised saline and closing the end with a stopcock. When using this technique, it is necessary to withdraw approximately 1 ml of blood/heparinised saline using the small "waste" syringe, prior to taking each sample. Likewise, about 1 ml of the heparinised saline solution must be introduced immediately after each sample has been withdrawn, to prevent the needle being blocked as a result of clotting.

Samples for plasma corticosteroid, prolactin and GH determinations are placed in lithium heparin-containing tubes, and, immediately after the test, these are centrifuged and the plasma separated and kept at 4°C (corticosteroids) or frozen (GH, prolactin) prior to assay.

INDEX